The
Financial
Management
of Hospitals

SIXTH EDITION

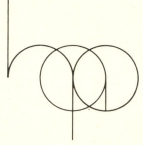

health administration press

HOWARD J. BERMAN
LEWIS E. WEEKS
STEVEN F. KUKLA

The Financial Management of Hospitals

SIXTH EDITION

HEALTH ADMINISTRATION PRESS
Ann Arbor, Michigan   1986

First Edition–November 1971, January 1973, July 1973
Second Edition–March 1974, November 1974, July 1975, June 1976
Third Edition–August 1976, November 1977, November 1978
Fourth Edition–September 1979, April 1980, July 1981
Fifth Edition–January 1982, July 1982, April 1983, March 1984, July 1984, May 1985,
         June 1986

90 89 88   8 7 6 5 4 3

Library of Congress Cataloging-in-Publication Data

Berman, Howard J.
   The financial management of hospitals.

   Bibliography: p.
   Includes index.
   1. Hospitals—Business management. 2. Hospitals—Finance. I. Weeks,
Lewis E. II. Kukla, Steven F., 1950–   . III. Title. [DNLM: 1. Economics,
Hospital. 2. Financial Management. WX 157 B516f]
RA971.3.B48   1986   362.1'1'0681   86-14861
ISBN 0-910701-18-0

Health Administration Press
A division of the Foundation of the
   American College of Healthcare Executives
1021 East Huron
Ann Arbor, Michigan 48104
(313) 764-1380

To Marilyn, Frances, and Virginia,
our wives,

for their patience and understanding
about the demands of time
this manuscript has taken.

Contents

PART IV
Resource Allocation Decisions:
Corporate Planning, Budgeting, and Control

PART V
Control and Analysis

PART VI
The Future

Foreword

When Howard Berman and Lew Weeks again did me the honor of asking me to write a foreword to this sixth and latest edition of *The Financial Management of Hospitals*, I was somewhat incredulous. After all, could there have been that long an interval since the fifth? In that edition I commented that since I had written the foreword in each of the preceding, Howard and Lew must have concluded that my doing so represented some sort of talisman, and not necessarily any profound contribution. But whatever their motivation, I am pleased to be a very modest piece of what is now a classic of its kind.

In authoring this new edition, Berman and Weeks are joined for the first time by Steven F. Kukla, a staff member of the American Hospital Association. His participation adds even more muscle to an already well-established and knowledgeable team.

When the first edition appeared 15 years ago, the authors likely had no idea that the book would prove to be so durable. However, that first effort obviously effectively addressed a real need and void in the field for both student and practitioner. Health administration educational programs were under criticism for not giving sufficient curricular emphasis to the financial concerns of the industry. Practitioners also felt the need for updating and new information in this area. Over the intervening years, and particularly recently, financial management capability has emerged as an even more critical concern as the field has undergone sweeping economic changes.

The authors have recognized these convolutions by the several succeeding editions, each of which has endeavored both to update prior text and to include new material pertinent to recent developments. This sixth edition well reflects such changes. There are major rewrites of the Blue

Cross and Medicare and Medicaid chapters and completely new chapters on cost accounting, financial analysis, and the future. Also updated are the bibliography and the acronyms section.

The fact that this is the sixth edition in 15 years speaks for itself as to the field's receptivity, and also to the authors' commitment to a publication that is contemporary in content and responsive to the academic and practitioner communities' changing needs. We are indebted to them for such a continuing effort.

ANDREW PATTULLO

Battle Creek, Michigan
June 14, 1986

Preface

The authors have been gratified by the reception and recognition that the previous editions of this work have received. We hope that this, the sixth edition, warrants the continued acceptance of both our colleagues and our students. It has been prepared with careful regard to their comments, criticisms, and vision of what could be achieved.

In writing this edition, we have revised and updated the fifth edition both to reflect the changing health care financial environment and to make the book a more complete reference and teaching document. Each chapter has been reviewed, and material has been added or modified as necessary. Statistical data have also been updated to reflect current performance and facts. In particular, Part II has been revised to reflect the near revolutionary changes that have taken place in hospital payment since the publication of the fifth edition. A new Part V has also been added to allow the subjects of management reporting, cost accounting, and financial analysis to be addressed more fully than in previous editions. The chapter on the future has been revised to reflect the implications of recent social and economic developments and changes in public attitudes. Finally, the bibliography has been changed to capture the growing body of literature.

As was so with previous editions, the responsibility for any errors or oversights must lie with the authors. The credit for any contributions that this work might make, however, must still accrue to our colleagues who have advised us and to our students who have taught us.

Particular appreciation must be expressed to all those who helped with the previous editions and to Maureen Graszer, Stephen Wood, Ronald Wacker, and the University of Chicago Hospital Administration classes of 1983, 1984, and 1985 for their help and advice in preparing this edition. At the Health Administration Press, Gene Regenstreif has been particularly helpful in the production of the book and Nancy Moncrieff in skillful editing of the manuscript.

Our sincere thanks to Andrew Pattullo for his interest and encouragement throughout the years.

HOWARD J. BERMAN
LEWIS E. WEEKS
STEVEN F. KUKLA

List of Acronyms

AA	Alcoholics Anonymous
AALL	American Association for Labor Legislation
AAPCC	Adjusted average per capita cost
AARP	American Association of Retired Persons
AB	Aid to the Blind
ABMT	Autologous bone marrow transplant
ACEP	American College of Emergency Physicians
ACHA	American College of Hospital Administrators
ACHE	American College of Healthcare Executives
ACP	American College of Physicians
ACR	Adjusted community rate
ACS	American College of Surgeons
ACTH	Adrenocorticotropic hormone
ADA	American Dental Association
ADAMHA	Alcohol, Drug Abuse, Mental Health Administration
ADC	Aid to Dependent Children
AFDC	Aid to Families with Dependent Children
AFDC-UP	Aid to Families with Dependent Children–Unemployed Parent
AFL-CIO	American Federation of Labor–Congress of Industrial Organizations
AFSCME	American Federation of State, County, and Municipal Employees
AHA	American Hospital Association
AHIP	Assisted Health Insurance Plan
AHPA	American Health Planning Association

AIA	American Institute of Architects
AICPA	American Institute of Certified Public Accountants
ALC	Alternate level of care
AMA	American Medical Association
AMI	American Medical International
AMRA	American Medical Records Association
ANA	American Nurses Association
ANHA	American Nursing Home Association (now American Health Care Association)
AOA	American Osteopathic Association
AOHA	American Osteopathic Hospital Association
APhA	American Pharmaceutical Association
APHA	American Public Health Association
APTD	Aid to the Permanently and Totally Disabled
ASIM	American Society of Industrial Medicine
ASO	Administrative service organization
AUPHA	Association of University Programs in Health Administration
BCA	Blue Cross Association
BCBSA	Blue Cross and Blue Shield Association
B&I	Business and Industry Loan Program
BMT	Bone marrow transplantation
BSA	Blue Shield Association
BUN	Blood urea nitrogen
CABG	Coronary artery bypass graft
CAP	Community action program, also Cost allocation program
CASH	Comprehensive audit system for hospitals
CAT	Computerized axial tomography
CBO	Congressional Budget Office
CCHP	Consumers Choice Health Plan
CCU	Coronary care unit
CD	Certificate of deposit
CDC	Centers for Disease Control
CEM	Consumer expenditures for personal health care
CEO	Chief executive officer
CFL	Commercial Facilities Loan Program
CFO	Chief financial officer
CHA	Canadian Hospital Association
CHAMPUS	Civilian Health and Medical Program for the Uniformed Services
CHA-US	Catholic Health Association–United States
CHIP	Comprehensive Health Insurance Plan
CHP	Comprehensive Health Planning Agency
CIR	Committee of Interns and Residents

CIS	Clinical information system
CMI	Case mix index
CMM	Comprehensive major medical
CMP	Competitive medical plan
COL	Cost of living
CON	Certificate of need
COO	Chief operating officer
COPD	Chronic obstructive pulmonary disease
COSTAR	Computer stored ambulatory record
C.P.A.	Certified Public Accountant
CPHA	Commission on Professional and Hospital Activities
CPI	Consumer price index
CRNA	Certified registered nurse anesthetist
CT	Computerized tomography
D.D.S.	Doctor of Dental Surgery
DES	Diethyl stilbestrol
DHEW	Department of Health, Education, and Welfare
DHHS	Department of Health and Human Services
DHSS	Department of Health and Social Services (Britain)
DNA	Deoxyribonucleic acid
D.O.	Doctor of Osteopathy
DOD	Department of Defense
DOL	Department of Labor
DOU	Diagnostic observation unit
DPI	Disposable personal income
DRG	Diagnosis-related group
ECF	Extended care facility
EDP	Electronic data processing
EEG	Electroencephalogram
EEOC	Equal Employment Opportunity Commission
EHI	Employees health insurance
EHIP	Employees health insurance plan
EKG	Electrocardiogram
EPO	Exclusive provider organization
EPSDT	Early and Periodic Screening, Diagnosis, and Treatment
ER	Emergency Room
ERISA	Employee Retirement Income Security Act
ESP	Economic Stabilization Program
ESRD	End stage renal disease
ESWL	Extracorporeal shock wave lithotripsy
FAH	Federation of American Hospitals (now Federation of American Health Systems)
FASB	Financial Accounting Standards Board

FDA	Food and Drug Administration
FDIC	Federal Deposit Insurance Corporation
FEC	Freestanding emergency clinic
FEHBP	Federal Employees Health Benefits Program
FERA	Federal Emergency Relief Administration
FHA	Federal Housing Administration
FHCIP	Federal Health Care Insurance Plan
FICA	Federal Insurance Contributions Act
FMCS	Federal Mediary and Conciliation Service
FMG	Foreign medical graduate
FmHA	Farmers Home Administration
FNMA	Federal National Mortgage Association
FSA	Flexible spending account
FTE	Full-time equivalent
GAO	General Accounting Office
GHAA	Group Health Association of America
GME	Graduate medical education
GNP	Gross national product
GP	General practitioner
HAS	Hospital Administrative Services
HCA	Hospital Corporation of America
HCFA	Health Care Financing Administration
HCPCS	HCFA's common procedure coding system
HCUP	Hospital Cost and Utilization Project
HEW	Department of Health, Education, and Welfare
HFMA	Healthcare Financial Management Association
HHS	Department of Health and Human Services
HI	Hospital insurance (Medicare A)
HIAA	Health Insurance Association of America
HIBAC	Health Insurance Benefits Advisory Council
HIMA	Health Industry Manufacturers Association
HIP	Health Insurance Plan of Greater New York
HIS	Hospital information system
HMO	Health maintenance organization
HPA	Health Policy Agenda for the American People
HPIC	Health Providers Insurance Company
HRA	Health Resources Administration
HRET	Hospital Research and Educational Trust
HSA	Health systems agency
HSP	Hospital specific portion
HUD	Department of Housing and Urban Development
ICCU	Intermediate coronary care unit
ICD-9-CM	International Classification of Disease, 9th Revision, Clinically Modified

ICRC	Infant care review committee
ICU	Intensive care unit
IHF	International Hospital Federation
ILGWU	International Ladies Garment Workers Union
IPA	Individual practice association
IPPB	Intermittent positive pressure breathing
IRR	Internal rate of return
IRS	Internal Revenue Service
IUD	Intrauterine device
IV	Intravenous
JCAH	Joint Commission on Accreditation of Hospitals
K-P	Kaiser-Permanente
LDR	Labor/delivery room
LOS	Length of stay
L.P.N.	Licensed practical nurse
MAC	Medical Administrative Corps
MAP	Medical Audit Program
MBO	Management by objectives
M.D.	Doctor of Medicine
MDC	Major diagnostic category
MEDEX	Training program for physician's assistants
MEDPAR	Medicare provider analysis and review
MESH	Medical Staff Hospital Organization
MET	Multiple employer trusts
MGMA	Medical Group Management Association
MI	Medical Insurance (Medicare Part B)
MIED	Maternal, infant early discharge
MIS	Management information system
MIT	Massachusetts Institute of Technology
MMIS	Medicaid management information system
MPI	Medical price index
MRE	Medical review entity
MRIS	Magnetic resonance imaging system
MSA	Medical Services Administration
NAFAC	National Association for Ambulatory Care
NAGE	National Association of Government Employees
NAHC	National Association for Home Care
NAHSE	National Association of Health Services Executives
NAPPH	National Association of Private Psychiatric Hospitals
NARD	National Association of Retail Druggists
NASA	National Aeronautics and Space Administration
NASW	National Association of Social Workers
NCHSR	National Center for Health Services Research
NHI	National health insurance

NHO	National Hospice Organization
NHS	National Health Service
NHSC	National Health Service Corps
NIH	National Institutes of Health
NLN	National League for Nursing
NLRB	National Labor Relations Board
NMA	National Medical Association
NME	National Medical Enterprise
NMR	Nuclear magnetic resonance
NOA	Notice of admission
N.P.	Nurse practitioner
NPN	Nonprotein nitrogen
NSF	National Science Foundation
NVU	Neurovascular unit
OAA	Old Age Assistance
OAI	Old Age Insurance
OASDI	Old Age, Survivors, and Disability Insurance
OASHDI	Old Age, Survivors, Health, and Disability Insurance
OASI	Old Age and Survivors Insurance
OB	Obstetrics
O.D.	Doctor of Optometry
OEO	Office of Economic Opportunity
OMB	Office of Management and Budget
OPD	Outpatient department
OPEIU	Office and Professional Employees International Union
OR	Operating room
ORSA	Operations Research Society of America
OSHA	Occupational Safety and Health Administration
OT	Occupational therapy
OTA	Office of Technology Assessment
P.A.	Physician's assistant
PAC	Preadmission certificate
PAHO	Pan American Health Organization
PARCOST	Ontario prescription price comparison plan
PAS	Professional Activities Study
PBGC	Pension Benefits Guaranty Corporation
PBI	Protein-bound iodine
PCN	Primary care network
PET	Positron emission tomography
PGP	Prepaid group practice
pH	Symbol used with numbers to express degrees of acidity-alkalinity
PHC	Primary health care

PHP	Prepaid health plan
PHS	Public Health Service
PIER	AHA Program for Institutional Effectiveness Review
PIP	Periodic interim payment
PIQuA	Private initiative in quality assurance
PKU	Phenylketonuria
PL	Public Law
PLA	Product line analysis
PMA	Pharmaceutical Manufacturers Association
PPA	Prudent purchaser agreement
PPO	Preferred provider organization
PPS	Prospective pricing system
PRIMEX	Training program for family nurse practitioners
p.r.n.	As circumstances require
PRO	Peer review organization
ProPAC	Prospective Assessment Commission
PRRB	Providers Reimbursement Review Board
PSRO	Professional standards review organization
PT	Physical therapy
QHMO	Qualified health maintenance organization
RBC	Red blood count
RCC	Ratio of costs to charges
RM	Risk management
RMP	Regional Medical Program
ROE	Report of eligibility
RVS	Relative value scale
RVU	Relative value unit
RWDSU	Retail, Wholesale, Department Store Union
SEC	Securities and Exchange Commission
SEIU	Service Employees International Union
SEP	Simplified Employee Pension Plan
SFR	Statement of financial requirements
SMI	Supplementary medical insurance
SMSA	Standard metropolitan statistical area
SNF	Skilled nursing facility
SPD	Summary plan description (under ERISA)
SPRI	Swedish Planning and Rationalization Institute
SRS	Social and rehabilitation service
SSA	Social Security Administration
SSI	Supplementary Security Income
SUR	Surveillance and utilization review
TCC	The Computer Company
TEFRA	Tax Equity and Fiscal Responsibility Act (1982)

THIS	Total hospital information system
TIP	Transplant Insurance Plan
Title XVIII	Medicare
Title XIX	Medicaid
TPA	Third party administrator
UAW	United Auto Workers
UB	Uniform billing
UCR	Usual, customary, reasonable
UHDDS	Uniform Hospital Discharge Data Set
UK	United Kingdom
UMW	United Mine Workers
UPRO	Utah Professional Review Organization
URC	Utilization review committee
USPHS	United States Public Health Service
USTF	Uniformed Services Treatment Facility
USW	United Steel Workers
VA	Veterans Administration
VCI	Variable cost insurance
VD	Venereal disease
VDT	Video display terminal
VE	Voluntary effort
VEBA	Voluntary Employees Beneficiaries Association
VHA	Voluntary Hospitals of America
VISTA	Volunteers in Service to America
VNA	Visiting Nurse Association
WBC	White blood count
WHO	World Health Organization
ZBB	Zero-base budget
ZEBRA	Zero balance reimbursement plan

PART

I

Introduction

Management progress begins
with an understanding of why,
and proceeds based on
a knowledge of how.

Seth

1

Financial Management

The notion that competent financial management is necessary for efficient and effective hospital operations is accepted as a truism by most administrators. Why, however, is competent financial management necessary? What is financial management's usefulness or value in hospital operations, and how can this usefulness be maximized?

Usually and erroneously, financial management is associated with the complex and often confusing world of accounting and seemingly esoteric tools (cash flow analysis, statements of sources and uses of funds, and budgets) which accompany the practice of accounting. It has been viewed historically as a specialized area of management, separate and apart from the general management of operations. This has been due primarily to the fact that

1. Financial management personnel have *failed to communicate* with operational management; they have not directed their efforts and reports to the needs of other managers and of the hospital in total.

2. Operational management has been focusing its attention on individual functions rather than concentrating and coordinating all aspects of the operation toward achievement of a common objective.

Thus, financial management traditionally has not been a part of the mainstream of operational management.

This traditional role, however, is changing, and financial management is rapidly becoming an integral component of total operational management. What is the operational benefit of this change? In order to answer not only this question but also those set out above, it is first necessary to define the objective of management.

OBJECTIVE OF MANAGEMENT

In the case of the commercial enterprise the objective of management is not difficult to identify. It is basically that of maximizing owner's wealth. Quite simply, management must administer the assets of the enterprise in order to obtain the greatest wealth for the owner; that is, management must maximize the value $E/R = W$, where "E" is the earning or profits from the assets, "R" is the capitalization rate or the subjective estimate of the likelihood of receiving the projected profits from the assets, and "W" is the value of the firm or the owner's wealth.

Given that management's objective is to maximize owner's wealth, the usefulness of financial management becomes clear. However, as indicated above, owner's wealth (W) is a function of the earnings (E) of the firm and the risk associated with the actual receipt of those earnings (R). Therefore, management's goal is to find that combination of E and R that will yield the highest possible value of W. To do this, management must use not only its general managerial skills, that is, planning, organizing, coordinating, motivating, and controlling to maximize E, but also its financial management skills to evaluate and select earnings streams and minimize R. Thus, if management is to maximize W, it must either be lucky or use financial tools and techniques.

In the case of a hospital, where the guidelines of return on investment and simple "bottom line" profitability either are not available or are not entirely meaningful, the objective of management is somewhat more difficult to define. If it is assumed that a hospital is needed, that is, the community is not overbedded, then intuitively one could suggest that the long-run objective of hospital management is to perpetuate the continued operation of the hospital by ensuring that total revenues at least equal total economic costs of operation. This objective, while pragmatic, is too limited in scope and definition to be managerially useful. It focuses on only one element of management's responsibilities, ignoring not only the basic function and purpose of the hospital, but also management's obligation to the community that is being served. Therefore, it is unacceptable and must be both expanded and modified.

Hospitals are vital community resources. As such, they must be managed for the benefit of the community. The objective of hospital management must be to provide the community with the services it needs, at a clinically acceptable level of quality, a publicly responsive level of amenity, and at the least possible cost.

Within this objective there are four points that should be noted. First, the objective implicitly includes the foregoing revenue versus cost equality goal, for the hospital must continue in existence if it is to provide services to the community. Second, it focuses the hospital not just on needed health services but rather on needed community services. It recognizes that the hospital is not just in the health or medical services business but rather in the human services business. This does not mean that the hospital should attempt to pursue an "all things to all people" strategy. In the current operating environment just the opposite is required. The current environment, however, also requires that the hospital reach out beyond the physical limits of its walls, bringing to the community a range of needed human services— not just traditional medical services.[1] Third, it applies equally well to not-for-profit (nonprofit or voluntary) and for-profit hospitals.[2] Finally, it both establishes management's responsibility to the community and provides a general set of operating criteria.

It should be noted that other objective functions have been suggested for hospital management. These alternatives range from the simple, but realistic, objective of employment security to profit maximization. Between these extremes are management goals, such as recovery of cost, output maximization, quality maximization, and cash flow maximization. While these various goals have been hypothesized, none has been subjected to vigorous empirical testing. Moreover, they all lack pragmatic insight into either the social/societal role of the hospital, the realities of hospital financing, or the intrinsically dynamic nature of a hospital's operating requirements. Nevertheless, they can be useful analytical devices; while not substituting for the strategic and planning value of the foregoing statement

---

[1] In conventional business terms, when the situation changes management must reconceptualize the nature of the firm's business. In the case of the hospital, the situation is changing rapidly. The above objective function reflects the changing environment and the demands and opportunities that are confronting the community resource known as the hospital.

[2] Throughout this century a portion of the nation's hospitals have, for federal tax purposes, been under for-profit ownership. It has been estimated that in 1928 there were 2,435 for-profit hospitals in the United States, 36% of all hospitals. By 1968 the number of for-profit hospitals had declined to 769, 11% of all hospitals. In the decade of the 1970s the number grew so that by 1982 there were 998 for-profit hospitals, equaling 14% of all hospitals and 8.2% of all beds. Importantly, not only did the number of for-profit hospitals increase but their industry structure changed, evolving for the most part from freestanding individual institutions owned by physicians to corporately owned hospital chains.

The increase in for-profit hospitals (now called investor-owned hospitals) was spurred by Medicare's recognition of a return on equity factor for such hospitals and by the growth in health insurance coverage and benefits. Investor-owned hospitals have shown the greatest market share increase in those states having the least regulation and the greatest increases in population, per capita income, and insurance coverage.

From a financial theory perspective, investor-owned hospitals represent an interesting "middle ground" between the purely commercial enterprise and the social enterprise of the nonprofit hospital. They are subject to the investment performance pressures of the commercial firm and the community responsibilities of the nonprofit hospital. The way these seemingly conflicting demands are harmonized is by tempering the notion of maximizing the short-run return to the owners. The operative goal of these hospitals is to provide the owners, within the constraints of the role of the hospital, an adequate return on their investment.

Given the above, the ideas, tools, and techniques discussed in this text are equally applicable to the for-profit and not-for-profit hospital.

of management's objective, they do provide an added dimension for understanding operational behavior.

VALUE OF FINANCIAL MANAGEMENT

Given this objective, the value of financial management can be readily seen. Primarily, financial management tools and techniques can aid management in providing the community with quality services at least cost by furnishing the data that are necessary for making intelligent capital investment decisions, by guiding the operations of certain hospital subsystems, and by providing the systems and data needed to monitor and control operations.

Financial management techniques, such as present value (discounted flow) analysis and internal rate of return analysis, can be used to determine the cost implications of the various capital investment opportunities available to a hospital. These techniques provide management with the quantitative data that are needed not only to develop capital budgets knowledgeably, but also to take advantage of investment opportunities that will reduce the cost of care.

Admittedly, cost is not the only factor that should be considered in hospital investment decisions. The needs of the community, the level of quality, and the capacity of the organization to achieve the various alternatives must also be weighed in the decision process. At times, these non-economic factors may transcend cost implications, and management may select other than the least cost alternative. However, if management is to make this decision wisely, it must be aware of the cost implications of the various alternative opportunities. This awareness can only be obtained through the use of the above financial management techniques.

Financial management tools and techniques also can aid management in a more direct way than just providing quantitative information for capital investment decision making. A hospital can be viewed as a complex system composed of a number of simple subsystems. Some of these subsystems, such as accounts payable and receivable management, cash and short-term investment management, and inventory management, are basically financial activities and can be operated at least cost through the use of such financial practices and techniques as: accounts receivable factoring, economic order quantity models, cash forecasting, and internal control procedures.

Additionally, financial management tools can help management to meet its objectives in a third way. Cost finding reports, expense and revenue budgets, and position and operating statements provide management with the information necessary to control internal operations.

Cost finding provides data on actual operational performance by cost center. This information can be compared to budgeted performance expectations to identify problem areas that require attention and to obtain an index of operational performance. These data, along with information provided via the position and operating statements, will also give management the material needed to evaluate and control the hospital's capital structure, that is, evaluate and control the proportion of capital obtained from various sources.

Cost finding is also of value to management in another way. If, over the long run, revenues are at least to equal expenses or costs, then management must, as accurately as possible, determine the costs of each revenue-producing area. Cost finding is the best available technique for accomplishing this. The data obtained through cost finding furnish not only the information necessary for negotiating equitable reimbursement rates with third party payers but also, when combined with a schedule of charges and a revenue budget, the information necessary for establishing an adequate charge structure. Obviously, both these functions must be carried out successfully if management is to ensure a revenue-expense equality and the continued existence of the hospital.

Thus, financial management can play a critical role in assisting management to achieve its operational objective (see Figure 1.1). Its usefulness, though mainly in the areas of cost control and reduction, is not limited to these factors. As has been indicated, financial management techniques are of help in assuring a revenue-expense equality. However, this and other uses of financial management tools are basically byproducts, flowing almost automatically from its primary cost and operational control values.

A Word of Clarification

A pause should be made at this time to clarify a point. The discussion so far in the book has focused on financial management and its importance in operating any type of enterprise. It should be made clear that throughout the chapter financial management rather than accounting was emphasized and that the importance of the financial manager and not that of the accountant was being stressed. The distinction being drawn may appear subtle and perhaps even unimportant. However, it is critical and deserves this moment of clarification to minimize future misunderstandings.

Financial management, as previously mentioned, is usually associated with the practice of accounting. However, though the two may be associated, they are not synonymous. Accounting can be described as the art of collecting, summarizing, analyzing, reporting, and interpreting, in monetary terms, information about the enterprise. This is an important function, but it is not financial management.

Financial management can be described as the art both of obtaining the funds that the enterprise needs in the most economic manner and of

FIGURE 1.1   Operational Value and Usefulness of Financial Management

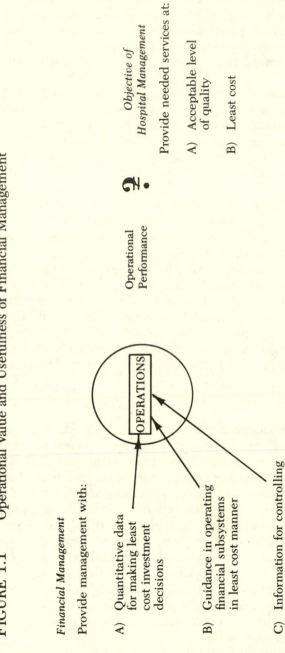

Financial Management

Provide management with:

A) Quantitative data for making least cost investment decisions

B) Guidance in operating financial subsystems in least cost manner

C) Information for controlling and evaluating operations

OPERATIONS

Operational Performance

2.

Objective of Hospital Management

Provide needed services at:

A) Acceptable level of quality

B) Least cost

Financial management provides data and management techniques that can assist management in guiding operational performance to meet the hospital's objective.

making the optimal use of those funds once obtained. Financial management can then be viewed as a decision process. Like all decision processes it needs information and facts if it is to function accurately, and certain techniques and tools if it is to function efficiently. Financial management techniques and tools provide the means for efficiency. The accounting system and the accountant provide the data needed for accuracy.

The two functions then are linked, with financial management building on accounting. Financial management utilizes accounting, and the information it produces, to determine how to operate the enterprise more effectively. The difference between the two can be viewed as one of scope, for financial management both includes and goes beyond accounting.

This difference in scope makes it important that we expand our horizon and not talk or think in terms of accounting only, but in terms of financial management and the financial manager. An accountant with an enlarged scope and perspective of operation can be a financial manager. However, accounting, by definition, cannot be financial management, for its goal is informational—not operational.

Financial management is accounting—plus. It is the use of the data generated by the accounting system for improved operations. In view of today's political climate and management environment, improved operations, and hence financial management, are necessities.

ORGANIZATION OF THE TEXT

The answers to the questions posed at the outset of this discussion should now be obvious. Competent financial management is a necessity for efficient hospital management, for it provides the information and tools necessary for controlling operations and reducing costs. The objective of this text is to acquaint the health services manager with both the potential that exists for improved operations through the use of the foregoing financial management tools and the mechanics of these tools.

It is neither expected nor hoped that an administrator will develop a sufficient facility with the tools and mechanics which will be discussed to perform personally the financial management function in his hospital. However, it is hoped that he will develop a sufficient familiarity and understanding of financial management to be cognizant of the need for competent financial management, to be aware of the tools and techniques that should be utilized, and to be able to evaluate the performance of his financial manager. It is to this end that the following text is designed.

Part I is intended to provide the reader with background material and an initial understanding of the financial environment in which a hospital exists. Chapter 2 sets out the accounting principles and conventions that apply to hospitals, and Chapter 3 discusses the internal organization that is necessary for effective financial management. Part II can also be considered to be background material, though of a somewhat different nature.

It is unusual to include a section on sources of operating revenue in a financial management text. However, hospitals maintain a unique operating relationship with their sources of revenue, that is, with third party purchasers of care. Hospitals, while treating many individual patients, are paid for services that they provide to these individuals by relatively few sources. These sources, because of their economic power, are able to affect substantially the financial status of an individual hospital by the method or procedure that they use to pay that hospital. Therefore, if one is to understand the financial parameters within which a hospital operates and within which financial management in general and working capital management in particular must function, it is necessary first to understand how hospitals are paid and what can be the effect of this payment mechanism.

Part II discusses in detail the nature of the hospital–third party relationship, the philosophies and payment guidelines of various third party cost-based reimbursement agreements, and the mechanics of determining hospital costs. Additionally, to cover the subject areas fully, the mechanics of rate setting is also examined in this part.

Part III builds on the foundation set out in Part II. It examines the operation of the financial subsystems of the hospital and the application and usefulness of financial management techniques in operating these systems in a least cost manner. The emphasis of this section is both on defining the nature, sources, and costs of working capital and on discussing how financial management techniques can be used not only to minimize a hospital's investment in working capital but also to maximize the return that can be obtained from those assets that must be so invested. Each component of working capital is examined, and the techniques for determining the optimal level of investment in each asset are explored. Also included in this section is a discussion of the management reports that are needed for effective evaluation, control, and guidance of working capital operations.

Part IV addresses operational resource allocation decisions. Its focus is on the corporate planning process, including strategic planning and marketing, operational planning, budgeting, and capital investment decision making. Its emphasis is not on mechanics but rather on providing a framework of management principles for making both short-term and long-run resource allocation decisions.

Part V is a section on operational control. It discusses first the principles, mechanics, and types of management report that are useful for monitoring, evaluating, and guiding operational performance on an ongoing basis. The second part of the section looks at financial analysis.

Part VI is a brief section that focuses on the future trends in hospital financing and on the nature of the operational environment that can be expected. Like all projections it is a bit speculative. Nevertheless, it serves to bring into an interesting perspective a variety of critical issues.

The organization of the text has been designed first to establish a working level of information about the internal and external financial environment of the hospital and then to build on that foundation, to examine specific financial management tools and processes and their application in hospital management. There is thus a pyramiding of subject matter and knowledge, culminating in an understanding of the skills necessary to evaluate the hospital's operational performance and financial position as well as to determine the nature of any needed changes or improvements.

SUGGESTED READINGS[3]

Anthony, Robert N. and Herzlinger, Regina E. *Management Control in Nonprofit Organizations.*

Berman, Howard J. "Financial Management: Necessity or Nicety?"

Cleverley, William O. *Financial Management of Health Care Facilities.*

Davis, Karen. "Economic Theories of Behavior in Nonprofit Private Hospitals."

Griffith, John R. *Quantitative Techniques for Hospital Planning and Control.*

Gross, Malvern J. and Warshauer, William, Jr. *Financial and Accounting Guide for Nonprofit Organizations.*

Silvers, J.B. "Identity Crisis: Financial Management in Health Care."

Silvers, J.B.; Zelman, William N.; and Kahn, Charles N. III (eds.). *Health Care Financial Management in the 1980s: Time of Transition.*

APPENDIX 1.A
CORPORATE TAX STATUS OF HOSPITALS

As has been indicated, the objective of this text is to acquaint the managers of both for-profit and nonprofit hospitals with the potential that exists for improved operations through the use of financial management tools and techniques. However, before going on, it should be made clear what is meant by "nonprofit." The simplest way to do this is to review the Internal Revenue Code, for nonprofit is a term that relates primarily to a hospital's tax status.

---

[3]Full publishing details for works cited in "Suggested Readings" will be found in Bibliography A or B at the end of this volume.

SUMMARY OF INTERNAL REVENUE CODE[4]

Corporate Taxation—Section 11

A. A tax is hereby imposed for each taxable year on the taxable income of every corporation.

B. The tax is to be progressive in nature ranging from 15% to 46% of taxable income.[5]

Exemption from Corporate Taxation—Section 501(c)(3)

A. Corporations and any community chest, fund, or foundation, organized and operated exclusively for religious, charitable, scientific, testing for public safety, literary, or educational purposes, or to foster national or international amateur sports competition or for the prevention of cruelty to children or animals are exempt from income taxes if no part of their net earnings goes to the benefit of any private shareholder or individual, no substantial part of their activities involves carrying on propaganda or otherwise attempting to influence legislation, and they do not attempt to participate or intervene in any political campaign.[6]

B. To qualify for an exemption under Section 501(c)(3), a hospital must meet the following requirements.[7]

---

[4]Internal Revenue Code of 1954 as amended to date.
[5]Corporate Tax Rate Table

| Taxable Income | | Tax Rate |
Over	Not Over	(%)
$ 0	$ 25,000	15
25,000	50,000	18
50,000	75,000	30
75,000	100,000	46
100,000	1,000,000	
1,000,000*		

*The Tax Reform Act of 1984 phases out the benefit of lower tax rates for corporations whose taxable income exceeds $1 million by increasing their tax by 5% of taxable income in excess of $1 million up to $1,405,000 or $20,250 whichever is less.

[6]A charitable organization presently jeopardizes its exempt status if a substantial part of its activities is propagandizing or otherwise attempting to influence legislation. Instead of application of a "substantial part of activities" test, a sliding scale limitation, based on a percentage of the organization's exempt purpose expenditures, may be used to determine appropriateness of tax exemption.

[7]It should be noted that in the original Code, a third requirement was also included, "operate to the extent of its financial ability for the benefit of those not able to pay for services." See Appendix 1.B for a discussion of how this requirement changed.

1. Be organized as a nonprofit, charitable organization whose purpose is caring for the sick
2. Not restrict the use of its facilities to a particular group of physicians or surgeons

Notification Requirements—Section 502

A. Organizations claiming exempt status under Section 501(c)(3) must comply with certain Internal Revenue Service notification requirements. An application for exempt status on Form 1023, when properly completed, constitutes the notice required.

B. A second notification is required of an organization claiming exempt status under Section 501(c)(3) if it is claiming public charity status.[8] An application for exempt status on Form 1023, when the appropriate portions are properly completed, constitutes the notice required.

Maintenance of Exemption—Section 503

A. A hospital, to maintain its tax exemption, must refrain from engaging in any prohibited financial transactions.

B. Prohibited financial transactions are defined as any transaction in which a Section 501(c)(3) corporation
   1. Lends any part of its income without receiving adequate security and interest
   2. Pays any compensation in excess of reasonable salary levels
   3. Makes any investments for more than adequate consideration
   4. Sells any assets for less than adequate consideration
   5. Subverts in any other manner substantial portions of its income or assets
   6. Makes any part of its services available on a preferential basis

C. If a hospital engages in any of these acts with an individual who is either an owner or an employee of the hospital, then it is engaging in a prohibited transaction and jeopardizes its tax exemption.

---

[8]The Tax Reform Act of 1969 created two general categories of exempt organizations with different rules and benefits for each: private foundations and other than private foundations (publicly supported organizations). "Other than private foundations" are organizations that receive a substantial portion of their receipts from direct or indirect contributions from the general public or from a governmental unit. Hospitals and medical research organizations related to hospitals are generally other than private foundations. As such, they are subject to a minimum of rules. Also, an individual donor can deduct contributions to publicly supported organizations up to 50% of adjusted gross income. (A 20% limit normally applies to contributions to private foundations.)

Information Return—Section 504

A. An annual return stating gross income, receipts, contributions, disbursements, and the like is required from 501(c)(3) organizations with the exception of: churches; the exclusively religious activities of religious orders; church or denomination sponsored foreign mission societies; and charitable organizations that normally have annual gross receipts of $25,000 or less.

B. The annual return of an exempt organization must be filed on Form 990—see Figure 1.A-1.

Unrelated Business Income—Sections 512 and 513[9]

A. Unrelated business income is the gross income derived by any exempt organization from any unrelated trade or business regularly carried out by it, less the deductions that are directly connected with the carrying on of such trade or business.

B. An unrelated trade or business is any trade or business the conduct of which is not substantially related to the exercise or performance by the hospital of its charitable purpose.

C. Income from several types of activity unrelated to patient care is not considered unrelated business income; for example,

1. Income from passive investment activities

2. Income derived from activities in which substantially all the work is performed without any compensation, such as a voluntarily operated gift shop, or from the sales of merchandise substantially all of which has been received by the hospital as gifts or contributions

3. Income derived from research

4. Income derived from activities that are carried out primarily for the convenience of patients or employees

D. Unrelated business income is taxed at the normal corporate tax rates.[10]

E. Exempt organizations with unrelated business income of more than $1,000 are required to file an income tax return on Form 990-T—see Figure 1.A-2.

---

[9]See "Bibliography of Rulings" at the end of this appendix.

[10]This is done to protect commercial enterprises from an unfair competitive advantage that nonprofit organizations might have if they were not required to pay taxes on the income derived from such activities.

FIGURE 1.A-1

Form **990**	**Return of Organization Exempt from Income Tax**	OMB No. 1545-0047
Department of the Treasury Internal Revenue Service	Under section 501(c) (except black lung benefit trust or private foundation), of the Internal Revenue Code or section 4947(a)(1) trust Note: You may be required to use a copy of this return to satisfy State reporting requirements. See instruction D.	**1984**

For the calendar year 1984, or fiscal year beginning , 1984, and ending , 19

Use IRS label. Other-wise, please print or type.	Name of organization	A Employer identification number (see instruction L)
	Address (number and street)	B State registration number (see instruction D)
	City or town, State, and ZIP code	C If address changed, check here ▶

D Check applicable box—Exempt under section ▶ ☐ 501(c) ( ) (insert number), OR ▶ ☐ section 4947(a)(1) trust   ☐ Check here if application exemption is pending

E Accounting method: ☐ Cash ☐ Accrual ☐ Other (specify) ▶

F Section 4947(a)(1) trusts filing this form in lieu of Form 1041, check here ▶ ☐ (see instruction C10).

G Is this a group return (see instruction J) filed for affiliates? . . . . . ☐ Yes ☐ No   If "Yes" to either, give four-digit group exemption number
Is this a separate return filed by a group affiliate? . . . . ☐ Yes ☐ No   (GEN) ▶

☐ Check here if your gross receipts are normally not more than $25,000 (see instruction B11). You do not have to file a completed return with IRS but should file a return without financial data if you were mailed a Form 990 Package (see instruction A). Some States may require a completed return.

☐ Check here if gross receipts are normally more than $25,000 and line 12 is $25,000 or less. Complete Parts I (except lines 13-15), III, IV, VI, and VII and only the indicated items in Parts II and V (see instruction I). If line 12 is more than $25,000, complete the entire return.

501(c)(3) organizations and 4947(a)(1) trusts must also complete and attach Schedule A (Form 990). (See instructions.)

Part I	**Statement of Support, Revenue, and Expenses and Changes in Fund Balances**	(A) Total	These columns are optional—see instructions	
			(B) Unrestricted/ Expendable	(C) Restricted/ Nonexpendable

Support and Revenue

1	Contributions, gifts, grants, and similar amounts received:			
	(a) Direct public support			
	(b) Indirect public support			
	(c) Government grants			
	(d) Total (add lines 1(a) through 1(c)) (attach schedule—see instructions)			
2	Program service revenue (from Part IV, line (f))			
3	Membership dues and assessments			
4	Interest on savings and temporary cash investments			
5	Dividends and interest from securities			
6	(a) Gross rents			
	(b) Minus: Rental expenses			
	(c) Net rental income (loss)			
7	Other investment income (Describe ▶)			
8	(a) Gross amount from sale of assets other than inventory . [Securities] [Other]			
	(b) Minus: cost or other basis and sales expenses			
	(c) Gain (loss) (attach schedule)			
9	Special fundraising events and activities (attach schedule—see instructions):			
	(a) Gross revenue (not including $_____ of contributions reported on line 1(a)) . . .			
	(b) Minus: direct expenses			
	(c) Net income (line 9(a) minus line 9(b))			
10	(a) Gross sales minus returns and allowances . . .			
	(b) Minus: Cost of goods sold (attach schedule) . .			
	(c) Gross profit (loss)			
11	Other revenue (from Part IV, line (g))			
12	Total revenue (add lines 1(d), 2, 3, 4, 5, 6(c), 7, 8(c), 9(c), 10(c), and 11).			

Expenses

13	Program services (from line 44(B)) (see instructions)			
14	Management and general (from line 44(C)) (see instructions) . . .			
15	Fundraising (from line 44(D)) (see instructions)			
16	Payments to affiliates (attach schedule—see instructions) . . .			
17	Total expenses (add lines 16 and 44(A))			

Fund Balances

18	Excess (deficit) for the year (subtract line 17 from line 12) . . .			
19	Fund balances or net worth at beginning of year (from line 74(A)) . .			
20	Other changes in fund balances or net worth (attach explanation) . .			
21	Fund balances or net worth at end of year (add lines 18, 19, and 20) . .			

For Paperwork Reduction Act Notice, see page 1 of the instructions.   Form **990** (1984)

FIGURE 1.A-1   Continued

Part II	Statement of Functional Expenses	All organizations must complete column (A). Columns (B), (C), and (D) are required for most section 501(c)(3) and (c)(4) organizations and 4947(a)(1) trusts but optional for others. (See instructions.)			
	Do not include amounts reported on lines 6(b), 8(b), 9(b), 10(b), or 16 of Part I.	**(A) Total**	**(B) Program services**	**(C) Management and general**	**(D) Fundraising**
	22 Grants and allocations (attach schedule)				
	23 Specific assistance to individuals				
	24 Benefits paid to or for members				
	25 Compensation of officers, directors, etc..				
	26 Other salaries and wages.				
	27 Pension plan contributions				
	28 Other employee benefits.				
	29 Payroll taxes				
	30 Professional fundraising fees				
	31 Accounting fees.				
	32 Legal fees				
	33 Supplies				
	34 Telephone				
	35 Postage and shipping				
	36 Occupancy				
	37 Equipment rental and maintenance				
	38 Printing and publications				
	39 Travel				
	40 Conferences, conventions and meetings				
	41 Interest				
	42 Depreciation, depletion, etc. (attach schedule). . .				
	43 Other expenses (itemize): **(a)** _____				
	(b) _____				
	(c) _____				
	(d) _____				
	(e) _____				
	(f) _____				
	44 Total functional expenses (add lines 22 through 43)				

Expenses (vertical label at left)

Part III	Statement of Program Services Rendered

List each program service title on lines (a) through (d); for each, identify the service output(s) or product(s) and report the quantity provided. Enter the total expenses attributable to each program service and the amount of grants and allocations included in that total. (See instructions for Part III.)

Expenses (Optional for some organizations—see instructions)

(a) _____

_____

_____

_____

(Grants and allocations $ _____)

(b) _____

_____

_____

_____

(Grants and allocations $ _____)

(c) _____

_____

_____

_____

(Grants and allocations $ _____)

(d) _____

_____

_____

_____

(Grants and allocations $ _____)

(e) Other program service activities (attach schedule)   (Grants and allocations $ _____)

(f) Total (add lines (a) through (e)) (should equal line 44(B))

FIGURE 1.A-1   Continued

Part IV	Program Service Revenue and Other Revenue (State Nature)	Program service revenue	Other revenue
(a)	Fees from government agencies		
(b)	....		
(c)	....		
(d)	....		
(e)	....		
(f)	Total program service revenue (enter here and on line 2)		
(g)	Total other revenue (enter here and on line 11)		

Part V	Balance Sheets	If line 12, Part I, and line 59 are $25,000 or less, you should complete only lines 59, 66, and 74 and, if you do not use fund accounting, line 73. If line 12 or line 59 is more than $25,000, complete the entire balance sheet. See instructions.

Note: Columns (C) and (D) are optional. Columns (A) and (B) must be completed to the extent applicable. Where required, attached schedules should be for end-of-year amounts only.	(A) Beginning of year	End of year		
		(B) Total	(C) Unrestricted/ Expendable	(D) Restricted/ Nonexpendable

Assets

45	Cash—non-interest bearing				
46	Savings and temporary cash investments				
47	Accounts receivable ▶ _____				
	minus allowance for doubtful accounts ▶ _____				
48	Pledges receivable ▶ _____				
	minus allowance for doubtful accounts ▶ _____				
49	Grants receivable				
50	Receivables due from officers, directors, trustees and key employees (attach schedule)				
51	Other notes and loans receivable ▶ _____				
	minus allowance for doubtful accounts ▶ _____				
52	Inventories for sale or use				
53	Prepaid expenses and deferred charges . . .				
54	Investments—securities (attach schedule)				
55	Investments—land, buildings and equipment: basis ▶ _____				
	minus accumulated depreciation ▶ _____ (attach schedule)				
56	Investments—other (attach schedule)				
57	Land, buildings and equipment: basis ▶ _____				
	minus accumulated depreciation ▶ _____ (attach schedule)				
58	Other assets ▶ _____				
59	Total assets (add lines 45 through 58)				

Liabilities

60	Accounts payable and accrued expenses				
61	Grants payable				
62	Support and revenue designated for future periods (attach schedule) .				
63	Loans from officers, directors, trustees and key employees (attach schedule)				
64	Mortgages and other notes payable (attach schedule) . . .				
65	Other liabilities ▶ _____ . . .				
66	Total liabilities (add lines 60 through 65)				

Fund Balances or Net Worth
Organizations that use fund accounting, check here ▶ ☐ and complete lines 67 through 70 and lines 74 and 75.

67	a. Current unrestricted fund				
	b. Current restricted fund				
68	Land, buildings and equipment fund				
69	Endowment fund				
70	Other funds (Describe ▶ _____)				

Organizations that do not use fund accounting, check here ▶ ☐ and complete lines 71 through 75.

71	Capital stock or trust principal				
72	Paid-in or capital surplus				
73	Retained earnings or accumulated income				
74	Total fund balances or net worth (see instructions)				
75	Total liabilities and fund balances/net worth (see instructions) . .				

FIGURE 1.A-1   Continued

Form 990 (1984)   Page **4**

Part VI List of Officers, Directors, and Trustees (List each officer, director, and trustee whether compensated or not.) (See instructions)

(A) Name and address	(B) Title and average hours per week devoted to position	(C) Compensation (if any)	(D) Contributions to employee benefit plans	(E) Expense account and other allowances
-----------------------------				

Part VII Other Information | Yes | No

76 Has the organization engaged in any activities not previously reported to the Internal Revenue Service? . . . . .
     If "Yes," attach a detailed description of the activities.

77 Have any changes been made in the organizing or governing documents, but not reported to IRS? . . . . .
     If "Yes," attach a conformed copy of the changes.

78 **(a)** Did the organization have unrelated business gross income of $1,000 or more during the year covered by this return?
     (b) If "Yes," have you filed a tax return on Form 990-T, Exempt Organization Business Income Tax Return, for this year?
     (c) If the organization has gross sales or receipts from business activities not reported on Form 990-T, attach a statement explaining your reason for not reporting them on Form 990-T.

79 Was there a liquidation, dissolution, termination, or substantial contraction during the year (see instructions)? . . . .
     If "Yes," attach a statement as described in the instructions.

80 Is the organization related (other than by association with a statewide or nationwide organization) through common membership, governing bodies, trustees, officers, etc., to any other exempt or nonexempt organization (see instructions)? . .
     If "Yes," enter the name of organization ▶ ---
     -- and check whether it is ☐ exempt **OR** ☐ nonexempt.

81 **(a)** Enter amount of political expenditures, direct or indirect, as described in the instructions . . ∟
     (b) Did you file Form 1120-POL, U.S. Income Tax Return for Certain Political Organizations, for this year? .

82 Did your organization receive donated services or the use of materials, equipment or facilities at no charge or at substantially less than fair rental value? . . . .
     If "Yes," you may indicate the value of these items here. Do not include this amount as support
     in Part I or as an expense in Part II. See instructions for reporting in Part III . . . . ▶ ∟

83 *Section 501(c)(5) or (6) organizations.*—Did the organization spend any amounts in attempts to influence public opinion about legislative matters or referendums (see instructions and Regulations section 1.162-20(c))? . . . . .
     If "Yes," enter the total amount spent for this purpose ∟

84 *Section 501(c)(7) organizations.*—Enter amount of:
     (a) Initiation fees and capital contributions included on line 12 . . . . ∟
     (b) Gross receipts, included in line 12, for public use of club facilities (see instructions) . . . ∟
     (c) Does the club's governing instrument or any written policy statement provide for discrimination against any person because of race, color, or religion (see instructions)? . . . .

85 *Section 501(c)(12) organizations.*—Enter amount of:
     (a) Gross income received from members or shareholders . . . . ∟
     (b) Gross income received from other sources (do not net amounts due or paid to other sources against amounts due or received from them) . . . . ∟

86 *Public interest law firms.*—Attach information described in instructions.

87 List the States with which a copy of this return is filed ▶ ---

88 During this tax year did you maintain any part of your accounting/tax records on a computerized system?. . .

89 The books are in care of ▶ -------------------------- Telephone No. ▶ ------------------------
     Located at ▶

Please Sign Here   Under penalties of perjury, I declare that I have examined this return, including accompanying schedules and statements, and to the best of my knowledge and belief it is true, correct, and complete. Declaration of preparer (other than taxpayer) is based on all information of which preparer has any knowledge.

▶ _____ | _____ | ▶ _____
   Signature of officer   Date   Title

Paid Preparer's Use Only

Preparer's signature ▶	Date	Check if self-employed ▶ ☐
Firm's name (or yours, if self-employed) and address ▶		ZIP code ▶

FIGURE 1.A-1   Continued

Schedule A. (Form 990). Supplementary Information; Sec. 501(c)(3) Organizations. (cont'd)

SCHEDULE A (Form 990) Department of the Treasury Internal Revenue Service	**Organization Exempt Under 501(c)(3)** (Except Private Foundation), 501(e), 501(f), 501(k), or Section 4947(a)(1) Trust Supplementary Information ▶ Attach to Form 990.	OMB No. 1545-0047

Name	Employer identification number

Part I Compensation of Five Highest Paid Employees
(Other than Officers, Directors, and Trustees—see specific instructions)

Name and address of employees paid more than $30,000	Title and average hours per week devoted to position	Compensation	Contributions to employee benefit plans	Expense account and other allowances

Total number of other employees paid over $30,000 . . . . ▶

Part II Compensation of Five Highest Paid Persons for Professional Services
(See specific instructions)

Name and address of persons paid more than $30,000	Type of service	Compensation

Total number of others receiving over $30,000 for professional services . . . . ▶

Part III Statements About Activities

		Yes	No
1	During the year have you attempted to influence national, State or local legislation, including any attempt to influence public opinion on a legislative matter or referendum? . . . . If "Yes," enter the total of the expenses paid or incurred in connection with the legislative activities $ _____ Complete Part VI of this form for organizations that made an election under section 501(h) on Form 5768 or other statement. For other organizations checking "Yes," attach a statement giving a detailed description of the legislative activities and a classified schedule of the expenses paid or incurred.		
2	During the year have you, either directly or indirectly, engaged in any of the following acts with a trustee, director, principal officer or creator of your organization, or any organization or corporation with which such person is affiliated as an officer, director, trustee, majority owner or principal beneficiary:		
	(a) Sale, exchange, or leasing of property?		
	(b) Lending of money or other extension of credit?		
	(c) Furnishing of goods, services, or facilities?		
	(d) Payment of compensation (or payment or reimbursement of expenses if more than $1,000)?		
	(e) Transfer of any part of your income or assets?		
	If the answer to any question is "Yes," attach a detailed statement explaining the transactions.		
3	Attach a statement explaining how you determine that individuals or organizations receiving disbursements from you in furtherance of your charitable programs qualify to receive payments. (See specific instructions.)		
4	Do you make grants for scholarships, fellowships, student loans, etc.?		

For Paperwork Reduction Act Notice, see page 1 of the separate instructions to this form.   Schedule A (Form 990) 1984

FIGURE 1.A-1   Continued

Schedule A. (Form 990). Supplementary Information; Sec. 501(c)(3) Organizations. (cont'd)

Schedule A (Form 990) 1984

Part IV   Reason for Non-Private Foundation Status (See instructions for definitions)

The organization is not a private foundation because it is (check applicable box; please check only **ONE** box):

5 ☐ ¹ A church, convention of churches, or association of churches. Section 170(b)(1)(A)(i).

6 ☐ ² A school. Section 170(b)(1)(A)(ii). (Also complete Part V, page 3.)

7 ☐ ³ A hospital or a cooperative hospital service organization. Section 170(b)(1)(A)(iii).

8 ☐ ⁴ A Federal, State or local government or governmental unit. Section 170(b)(1)(A)(v).

9 ☐ ⁵ A medical research organization operated in conjunction with a hospital. Section 170(b)(1)(A)(iii). **Enter name, city, and State of hospital ▶** ....

10 ☐ ⁶ An organization operated for the benefit of a college or university owned or operated by a governmental unit. Section 170(b)(1)(A)(iv). (Also complete Support Schedule.)

11 ☐ ⁷ An organization that normally receives a substantial part of its support from a governmental unit or from the general public. Section 170(b)(1)(A)(vi). (Also complete Support Schedule.)

12 ☐ ⁸ An organization that normally receives: (a) no more than 1/3 of its support from gross investment income and unrelated business taxable income (less section 511 tax) from businesses acquired by the organization after June 30, 1975, and (b) more than 1/3 of its support from contributions, membership fees, and gross receipts from activities related to its charitable, etc., functions—subject to certain exceptions. See section 509(a)(2). (Also complete Support Schedule.)

13 ☐ ⁹ An organization that is not controlled by any disqualified persons (other than foundation managers) and supports organizations described in (1) boxes 5 through 12 above or (2) section 501(c)(4), (5), or (6) if they meet the test of section 509(a)(2). See section 509(a)(3).

Provide the following information about the supported organizations. (See instructions for Part IV, box 13.)

(a) Name of supported organizations	(b) Box number from above

14 ☐ ⁰ An organization organized and operated to test for public safety. Section 509(a)(4). (See specific instructions.)

Support Schedule (Complete only if you checked box 10, 11, or 12 above) Use cash method of accounting.

Calendar year (or fiscal year beginning in) ▶	(a) 1983	(b) 1982	(c) 1981	(d) 1980	(e) Total
15 Gifts, grants, and contributions received. (Do not include unusual grants. See line 28.)					
16 Membership fees received					
17 Gross receipts from admissions, merchandise sold or services performed, or furnishing of facilities in any activity that is not a business unrelated to the organization's charitable, etc., purpose.					
18 Gross income from interest, dividends, amounts received from payments on securities loans (section 512(a)(5)), rents, royalties, and unrelated business taxable income (less section 511 taxes) from businesses acquired by the organization after June 30, 1975					
19 Net income from unrelated business activities not included in line 18					
20 Tax revenues levied for your benefit and either paid to you or expended on your behalf					
21 The value of services or facilities furnished to you by a governmental unit without charge. Do not include the value of services or facilities generally furnished to the public without charge					
22 Other income. Attach schedule. Do not include gain (or loss) from sale of capital assets					
23 Total of lines 15 through 22					
24 Line 23 minus line 17					
25 Enter 1% of line 23					

26 Organizations described in box 10 or 11:
   (a) Enter 2% of amount in column (e), line 24 ....
   (b) Attach a list (not open to public inspection) showing the name of and amount contributed by each person (other than a governmental unit or publicly supported organization) whose total gifts for 1980 through 1983 exceeded the amount shown in 26(a). Enter the sum of all excess amounts here ....

(continued on page 3)

FIGURE 1.A-1   Continued

Schedule A. (Form 990). Supplementary Information; Sec. 501(c)(3) Organizations. (cont'd)

Schedule A (Form 990) 1984

Page **3**

Part IV	Support Schedule (continued)(Complete only if you checked box 10, 11, or 12 on page 2)

27 Organizations described in box 12, page 2:

   (a) Attach a list, for amounts shown on lines 15, 16, and 17, showing the name of, and total amounts received in each year from each "disqualified person," and enter the sum of such amounts for each year:

   (1983)................(1982)................(1981)................(1980)................

   (b) Attach a list showing, for 1980 through 1983, the name and amount included in line 17 for each person (other than "disqualified persons") from whom the organization received more, during that year, than the larger of: the amount on line 25 for the year or $5,000. Include organizations described in boxes 5 through 11 as well as individuals. Enter the sum of these excess amounts for each year:

   (1983)   (1982)   (1981)   (1980)

28 For an organization described in boxes 10, 11, or 12, page 2, that received any unusual grants during 1980 through 1983, attach a list (not open to public inspection) for each year showing the name of the contributor, the date and amount of the grant, and a brief description of the nature of the grant. Do not include these grants in line 15 above. (See specific instructions.)

Part V	Private School Questionnaire

To Be Completed ONLY by Schools that Checked Box 6 in Part IV

		Yes	No
29	Do you have a racially nondiscriminatory policy toward students by statement in your charter, bylaws, other governing instrument, or in a resolution of your governing body?		
30	Do you include a statement of your racially nondiscriminatory policy toward students in all your brochures, catalogues, and other written communications with the public dealing with student admissions, programs, and scholarships? . . .		
31	Have you publicized your racially nondiscriminatory policy by newspaper or broadcast media during the period of solicitation for students or during the registration period if you have no solicitation program, in a way that makes the policy known to all parts of the general community you serve?.		
	If "Yes," please describe; if "No," please explain. (If you need more space, attach a separate statement.)		
32	Do you maintain the following:		
(a)	Records indicating the racial composition of the student body, faculty, and administrative staff?.		
(b)	Records documenting that scholarships and other financial assistance are awarded on a racially nondiscriminatory basis?.		
(c)	Copies of all catalogues, brochures, announcements, and other written communications to the public dealing with student admissions, programs, and scholarships?.		
(d)	Copies of all material used by you or on your behalf to solicit contributions?		
	If you answered "No," to any of the above, please explain. (If you need more space, attach a separate statement.)		
33	Do you discriminate by race in any way with respect to:		
(a)	Students' rights or privileges?.		
(b)	Admissions policies?.		
(c)	Employment of faculty or administrative staff?		
(d)	Scholarships or other financial assistance (see instructions)?.		
(e)	Educational policies?		
(f)	Use of facilities?		
(g)	Athletic programs?		
(h)	Other extra-curricular activities?		
	If you answered "Yes," to any of the above, please explain. (If you need more space, attach a separate statement.)		
34 **(a)**	Do you receive any financial aid or assistance from a governmental agency?		
(b)	Has your right to such aid ever been revoked or suspended?		
	If you answered "Yes," to either 34(a) or (b), please explain using an attached separate statement.		
35	Do you certify that you have complied with the applicable requirements of sections 4.01 through 4.05 of Rev. Proc. 75-50, 1975-2 C.B. 587, covering racial nondiscrimination? If "No," attach an explanation (see instructions for Part V) . . .		

FIGURE 1.A-1   Continued

Schedule A. (Form 990). Supplementary Information; Sec. 501(c)(3) Organizations. (cont'd)

Part VI Lobbying Expenditures By Public Charities (See Instructions)
(To be completed ONLY by an eligible organization that filed Form 5768.)

Check here ▶ **(a)** ☐   If the organization belongs to an affiliated group (see instructions).
Check here ▶ **(b)** ☐   If you checked (a) and "limited control" provisions apply (see instructions).

	(a) Affiliated group totals	(b) To be completed for ALL electing organizations
Limits on Lobbying Expenses		
36 Total (grassroots) lobbying expenses to influence public opinion		
37 Total lobbying expenses to influence a legislative body		
38 Total lobbying expenses (add lines 36 and 37)		
39 Other exempt purpose expenses (see Part VI instructions)		
40 Total exempt purpose expenses (add lines 38 and 39) (see instructions).		
41 Lobbying nontaxable amount. Enter the smaller of $1,000,000 or the amount determined under the following table—		

If the amount on line 40 is—	The lobbying nontaxable amount is—
Not over $500,000	20% of the amount on line 40. . . . .
Over $500,000 but not over $1,000,000 . . .	$100,000 plus 15% of the excess over $500,000 . . .
Over $1,000,000 but not over $1,500,000 . . .	$175,000 plus 10% of the excess over $1,000,000 . . .
Over $1,500,000.	$225,000 plus 5% of the excess over $1,500,000 . . .

	(a)	(b)
42 Grassroots nontaxable amount (enter 25% of line 41)		
(Complete lines 43 and 44. File Form 4720 if either line 36 exceeds line 42 or line 38 exceeds line 41.)		
43 Excess of line 36 over line 42		
44 Excess of line 38 over line 41		

4-Year Averaging Period Under Section 501(h).

(Some organizations that made a section 501(h) election do not have to complete all of the five columns below. See the instructions for lines 45-50 for details.)

(Line references below are to column (b) of Part VI, Schedule A (Form 990) for the respective tax year)	Lobbying Expenses During 4-Year Averaging Period				
Calendar year (or fiscal year beginning in) ▶	(a) 1984	(b) 1983	(c) 1982	(d) 1981	(e) Total
45 Lobbying nontaxable amount (see instructions)					
46 Lobbying ceiling amount (150% of line 45(e))					
47 Total lobbying expenses (see instructions)					
48 Grassroots nontaxable amount (see instructions)					
49 Grassroots ceiling amount (150% of line 48(e))					
50 Grassroots lobbying expenses (see instructions)					

FIGURE 1.A-2

Form 990-T. Exempt Organization Business Income Tax Return.

Form **990-T**	**Exempt Organization Business Income Tax Return**	OMB No. 1545-0687
Department of the Treasury Internal Revenue Service	(Under Section 511 of the Internal Revenue Code) For calendar year 1984 or other tax year beginning .... 1984, and ending 19	**1984**

Name of organization	**A** Employer identification number (employees' trust see instruction for Block A)
Address (number and street)	
City or town, State, and ZIP code	**B** Enter unrelated business activity codes from page 10 of instructions

C Check box if address changed . . . . . ▶ ☐ **D** Exempt under section . . . . . ▶ 501 ( ) ( )

E Check applicable box . . ▶ ☐ Corporation ☐ Trust ☐ Section 401(a) trust

F Group exemption number (see instructions for Block F) ▶

If the unrelated trade or business gross income is $10,000 or less, complete only page 1, Part III on page 2, and sign the return. Complete all applicable parts of the form (except lines 1 through 4) if unrelated trade or business gross income is over $10,000.

Taxable Income	1 Unrelated trade or business gross income (state sources ▶ ....)	**1**
	2 Deductions (complete Parts I and II instead of lines 1, 2, 3 and 4 if you have gross income over $10,000) .	**2**
	3 Unrelated business taxable income before specific deduction (subtract line 2 from line 1)	**3**
	4 Specific deduction (see instructions)	**4**
	5 Unrelated business taxable income (subtract line 4 from line 3 or enter amount from line 33, page 2) .	**5**
Tax Computation	**Organizations Taxable as Corporations (See Instructions for Tax Computation)**	
	6 (a) Check if you are a member of a controlled group (see sections 1561 and 1563) . . . . . ☐	
	(b) If checked, see instructions and enter your share of the $25,000 in each taxable income bracket:	
	(i) $ .... (ii) $ .... (iii) $ .... (iv) $	
	7 Income tax on amount on line 5, above. Check here ▶ ☐ if alternative tax from Schedule D (Form 1120) is used.	**7**
	Trusts Taxable at Trust Rates (See Instructions for Tax Computation)	
	8 Enter the tax from the tax rate schedule in the instructions on the amount on line 5	**8**
	9 (a) Foreign tax credit (corporations attach Form 1118, trusts attach Form 1116) . **9(a)**	
	(b) Other credits (see instructions) . . . . **9(b)**	
	(c) General business credit.— Check if from **9(c)**	
	☐ Form 3800 ☐ Form 3468 ☐ Form 5884 ☐ Form 6478	
Total Income Tax	10 Total (add lines 9(a) through 9(c))	**10**
	11 Subtract line 10 from line 7 or line 8	**11**
	12 Tax from recomputing prior year investment credit (attach Form 4255)	**12**
	13 Minimum tax on tax preference items (Corporations only– see instructions)	**13**
	14 Alternative minimum tax (Trusts only–see instructions)	**14**
	15 Total tax (add lines 11 through 14)	**15**
	16 Credits and payments:	
	(a) Tax deposited with Form 7004 or Form 2758 . . . . **16(a)**	
	(b) Foreign corporations—Tax paid or withheld at the source (see instructions) . **16(b)**	
	(c) Credit from regulated investment companies (attach Form 2439) . **16(c)**	
	(d) Credit for Federal tax on gasoline and special fuels (attach Form 4136) **16(d)**	
	(e) Other credits and payments (see instructions) . . . . . . **16(e)**	
	(f) Total credits and payments (add lines 16(a) through 16(e))	**16(f)**
	17 **TAX DUE** (subtract line 16(f) from line 15). See instructions for depositary method of payment . ▶	**17**
	18 **OVERPAYMENT** (subtract line 15 from line 16(f)) . . . . ▶	**18**

Please Sign Here	Under penalties of perjury, I declare that I have examined this return, including accompanying schedules and statements, and to the best of my knowledge and belief, it is true, correct, and complete. Declaration of preparer (other than taxpayer) is based on all information of which preparer has any knowledge.		
	▶ Signature of officer	Date	▶ Title

Paid Preparer's Use Only	Preparer's signature ▶	Date	Check if self-employed ☐	Preparer's social security no.
	Firm's name (or yours, if self-employed) and address		E.I. No. ▶	
			ZIP code ▶	

For Paperwork Reduction Act Notice, see page 1 of instructions. Form **990-T** (1984)

10/84 page 724,663

FIGURE 1.A-2 Continued

Form 990-T. Exempt Organization Business Income Tax Return. (cont'd)

Form 990-T (1984)   Page **2**

Part I — Unrelated Trade or Business Income

1 (a) Gross receipts or sales _____ (b) Less returns and allowances _____ Balance ▶	1(c)	
2 Cost of goods sold and/or operations (Schedule A)	2	
3 Gross profit (subtract line 2 from line 1(c))	3	
4 (a) Capital gain net income (attach separate Schedule D) (see instructions)	4(a)	
(b) Net gain or (loss) from Part II, Form 4797 (attached)	4(b)	
(c) Capital loss deduction for trusts	4(c)	
5 Income or (loss) from partnerships (attach statement)	5	
6 Rent income (Schedule C)	6	
7 Unrelated debt-financed income (Schedule E, line 2)	7	
8 Investment income of a section 501(c)(7) or (9) organization (Schedule F)	8	
9 Interest, annuities, royalties, and rents from controlled organizations (Schedule G) . .	9	
10 Exploited exempt activity income (Schedule H)	10	
11 Advertising income (Schedule I, Part III, Column A)	11	
12 Other income (see instructions for line 12—attach schedule)	12	
13 TOTAL—Unrelated trade or business income (add lines 3 through 12)	13	

Part II — Deductions Not Taken Elsewhere
(Except for contributions, deductions must be directly connected with the unrelated business income.)

14 Compensation of officers, directors, and trustees (Schedule J)	14	
15 Salaries and wages	15	
16 Repairs (see instructions)	16	
17 Bad debts (see instructions)	17	
18 Interest (attach schedule)	18	
19 Taxes	19	
20 Contributions (see instructions)	20	
21 Depreciation (attach Form 4562) 21		
22 Less depreciation claimed in Schedule A and elsewhere on return . . . . 22(a)	22(b)	
23 Depletion	23	
24 (a) Contributions to deferred compensation plans (see instructions)	24(a)	
(b) Employee benefit programs (see instructions)	24(b)	
25 Other deductions (attach schedule)	25	
26 TOTAL DEDUCTIONS (add lines 14 through 25)	26	
27 Unrelated business taxable income before allowable advertising loss (subtract line 26 from line 13) .	27	
28 Advertising loss (Schedule I, Part III, Column B)	28	
29 Unrelated business taxable income before net operating loss deduction (subtract line 28 from line 27) .	29	
30 Net operating loss deduction (see instructions)	30	
31 Unrelated business taxable income before specific deduction (subtract line 30 from line 29)	31	
32 Specific deduction (see instructions for line 4 of page 1)	32	
33 Unrelated business taxable income (subtract line 32 from line 31. Enter here and on page 1, line 5 . . .	33	

SCHEDULE A—COST OF GOODS SOLD AND/OR OPERATIONS
(See Instructions for Part I, line 2)

Method of inventory valuation (specify) ▶

1 Inventory at beginning of year	1	
2 Purchases	2	
3 Cost of labor	3	
4 Other costs (attach schedule)	4	
5 TOTAL—Add lines 1 through 4	5	
6 Inventory at end of year	6	
7 Cost of goods sold and/or operations. Subtract line 6 from line 5. (Enter here and on line 2, Part I.) . . .	7	

Part III — Statements Regarding Certain Activities and Other Information

	Yes	No
1 At any time during the tax year, did you have an interest in or a signature or other authority over a bank account, securities account, or other financial account in a foreign country (see page 9 of the instructions for exceptions and filing requirements for TD F 90-22.1)?		
If "Yes," write in the name of the foreign country _____		
2 Were you the grantor of, or transferor to, a foreign trust which existed during the current tax year, whether or not you had any beneficial interest in it? If "Yes," you may have to file Forms 3520, 3520-A, or 926.		

The books are in care of ▶   Telephone number ▶

FIGURE 1.A-2 Continued

Form 990-T. Exempt Organization Business Income Tax Return. (cont'd)

Form 990-T (1984)   Page **3**

SCHEDULE C—RENT INCOME FROM REAL PROPERTY AND PERSONAL PROPERTY LEASED WITH REAL PROPERTY
(See Instructions for Part I, line 6)

1. Description of property	2. Rent received or accrued	3. Percentage of rent for personal property
		%
		%
		%
		%
		%

4. Complete for any item if the entry in column 3 is more than 50%, or if the rent is based on profit or income		5. Complete for any item if the entry in column 3 is more than 10% but not more than 50%		
(a) Deductions directly connected (Attach schedule)	(b) Income includible (Column 2 minus column 4(a))	(a) Gross income reportable (Column 2 x column 3)	(b) Deductions directly connected with personal property (Attach schedule)	(c) Income includible (Column 5(a) minus column 5(b))

Add columns 4(b) and 5(c) and enter total here and on line 6, Part I, page 2 . . . .

SCHEDULE E—UNRELATED DEBT-FINANCED INCOME (See Instructions for Part I, line 7)

1. Description of debt-financed property	2. Gross income from or allocable to debt-financed property	3. Deductions directly connected with or allocable to debt-financed property	
		(a) Straight-line depreciation (Attach schedule)	(b) Other deductions (Attach schedule)
1			

4. Amount of average acquisition indebtedness on or allocable to debt-financed property (Attach schedule)	5. Average adjusted basis of or allocable to debt-financed property (Attach schedule)	6. Percentage which col. 4 is of col. 5	7. Gross income reportable (Column 2 x column 6)	8. Allocable deductions (Column 6 x total of columns 3(a) and 3(b))	9. Net income or (loss) includible (Column 7 minus column 8)
		%			
		%			
		%			
		%			

2 Total (enter here and on line 7, Part I, page 2) . . . .
3 Total dividends-received deductions included in column 8 . . . .

SCHEDULE F—INVESTMENT INCOME OF A SECTION 501(c)(7) OR (9) ORGANIZATION
(See Instructions for Part I, line 8)

1. Description	2. Amount	3. Deductions directly connected (Attach schedule)	4. Net investment income (Column 2 minus column 3)	5. Set-asides (Attach schedule)	6. Balance of investment income (Column 4 minus column 5)

Total (enter here and on line 8, Part I, page 2) . . . .

SCHEDULE G—INCOME (ANNUITIES, INTEREST, RENTS AND ROYALTIES) FROM CONTROLLED ORGANIZATIONS
(See Instructions for Part I, line 9)

1. Name and address of controlled organization(s)	2. Gross income from controlled organization(s)	3. Deductions of controlling organization directly connected with column 2 income (Attach schedule)	4. Exempt controlled organizations		
			(a) Unrelated business taxable income	(b) Taxable income computed as though not exempt under sec. 501(a), or the amount in col. (a), whichever is more	(c) Percentage which col. (a) is of col. (b)
					%
					%
					%

5. Nonexempt controlled organizations			6. Gross income reportable (Column 2 x column 4(c) or column 5(c))	7. Allowable deductions (Column 3 x column 4(c) or column 5(c))	8. Net income includible (Column 6 minus column 7)
(a) Excess taxable income	(b) Taxable income, or amount in column (a), whichever is more	(c) Percentage which col. (a) is of col. (b)			
		%			
		%			
		%			

Total (enter here and on line 9, Part I, page 2) . . . .

10/84 page 724,665

FIGURE 1.A-2   Continued

Form 990-T. Exempt Organization Business Income Tax Return. (cont'd)

SCHEDULE H—EXPLOITED EXEMPT ACTIVITY INCOME, OTHER THAN ADVERTISING INCOME
(See Instructions for Part I, line 10)

1. Description of exploited activity	2. Gross unrelated business income from trade or business	3. Expenses directly connected with production of unrelated business income	4. Net income from unrelated trade or business (Column 2 minus column 3)	5. Gross income from activity that is not unrelated business income	6. Expenses attributable to column 5	7. Excess exempt expenses (Column 6 minus column 5, but not more than column 4)	8. Net income includible (Column 4 minus column 7)

Total (enter here and on line 10, Part I, page 2) . . . .

SCHEDULE I—ADVERTISING INCOME AND ADVERTISING LOSS (See Instructions for Part I, line 11)

Part I   Income from periodicals reported on consolidated basis

1. Name of periodical	2. Gross advertising income	3. Direct advertising costs	4. Advertising gain or loss (col. 2 minus col. 3). If loss, enter in col. B, Part III. Do not complete cols. 5, 6 and 7. If gain, complete cols. 5, 6 and 7.	5. Circulation income	6. Readership costs	7. If col. 5 exceeds col. 6, enter in col. A, Part III, the gain shown in col. 4. If col. 6 exceeds col. 5, subtract col. 6 plus col. 3 from col. 5 plus col. 2. Enter gain in col. A, Part III.

Totals . . . .

Part II   Income from periodicals reported on a separate basis

Part III   Column A—Advertising Income

(a) Enter "consolidated periodical" or names of non-consolidated periodicals	(b) Enter total amount from column 4 or 7, Part I, and amounts listed in cols. 4 and 7, Part II
Enter total here and on line 11, Part I, page 2	

Part III   Column B—Advertising Loss

(a) Enter "consolidated periodical" or names of non-consolidated periodicals	(b) Enter total amount from column 4, Part I, and amounts listed in column 4, Part II
Enter total here and on line 28, Part II, page 2	

SCHEDULE J—COMPENSATION OF OFFICERS, DIRECTORS, AND TRUSTEES

1. Name	2. Title	3. Percent of time devoted to business	4. Compensation attributable to unrelated business
		%	
		%	
		%	
		%	
		%	
		%	

Total (enter here and on line 14, Part II, page 2) . . . .

Thus, nonprofit does not mean that a hospital cannot earn a profit. Rather, it simply means that no part of the hospital's net earnings (profit) can inure either directly or indirectly to the benefit of any private individual. It is in this sense that the term is used in this text.[11]

BIBLIOGRAPHY OF REVENUE RULINGS AND CASES[12]

1. *Revenue Ruling 57-313*
   A medical research foundation's illustration and electroencephalography department brought in 75% of its revenues. The income source was so disproportionate to the foundation's exempt activities that it was classified unrelated business.

2. *Revenue Ruling 66-323*
   A community blood bank that sold blood and blood components to commercial laboratories was conducting unrelated business. (Revenue Ruling 66-323 was modified by Revenue Ruling 78-145.)

3. *Revenue Ruling 68-374*
   A hospital pharmacy, although its sales were primarily to hospital patients, was also open to the general public and derived a small percentage of its income from frequent and continuous sales to walk-in customers. Since those sales were regularly carried on, they were considered unrelated trade or business according to Section 512 of the Internal Revenue Code.

4. *Revenue Ruling 68-375*
   The sale of pharmaceutical supplies by a tax-exempt hospital to private patients of physicians with offices in a hospital-owned medical building constituted unrelated trade or business.

5. *Revenue Ruling 68-376*
   This ruling illustrates six situations in which purchasers of pharmaceutical supplies from a hospital were considered patients of that hospital; therefore, these pharmaceutical sales were considered related to the exempt purpose of the hospital.

6. *Revenue Ruling 68-550*
   Income from providing a mailing service for other organizations was classified as income from unrelated business, although the mailing equipment was used for exempt activities.

---

[11]The foregoing is not intended to be a complete discussion of tax law or regulations. Hospitals should retain competent tax counsel and regularly consult with that counsel.

[12]This material is excerpted from an American Hospital Association Technical Advisory Bulletin, "Unrelated Business Income of Tax-Exempt Health Care Institutions." Copyright of the same title. Used with permission.

7. *Revenue Ruling 69-69*
   An exempt cultural organization's leasing of a studio apartment was not necessary to further the organization's exempt purpose and was held to be not related.

8. *Revenue Ruling 69-267*
   The operation of a gift shop patronized by patients, visitors making purchases for patients, and employees by a Section 501(c)(3) hospital does not constitute unrelated trade or business under Section 513 of the Internal Revenue Code.

9. *Revenue Ruling 69-268*
   The operation of a cafeteria and coffee shop primarily for employees and medical staff by a Section 501(c)(3) hospital does not constitute unrelated trade or business under Section 513 of the Internal Revenue Code.

10. *Revenue Ruling 69-269*
    The operation of a parking lot for patients and visitors only by a Section 501(c)(3) hospital does not constitute unrelated trade or business under Section 513 of the Internal Revenue Code.

11. *Revenue Ruling 69-463*
    The leasing of its adjacent office building and the furnishing of certain office services by an exempt hospital to a hospital-based medical group are not unrelated trade or business under Section 513 of the Internal Revenue Code.

12. *Revenue Ruling 69-464*
    Leases of office spaces by an exempt hospital to members of its medical staff who contribute importantly to the performance of hospital functions are not considered business leases within the meaning of Section 514 of the Internal Revenue Code.

13. *Revenue Ruling 69-633*
    The court took the position that the sale of laundry services to other hospitals is not an activity substantially related to the performance of the selling hospital's exempt purpose and is therefore unrelated trade or business.

14. *Revenue Ruling 73-127*
    An exempt organization's operation of a retail grocery store as part of its therapeutic program for emotionally disturbed adolescents, where the store was almost entirely staffed by adolescents and was conducted on a scale no larger than reasonably necessary for performance of the organization's exempt functions, was not unrelated business income.

15. *Revenue Ruling 73-424*
    Income derived by an exempt organization from the sale of advertising in its annual yearbook was held to be unrelated business taxable income.

16. *Revenue Ruling 75-200*
    Income from the sale of advertising by the paid staff of an exempt organization during a four-month period was held to be income from unrelated trade or business regularly carried on because of the possible similarity to commercial sales practices.

17. *Revenue Ruling 75-201*
    The sale of advertising by volunteers of an exempt organization, which raised funds for a symphony orchestra and published an annual concert book distributed at the orchestra's annual charity ball, was not a business regularly carried on according to Section 512 and therefore was related business income.

18. *Revenue Ruling 75-33*
    The rental of dormitory rooms by an exempt organization is substantially related to the basis for the organization's exemption and is not unrelated trade or business within the meaning of Section 513 of the Internal Revenue Code.

19. *Revenue Ruling 78-43*
    The operation of a travel tour program by a university alumni association under which the association is paid a fee by the travel agents on a per person basis is an unrelated trade or business.

20. *Revenue Ruling 78-435*
    The sale of hearing aids to its patients by an exempt hospital, which has as its primary activity the rehabilitation of the handicapped, including those with hearing deficiencies, does not constitute unrelated trade or business under Internal Revenue Code Section 513.

21. *Private letter ruling (LTR 7843126, July 31, 1978)*
    A physical and respiratory therapy service provided by one hospital to patients of another hospital was substantially related to the hospital's exempt purpose and did not produce unrelated business taxable income.

22. *Carle Foundation vs. U.S., Civil No. 75-2-148 (D.C.E.D. Ill., March 30, 1978)*
    The court determined that pharmacy sales by the Carle Foundation to the nonpatient public constituted unrelated business.

APPENDIX 1.B
REVENUE RULING 69-545[13]

Revenue Ruling 69-545 contains two examples of hospitals—one operating as a public charity and the other as a private facility. The examples illustrate whether a nonprofit hospital that claims exemption under Sec. 501(c)(3) operates to serve a public interest rather than a private interest.

Advice has been requested whether the two nonprofit hospitals described below qualify for exemption from federal income tax under section 501(c)(3) of the Internal Revenue Code of 1954. The articles of organization of both hospitals meet the organizational requirements of section 1.501(c)(3)-1(b) of the Income Tax Regulations, including the limitation of the organizations' purposes to those described in section 501(c)(3) of the Code and the dedication of their assets to such purposes.

SITUATION 1

Hospital A is a 250-bed community hospital. Its board of trustees is composed of prominent citizens in the community. Medical staff privileges in the hospital are available to all qualified physicians in the area, consistent with the size and nature of its facilities. The hospital has 150 doctors on its active staff and 200 doctors on its courtesy staff. It also owns a medical office building on its premises with space for 60 doctors. Any member of its active medical staff has the privilege of leasing available office space. Rents are set at rates comparable to those of other commercial buildings in the area.

The hospital operates a full-time emergency room, and no one requiring emergency care is denied treatment. The hospital otherwise ordinarily limits admissions to those who can pay the cost of their hospitalization, either themselves, or through private health insurance, or with the aid of public programs such as Medicare. Patients who cannot meet the financial requirements for admission are ordinarily referred to another hospital in the community that does serve indigent patients.

The hospital usually ends each year with an excess of operating receipts over operating disbursements from its hospital operations. Excess funds are generally applied to expansion and replacement of existing facilities and equipment, amortization of indebtedness, improvement in patient care, and medical training, education, and research.

SITUATION 2

Hospital B is a 60-bed general hospital that was originally owned by five doctors. The owners formed a nonprofit organization and sold their

---

[13]Also released as Technical Information Release 1022, dated October 8, 1969.

interests in the hospital to the organization at fair market value. The board of trustees of the organization comprises the five doctors, their accountant, and their lawyer. The five doctors also make up the hospital's medical committee and thereby control the selection and the admission of other doctors to the medical staff. During its first five years of operations, only four other doctors have been granted staff privileges at the hospital. The applications of a number of qualified doctors in the community have been rejected.

Hospital admission is restricted to patients of doctors holding staff privileges. Patients of the five original physicians have accounted for a large majority of all hospital admissions over the years. The hospital maintains an emergency room, but on a relatively inactive basis, and primarily for the convenience of the patients of the staff doctors. The local ambulance services have been instructed by the hospital to take emergency cases to other hospitals in the area. The hospital follows the policy of ordinarily limiting admissions to those who can pay the cost of the services rendered. The five doctors who made up the original medical staff have continued to maintain their offices in the hospital since its sale to the nonprofit organization. The rental paid is less than that of comparable office space in the vicinity. No office space is available for any of the other staff members.

RULING

Section 501(c)(3) of the Code provides for exemption from federal income tax of organizations organized and operated exclusively for charitable, scientific, or educational purposes, no part of the net earnings of which inures to the benefit of any private shareholder or individual.

Section 1.501(c)(3)-1(d)(1)ii of the regulations provides that an organization is not organized or operated exclusively for any purpose set forth in section 501(c)(3) of the Code unless it serves a public rather than a private interest.

Section 1.501(c)(3)-1(d)(2) of the regulations states that the term "charitable" is used in section 501(c)(3) of the Code in its generally accepted legal sense.

To qualify for exemption from federal income tax under section 501(c)(3) of the Code, a nonprofit hospital must be organized and operated exclusively in furtherance of some purpose considered charitable in the generally accepted legal sense of that term, and the hospital may not be operated, directly or indirectly, for the benefit of private interests.

In the general law of charity, the promotion of health is considered to be a charitable purpose: "Restatement (Second), Trusts," sec. 368 and sec. 372; "IV Scott on Trusts" (3rd ed. 1967), sec. 368 and sec. 372. A nonprofit organization whose purpose and activity are providing hospital care is promoting health and may, therefore, qualify as organized and operated in furtherance of a charitable purpose. If it meets the other requirements of section 501(c)(3) of the Code, it will qualify for exemption from federal income tax under section 501(a).

Since the purpose and activity of Hospital A, apart from its related educational and research activities and purposes, are providing hospital care on a nonprofit basis for members of its community, it is organized and operated in furtherance of a purpose considered charitable in the generally accepted legal sense of that term. The promotion of health, like the relief of poverty and the advancement of education and religion, is one of the purposes in the general law of charity that is deemed beneficial to the community as a whole even though the class of beneficiaries eligible to receive a direct benefit from its activities does not include all members of the community, such as indigent members of the community, provided that the class is not so small that its relief is not of benefit to the community: "Restatement (Second), Trusts," sec. 368, comment (b) and sec. 372, comments (b) and (c); "IV Scott on Trusts" (3rd ed. 1967), sec. 368 and sec. 372.2. By operating an emergency room open to all persons and by providing hospital care to all those persons in the community able to pay the cost thereof either directly or through third party reimbursement, Hospital A is promoting the health of a class of persons that is broad enough to benefit the community.

The fact that Hospital A operates at an annual surplus of receipts over disbursements does not preclude its exemption. By using its surplus funds to improve the quality of patient care, expand its facilities, and advance its medical training, education, and research programs, the hospital is operating in furtherance of its exempt purposes.

Furthermore, Hospital A is operated to serve a public rather than a private interest. Control of the hospital rests with its board of trustees, which is composed of independent civic leaders. The hospital maintains an open medical staff, with privileges available to all qualified physicians. Members of its active medical staff have the privilege of leasing available space in its medical building. (For more information see Revenue Ruling 69-464.) It operates an active and generally accessible emergency room. These factors indicate that the use and control of Hospital A are for the benefit of the public and that no part of the income of the organization is inuring to the benefit of any private individual nor is any private interest being served.

Accordingly, it is held that Hospital A is exempt from federal income tax under section 501(c)(3) of the Code.

Hospital B is also providing hospital care. However, to qualify under section 501(c)(3) of the Code, an organization must be organized and operated *exclusively* for one or more of the purposes set forth in that section. Hospital B was initially established as a proprietary institution operated for the benefit of its owners. Although its ownership has been transferred to a nonprofit organization, the hospital has continued to operate for the private benefit of its original owners who exercise control over the hospital through the board of trustees and the medical committee. They have used their control to restrict the number of doctors admitted to the medical staff, to enter into favorable rental agreements with the hospital, and to limit emergency room care and hospital admission substantially to their own patients. These facts indicate that the hospital is operated for the private benefit of its original owners, rather than for the exclusive benefit of the public. See "Sonora Community Hospital v. Commissioner," 46 T.C. 519 (1966), aff'd 397 F.2d 814 (1968).

Accordingly, it is held that Hospital B does not qualify for exemption from federal income tax under section 501(c)(3) of the Code. In considering whether a nonprofit hospital claiming such exemption is operated to serve a private benefit, the Service will weigh all the relevant facts and circumstances in each case. The absence of particular factors set forth above or the presence of other factors will not necessarily be determinative.

Even though an organization considers itself within the scope of Situation 1 of the Revenue Ruling, it must file an application on Form 1023, Application for Recognition of Exemption (see Figure 1.B-1), to be recognized by the Service as exempt under section 501(c)(3) of the Code. The application should be filed with the District Director of Internal Revenue for the district in which is located the principal place of business or principal office of the organization. See section 1.501.(a)-1 of the regulations.

Revenue Ruling 56-185, C.B. 1956-1, 202 sets forth requirements for exemption of hospitals under section 501(c)(3) more restrictive than those contained in this Revenue Ruling with respect to caring for patients without charge or at rates below cost. In addition, the fourth requirement of Revenue Ruling 56-185 is ambiguous in that it can be read as implying that the possibility of shareholders or members sharing the assets of a hospital upon its dissolution will not preclude exemption of the hospital as a charity described in section 501(c)(3) of the Code. Section 1.501(c)(3)-1(b)(4) of the regulations promulgated subsequent to Revenue Ruling 56-185 makes it clear, however, that an absolute dedication of assets to charity is a precondition to exemption under section 501(c)(3) of the Code.

Revenue Ruling 56-185 is hereby modified to remove therefrom the requirements relating to caring for patients without charge or at rates below cost. Furthermore, requirement 4 has been modified by section 1.501(c)(3)-1(b)(4) of the regulations.

It is interesting to note that, though Revenue Ruling 69-545 eliminated the requirement relating to caring for patients without charge from the exemption qualification criteria, the gap has, at least, been partially filled by revisions to Title 42 of the Public Health Act. The thrust of the revisions to Part 53 (Grants, Loans and Loan Guarantees for Construction and Mod-

FIGURE 1.B-1   IRS Form 1023, Schedule D

Schedule D.—Hospitals and Medical Research Organizations

☐ Check here if you are claiming to be a hospital and complete the questions in Part 1 of this Schedule.

☐ Check here if you are claiming to be a medical research organization operated in connection with a hospital and complete the questions in Part II of this Schedule.

Part I.—Hospitals

1 (a) How many doctors are on the hospital's courtesy
        staff? ....

   (b) Do such doctors include all the doctors in the
        community? ....☐ Yes   ☐ No

        If "No," please give the reasons why and explain
        how the courtesy staff is selected.

2 Composition of board of directors or trustees. (If more
   space is needed, attach schedule.)

Name and address	Occupation

3 (a) Does the hospital maintain a full-time
        emergency room? ....☐ Yes   ☐ No

   (b) What is the hospital's policy as to administering emergency services to persons without apparent means to pay?

   (c) Does the hospital have any arrangements with police, fire, and voluntary ambulance services as to the delivery or admission of emergency cases? ....☐ Yes   ☐ No

        Please explain.

FIGURE 1.B-1   Continued

4   (a) Does or will the hospital require a deposit from per-
       sons covered by Medicare or Medicaid in its admis-
       sion practices? .... ☐ Yes   ☐ No

       If "Yes," please explain.

    (b) Does the same deposit requirement apply to all
       other patients? .... ☐ Yes   ☐ No

       If "No," please explain.

5   Does or will the hospital provide for a portion of its
    services and facilities to be used for charity patients? . ☐ Yes   ☐ No

    Please explain (include data as to the hospital's past
    experience in admitting charity patients and arrange-
    ments it may have with municipal or governmental
    agencies for absorbing the cost of such care).

6   Does or will the hospital carry on a formal program of
    medical training and research? .... ☐ Yes   ☐ No

    If "Yes," please describe.

7   Does the hospital provide office space to physicians car-
    rying on a medical practice? .... ☐ Yes   ☐ No

    If "Yes," attach a list setting forth the name of each
    physician, the amount of space provided, the annual
    rent (if any), and the expiration date of the current lease.

Part II.—Medical Research Organizations

1   Name the hospital(s) with which you have a relationship
    and describe the relationship(s).

Continued

FIGURE 1.B-1   Continued

2   Describe your present and proposed (indicate which) medical re-
    search activities showing the nature of such activities and the amount
    of money which has been or will be spent in carrying them out. (Di-
    rect conduct of medical research does not include grants to other
    organizations.)

3   Attach a statement of assets showing the fair market value of your
    assets and the portion of such assets directly devoted to medical
    research.

ernization of Hospitals and Medical Facilities) Subpart L (Community
Service; Services for Persons Unable to Pay; Nondiscrimination) can be
summarized as requiring that institutions receiving—or having received—
Hill-Burton assistance are obligated to make available a reasonable volume
of services to persons unable to pay.[14] Compliance with this requirement
is presumed if the institution

1. Either budgets for the support of, and makes available on request,
   uncompensated services at a level not less than the lesser of 3% of
   operating costs or 10% of all federal assistance provided under the
   Act; or

2. Certifies that it will not exclude any person from admission on the
   ground that such person is unable to pay.

[14]*Federal Register,* Vol. 37, No. 142, July 22, 1972 and *Federal Register,* Vol. 40, No. 194,
October 6, 1975: operates to serve a public interest rather than a private interest.

CHAPTER

2

Accounting Principles
for Hospitals

It is somewhat unusual to begin a text on financial management with a discussion of accounting principles, and one may ask "Why do so here?" The answer, quite simply, is that if hospital managers are to understand the value of financial management for improved hospital operations and feel comfortable in its use, they must have a full understanding of the financial workings of the hospital. The best way to obtain such an understanding is to begin with a review of the objectives of financial reporting and the related accounting principles.

An understanding of these is critical to the knowledgeable use of financial data, for they determine the nature and character of the financial information that the manager receives. Therefore, if a manager is to be able to understand and properly evaluate and utilize financial data, he must first understand the objectives that guide the collection and presentation of these data.

The purpose of this chapter is thus twofold. First, it is to review and point out the differences and similarities between commercial and hospital accounting practices. Some of the material that will be discussed should be familiar. Therefore, little attention will be devoted to the mechanical workings or applications of these principles, for they should already be understood. However, those readers with questions as to mechanics or applications should consult any familiar beginning or intermediate accounting text.

The second objective of this chapter is to provide some familiarity with, and orientation to, the financial environment of the hospital. Thus, attention will be devoted to the unique features of hospital accounting.

OBJECTIVES OF FINANCIAL REPORTING

The objectives of financial reporting are summarized in the Financial Accounting Standards Board (FASB) Statement of Financial Accounting Concepts No. 1:

1. Financial reporting should provide information that is useful to present and potential investors, creditors, and other users in making rational investment, credit, and similar decisions.

2. Financial reporting should provide information about the economic resources of an enterprise, the claims to those resources, and the effects of transactions, events, and circumstances that change resources.

3. Financial reporting should provide information about an enterprise's financial performance during a period.

4. Financial reporting should provide information about how an enterprise obtains and spends cash, about its borrowing and repayment of borrowing, about its capital transactions, and about other factors that may affect its liquidity or solvency.

5. Financial reporting should provide information about how management of an enterprise has discharged its stewardship responsibility for the use of enterprise resources.

6. Financial reporting should provide information that is useful to managers and directors in making decisions in the interest of owners.

The emphasis of these objectives is on the information needs of external users common to for-profit, publicly held enterprises. However, one may substitute the terms hospital for enterprise and community for owners, and the objectives are equally applicable.

Management must also incorporate the same objectives into its own information requirements. Ideally, management must have a detailed understanding of the past, present, and future, the internal and external pressures on the enterprise. Management's needs are also more detailed than those of the external user groups and are certainly more urgent with respect to their required timing.

BASIC ACCOUNTING CONCEPTS

Accounting practices have developed over a long period of years. During this time, several basic concepts have been accepted and adopted by accountants as fundamental guides that define the manner in which accounts should be kept. The need for such guides should be quite easily understood.

Without general rules or guides for the recording of business transactions and the preparation of accounts, it would be impossible for accounting information to be understandable and useful to various parties. This would be the case, for there would be no common basis for recording transactions. Similar transactions, if accounting records are to be understood, must yield, at least in terms of the accounting records, similar results. If this end is to be attained, certain basic concepts must be used in preparing accounting records. Thus, over the years accountants have adopted a basic body of theory that is used as a guide for preparing all accounting records. In this way uniformity is obtained, and accounting records are understandable and useful to all persons who need them.

Presented below are six basic accounting principles or concepts with which managers should be familiar and that they should understand if they are to be able to use accounting data and reports. It should be pointed out that accounting is not a static art. Some of these principles are continually being questioned and reviewed and, in time, will be modified. However, they are currently the accepted guide, and while the reader may question the propriety of some, he or she should, at this point, accept and attempt to understand these principles to be able to utilize accounting data and financial reports knowledgeably.

ENTITY CONCEPT

For accounting purposes the hospital or, for that matter, any other business is personified and viewed as an entity capable of taking economic actions. Thus, the accountant considers the hospital as an entity that is separate and distinct from its employees, contributors, and governing board. Accounts are kept for the business entity—not for the persons associated with the entity—and reflect the events that affect the business.

As a corollary to the entity concept, accountants have also assumed that the entity will be one of continuing activity—it will be a going concern with an almost indefinite life. The persons associated with the entity may come and go, but the entity will remain.[1] Thus, in preparing statements and reports, the accountants' method and valuations should reflect the continuity assumption instead of the assumption that the entity will be liquidated and that its assets and liabilities should be valued at their liquidation price.

---

[1] It should be noted that the continuity concept does not imply permanence of existence. Rather, it assumes that the entity will continue in existence long enough to carry out current plans and meet contracted commitments.

TRANSACTIONS CONCEPT

Given that a hospital is an accounting entity, the results of all trans-actions affecting that entity must be included in the accounting records and reports. The value and need for this general rule should be quite clear. If accounting data and reports are to be dependable and valid, all transactions of the entity must be included. If this is not done, then the accounting records can be manipulated to describe any operational picture that is de-sired. Therefore, complete recording and disclosure of all transactions is necessary if an accurate presentation of financial condition is to be obtained.

However, the necessity of reporting all transactions does not necessar-ily mean that all transactions must be reported on an individual basis. Individualized reporting could result in financial reports being too cum-bersome to be useful management tools. Therefore, it is acceptable re-porting practice to summarize transactions—as long as the effect of every transaction is reported and a "fair" statement of financial condition is presented.

COST VALUATION CONCEPT

The previous discussion sets forth as a general rule that all transactions must be included in the accounting record. The question that can be raised at this point is: At what value should these transactions be recorded? This is perhaps one of the most difficult questions facing accountants, for a num-ber of values exist for any given asset or liability: sale price, replacement cost, purchase price, to name a few. Faced with this dilemma, accountants and others have found that cost, or the price paid to acquire an item, is generally the most useful basis of valuation for purposes of the permanent accounting record.

Admittedly, the use of this cost as the basis for valuation has some drawbacks. Over time, especially during periods of fluctuating prices, the value of an item can vary substantially. In this situation, the accounting value of an item will only accurately reflect the value of an item as of the time it is acquired and will not show its current worth. Also, cost valuation requires that something of value be given up for an item in order for that item to be recorded in the account. This means, therefore, that the intan-gible assets of an enterprise, such as the skill of management, reputation, and special expertise, are generally not included in accounting records.[2]

---

[2]It should be noted that tangible assets may, from time to time, be obtained as contri-butions or donations. In such cases, in order to avoid understating the worth of the enterprise, these assets should be recorded in the accounts even though, in the usual sense, nothing of value has been given up to obtain the assets. In instances of this nature, accountants have assumed that the basis of valuation or cost is equal to the fair market value of the assets as of the time they are received. Intangible assets are also occasionally valued in the accounting

Recognizing these problems of cost valuation, some have argued that a different basis should be used—a basis that shows at all times the current value of the operation. However, there are several compelling reasons for the continued use of a historical cost basis of valuation.

Cost has the important advantage over all other bases of valuation in that it is determinable, definite, objective, and verifiable. Cost is the only basis of valuation that is definite and not a matter of conjecture or opinion. If sale or replacement cost were used as the basis for valuation of any item, not only would value be subject to varying opinions and judgments, but also the determination of a value for each item at the end of the accounting period would be a costly and laborious task with questionable benefits in view of the costs involved. Thus, if accounting reports are to provide consistent and factual figures, cost should be used as the basis of valuation.

In addition to the permanent accounting reports based on cost, management may feel that it is desirable to prepare supplementary reports designed to reflect price level change. This approach to the asset valuation problem not only allows for the benefits of cost valuation to be retained, but also allows for the effects of price level changes to be reflected in the accounting reports. In this way, the advantages of cost valuation and the potential advantages of price level adjustments to cost are both available.[3]

DOUBLE ENTRY CONCEPT

The accounting records should not only reflect, on a cost basis, all transactions of the entity, but also be constructed in such a manner as to reflect the two aspects of each transaction, that is, the change in asset forms or the change in assets, and the change in the source of financing—liabilities. For example, if a hospital purchases an automobile for cash, not only must the cash account be adjusted, but also an entry must be made to show the acquisition of a fixed asset. If the hospital had borrowed funds to finance the car, two entries would still have to be made. One entry would have to be made to show the acquisition of the fixed asset, and another entry would have to be made to reflect the source of financing, that is, the liability that was incurred. Thus, if the accounting records are to reflect fully the effect of any given transaction, two entries must be made.

---

records by means of a "goodwill" entry which is equal to the difference between the accounting value and the price paid for a business as a whole. This entry, however, is generally not found in nonprofit hospital accounting records.

[3]Statement of Financial Accounting Standards No. 33, *Financial Reporting and Changing Prices*, issued by the FASB requires the effects of changing prices to be presented as supplementary information in published annual reports of certain public enterprises that have either (1) inventories and property, plant and equipment (before deducting accumulated depreciation) amounting to more than $125 million; or (2) total assets amounting to more than $1 billion (after deducting accumuled depreciation).

Accounting records, therefore, are constructed on the basis of a double entry system, with every transaction affecting at least two items. This is a concept with which all should be familiar, for it is really no more than just requiring that the debit entries balance the credit entries.

ACCRUAL CONCEPT

Just as the cost valuation concept provides the guide for recording assets and liabilities, the accrual concept provides the guide for accounting for revenues and expenses. The accrual concept can be more easily understood if it is viewed not as a theoretical concept, but rather as a system of accounting—a system that requires that revenue be recorded in the accounts when realized and that expenses be recorded in the period in which they contribute to operations.

The desirability of handling revenues and expenses in this manner should be clear. As was discussed earlier, accounting records and reports should accurately reflect the effects of all transactions. However, in any given accounting period, net income represents the results of all transactions or operations within that period. Thus, the accounting records should also accurately reflect net income. To do this, the records must include only those revenues and expenses that apply to the given period and exclude all revenues and expenses that result from transactions of other accounting periods.

This matter of properly allocating income and expenses to the appropriate fiscal period is often a difficult problem to accountants. Faced with this problem, accountants have developed two rules to aid them in allocating revenues and expenses. Simply stated, these rules are: (1) revenues and losses should be recorded in the period in which they are realized; and (2) expenses should be recorded in the period in which they contribute to operations.

These two guides provide objectives tests for determining when revenues and expenses should be recorded. Realization of a revenue or loss means that the gain or loss must be definitely established and the amount must be determined before an accounting entry is made. Thus, for example, assets must be sold before the gain or loss from holding the assets is entered into the accounting record.

In allocating expenses, a somewhat different guide is used. As has been stated above, expenses are recognized in the period during which they contribute to operations. This notion can be illustrated by assuming that employees are paid in January for work performed in December. Using the contribution test, the expense should be allocated to December, the month in which the contribution to operations was made, not to January. Thus, the expense should be recognized and recorded in the accounts not when the wages are paid, but rather when the work is done.

The use of these two rules allows accountants to allocate revenues and expenses to the proper accounting period. In this way, the accounting reports accurately present the operating results of the period.

MATCHING CONCEPT

The use of the realization and contribution rules allows accounting to bring together related income and expenses in an accurate manner in the same accounting period. However, if the results of a particular operation are to be described objectively, not only must income and expenses of the same accounting period be brought together, but also associated revenues and expense items must be matched in order properly to determine net income.

If it were not necessary to match related items of revenue and expense, then it would be possible to manipulate income from different types of activity to produce whatever type of operating picture is desired. Thus, the necessity of matching is similar to the necessity for including the results of all transactions in the accounts. Only by matching expenses against related revenues can the results of a particular operating activity be accurately and objectively presented.

ACCOUNTING CONVENTIONS

The foregoing concepts should not be regarded as infallible rules to be followed in every situation. Instances may arise wherein it would be desirable to make certain exceptions in the application of these concepts. Additionally, in practice, the above concepts are modified by certain conventions, the most important of which are: relevance, reliability, neutrality, materiality, comparability, conservatism, costs and benefits, and industry practices.

RELEVANCE

Accounting is not intended to capture information from an infinite and unstructured range of sources. The information must be logically related to management decisions and to future viability to be relevant. Accounting information can be relevant either by improving the decision maker's ability to predict a future occurrence or by confirming an earlier judgment. In both situations, the relevance of the information contributes to the ultimate certainty of the decision and its potential outcomes. Therefore, to be truly relevant to both external users and management, accounting information must be capable of helping users to form a more precise prediction of their past or future efforts.

Timeliness is a necessary aspect of relevance. Untimely data are irrelevant because they have no capacity to influence decisions. If information is not available when it is needed or becomes available only after it no longer has any value, it lacks relevance.

RELIABILITY

That information is to be reliable as well as relevant is a notion that is central to both accounting and decision making. In being reliable, accounting information warrants only what it purports to represent—verifiable information for establishing informed decisions.

Reliability does not guarantee certainty in decision making. Accounting merely functions as a means of representing the economic decisions and financial condition of the enterprise through the selection of alternative, yet generally accepted methodologies. Given the vastness in the range of user objectives, presentation options, and the limitations of accounting conventions, it is not possible to assure that accounting information will provide "perfect knowledge."

NEUTRALITY

Neutrality simply means that the process of choosing between alternative accounting presentations should be a function of the relevance and reliability of the information as opposed to a desire to attain a predetermined result. This, of course, is difficult to reconcile with actual accounting practice. Both management and ownership have a bias in the message they wish to convey to the potential users of financial information. Differing accounting presentations can add to or detract from the delivery of that message.

MATERIALITY

Accounting is not intended to be an abstract academic exercise. Rather, it should be a useful tool for management's evaluation and control of operations. Thus, the accounting report should not attempt to reflect a great number of events that are so insignificant that the work and cost of recording them are not justified by the benefit received. For example, the matching principle requires that expenses be matched against related revenue. However, in a large operation, such as a hospital, an insignificant amount of revenue may be obtained from the selling of scrap material. Strict adherence to accounting theory would require that the expenses involved in collecting and selling such scrap material be offset against the revenues obtained. However, unless the revenues from the sale or the expenses related to those revenues are of real importance, it is neither particularly helpful nor necessary to adhere strictly to theory. The point involved here is one of materiality.

Materiality, however, is counterbalanced by the notion of full disclosure. This notion requires that significant data be accurately and completely reflected in the accounting reports. Thus, it is difficult to give any firm guidelines as to what is material or immaterial. Materiality varies with the relative amount and relative importance of the transactions being considered. One's decisions should be based upon common sense and a judgment of the relative importance of the transaction to the total operation.

COMPARABILITY

If the full benefits of accounting reports are to be obtained, one must be able to compare reports across similar organizations and between years. To attain such comparability, the reports must be prepared on a consistent basis. Without consistency, the value and usefulness of accounting reports are severely limited. Thus, accountants place considerable emphasis on consistency, and changes in the methods of keeping accounts or deviations from generally accepted principles should not be made without careful consideration.

CONSERVATISM

Historically, accountants have interpreted conservatism as a "command to err" in the direction of understatement of either net income or asset valuation. Only recently has the accounting profession realized that this introduces a performance bias that conflicts with the other accounting conventions. Conservatism is now to be applied in conjunction with the measurement of the uncertainty attached to the decision alternatives of a specific situation. If the value of an asset or an income item is in doubt and any of the possible estimates is equally likely to occur, then conservatism dictates the selection of the least optimistic estimate. If any estimate is more likely to occur than the others, then conservatism is not applicable to the situation.

COSTS AND BENEFITS

Accounting practitioners have come to realize that more data, or even more detail, will likely increase the relevance and reliability of the accounting information presented. However, more data are available only by expending resources and incurring assembly costs. The time and costs invested in data collection take operating resources and funds away from productive investment. Therefore, they must be offset by an equal or greater benefit if they are to be cost justifiable.

Many times, the benefits of additional information are not measurable in monetary terms. Will creditors lend more? Will management become more operationally efficient? Will a decision become more certain? The evaluation of the cost/benefit relationship of accounting information can be extremely subjective. In addition, management does not entirely control the data demands of the external users. Management's decisions in this area are being influenced increasingly by the operational needs and data demands of owners, creditors, and government.

In addition to the above conventions, various industries also may have unique accounting practices that affect the way accounting records are kept and reports are presented. The hospital industry is one such industry. The remainder of this chapter will be devoted to discussing the particular accounting conventions of the hospital industry.

HOSPITAL ACCOUNTING

The foregoing concepts and conventions have been developed primarily for use by profit-making enterprises. These guidelines, however, are equally applicable to hospitals and hospital accounting. Hospitals, though differing in orientation from commercial enterprises, are still a form of business. Therefore, the principles of sound business management, such as the above accounting guides or rules, are just as applicable to hospitals as they are to General Electric, Ford Motor Company, Consolidated Edison or any other commercial enterprise. The nonprofit operating philosophy of most hospitals should neither constitute an excuse nor be used as a justification for irresponsible management or accounting practices. Hospital accounting practices should thus be based upon the above rules and conventions.

In addition to these generally recognized accounting conventions, hospitals have been influenced by their operating environment. Because of the unique financing relationship between traditional hospital payment methodologies and operating costs, hospitals have adopted several accounting conventions unique to themselves.

ADJUSTMENTS FOR CONTRACTUAL ALLOWANCES

Because of the influences of cost-based reimbursement and the differing payment levels of third party payers, hospitals have adopted an accounting convention that reconciles the hospital's public price list for its services to the payment received from non–charge basis payers. This convention utilizes a general ledger account entitled "Adjustments for Contractual Allowances." The purpose of this account is to record the aggregate difference between the hospital's billed charges and the amount actually received as payment from third party payers. The transactions recorded in this account are analogous to the sales discounts provided by commercial business, with one notable difference. In a commercial business, management determines the level of any discounts. While this type of management activity is increasing as hospitals engage in more direct contracting under preferred provider agreements, governmental payers are the primary source of the contractual allowances recorded. Both Medicare and Medicaid continue to receive large discounts as a result of their ability to set their payment levels unilaterally.[4]

Currently, the continued use of this convention is being debated. Some practitioners argue that the account serves no benefit to the financial statement user and is even misleading because of the differing policies of individual hospitals in price discounting, cost shortfalls, bad debts, and charity care. That may be, however, the specific value of this account. The Allowance for Contractuals provides creditors and management with a readily available measurement of the markup that is incorporated in the hospital's prices to cover expenses unrecognized or not allowed by individual payers.

FUND ACCOUNTING

Many hospitals utilize fund accounting to comply with the stewardship responsibilities imposed by philanthropic donations. Quite simply, fund accounting requires that a hospital maintain a separate set of accounting records for each distinct phase of financial activity, function, or responsibility. This means that a single hospital may have four or five sets of records or books, as opposed to the one set generally used by a commercial enterprise.

One way to conceptualize what is involved in fund accounting is to view the hospital as an operating company with several divisions. Each division operates as an entity with its own accounts and profit objective and deals with the other divisions, in the same manner, as if they were completely separate operations. Similarly, in fund accounting each distinct phase of financial activity is handled as if it were a separate accounting entity with its own particular objective and purpose. The accounts within each fund are self-balancing, that is, debits equal credits, and can be used to produce balance sheets and income statements. Interfund transactions, though in reality being within the same total entity, are handled in principle as though they involved entirely separate enterprises. Thus, fund accounting is a technique for establishing, within a single hospital, separate ac-

---

[4]It is also possible, under the fixed price arrangements currently being established, for the actual payment made to be greater than the sum of the hospital's charges on a procedural basis. This occurs when the unit of payment is an aggregate measure of services, that is, discharges or visits. The effect on the Adjustments for Contractual Allowances is a positive addition to the hospital's gross revenue. This is more likely to occur in individual cases than in the total hospital revenues.

counting subentities, each representing a distinct phase of financial operations or managerial responsibility.

Generally, fund accounting incorporates the following:

Unrestricted Fund	Fund used to account for all the resources, obligations, and capital not restricted to a particular purpose by an external authority. This fund is available for the regular day-to-day operations of the hospital;
Endowment Fund	Fund used to account for donor-restricted assets given to the hospital, the principal amount of which is to be maintained intact and only the income from which is expendable;
Plant Fund	Fund used to account for the hospital's investment in buildings, land, equipment, and reserves to replace these assets, as well as related long-term debts;
Specific Purpose Fund	Fund used to account for cash or other current assets restricted to the financing of specific activities;
Construction Fund	Fund used to account for transactions related to the acquisition or construction of new plant assets.

Though the American Hospital Association recommends the above major funds, its guidelines are flexible. A particular hospital may never need to use the Specific Purpose Fund and may only periodically need the Construction Fund. Conversely, some hospitals may need additional funds to account properly for certain actions of their governing board. Therefore, a hospital's fund accounting system can and should be custom tailored to meet its own unique needs and should not be unduly bound by the above guidelines.

Many hospital accounting authorities question the need for fund accounting.[5] Fund accounting was adopted by hospitals as a response to a

---

[5]The American Institute of Certified Public Accountants (AICPA) has also raised the question of the necessity of fund accounting. The AICPA has noted that reporting on a fund accounting basis may be helpful where needed to achieve a proper segregation and presentation of unrestricted resources from those resources over which the board has little, if any, discretion because of externally imposed restrictions. If an organization has restricted resources and elects not to report on a fund accounting basis, disclosure of all material restrictions should be made.

need that arose early in their development as community institutions. Hospitals, because of their objective of service to the community, are often the recipients of large gifts and endowments that are given as trusts to be used for specific purposes. Acceptance of such gifts places a hospital in a fiduciary position wherein it is legally obligated to conform to the restrictions placed upon the use of the donated funds. To carry out this obligation, it was felt that there was a need for a separate accounting for those assets whose use was to be limited to particular activities or functions. Fund accounting was developed to provide for this accounting need.

Fund accounting presentations appear in hospital financial statements in varying degrees of detail. Figure 2.1 illustrates the current convention. Aggregate unrestricted funds, restricted funds, and special purpose funds are shown on the balance sheet. The "Statement of Changes in Fund Equities" presents the details of those transactions that contributed to change in the fund balances over the prior two reporting periods. The hospital's income statement contains no fund information. It is presented as an all-inclusive operating statement.

The critical factors for the hospital manager to realize and understand are the following:

1. That fund accounting is a commonly used hospital accounting system
2. That fund accounting requires the creation of a separate accounting entity for each distinct financial activity or responsibility of the hospital
3. That a hospital's fund accounting system should be designed to meet its own unique situation, that is, if the organization structure is appropriate, funds should be merged—such as the operating and plant funds—or, if necessary, additional funds should be created

The mechanics of fund accounting will be left to the accountants and hospital accounting texts. Readers with questions as to mechanics should consult any hospital accounting text such as *Introduction to Hospital Accounting* by Seawell (See Suggested Readings).

FUNDED DEPRECIATION

Management's stewardship responsibilities have also resulted in the establishment of a unique method for accumulating funds for asset acquisition. The practice of "funded depreciation" attempts to allocate cash into the plant fund. The cash is then imprested for capital expansion or replacement. The level of the funding is generally a function of the hospital's current depreciation expense. Because depreciation expense is set at historical cost levels, the cash is invested in interest-yielding securities to earn additional funds that may offset some of the effects of inflation. In some instances, the funds are also lent to the hospital's operating fund for short

FIGURE 2.1

Caryn Memorial Hospital and Health Center
Balance Sheets, December 31, 1984 and 1983

Assets	1984	1983
		UNRESTRICTED
Current assets:		
Cash	$ 74,418	135,296
Accounts receivable, less estimated uncollectibles of $749,302 in 1984 and $757,880 in 1983	4,372,116	4,538,245
Due from third party payers	666,930	458,659
Other receivables	270,521	32,581
Inventories	310,518	315,128
Prepaid expenses	90,517	7,328
Total current assets	5,785,020	5,487,237
Property, plant, and equipment, at cost, less accumulated depreciation of $6,186,048 in 1984 and $5,615,377 in 1983	6,505,496	6,777,786
Other assets:		
Cash—Board-designated	—	10,329
Deferred Medicare receivable	130,526	144,826
Lease deposits	10,266	6,357
Deferred charges	32,526	32,526
Total other assets	173,318	194,038
	$12,463,834	12,459,061
		RESTRICTED
		Specific Purpose
Cash	$ —	827
Investments, at cost, which approximates market value	368,962	698,912
Due from unrestricted funds	555,416	878,593
Total	$ 924,378	1,578,332
		Plant Replacement and
Cash	78,273	8,003
Pledges receivable	1,335,967	—
Due from unrestricted funds	283,023	389,889
Preconstruction costs	209,889	—
	$ 1,907,152	397,892

See accompanying notes to financial statements.

Liabilities and Fund Balances	1984	1983
FUNDS		
Current liabilities:		
Accounts payable	$ 2,179,857	1,870,266
Accrued expenses	329,488	423,219
Accrued payroll and related withholdings	1,226,326	1,366,188
Accrued vacation pay	239,236	293,187
Refunds due to patients	193,305	176,681
Current installments of pension liability	396,493	157,072
Current installments of long-term debt	276,324	298,970
Current installments of obligations under		
capital lease agreements	173,354	150,566
Notes payable	125,000	184,000
Due to third party payers	754,508	562,908
Due to specific purpose funds	555,416	878,593
Due to plant replacement and expansion fund	283,023	389,889
Total current liabilities	6,732,330	6,751,539
Long-term debt:		
Obligations under capital lease agreements,		
net of current installments	324,795	348,450
Long-term debt, net of current installments	1,794,210	1,800,934
Pension liability, net of current installments	326,922	566,937
Total long-term debt, net		
of current installments	2,445,927	2,716,321
Fund balances	3,285,577	2,991,201
	$12,463,834	12,459,061
FUNDS		
Fund		
Insurance premium payable	$ —	292,500
Reserve for estimated malpractice claims		
payable	924,378	1,285,832
Total	$ 924,378	1,578,332
Expansion Fund		
Fund balance	$ 1,907,152	397,892

FIGURE 2.1   Caryn Memorial Hospital and Health Center Statements of Revenues and Expenses, Years Ended December 31, 1984 and 1983

	1984	1983
Patient service revenues:		
Routine service revenues	$18,035,221	17,052,709
Ancillary department revenues	12,418,896	10,701,798
	30,454,117	27,754,507
Less contractual allowances and provision for uncollectible accounts	9,660,194	9,466,099
Net patient service revenues	20,793,923	18,288,408
Other operating revenues	868,904	487,072
Total operating revenues	21,662,827	18,775,480
Operating expenses:		
Professional care of patients	11,695,442	10,076,627
General services	3,475,242	3,164,131
Administrative and fiscal services	3,048,481	2,633,452
Employee health and welfare benefits	2,782,786	2,368,028
Depreciation	570,671	561,327
Total operating expenses	21,572,622	18,803,565
Income (loss) from operations	90,205	(28,085)
Nonoperating revenue:		
Unrestricted gifts and bequests	216,518	113,786
Investment income	1,457	6,003
Total nonoperating revenue	217,975	119,789
Excess of revenues over expenses	$ 308,180	91,704

See accompanying notes to financial statements.

FIGURE 2.1   Caryn Memorial Hospital and Health Center
Statements of Changes in Fund Balances, Years Ended
December 31, 1984 and 1983

	Unrestricted Funds	Plant Replacement and Expansion Fund
Balances, December 31, 1982	$2,717,197	563,842
Excess of revenues over expenses	91,704	—
Restricted gifts and bequests	—	12,000
Payment for debt service	315,427	(315,427)
Additions to property, plant, and equipment	423,053	(423,053)
Funding of depreciation	(560,530)	560,530
Donated equipment	4,350	—
Balances, December 31, 1983	2,991,201	397,892
Excess of revenues over expenses	308,180	—
Restricted gifts and bequests	—	1,495,456
Payment for debt service	409,273	(409,273)
Additions to property, plant, and equipment	147,594	(147,594)
Funding of depreciation	(570,671)	570,671
Balances, December 31, 1984	$3,285,577	1,907,152

See accompanying notes to financial statements.

periods to earn a return while providing short-term operating capital to the hospital.

HOSPITAL CHART OF ACCOUNTS

In addition to fund accounting, the American Hospital Association recommends that a hospital adopt a chart of accounts, that is, an account classification system uniform across the hospital's organizational departments. A chart of accounts is actually nothing more than a listing of the account titles, with numerical symbols, for all the asset, liability, capital, revenue, and expense accounts of a hospital.

The notion of what a chart of accounts is can be understood most easily by examining a sample chart of accounts. Table 2.1 is an excerpt from the chart of accounts of a particular hospital. As can be seen in the right-hand column, all the journal account titles that the hospital has for each category of assets are listed. The left-hand column lists the numerical classification code for each account. A complete chart of accounts would contain a listing, each with its corresponding account number, of all the journal accounts of the hospital.

Table 2.2 is a summary of the overall numbering system suggested by the American Hospital Association. As can be seen from the table, the three numbers at the left of the decimal point indicate the control or primary account classification, and the two digits to the right indicate the secondary account classification. For example, account number 111.20 from Table 2.1 can be translated as below. Thus, the account numbers indicate, to the experienced reader, that the account is not only an asset account in the Operating Fund, but also that the asset is a temporary investment. The fourth and fifth digits further specify the identity of the account, that is, indicate that it is a bank savings.

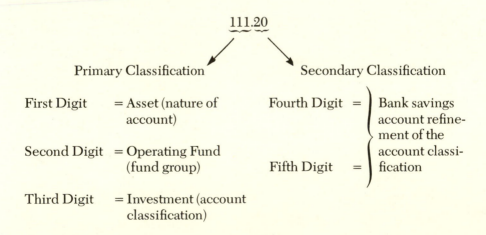

TABLE 2.1   Sample Chart of Accounts

Assets:
Operating Fund

110.00–110.49	*Cash*	
	110.00	Cash on Deposit—General Fund
	110.10	Cash on Deposit—Payroll
	110.20	Cash on Deposit—Supplies and Expense
110.50–110.99	*Cash Imprest Funds*	
	110.50	Cashiers Change Fund
	110.51	Cafeteria Change Fund
	110.52	Nightbox
	110.53	X-ray Change Fund
	110.60	Brink's Revolving Change Fund
	110.70	Laboratory Machine Fund
	110.80	U.S. Post Office—Stamp Fund
111.00–111.99	*Investments*	
	111.20	Savings R. and M. Friedman Bank
112.00–112.09	*Accounts and Notes Receivable*	
	112.00	Accounts Receivable—Inpatients
	112.01	Accounts Receivable—Outpatients
112.10–112.19	*Allowance for Uncollectable Receivables*	
	112.10	Allowance for Doubtful Accounts
	112.11	Allowance for Blue Cross Adjustments
	112.12	Allowance for Medicare Adjustments
112.20–112.29	*Recoveries of Accounts Written Off*	
	112.20	Other Accounts Receivable—Suspense
	112.21	Allowance for Bad Debts—Suspense
112.30–112.39	*Other Receivables*	
	112.30	Tuition Receivable
	112.31	Taxes Receivable—Current
	112.32	Accounts Receivable—X-ray Room Rent
	112.33	Accounts Receivable—Clearance

TABLE 2.2   Summary—Numerical Coding System—Primary Classification

110–196 Assets	110–114	Operating Fund
	120–122	Specific Purpose Fund
	130–132	Endowment Fund
	140–146	Plant Fund
	150–155	Construction Fund
	160–196	Other Funds
217–298 Liabilities	217	Operating Fund
	227	Specific Purpose Fund
	237–238	Endowment Fund
	247–248	Plant Fund
	257–258	Construction Fund
	267–298	Other Funds
219–299 Capital Accounts	219	Operating Fund
	229	Specific Purpose Fund
	239	Endowment Fund
	249	Plant Fund
	259	Construction Fund
	269–299	Other Funds
310–599 Revenue Accounts	310–499	Patient Service Revenue
	500–529	Deductions from Revenue
	530–599	Other Revenue
600–999 Expense Accounts	600–699	Nursing Service
	700–799	Other Professional Services
	800–899	General Services
	900–949	Fiscal Services
	950–979	Administration Services
	980–999	Unassigned Expenses

Summary—Logic of Coding System

Asset, Liability, and Capital Accounts	Revenue and Expense Accounts

Primary Classification

First digit	Nature of account, for example, asset, liability, capital	Nature of revenue and expense accounts—classified by unit, for example,
Second digit	Fund Group	
Third digit	Account classi-fication, for example, cash, inventory, revenue by nursing unit	402—Laboratory-Clinical 435—Anesthesiology 601—Nursing Service–Administration 735—Anesthesiology

TABLE 2.2   Continued

Secondary Classification	
Fourth Digit	Additional classification codes available for use as needed, to provide for refinement of the
Fifth Digit	primary classification.

The internal operational value of a chart of accounts is twofold. First, a chart of accounts, through the use of numerical account titles, facilitates the performance of the entire accounting process, from the collection of data to the presentation of reports, not only by saving clerical time and effort, but also by reducing the number of errors. Also, the chart of accounts, by requiring the systematic organization of accounts, provides the basis for management control of operations through responsibility accounting and management by objectives. Thus, a chart of accounts is a basic and necessary element in any accounting system and should be utilized by all hospitals.

Admittedly, no two hospitals are exactly alike. It follows, therefore, that no two hospitals will have exactly the same charts of accounts. In designing its chart of accounts, the American Hospital Association was well aware of this problem and designed a system that is flexible enough to meet the specific requirements of all hospitals while still maintaining a basic uniformity for the recording and reporting of financial data. The recommended chart of accounts provides the basis for operational accountability, comparability, and control while at the same time being sufficiently general to be a useful guideline for all hospitals.

There is little value, at this point, in discussing the recommended chart of accounts in more detail. Those readers who desire additional information should refer to the American Hospital Association's publication entitled *Chart of Accounts for Hospitals*. For the moment, the hospital manager should just be aware of and understand the internal operational values of a chart of accounts.

Third party payment methodologies have also influenced the manner in which hospitals maintain their internal accounting records. Until the inception of prospective fixed price payment, a large portion of hospital payments were made based on the costs incurred by the hospital in providing its services. As a result, the procedure utilized to allocate and apportion costs to the different revenue-producing cost centers was extremely important. Revenue maximization was accomplished by channeling costs into those service departments in which the cost-basis payers' participation was the greatest. The full mechanics of cost allocation and cost apportionment are discussed in Chapter 5. A further discussion of the more recent developments in hospital cost accounting is provided in Chapter 21.

SUGGESTED READINGS

American Hospital Association. *Chart of Accounts for Hospitals.*

American Hospital Association. *Managerial Cost Accounting.*

American Institute of Certified Public Accountants. *Hospital Audit Guide.*

Davidson, Sidney; Schindler, James S.; and Weil, Roman L. *Fundamentals of Accounting.*

Financial Accounting Standards Board. Statements on Financial Accounting Concepts, Nos. 1, 3, and 4.

Foyle, William R. "Merge the Plant and General Funds—Why Not?"

Hay, Leon F. *Accounting for Government and Nonprofit Entities, Sixth Edition.*

Moyer, C.A. and Mautz, R.K. *Intermediate Accounting: A Functional Approach.*

Seawell, L. Vann. *Hospital Accounting and Financial Management,* Chapters 1 and 3.

Seawell, L. Vann. *Hospital Financial Accounting: Theory and Practice.*

Seawell, L. Vann. *Introduction to Hospital Accounting.*

3

Financial Organization: The Hospital

A well-managed hospital operation is generally not the result of individual genius or effort. Rather, it is the product of the efforts and intellects of a group of individuals organized to function in concert. Organization provides the mechanism for allocating responsibilities and channeling efforts so that not only will all necessary tasks be performed, but also all work will be coordinated and controlled to achieve the objectives of the hospital in the most efficient and effective manner. Sound organization in all areas is thus one of the critical elements necessary for effective management. (See Appendixes 3.A and 3.B.)

Sound organization can take many forms. There is no single right or proper organization structure that can be recommended for all hospitals. The type of organization plan best suited for any given hospital depends on the size and characteristics of the operation, the probabilities and nature of any future expansion or changes in function, and the personality and style of the hospital's management group. However, certain patterns of organization have been found to be practicable, and certain guiding principles can be applied to almost all situations.

The purpose of this chapter is to examine these principles and practices as they relate to the financial organization structure of a hospital. Admittedly, they will not be ideally applicable in all situations. However, they do provide the basis for the financial organization of a hospital and should be understood if the reader is to obtain a working knowledge of hospital financial management.

ORGANIZATION STRUCTURE

The governing board of a voluntary hospital is vested by law with the ultimate authority and responsibility for managing all of the hospital's business. Therefore, the governing board is responsible for all phases of hospital operations, including financial operations. Thus, as is indicated in Figure 3.1, the financial organization structure of a hospital begins with the governing board.

The governing board itself, however, does not personally manage a hospital's financial operations. Rather, it generally utilizes the same basic staff/line combination approach that it employs to carry out many of its other responsibilities. That is, not only does it delegate line responsibility for the actual management of financial operations to certain hospital employees, but also it generally delegates the responsibility for ensuring that financial operations are properly managed to a committee of trustees that acts in a staff capacity to the board. Thus, line responsibility for financial operations is delegated to administration (the chief executive officer), and a finance committee is usually appointed to ensure that financial operations are performed appropriately.

The finance committee acts as the control or "check" in a hospital's system of financial checks and balances. It is responsible for overseeing the financial operations and position of the hospital, ensuring that adequate working and long-term capital are available, and for advising the board on all fiscal and investment matters.[1]

In addition to the finance committee, the board usually appoints or elects one of its members to serve as the hospital's treasurer. In a commercial enterprise the treasurer is generally a full-time employee of the firm whose function is primarily custodial. He is responsible for safeguarding the assets of the firm, supervising the receipt and disbursement of cash, and ensuring that the operation is adequately financed. As the custodian of the firm's assets, he counterbalances the chief financial officer, who controls the process by which assets are handled, to provide an adequate system of financial checks and balances.

The financial structure of the hospital, due to legal and philosophical constraints as well as pragmatic realities, has not developed in the same manner as that of the commercial corporation. The treasurer, as a member of the governing board, is usually not an employee of the hospital and does not devote his full time to the day-to-day management of the hospital's financial operations. Also, the duties traditionally assigned to the treasurer

---

[1]Some hospitals may have a separate budget committee to review the budget and examine any deviation, a separate audit committee to review the annual audit and oversee the performance of the independent auditors, and a building fund committee to raise certain long-term capital. However, these functions can, if desired, be performed by the finance committee or by subcommittees of the finance committee.

FIGURE 3.1   Financial Organization Structure—Voluntary General Hospital

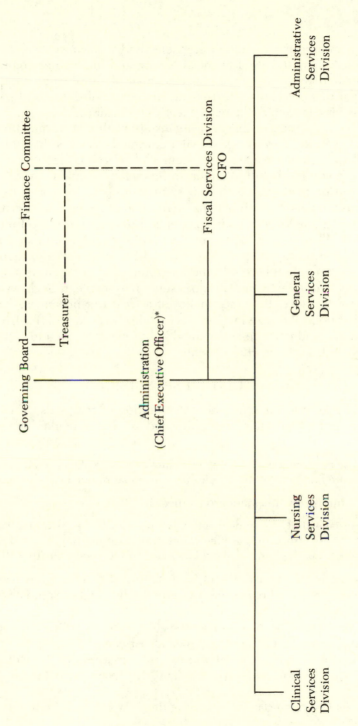

*It is common to find organization structures with a chief operating officer (COO). In such instances, the COO and the CFO typically report directly to the CEO.

in a commercial corporation are delegated, in a hospital corporation, to administration, the chief financial officer, and the finance committee. The hospital treasurer serves as the chairman of the finance committee and through this mechanism carries out his custodial duties and provides the means for a system of financial checks and balances.

This approach to financial organization, though commonly used, obviously can be questioned. It may be argued that it is difficult, if not impossible, to obtain an adequate system of checks and balances if the treasurer is not devoting his full attention to financial operations. Additionally, the case can be made that as the size of the hospital increases, the custodial and cash management functions increase and become more critical. Thus, a full-time employee-treasurer is needed to carry out these functions adequately. Whether these arguments are valid or not is a moot point, for, as has been indicated, there is no single right or proper organization structure. There is nothing inherent in the foregoing plan to preclude summarily its usefulness or effectiveness. It does seem reasonable, though, to expect that at some size level the employment of a treasurer becomes advantageous. At what point this size level is reached, however, will differ from hospital to hospital and must be determined individually by each institution, based on the costs and potential benefits.

LINE RESPONSIBILITY

The Joint Commission on Accreditation of Hospitals, in its standards for accrediting hospitals, has established as a basic standard or requirement that:

> The governing body, through its chief executive officer, shall provide for the control and use of the physical and financial resources of the hospital.

It interprets this standard as meaning that:

> Responsibility for implementing the policies of the governing body relative to the control and the effective utilization of the physical and financial resources of the hospital should be given to the chief executive officer.

Thus, the line responsibility or the responsibility for actually managing the day-to-day financial operation lies with the hospital's administrator or chief executive officer.[2]

It is impossible, however, for the chief executive officer or administrator to exercise personal supervision over all aspects of the hospital's operations. The demands, both internal and external, that require the administrator's personal attention and expertise, and the technical nature of operations

---

[2]Joint Commission on Accreditation of Hospitals, *Standards for Accreditation of Hospitals*, p. 7.

have increased to the point that the administrator must delegate the personal supervision and management of many tasks to members of his staff. Thus, the direct supervision of financial operations is delegated to the chief financial officer.[3]

The fact that the administrator delegates the day-to-day responsibility for financial management does not mean that he can or should ignore this phase of operations. He should actively involve himself in all financial policy, capital investment, and capital financing decisions. However, the day-to-day supervision and management of financial operations should be left to the chief financial officer (CFO), with the chief executive officer satisfying himself, through various reporting and control mechanisms, that the hospital's financial objectives are being achieved and that the CFO is properly carrying out his responsibilities.

As the party with the direct responsibility for financial management, the CFO, regardless of his actual title, is the hospital's chief financial officer and occupies the most critical line position in the hospital's financial organization structure. Historically, the role and managerial value of the CFO have been inappropriately defined, focusing on bookkeeping and business office management instead of on management accounting and financial management. Thus, the managerial value and usefulness of both the CFO and financial management have been deemphasized. Often, neither the administrator nor the governing board realized the value of financial planning and data or the significance of the financial manager's potential contribution. Consequently, the financial management found in hospitals in the past has been often inadequate and at times nonexistent.

However, the pendulum is now swinging in the other direction. Pressures from purchasers (business) and other third party payers, government agencies, and the public, regarding both hospital costs and the efficacy of hospital management, have caused both administrators and trustees to realize the need and value of quality financial management and the necessity of having a qualified CFO as an executive officer at the policy-making level. Thus, it is reasonable to expect that the management role and function of the CFO will become increasingly important in the future.

What, though, are the function and role of the CFO? If an administrator is to be able to satisfy himself that the controller is properly carrying out his financial management responsibilities, he must first be familiar with and understand the CFO's function. Therefore, a discussion of the specific functions of the CFO is germane at this point.

---

[3]The title of the chief financial officer will vary from hospital to hospital. In some institutions, the position may be identified as the controller. In others, it may be the vice president of fiscal services. As a rule of thumb, the function should carry a title that is generally similar to that of other line managers.

CHIEF FINANCIAL OFFICER'S FUNCTIONS

The Committee on Ethics and Eligibility Standards of the Financial Executives Institute has defined the CFO's function as follows:

1. To establish, coordinate, and maintain, through authorized management, an integrated plan for the control of operations. Such a plan would provide, to the extent required in the business, cost standards, expense budgets, sales forecasts, profit planning, and programs for capital investment and financing, together with the necessary procedures to effectuate the plan.

2. To measure performance against approved operating plans and standards and to report and interpret the results of operations to all levels of management. This function includes the design, installation, and maintenance of accounting and cost systems and records, the determination of accounting policy, and the compilation of statistical records as required.

3. To measure and report on the validity of the objectives of the business and on the effectiveness of its policies, organization structure, and procedures in attaining those objectives. This includes consulting with all segments of management responsible for policy or action concerning any phase of the operation of the business as it relates to the performance of this function.

4. To report to government agencies, as required, and to supervise all matters relating to taxes.

5. To interpret and report on the effect of external influences on the attainment of the objectives of the business. This function includes the continuous appraisal of economic and social forces and of government influences as they affect the operations of the business.

6. To provide protection for the assets of the business. This function includes establishing and maintaining adequate internal control and auditing, and assuring proper insurance coverage.

The Committee's definition is designed primarily for the controller of a commercial firm. However, the generic problems of management do not vary significantly between industries. Admittedly, hospitals differ in some respects from their commercial counterparts, but the basic problems of planning and organizing operations, obtaining adequate financing, controlling costs, and measuring and reporting performance are the same in all instances. Thus, the above definition is sufficiently broad in concept to be applicable to the hospital CFO.

To simplify discussion of the controller's function it may be advisable to recast the above definition into a more functionally oriented listing. Although there is some overlap between categories, the controller's primary or basic functions and activities can be set out as follows:

THE PLANNING FUNCTION

The development and maintenance of an integrated budget or plan of operations are often felt to be the major and most critical functions of the CFO. The objective of a hospital can generally be stated as that of providing its community with the services that it needs at an acceptable level of quality and at the least possible cost. This is a complex goal that cannot be achieved unless the efforts of all departments are carefully coordinated and planned. Planning is, thus, a necessity for effective operations. However, it should be understood at the outset that the plan is the hospital's plan, not the CFO's, and that all members of management must participate in the development of the plan and support its objective.

The CFO's role in planning should be one of educating management to the need for a plan, coordinating the preparation of the plan, examining and testing the plan for adequacy and accuracy, and translating the final plan into financial terms. The CFO is only a counselor and coordinator. The responsibility for planning for each separate operational function must lie with the appropriate department head and administrator.

THE RECORDING FUNCTION

The systematic recording of financial transactions is commonly viewed as, and traditionally has been, the principal function of the hospital CFO. Pressures for improved financial management, though, are forcing the CFO to delegate the actual performance of this function to the accounting specialist members of his staff, and to devote his own time and energies to more comprehensive financial problems. Nevertheless, the CFO is still responsible for ensuring that all financial transactions are accounted for and that accurate records are maintained. Thus, although he may delegate actual performance of this activity, he should carefully supervise its accomplishment.

The various specific aspects or components of the recording function are discussed further in the following section.

THE MEASURING FUNCTION

Management needs to have information available from the measurement and evaluation of the actual operational performance so that the hospital's objectives can be met and its plan of operations carried out. This function can perhaps be understood most easily if it is viewed as the feedback loop and monitor for the planning function. The planning function sets the standards for operations, and the measuring function ascertains and analyzes the level of actual performance. The results of these two functions can be compared to determine the extent of any deviation between planned and actual performance, and the nature of any necessary corrective action. Together, these functions—along with the reporting function—provide the basis for management control of operations.

It should be noted that the CFO does not personally enforce control of operations. Rather, his role is one of assisting functional management—just as it is in planning—by providing the information needed to control operations and to achieve the desired objectives and level of performance. To perform this role properly, not only should the CFO provide measures of actual performance, but also he should assist in evaluating performance and review the mechanism by which data are gathered. Thus, he can assure that sufficient data are available and that they are being provided on a timely basis.

THE REPORTING FUNCTION

Viewed from an internal management standpoint, the reporting function is closely related to the planning and measuring functions. Without reporting, planning operations and measuring actual performance are exercises in futility. Reporting is the mechanism by which information is communicated and planning and measuring are brought together to provide the basis for controlling operations. Effective control is impossible without an appropriate and efficient reporting system.

The CFO's reporting responsibilities, however, go beyond just the preparation and presentation of figures, charts, and other reports. To be effective, the CFO must also interpret the presented information so that its meaning and implications are understandable to all members of management. This aspect of the reporting function is critical, for without interpretation the managerial usefulness of reports is, at best, limited. Thus, if management is to obtain the information necessary to direct and control operations, the CFO must not only provide information, but also analyze or interpret the data so that their managerial usefulness is clear.

In addition to the above internal responsibilities, the reporting function also carries with it external reporting obligations, for example, cost reports for third party payers, informational returns for the Internal Revenue Service, financial reports for lenders, trustees, and the public. These reports, though of marginal internal management value, are important for the overall well-being and operation of a hospital. The CFO, therefore, to fulfill his reporting function adequately, must carry out both its internal and external aspects.

THE ADVISING FUNCTION

The advisory function of the CFO is closely linked to the reporting function and actually can be considered as a component of that function. However, because of the significance of the contribution that the CFO can make through the proper exercise of this function, it is specifically set out to emphasize its importance.

Through measuring and reporting on the validity of the institution's objectives and on the effectiveness of its policies, organization, and procedures in achieving those objectives, the CFO can not only force management to evaluate the hospital's current operational status, but also aid in the establishment of future operating policies. Additionally, the CFO, by analyzing the impact of external political and economic factors, can advise management as to what actions must be taken to achieve the desired operational goals. Thus, the CFO occupies a unique position as a counselor to management, responsible both for ensuring that total operational achievements are periodically evaluated and for aiding in the establishment of future operational guidelines.

THE RECORDING FUNCTION: FURTHER DISCUSSION

As has been indicated, the recording function has been in the past the principal activity of the hospital CFO. The major items included in this function have been (1) the development and operation of the hospital's general accounting system; (2) the design and custody of all of the books, records, and forms needed to record financial transactions; and (3) the development and installation of an adequate system of internal control. The first two items are of a technical accounting nature and as such are not really appropriate to this text. Readers wishing detailed information in these areas should consult any basic accounting text, such as *Hospital Financial Accounting: Theory and Practice* by L. Vann Seawell. The third item, however, is basic to sound financial management and merits further discussion here.

Internal control has been defined by the Committee on Auditing Procedures of the American Institute of Certified Public Accountants as:

> the plan of organization and all of the coordinate methods and measures adopted within a business to safeguard its assets, check the accuracy and reliability of its accounting data, promote operational efficiency, and encourage adherence to prescribed managerial policies.

Thus, internal control involves not only the control or safeguarding of assets, but also the plan of organization and all the methods and procedures that relate to operational efficiency. In a broad sense, therefore, internal control can be viewed as including two basic types or areas of control—accounting control and administrative control.

Accounting control is concerned mainly with safeguarding the assets of the hospital and assuring the reliability of the financial records. Administrative control is concerned mainly with operational efficiency and adherence to managerial policies. It should be noted, though, for purposes of internal management, that the two areas are interrelated and both are needed if control is to be achieved.

The Committee on Auditing Procedures specifies four items that are necessary for a satisfactory control system:[4]

1. A plan of organization that provides an appropriate segregation of functional responsibilities

2. A system of authorization and record procedures adequate to provide accounting control over assets, liabilities, revenues, and expenses

3. Sound practices to be followed in performance of the duties and functions of each of the organizational departments

4. A degree of quality of personnel commensurate with responsibilities

ORGANIZATION PLAN

As has been discussed earlier, there is no single right or proper organization structure for all hospitals. However, regardless of the specific organization plan adopted, certain basic principles of organization are applicable in all cases. Specifically, the organization structure should establish clear lines of authority and responsibility, create independence of operation, demark custodial and record-keeping responsibilities, ensure that an individual is not responsible to more than one person, and provide for proper spans of control. These organizational features are essential not only for internal control, but also for effective operational management.

ACCOUNTING PROCEDURES

A formal system of authorization and record procedures is as critical for internal control as is a sound organization plan. Procedures provide the prescribed manner by which all types of transaction should be handled, including the records, forms, and accounts to be used and the authorization or approvals that are needed. Authorizations are of particular importance, for they provide not only the checks and balances needed to control any

---

[4]Committee on Auditing Procedures, *Auditing Standards and Procedures,* "Statement on Auditing Procedures, No. 33," 1963, p. 27.

given procedure but also, when combined with the proper forms, the documentation necessary for both the accounting records and external audits. Thus, in essence, procedures and authorizations are complementary. That is, procedures specify a given process, and authorizations provide the mechanism for ensuring that the process or procedures are properly carried out. Together, they provide the basis for accounting control.

OPERATING PRACTICES

In addition to formal accounting procedures, a sound system of operating practices and authorizations is requisite for effective internal control. Just as accounting procedures provide the mechanism for ensuring that transactions are documented and that accounting records are adequate, operating procedures provide the means for ensuring that transactions proceed efficiently and that proper checks and balances exist.

Fundamental to sound operating procedures are such practices as

1. Obtaining competitive bids from suppliers
2. Matching packing slips against purchase orders and suppliers' invoices
3. Prenumbering all forms and checks
4. Maintaining individual records of all capital assets
5. Separating custodial and record-keeping responsibilities
6. Requiring dual signatures on checks
7. Reconciling general and subsidiary ledgers

A complete listing of all of the practices that should be employed to assure proper internal control of operations is beyond the scope of this text. Readers desiring additional information in this area should consult the American Hospital Association's manual, *Internal Control of Hospital Finances: A Guide for Management.*

QUALITY PERSONNEL

The final, and perhaps the most important, factor necessary for internal control is an adequate number of qualified personnel who are capable of carrying out established procedures and practices in an efficient manner. Organization plans and procedural manuals are inanimate. They cannot, in themselves, perform the various tasks that they prescribe; only people can vitalize procedures. Therefore, if procedures are to be carried out properly and if internal control is to be more than just charts and manuals, the employees of the hospital must be of the quality and possess the skills necessary to carry out their tasks in the prescribed manner. Without adequate personnel, it is impossible to operate an effective system of internal control.

It should be noted, however, that though qualified personnel are necessary in all areas, the internal auditor is the key employee in any internal control system. Not only is the internal auditor responsible for protecting the hospital's assets against fraud, error, and loss, but his functions also include

1. Reviewing and appraising the soundness, adequacy, and application of accounting, financial, and operating controls

2. Ascertaining the extent of compliance with established policies, plans, and procedures

3. Ascertaining the reliability of accounting and other data developed within the organization

4. Appraising the quality of performance in carrying out assigned responsibilities[5]

He is, in effect, the man who monitors the internal control system, assuring both that it is functioning and that it is functioning properly.

In order to perform this task, he should occupy a staff position and report directly to executive management, for example, the chief financial officer, the chief operating officer, or the chief executive officer. In this way he will have the organizational independence to avoid conflicts of interest and the freedom to appraise operations objectively.

CHECKLIST

In addition to the above basic characteristics, the American Hospital Association has suggested that the following checklist can be used to appraise the adequacy of an internal control system.[6]

1. Does the hospital have a current organization chart?

2. Are the accounting and treasury functions satisfactorily defined and segregated?

3. To whom does the chief accounting officer report?

4. Does the hospital have an internal auditor? To whom does he report? Outline briefly the scope of the internal audit work.

5. Is a chart of accounts used?

6. Is a current accounting manual used?

---

[5]Institute of Internal Auditors, "Statement of the Responsibilities of the Internal Auditor," New York, 1967.

[6]American Hospital Association, *Internal Control, Internal Auditing, and Operations Auditing for Hospitals,* pp. 10–11.

7. Are monthly statements to management prepared and furnished, along with supporting analyses and explanatory comments?

8. Are the monthly statements—relative to material variances from standards, budgets, or prior periods—discussed with the board of directors, executive committee, treasurer, department heads?

9. Are costs and expenses under budgetary control?

10. Has the general policy concerning insurance coverage been defined by the board of directors? Is the insurance coverage periodically reviewed by a responsible officer or employee?

11. Are journal entries (a) adequately explained and supported and (b) approved by a responsible employee?

12. Are all employees required to take annual vacations? Have provisions been made for the temporary reassignment of duties in the absence of an employee on vacation?

13. Does a responsible employee maintain a calendar or follow-up file on such matters as the due dates of tax returns and special reports and the expiration dates of the period of limitations on tax refund claims?

14. What is the hospital's policy concerning its key employees (such as purchasing agents, department or division managers) having any direct or indirect ownership or profit participation in outside business enterprises with which the hospital does business? What procedures are followed to determine that such a policy is being complied with?

Readers desiring a detailed discussion of policies and procedures relative to any of the above items should refer to the previously mentioned American Hospital Association manual.

INDEPENDENT AUDITORS

In addition to an internal auditor, prudent management requires that the hospital utilize an external independent auditor.

An independent auditor differs from an internal auditor in that

1. He is not an employee of the hospital;

2. His primary concern is not the needs of internal management, but rather the needs of external agencies and organizations;

3. His review of operations is limited to basically financial matters;

4. He is only incidentally concerned with the detection and prevention of fraud; and

5. His examination of the hospital is periodic as opposed to continuous.

The value and usefulness of an independent auditor lie as much in business convention as they do in operational control.

The opinion of an independent auditor, concerning the financial statements of a hospital, is the best possible indication of whether persons who are not associated with the hospital may justifiably rely upon those statements in making financial decisions.[7] The assumed need for such an opinion is derived from an implicit value judgment concerning the self-interest and character of internal management.

Whether this value judgment is valid is a moot point. Audited financial statements, bearing an independent opinion, have come to be commonly accepted both as being credible and as containing data that can be freely relied upon by the external agencies and organizations. This position and this philosophy are recognized by the federal government under the Medicare program, by Blue Cross plans, and by state governments under their rate review and public disclosure programs.

An independent auditor is also of value in terms of operational control. Due to his financial and attitudinal independence from the hospital—he is not an employee of the hospital and his code of ethics requires independent thought and action—he provides a check and balance, at least in regard to financial matters, on both the internal auditor and the entire concern. The value of this "fail-safe" mechanism is obvious and in itself justifies the use of an independent auditor.

In selecting an auditor, careful consideration should be given to technical competence and independence. At a minimum, the auditor should be a certified public accountant. Admittedly, certification does not guarantee technical competence. However, it is evidence that, at least at one point in time, he has demonstrated his qualifications to render competent service. Hence, certification should be considered a basic requisite for selection.

The matter of the auditor's independence must also be weighed in the selection process. The auditor must be financially independent of his client in that "Any direct financial interest or material indirect financial interest is prohibited as is any relationship to the client, such as . . . voting trustee, director, officer, or key employee."[8] He also must be independent in terms of his fee not being contingent upon his findings or the results of his service. Last, the auditor's independence must not be compromised by his being selected by the very persons whose work he would be reviewing. In operational terms this means that the governing board, or one of its committees—such as the finance committee or audit committee with the approval

---

[7]Stettler, Howard F., *Systems Based Independent Audits*, 1967, p. 1. See also American Institute of CPA, *Hospital Audit Guide*, 1972.

[8]American Institute of Certified Public Accountants, "Code of Ethics," Article 101.

of the board—as opposed to the chief executive officer or the CFO, should select the auditor.

AUDIT COMMITTEE AND THE AUDIT

As just mentioned, the independent auditor might be selected by the audit committee of the board. Audit committees are relatively recent organizational developments. In commercial firms they have been the outgrowth of increased governmental and public interest in financial reporting due to the incidence of questionable or illegal payments and unexpected financial failures. To provide closer scrutiny of management as well as to afford additional protection to nonofficer directors and stockholders, the device of the audit committee was created. In 1970 only about one-third of the nation's major commercial corporations used audit committees. By the middle of the decade more than 85% had instituted audit committees.

The hospital field can draw a useful lesson from the experience and actions of these commercial corporations. The audit committee can be a useful mechanism for assuring the existence and proper functioning of the checks and balances in the hospital's financial systems. It is a committee with a broad but at the same time limited focus, charged with assuring that the independent auditor is doing his job and that management is using "due care" in establishing and maintaining effective internal accounting practices and high standards of financial reporting.

In terms of logistics and mechanics, the audit committee should function and be supported like any other board committee. Meetings should be formally scheduled, annotated agenda should be prepared and distributed prior to the meetings, staff support by both the independent auditor and the fiscal services division should be provided, and opportunities for executive sessions both with and without the independent auditor should be included as part of the normal agenda.

Typically, the committee should meet at least twice a year. The first meeting should address the scope of the audit, with particular attention to identifying areas of audit emphasis and financial matters of concern to the directors. The second meeting should be held after the audit is completed and focus on reviewing the financial statements, the management letter provided by the auditor, and any other comments the auditor might have. Obviously, depending on the scope of the audit and the audit findings, additional meetings might be needed either during or after the audit. The audit committee should report either directly to the finance committee or to the board as a whole.

With respect to the audit itself, it is basically a series of accounting procedures designed to test, on a selected basis, the financial transactions of the firm—to form an opinion on the accuracy and reliability of the hospital's financial statements. Importantly, it is not an examination of every transaction. The end result of the audit is an expression of opinion by the independent auditor.

The auditor's opinion can be unqualified, indicating that the financial statements were prepared in accord with generally accepted accounting practice and that they fairly represent the financial position of the hospital. Alternatively, the auditor can offer a qualified opinion. In a qualified opinion the auditor takes exception to some specific aspect of the financial statements or notes some contingency, for example, significant outstanding litigation, that might affect the financial statements. In extreme cases the auditor might provide an adverse opinion, stating that the statements do not fairly represent the financial position of the hospital. Adverse opinions are usually the result of material differences between the hospital's accounting practices and generally accepted accounting practices or uncertainties about future events that might materially affect the financial statements. When an auditor is unable to form an opinion, a disclaimer of opinion is provided. A disclaimer of opinion results for example when the scope of the audit is too limited to allow for an informed opinion to be offered.

Obviously, any adverse opinion or disclaimer detracts from the credibility of the financial statements and should be of concern not only to management but also to the audit committee and the board. The reasons for any qualification should be understood and corrective actions, if needed, should be taken, for example, increase contingency reserves for outstanding litigation, revise accounting practices, or improve internal control procedures.

CONCLUSION

Given the foregoing material, one should have a general understanding of the functional responsibilities of the CFO. This understanding can be clarified further by examining the organization chart pictured in Figure 3.2.

Figure 3.2 illustrates the broad scope and importance of the CFO's responsibilities. If a CFO is to carry out these responsibilities properly, he must possess not only a knowledge of accounting principles and procedures, but also the ability to interpret and analyze accounting and statistical data, communicate with and motivate employees and other managers, and utilize accounting data not as ends in themselves, but rather as the means to effective financial and hospital management. The CFO, thus, must be more than just an accountant. He must have both the imagination to convert static accounting data into management information and the technical skill to employ such information as an aid in managing not only the financial operations of the hospital, but also total operations.

The CFO obviously occupies a key position in the organization struc-

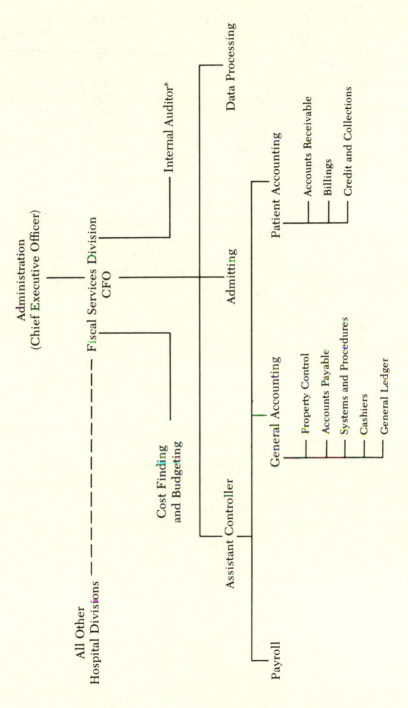

FIGURE 3.2   Organization Chart Fiscal Services Division

Administration
(Chief Executive Officer)

All Other
Hospital Divisions — — — — — — — Fiscal Services Division
CFO

Internal Auditor*

Data Processing

Admitting

Patient Accounting

Accounts Receivable

Billings

Credit and Collections

Cost Finding
and Budgeting

Assistant Controller

General Accounting

Property Control

Accounts Payable

Systems and Procedures

Cashiers

General Ledger

Payroll

*The internal auditor could also report to the chief executive officer or to a chief operating officer.

ture of the hospital. The demands upon a chief executive officer's time and the specialized technical complexities of financial operations prohibit an administrator from personally supervising day-to-day financial operations. Therefore, to fulfill his fiscal responsibilities properly, an administrator must obtain the services of a competent CFO and ensure that the CFO adequately carries out functions of his position. The remainder of this text is devoted to providing an administrator with the background and knowledge necessary to aid him in evaluating both a CFO's performance and the financial condition of a hospital.

SUGGESTED READINGS

Allcorn, Seth. *Internal Auditing for Hospitals.*

American Institute of Certified Public Accountants. *Hospital Audit Guide.*

Caruana, Russell A. *A Guide to Organizing the Hospital's Fiscal Services Division.*

Heckert, J. Brooks and Willson, James D. *Controllership,* Chapters 1, 2, and 6.

Linklater, R. Bruce. *Internal Control of Hospital Finances: A Guide for Management.*

Murphy, Thomas. "The Hospital Treasurer and Controller: Duties and Responsibilities."

Seawell, L. Vann. *Hospital Financial Accounting: Theory and Practice,* Chapters 1 and 5.

Shelton, Robert M. "The Hospital Financial Manager Today."

Taylor, Philip J. and Nelson, Benjamin O. *Management Accounting for Hospitals,* Chapters 1 and 12.

Tonkin, G.W. "The Controller's Role on the Management Team."

APPENDIX 3.A
ILLUSTRATIVE HOSPITAL ORGANIZATION CHARTS

As has been discussed, there is no single right or proper organization structure. To illustrate this point, several alternative organization structures are presented on the following pages.

ALTERNATIVE 1   Smaller Hospitals

Revenue account numbers
are shown at left in
italics (310).
Expense account numbers
are shown at right (610).

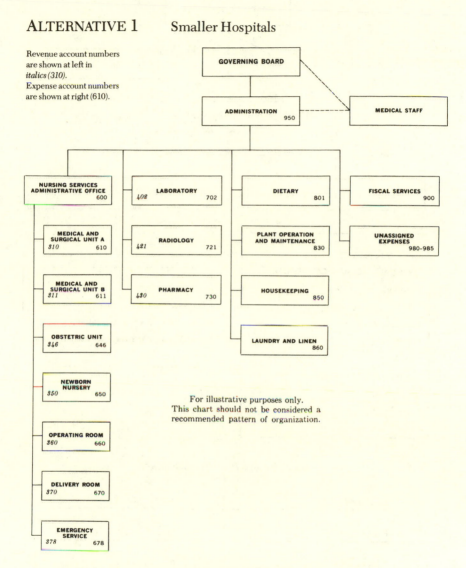

For illustrative purposes only.
This chart should not be considered a
recommended pattern of organization.

Source: Reprinted with permission from *Chart of Accounts for Hospitals*, published by the American Hospital Association.

ALTERNATIVE 2

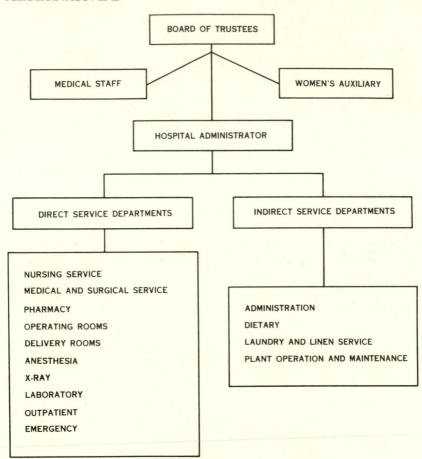

BOARD OF TRUSTEES

MEDICAL STAFF

WOMEN'S AUXILIARY

HOSPITAL ADMINISTRATOR

DIRECT SERVICE DEPARTMENTS

INDIRECT SERVICE DEPARTMENTS

NURSING SERVICE

MEDICAL AND SURGICAL SERVICE

PHARMACY

OPERATING ROOMS

DELIVERY ROOMS

ANESTHESIA

X-RAY

LABORATORY

OUTPATIENT

EMERGENCY

ADMINISTRATION

DIETARY

LAUNDRY AND LINEN SERVICE

PLANT OPERATION AND MAINTENANCE

DETAIL OF ADMINISTRATIVE DEPARTMENT

ACCOUNTING	ADMITTING
PURCHASING	CREDIT AND COLLECTION
PUBLIC RELATIONS	PERSONNEL
GENERAL CLERKS	STOCKKEEPING

Source: L. Vann Seawell, "Practice Hospital Organization Chart," *Principles of Hospital Accounting*, Physicians' Record Co., 1960, p. 329. Reprinted with permission.

ALTERNATIVE 3

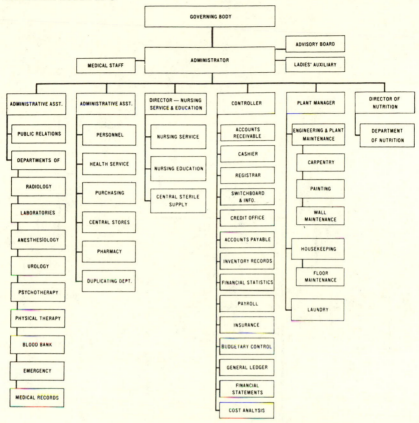

DIVISION OF BUSINESS ADMINISTRATION

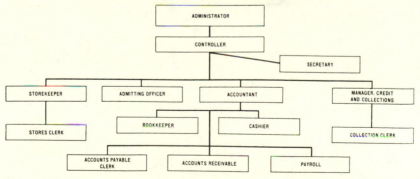

Source: L. Vann Seawell, "Organization Chart," *Hospital Accounting and Financial Management,* Physicians' Record Co., 1964, p. 14. Reprinted with permission.

ALTERNATIVE 4

GENERAL ORGANIZATION

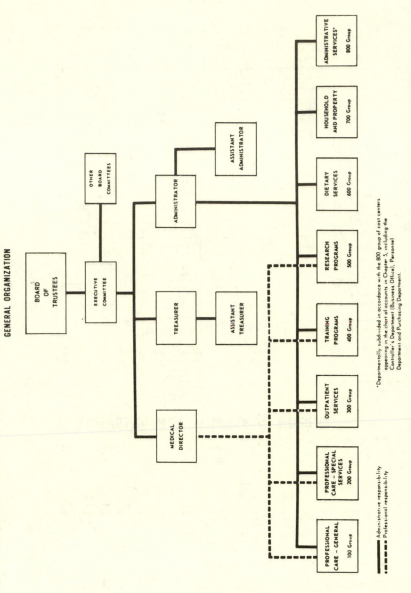

Source: Philip J. Taylor and Benjamin O. Nelson, *Management Accounting for Hospitals*, 1964. Philadelphia: W.B. Saunders Company. Reprinted with permission.

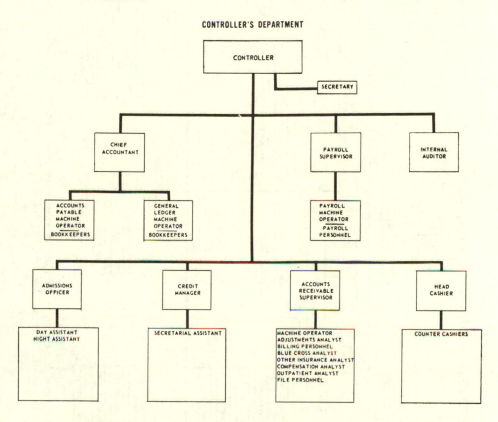

CONTROLLER'S DEPARTMENT

CONTROLLER

SECRETARY

CHIEF ACCOUNTANT — PAYROLL SUPERVISOR — INTERNAL AUDITOR

ACCOUNTS PAYABLE MACHINE OPERATOR / BOOKKEEPERS

GENERAL LEDGER MACHINE OPERATOR / BOOKKEEPERS

PAYROLL MACHINE OPERATOR / PAYROLL PERSONNEL

ADMISSIONS OFFICER — CREDIT MANAGER — ACCOUNTS RECEIVABLE SUPERVISOR — HEAD CASHIER

DAY ASSISTANT
NIGHT ASSISTANT

SECRETARIAL ASSISTANT

MACHINE OPERATOR
ADJUSTMENTS ANALYST
BILLING PERSONNEL
BLUE CROSS ANALYST
OTHER INSURANCE ANALYST
COMPENSATION ANALYST
OUTPATIENT ANALYST
FILE PERSONNEL

COUNTER CASHIERS

Source: Philip J. Taylor and Benjamin O. Nelson, *Management Accounting for Hospitals,* 1964. Philadelphia: W.B. Saunders Company. Reprinted with permission.

ALTERNATIVE 5　　Manufacturing Corporation

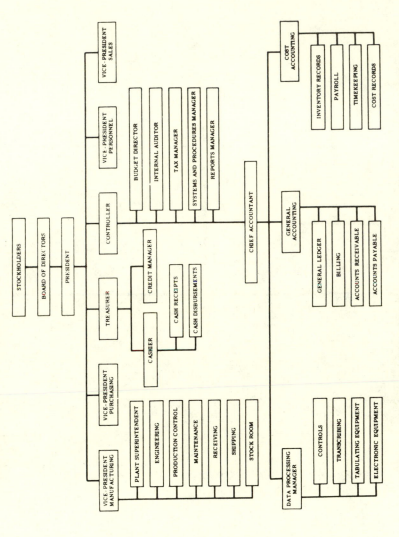

Source: Howard F. Stettler, *Systems Based Independent Audits* © 1967. Reprinted by permission of Prentice-Hall, Inc., Englewood Cliffs, N.J.

ALTERNATIVE 6   Manufacturing Corporation

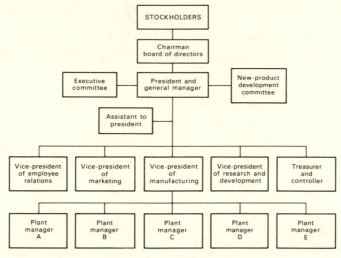

Source: From *Management Theory and Practice, Fourth Edition* by Ernest Dale, copyright 1978. Used with the permission of McGraw-Hill Book Company.

ALTERNATIVE 7   Manufacturing Corporation

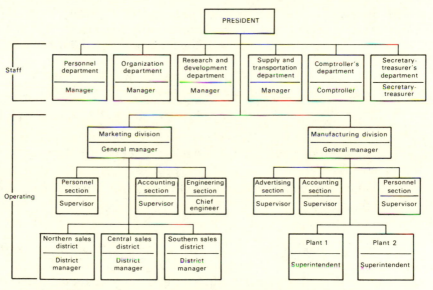

Source: "From *The Management Guide* prepared by George Lawrence Hall with the assistance of other members of the department on organization, Standard Oil Company of California; 2nd ed. edited by Franklin E. Drew and George Lawrence Hall, Standard Oil Company of California, March 1956, p. 35. Now out of print," as reproduced in Ernest Dale, *Management Theory and Practice, Second Edition,* copyright 1969 by McGraw-Hill Book Company.

APPENDIX 3.B
ALTERNATIVE CORPORATE ORGANIZATION STRUCTURES[9]

Figure 3.1 depicted the traditional single corporation approach to hospital organization. Until relatively recently this model was the common form of hospital corporate organization. However, in the 1970s hospitals began to examine alternatives to this traditional approach. The driving forces behind this movement have been several. The principal factor, though, has been a recognition that in many environments

1. Nonprofit hospitals will no longer be able to rely on patient care revenue as either their sole or their primary source of discretionary income;

2. Freestanding, fee-for-service hospitals will find, due to expanded regulatory controls, that it is increasingly difficult to operate successfully; and

3. Hospitals that are adaptive and responsive to change will have a greater likelihood of being able to operate successfully.

As a result of these pressures, hospitals have reassessed and are continuing to reassess their form of legal organization structure. In many instances this assessment has resulted in hospitals' adopting new legal structures designed to: protect present and future assets; facilitate the development of new services and activities; maximize patient care and other operating as well as nonoperating income; and attract additional funds through philanthropy.

Generically, the organization structure alternatives being utilized fall into four models:

1. Hospital corporation with a subsidiary controlled development foundation

2. Hospital corporation with a sister, quasi-independent development foundation

3. Hospital corporation with a wholly independent development foundation

4. Parent holding company structure

Each of these models has various advantages and limitations. In all instances, however, their goal is to enable the hospital to cope and compete better as an economic entity. In deciding which, if any, of these models to utilize, the hospital should seek the advice of both its corporate counsel and its tax advisor. Each of these models is illustrated below.

---

[9]The material for this appendix was drawn from "Legal Issues for Diversification and Divestiture," a speech by Ross E. Stromberg, Esq., and is reprinted with his permission.

ALTERNATIVE 1   Hospital Corporation with a
Subsidiary Controlled Development
Foundation

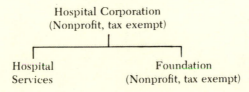

Hospital Corporation
(Nonprofit, tax exempt)

Hospital
Services

Foundation
(Nonprofit, tax exempt)

ALTERNATIVE 2   Hospital Corporation with a Sister,
Quasi-Independent Development
Foundation

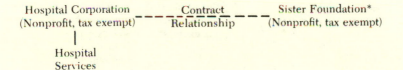

Hospital Corporation
(Nonprofit, tax exempt)

Contract
Relationship

Sister Foundation*
(Nonprofit, tax exempt)

Hospital
Services

*The foundation has an independent board, with the hospital not in explicit
control; that is, the hospital has less than 50% control over the foundation's
board. The hospital, however, has considerable de facto control. Also, the
hospital is the sole beneficiary of the foundation.

ALTERNATIVE 3   Hospital Corporation with a Wholly Independent Development Foundation

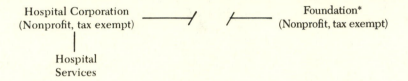

Hospital Corporation
(Nonprofit, tax exempt)

Hospital
Services

Foundation*
(Nonprofit, tax exempt)

ALTERNATIVE 4   Parent Holding Company Structure

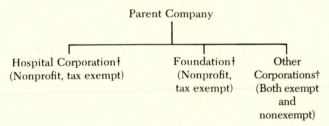

Parent Company

Hospital Corporation†
(Nonprofit, tax exempt)

Foundation†
(Nonprofit,
tax exempt)

Other
Corporations†
(Both exempt
and
nonexempt)

*The foundation is completely independent of the hospital, with no crossover board members or corporate officers. Moreover, the hospital is one of several possible beneficiaries.

†Each subsidiary corporation has its own board. Membership of the various boards can be the same.

Sources of
Operating Revenue

Introduction:
The Past Is Prologue

It is somewhat unorthodox to include in a text on financial management a discussion of the sources of operating revenue available to a firm. However, in the case of hospital financial management, if a complete understanding of the hospital's financial environment is to be obtained, this approach may be the best way to start, for a unique relationship exists between hospitals and the actual payers for care.

Hospitals, though treating many individual patients, are paid for the services that they provide by relatively few sources. These sources, because of their relative economic power, are able to affect the financial status of an individual hospital substantially by their payment methods or procedures. Therefore, it seems advisable, before examining the application of financial management tools and techniques to hospital management, first to consider how hospitals are paid.

By way of introduction, it is instructive to begin by looking backward. Like many complex phenomena, the beginnings of the current patterns of hospital payment are difficult to trace. The history of the present financing system reflects both an overlapping of ideas—as different people in different geographic areas were attempting to solve the same problems at the same time—and a rediscovery—under new circumstances—of previously tried mechanisms. However, out of this image, a thread of logic which portrays a reasonable systematic development process can be deciphered.

Prior to the turn of the century, most hospitals billed and were paid on what would be now called an all-inclusive rate. That is, hospitals charged all patients the same daily rate. This single rate covered all services that the hospital provided.

By today's standards, this sort of flat rate approach is admittedly simplistic. However, when viewed in the context of times—when hospitals provided only limited services and had an undifferentiated product—the approach not only provided for equity but also represented an administratively sound way to operate.

The flat rate approach served as a workable mechanism until hospitals began to provide more complex and differentiated products. The development of specific techniques in surgery, the increased use of anesthesia, and the discovery of the Roentgen ray enabled the hospital product to be improved and different products to be provided to different patients. As a result, hospitals established a system of special service charges; patients who used particular services paid separately for them. The intent of the special service charge system was simply to maintain equity between patients who used particular services and those who did not.

Special services and special service charges grew in variety and amount with the introduction of laboratory services, physical therapy, drugs, and so forth. By the 1920s, it was not unusual for a patient's total amount of special service charges to exceed the regular daily service charges.

The growth in special service charges, combined with a general increase in hospital charges, resulted in adverse public reaction to both hospital costs and the à la carte approach to billing. As a result of this reaction, the hospital industry began to reconsider—as a means of spreading costs among patients—the practicability of an all-inclusive rate financing system.

The early use of the inclusive rate system in the 1920s applied only to certain special services such as laboratory examinations. A few years later the principle was applied to certain admissions by diagnosis such as tonsillectomies and maternity service. In the early 1930s, all-inclusive rates were established by some hospitals for all inpatients. These rates varied only as to the length of stay of the patient and the type of accommodations occupied.

While the industry, in general, was moving back to an all-inclusive rate payment mechanism, a complementary—and perhaps, more important—innovation was being introduced in Ohio. In 1919, the state of Ohio introduced, for purposes of workmen's compensation payment, the concept of an all-inclusive rate based on audited costs. The significance of this concept should not be lost, for it provided half the foundation for over 40 years of hospital payment systems. With the introduction of "audited costs," the basis of payment to hospitals not only shifted in terms of decision loci, but also in terms of reliance on objective quantifiable data—cost.

In the early 1920s, the state of Pennsylvania implemented a variation of the Ohio mechanism by paying hospitals on the basis of the estimated cost per day. In the 1930s, the federal government first became involved, through the Children's Bureau, in hospital care reimbursement. Like Ohio, the federal government also added an innovation. In this instance, the concept was that of "reimbursable cost." That is, as opposed to full hospital costs, the Children's Bureau only paid the costs per day that were applicable to patient care, excluding costs that were not for direct patient care, that is, administrative and benefits.

With the introduction of the notion of reimbursable costs, the other half of the payment system foundation was in place. Throughout the next four decades, with the exception of the period in the 1930s when Blue Cross plans were getting started and a flat rate system was used, a variety of retrospective, prospective, incentive, and disincentive systems were used to pay hospitals. Similarly, the methods of calculating costs and obtaining increased uniformity of calculation among hospitals evolved. While each of these systems and methods built upon and differed from the others, central to each—as well as to the current system—has been and is the notion of audited reimbursable cost.

It is this foundation upon which the following chapters should be considered.

4

Sources of Revenue

INTRODUCTION

Hospitals are big business. In fact, hospitals are one of the biggest industries in the country. The operation and management of a hospital, however, are in many ways unlike those of other businesses. The distinction between the operation of hospitals and commercial enterprises is particularly apparent in regard to the sources of the revenues that are obtained to support the institution.

With most businesses the source of revenue is the sale of goods or services. The nonhospital business buys or manufactures goods or provides services at a certain price and sells those products in a competitive or quasi-competitive market at prices that it hopes will return a profit. Most businesses are run for profit, which tends to challenge management and to force it to produce efficiently and competitively in order to return a profit to the owners.

At one time hospitals were maintained basically to care for the critically or chronically ill and depended on benefactors and philanthropists to finance any deficits. Today, due to increased utilization of hospitals and greater costs of operation, the benefactor alone cannot subsidize hospital operations. He may furnish capital funds at some time in his life to erect a hospital building to bear his name, but taxes have eaten into his income to such a degree that he no longer stands ready at each year-end to make up the hospital's operating losses.

Most of today's hospitals are not managed as profit-making, competitive institutions and, as stated, they generally do not have philanthropists who will make up their deficits. Today, voluntary hospitals depend on "third parties" as their major source of revenue.

Who is a third party? The third party (besides the hospital and patient who are the first two parties) is Blue Cross, the commercial insurance company, Medicare, Medicaid, workers' compensation, or any agent other than the patient who contracts to pay all or part of a patient's hospital bill. A third party is the major source of revenue for the hospital, is a sure source of revenue, and is a party that can be depended upon to pay its bill within a certain payment system and within a reasonably constant time period. Therefore, the third party is a highly important factor in the operation of a hospital.

The share of total hospital expenses paid by the third party will vary from area to area and from hospital to hospital. On average, however, one can think of hospital revenues (collections, not charges) as coming predominantly from third parties.

The major purchasers of hospital care today, Blue Cross, the federal government (principally Medicare and Medicaid), insurance firms, and HMOs, usually pay on a "cost," "cost-plus," "contract," "DRG," or "capitation" basis because they say they are wholesale buyers of care. The remainder of the purchasers of hospital care pay at rates higher than the aforementioned reimbursement formulas. Some of these higher charges are partially covered by commercial insurance policies, which pay certain indemnities for specified services. Any balance beyond the stated indemnities would be charged directly to the patient. The same is true for "deductibles" and services beyond those allowed under a third party policy.

On the face of it, this method of charges and payments seems plausible and quite fair. As indicated earlier, most voluntary community hospitals are not operated for profit. In fact, they are classified as not-for-profit. Under this not-for-profit arrangement, the major portion of third party contracts calls for reimbursements ultimately based on allowable costs. The self-pay patient pays the balance, which might seem his just share.

Unfortunately, Mr. Self-Pay Patient is in a very uncomfortable position where he is unable to do much to protect himself against the uncontrolled explosion in the price of hospital care.

He purchases services at retail in a system where all the other major payers for care purchase services at cost or very slightly above cost. However, the problem is not that the third party purchasers pay cost, but rather that cost as defined by the purchasers is neither total accounting cost nor economic cost. Thus, what is not allowed as cost by third party payers must be paid by someone else and that someone else is the only one left, Mr. Self-Pay, who must pay the highest rate of all.

The last point is critical and deserves further clarification. In accounting terms, cost can be defined as any release of value. That is, a cost is incurred any time something of value—usually money—is given up to obtain something else. Thus, cost is equal to the money given up to obtain labor and capital necessary to operate the hospital and treat patients. This definition of cost would probably be accepted in theory by both hospitals and third parties. However, third parties do not feel that this approach represents an equitable basis for paying hospitals. Instead, they suggest there are two types of cost: the full cost defined above (the total cost incurred in operating the hospital); and reimbursable cost, which differs from full cost in that it does not include all the cost involved in operating the hospital. Every hospital has many legitimate costs that might not be evident to one unfamiliar with the administration of a hospital.

A hospital is a complex organization with problems peculiar to its field. It develops expenses in its operation, some of which may seem only tangential to the care of patients, yet which can be pointed to as part of the total process of medical and nursing care. The legitimacy of some of these costs has been rejected by the large third party purchasers of care who feel the costs are not directly related to the care their clients are receiving, that they are not directly related to any of the nursing, medical, or paramedical services they are purchasing.

Over the years, the justification for allowing the so-called tangential or peripheral costs under the reimbursement formulas has been debated by the hospitals, Blue Cross, and government. Some of the costs have been allowed; others have been disallowed or are still under discussion. In the meantime, the costs being debated are still being incurred by hospitals and are still being paid by Mr. Self-Pay.[1]

It has been mentioned, but bears repeating, that not all of the expenses a hospital incurs are considered allowable costs and consequently Mr. Self-Pay, from whom 10% to 12% of the hospital's revenue comes, must pay the disallowed costs if the hospital can find no other source of payment.

DEBATED AREAS OF HOSPITAL COSTS

A discussion of the debated areas of hospital costs should illustrate and clarify the problem.

DEPRECIATION OF BUILDINGS AND EQUIPMENT

Depreciation could be said to be merely a recognition that things wear out and need to be replaced. If allowance is made for this depreciation and the money value is set aside, with price levels constant, then the buildings and equipment can be replaced as they wear out. This is simplified language.

---

[1]Some commercial firms are operating under another set of rules that allows them to offer protection on a defined benefit basis or on a wide coverage basis, such as the major medical policy, with a deductible factor—both conditions under rates based on actuarial figures.

Unfortunately, depreciation cannot be discussed with such simplified language. Depreciation is an expense of doing business, whether in a supermarket or in a community hospital. There is no question in the mind of the supermarket operator that depreciation of buildings and movable equipment is a real cost of doing business, but the hospital has often in the past had to debate whether depreciation should be an allowable cost under third party reimbursement formulas.

For the most part, third parties now accept and recognize depreciation as a legitimate operating expense and allow its inclusion in the reimbursement formula. This acceptance, however, has not ended the controversy surrounding depreciation, for hospitals and third parties now have shifted the debate from whether depreciation should be considered as a legitimate operating expense to what the conditions should be for accepting it as an expense. The conditions or debatable points are likely to be: whether the amount to be depreciated should be the historical (original) cost or the replacement cost of the buildings and equipment; what the estimated life of the items should be; and what the method of computing depreciation should be. Historical cost generally is and should be used in calculating depreciation in reimbursement formulas; estimated life of buildings and equipment is determined by past practice and by rulings of the Internal Revenue Service; and the actual depreciation is computed by a method agreeable to both parties.[2, 3]

Three of the common methods of computing depreciation are: straight line; sum-of-the-years in digits; and double declining balance. The last two methods are often referred to as accelerated depreciation. In the first two methods the sum to be depreciated would be the historical cost less the

---

[2]The argument for the use of historical cost rather than replacement cost for computing depreciation can be based on the definition of depreciation. The historical cost method is correct if depreciation is considered as a means of allocating previously incurred costs to the proper time periods during which the facilities are used up. Replacement of worn-out facilities should be a separate problem. Replacement can be financed from the depreciation fund without being related to the method of computing depreciation.

[3]Though historical cost has been the traditional standard for reporting asset values and computing depreciation, the Securities and Exchange Commission (SEC) in 1976 adopted regulations that would require certain companies to disclose replacement cost information in financial statements filed with the Commission. The SEC's ruling initially applies only to public corporations that have inventories and gross property, plant, and equipment that aggregate more than $100 million and that comprise more than 10% of assets.

Such companies are required to disclose the estimated current replacement cost of inventories and productive capacity at the end of each fiscal year for which a balance sheet is required and the approximate amount of cost of sales and depreciation based on replacement cost for the two most recent full fiscal years.

The SEC's initial efforts, though appropriately flexible—and allowing for imprecision, are an attempt to assure that financial reports reflect current business economics. More important, the SEC's initiative sets a new precedent that, if extended, not only can radically change financial reporting and corporate management behavior—but also, if extended to the full health industry, can have profound implications on health planning and hospital payment.

estimated salvage value, and would be computed over the "lifetime" by an agreed upon method. The third method depreciates the *total* historical cost leaving a balance at the end of the period, which would be an amount similar to the salvage value allowed under the other methods.

The straight line method of calculating depreciation is to divide the cost of the item to be depreciated less the salvage value by the number of years of estimated life. For example, a $60,000 item with a salvage value of $5,000 would leave a balance of $55,000 for depreciation. If the estimated life is ten years, the depreciation allowed each year is one-tenth of the balance after subtracting the salvage value, or $5,500.

Under the sum-of-the-years digit method, the amount to be depreciated is multiplied by a fraction made up of a numerator to equal the number of years of estimated life remaining and a denominator equal to the sum of the total years of life. Using the same set of figures as in the first example, depreciation by the sum-of-years method is computed as follows: the first year,

$$\$55,000 \times \frac{10 \text{ (Years of estimated life remaining)}}{55 \text{ (Sum of total years } 10 + 9 + 8 + 7 + 6 + 5 + 4 + 3 + 2 + 1 = 55)} = \$10,000;$$

the second year,

$$\$55,000 \times \frac{9}{55} = \$9,000;$$

the third year the fraction would be

$$\frac{8}{55}$$

and so on.

With the double declining method, depreciation is figured by dividing the total historical cost by half the number of estimated years of life the first year; thereafter, each year divide the remaining balance by half of the total years of life. In the example used before, figuring by the double declining balance method, the depreciation the first year is computed by dividing $60,000 by 5 (half the estimated life years), or $12,000, leaving a balance of $48,000. The second year the $48,000 is divided by 5 to give a depreciation of $9,600, leaving a balance of $38,400, and so on.

The method of depreciation that a hospital can use under the cost and cost-plus formulas of reimbursement must be negotiated in many cases because there are differences in the depreciation rates by the accelerated methods (the sum-of-the-years digit method and the declining balance method) from the straight line method, particularly in the first five years.

Table 4.1 illustrates the differences and the management implications of the accelerated methods.

During times of rising price levels, it is important to recover capital costs through depreciation as quickly as possible so that the hospital's capital funds can be reinvested to protect against the lower purchasing power caused by inflation and rising price levels. The usefulness of accelerated depreciation to gain this protection becomes apparent when one realizes that depreciation funds can be invested or used immediately for capital purposes in dollars that reflect current value. If it is necessary to wait a few years longer to receive depreciation funds, and prices rise, the funds obtained through depreciation will buy less. Therefore, during periods of rising prices it is important for the hospital to depreciate its buildings and equipment at accelerated rates in order to have depreciation funds with the greatest possible purchasing power for replacement purposes.

DEBT PRINCIPAL AS AN ALLOWABLE COST

Hospitals, as do individuals, often buy buildings, land, and major equipment on deferred payments. The purchase is usually financed under a plan providing for payments on the principal, plus an interest charge on the unpaid balance, much as an individual finances the purchase of a home. The individual certainly thinks of the monthly payment on his home as an expense for which he must budget and plan. The hospital must also make provisions to meet the principal and interest payments on its debt. However, considering the hospital's payment as an allowable expense in the cost reimbursement formulas raises an interesting question that reasonably can be asked: should payments on debt be an allowed cost under reimbursement formulas for hospital care?

In the previous section depreciation was shown as a method of recovering the historical cost, less salvage value, of buildings and equipment over the estimated lifetime of the items. Thus, depreciation compensates the hospital for the expense of purchasing buildings and equipment. If the payments on the principal of the debt were allowed as an expense, and if an expense item were also allowed for depreciation on buildings and equipment, then there would be two allowances (double allowance) for the cost of buildings and equipment. If depreciation is the route used to allow for the cost of buildings and equipment, as it should be, then there is an orderly method to recover the cost of buildings and equipment over the estimated lifetime of those items, no matter how they were acquired: by cash, by deferred payments, or by gifts. Thus, there is no need for additional funds to amortize debt because funds for this purpose are provided through depreciation expense payments.

Debt principal payments are not recognized as allowable cost by either Blue Cross or the federal government. Accelerated depreciation, with de-

TABLE 4.1 Depreciation by Three Methods

Historical Cost $60,000
Salvage Value $ 5,000
Net Cost to be Depreciated $55,000

Historical Cost to be Depreciated $60,000

| Straight Line | | | Sum-of-Years Digit | | | | Double Declining Balance | | |
Deprec. Year	Depreciation Amt. This Yr.	Deprec. to Date	Deprec. Year	Est. Life	Depreciation Amt. This Yr.	Deprec. to Date	Deprec. Year	Depreciation Amt. This Yr.	Deprec. to Date
1	$5,500	$ 5,500	1	10	$10,000	$10,000	1	$12,000	$12,000
2	$5,500	$11,000	2	9	$ 9,000	$19,000	2	$ 9,600	$21,600
3	$5,500	$16,500	3	8	$ 8,000	$27,000	3	$ 7,680	$29,280
4	$5,500	$22,000	4	7	$ 7,000	$34,000	4	$ 6,144	$35,424
5	$5,500	$27,500	5	6	$ 6,000	$40,000	5	$ 4,915	$40,339
6	$5,500	$33,000	6	5	$ 5,000	$45,000	6	$ 3,932	$44,271
7	$5,500	$38,500	7	4	$ 4,000	$49,000	7	$ 3,146	$47,417
8	$5,500	$44,000	8	3	$ 3,000	$52,000	8	$ 2,517	$49,934
9	$5,500	$49,500	9	2	$ 2,000	$54,000	9	$ 2,013	$51,947
10	$5,500	$55,000	10	1	$ 1,000	$55,000	10	$ 1,611	$53,558

preciation funded, should be the method of accounting for the cost of buildings and equipment. It would seem that anyone arguing for double allowance
is in an untenable position.

The special problem of how to cover the need for extra capital for
facilities, for added services, or for the acquisition of additional land is
discussed below in "Plus Factor as an Allowable Cost."

EDUCATION AS AN ALLOWABLE COST

Education is an expense item in hospitals that varies greatly with the
size of the hospital and the services it offers. Some small hospitals spend
little or nothing in this area. At the other extreme, the large university
teaching hospital has training expenses for medical students, residents, and
nurses in addition to medical faculty costs, paramedical training courses,
continuing education, and other hospital in-service activities. For purposes
of the reimbursement formulas, reasonable net costs are allowed for approved patient-related educational purposes. The net cost is the balance
after grants, scholarships, and other monies paid in support of the educational programs have been deducted from the total expense incurred. This
approach to paying educational costs is quite reasonable. The only debatable point here is the relation of the cost to the patient. The administrator
should consider educational programs necessary to the operation of his
hospital as patient-related, for the prime purpose of the institution is to give
the best possible care to the patient.

RESEARCH AS AN ALLOWABLE COST

Research has the same criteria for acceptance as an allowable cost
under reimbursement formulas as education: the research expense should
be net expense after deduction of grants, gifts for research, and other monies
designated for research; and the research must be patient-related. Patient
relationship is sometimes more difficult to interpret with research than with
education because research, by nature, might seem to be more "pure" than
"applied." If the hospital determines that the research it approves is pragmatic, the administrator should insist that it is patient-related and that the
net expense be allowed as a reimbursable cost. Research is a necessary
ingredient of a dynamic process such as the provision of health care and
should be allowed in total as a reimbursable expense.

BAD DEBTS AS ALLOWABLE COST

Blue Cross and Medicare (as well as other government programs) buy
and pay for hospital service according to an arrangement agreed upon by
the buyer and provider of the services. The agencies buying services pay
for all they buy at an agreed rate so, at least in theory, there are no bad

debts in this contractual relationship. Although bad debts may not arise directly from the hospital–third party relationship, there are at least two attitudes about the third party's responsibilities for bad debts. One attitude might be: if the hospital has bad debts resulting from services furnished to self-pay patients, it cannot expect Blue Cross or Medicare to consider the bad debts as an allowable cost in its reimbursement formula. However, there is a possible exception in which bad debts occur in third party relationships. If Blue Cross or Medicare deducts certain amounts from the benefits of patients (according to contract or agreement), the hospital must bill the patient directly for the deducted amounts. These deducted amounts are difficult and costly to collect and often become bad debts. There is some justification for the allowance of this kind of bad debt as an expense item under the payment formula.

A second attitude might be that a hospital must be financially viable in order to furnish Blue Cross subscribers and Medicare clients with services on a cost basis. Furthermore, the hospital cannot remain in a viable state if all its real costs are not met. Therefore, aside from overcharging the self-pay patient and/or depending on fund drives or benefactors to pay off bad debts and some of the other real costs that have been disallowed in reimbursement formulas, the hospitals are going to have to insist that the third party purchasers of care pay their fair shares of all the real operating costs.

INTEREST EXPENSE AS AN ALLOWABLE COST

Interest expense is generally recognized as a legitimate claim. However, the term "net interest" is used in reimbursement negotiations to mean the interest expense a hospital incurs less any interest the hospital receives on investments. For accounting purists, it is an abhorrent practice to combine the two in this manner. Nevertheless, there is no disagreement that interest paid is an expense, and that interest earned generally should be credited against operating expenses by proper accounting methods. However, the two are discrete and different items and deserve to be so treated.

Interest paid by the hospital for purposes agreed on as legitimate by the hospital and the third party should be allowed as an expense. Interest earned by the hospital should be considered separately from interest paid—not as a bookkeeping item only—but on the characteristics of each transaction of business producing interest or dividends. For example, under the present Medicare reimbursement formula, interest earned on investments of funds from the depreciation account can be added to that account without deducting any part of the earnings from the allowance (under the reimbursement formula) for the interest the hospital pays on its obligations. In the same manner, interest or dividends earned on investments from other special purpose funds should be credited to those funds.

Interest paid by the hospital is an expense. Interest earned by the hospital can be revenue or it can be money paid into an account for a special purpose. Special purpose funds, in the final analysis, are eventually used to support the hospital's health care delivery system and furnish needed dollars that will not be requested from Blue Cross, Medicare, or the public. There are several ways the interest-earned dollars flow through the system, but ultimately the patient benefits. Net interest is a fiction and as such should be dropped from discussions of the very real problems faced in providing quality hospital care.

FREE SERVICE, ALLOWANCES, OR DISCOUNTS AS ALLOWABLE COSTS

These items are considered under the heading of revenue rather than cost by Blue Cross and the government, even though the hospital would prefer to include them as expenses. A service being furnished at a discount (or free) is a service being furnished at a rate agreed upon by the hospital and the other party, whether the party be an employee, a staff physician, a student, or an indigent patient. The hospital would like to include all discounts and allowances as costs recoverable from Blue Cross and the government, as well as from the private patient.

It would seem fair to consider discounts and allowances as deductions from the prices charged patients or other purchasers. Therefore, the revenue is reduced, not an expense incurred, when services or goods are sold at reduced prices.

Free service, whether it be charity or an unpaid bill that must be charged off, represents a cost. Someone must pay for that cost which is inescapable in operating a general hospital. Since it is a kind of cost that is always present, it would seem fair to spread the payment of this cost to all who use the hospital. Presently, the self-pay patient pays the costs that no one else wants to assume or that cannot be met by contributions or other nonoperating sources of revenue.

PLUS FACTOR AS AN ALLOWABLE COST

A better term should be coined than plus factor for a necessary cost element now to be discussed so it will not be confused with the cost-plus allowed under certain Blue Cross contracts for certain unforeseen costs or contingencies. Besides cost-plus there is need for another plus factor, a certain small percentage of the capital invested in the hospital plant that would be allowed each year for growth, for increases in the cost of replacement of existing facilities and equipment, and for keeping abreast of the state of the art. This in no way implies that the plus factor should be sufficient for large building programs or for added services; it should be sufficient merely to ensure that the hospital does not fall behind with its present facilities. This plus factor is not acceptable to the third parties, but it is an economic cost and a reality of need that will not disappear and that should be viewed as a reasonable and necessary cost of operation.

THE POSITION OF THE
AMERICAN HOSPITAL ASSOCIATION

The AHA has issued four documents of historical importance in the past 23 years which have had a direct bearing on the question of hospital revenues. The first publication was "Principles of Payment for Hospital Care," revised in 1963; the second was *Statement on the Financial Requirements of Health Care Institutions and Services* in 1969; the third was the *Financial Requirements of Health Care Institutions and Services* in 1977; the fourth was a restatement of the 1969 and 1977 documents in 1979.

In "Principles," the Association addressed itself to several of the questionable items of expense for which hospitals request allowance as cost in the Blue Cross and government reimbursement formulas. By 1969, the evolution in the thinking of AHA was evident. Although the same questions of allowable costs were included, the descriptive words were different. In 1969, the AHA was now looking at the relationship of the health care institution and the wholesale purchaser of services from a wider perspective—even a more philosophic frame of reference. The 1977 policy document reaffirms and updates the 1969 *Statement on the Financial Requirements of Health Care Institutions and Services*, emphasizing that all purchasers of health care must recognize and share fully in the total financial requirements of institutions providing care. It also highlights the concept of the institution needing, as a capital requirement, adequate reserves. The 1979 statement contains a new definition of financial requirement.

The Association was talking about "the health care institution" instead of the "hospital," was recommending areawide planning, and was speaking of the purchaser meeting "the full financial requirements of the providers." Many of the words were changed in 1969 from those of the 1963 "Principles" which might have had bad connotations for the major purchasers. The new view was wider and more prospective; it was an attempt to consider the hospital financial system as an entity rather than the sum of several diverse pieces.

The four documents will be discussed in detail because they deal with problem areas that affect the solvency of almost all hospitals.

PRINCIPLES OF PAYMENT
FOR HOSPITAL CARE, 1963

The American Hospital Association, in this document, discussed the problems its member hospitals faced in being reimbursed for hospital care

given to Blue Cross subscribers or to patients whose care was paid for by
a government agency. The summary of the major recommendations given
below indicates a need for both a change in the hospital–third party contracts and a change in the attitudes on several of the debatable issues already discussed in this chapter.

The recommendations included

1. The amount and method of payment to hospitals should ensure
   fair and adequate payment for the provider of service; that essential
   services be maintained; and that encouragement be given to develop higher standards of service. (This was a good general statement to serve as a preamble.)

2. Agencies purchasing hospital services should pay the costs incurred in providing the services, and total payments should not
   exceed total hospital charges for those services during the accounting period. (Again, a generalization that costs incurred in providing
   services should be paid, but that payments should not exceed regular hospital charges.)

3. There should be a uniform reimbursement rate for similar services
   for all third party agencies.

4. Third parties should not be expected to pay for a portion of the
   cost of a specific case that has been or will be paid from other
   revenues. (As an example, the care of a traffic accident victim might
   be totally or partially paid for as an automobile insurance benefit.
   This is accepted practice.)

5. Charges to self-pay patients should be based upon and reasonably
   related to costs. (Strangely enough, in a commentary on this point,
   it was stated that charges to self-pay patients should not be less
   than composite cost. In practice, the self-pay patient usually pays
   more than the cost allowed under the reimbursement formulas.)

6. Hospitals furnishing services to beneficiaries of third party purchasers should make essential facilities and high quality service
   available with "due regard to economy and efficiency." (This is a
   necessary point for a document of this kind, even if it is self-evident.)

7. "Rates of payment should reflect current hospital costs," thus making it necessary that providers and buyers of hospital service have
   a workable method of compensating for changing costs. (A formula
   is necessary to compensate for changing costs because in some
   instances the periods for reconciling accounts under the reimbursement formulas can be several months or a year apart. If costs
   should change rapidly, as they often do, a hospital could be caught
   with a rate of payment well below actual cost.)

8. Payments to different hospitals for the same service may differ because of variation of costs reflecting occupancy rate, hospital design and equipment, medical staff, employees' salaries, services offered, location of hospital (urban, rural, suburban), and other details. (This difference of conditions in hospitals, which may vary the cost of providing the same service, is understood and accepted.)

9. "The determination of reimbursable cost requires acceptance and use of uniform definitions, accounting, statistics and reporting"— preferably using AHA financial publications as guides. (If there is to be a uniform method of computing reimbursable cost, there certainly should be uniformity in accounting and record keeping.)

10. The principle of average cost per inpatient day should be applied in reimbursement cost formulas when the patients for whom a third party contracting agency is responsible are average for the hospital. This makes it necessary to take into consideration accommodations (private, semiprivate, ward), type of unit or service (obstetrics, medical, surgical, chronic care), and other special conditions. (This is another reasonable recommendation pointed toward all parties being treated alike in charges for service whether the patient's care is being paid under Blue Cross, Medicare, or self-pay plans.)

11. Expenditures for medical research, "over and beyond the usual care of patients," should not be included in reimbursable cost. (This would seem to necessitate definition of allowable net expense for medical research, including what medical research is related to patient care and what is not. This might be a problem difficult to negotiate in some instances.)

12. The net cost of medical, nursing, and other related education should be an allowable cost. (This was discussed earlier in the chapter where net cost was determined by subtracting grants, tuition allowances, and other monies designated for education from the total cost of education.)

13. Bad debts, unpaid costs of the indigent and medically indigent, and courtesy allowances should not be included in reimbursable cost but should be considered as deductions from earned income. (The authors have taken a view different from AHA on this point. Earlier in the chapter bad debts and other unpaid costs were called costs that should be allowed in the reimbursement formulas; discounts were considered reductions in revenue, but not an allowable cost.)

14. Ordinary remodeling should be charged against maintenance repairs as an expense item; remodeling that enhances capital value

should be capitalized and, therefore, not included in reimbursable costs. (This should not be controversial.)

15. Net interest (as explained earlier in the chapter) at a reasonable rate incurred on capital or other indebtedness should be allowed in determining reimbursable costs. (This, too, is generally acceptable.)

16. Expenses incurred by hospitals providing services of sisters or other members of religious orders should be allowed as operating expenses at rates no greater than those paid employees for similar work. (This is common practice.)

17. Income received from government agencies, foundations, and others to support projects or pay salaries of special employees who ordinarily would not be employed by the hospital should be deducted from expenses in determining reimbursable cost. (Hospitals should not oppose this reasonable recommendation.)

18. A separate cost for the nursery care of newborns should be allowed. (This recommendation of a separate cost center for nursery care of newborns was prompted by instances in which nursery care is a substantial unit of care and the special costs involved might influence the average cost of care of the whole hospital. By separating costs of the nursery, other patient costs could be figured more fairly.)

19. Depreciation of buildings and equipment should be allowed (and be used for capital purposes) in accordance with the recommendations of AHA's *Uniform Chart of Accounts and Definitions for Hospitals.* (The AHA believes its rates of depreciation have become standard, and this is probably true.)

20. Expenses for inpatient and outpatient services should be segregated. (This is necessary because of the difference in Blue Cross reimbursement rates for inpatients and outpatients, and because cost factors and conditions in the two sectors are different, thus affecting any cost analysis.)

21. Hospitals should not be required to use funds from endowment funds or restricted gifts to reduce third party payments. (This is a reiteration of the principle that third parties who purchase hospital service on a cost-based formula should pay the total costs of providing that service, thus obviating a need for the hospital to supplement the third party payment from any source.)

22. Income from endowment funds or gifts designated for the care of specific groups of third party beneficiaries should be used to reduce third party payments for persons in such groups. (This is a fair proposal.)

23. "Hospitals should not be required to use net income from non-patient service to reduce third party payments." (Net income from rental of office space or from sharing of facilities with other organizations might be considered a revenue different from interest received on investments. However, a question might arise as to whether net income from nonpatient services should not indirectly reduce the charges to all classes of purchasers, although certainly not to third party payers alone.)

24. The AHA "Principles" also include the obligations of the parties, as applicable: to keep and make available adequate records; to furnish satisfactory service and payment; to make reports in the form and at the time agreed upon; to make studies of factors of the services provided in order to promote quality of care and economy of cost; and for the hospitals to act in association to develop more uniform standards and practices.

All the points noted in the AHA "Principles" are pertinent and deserve consideration and study by all parties concerned on a continuing basis, for the administration of a hospital and the care of its patients are fluid, ever-changing processes.

STATEMENT ON THE FINANCIAL REQUIREMENTS OF HEALTH CARE INSTITUTIONS AND SERVICES, 1969

The *Statement* proposes a program that would provide proper financing of the health care system and calls for the system to accept "the community's right to insist on proper planning within that system." The *Statement* is labeled as a set of general guidelines and is couched in rather euphemistic terms to sweeten the words previously used to describe some of the debated elements of reimbursement formulas.

It is important for the reader to note how the AHA stresses the responsibility of all purchasers of care to bear their proportionate shares of the operating and capital costs of the health care institutions, and how the community and the area planning agencies are considered participating partners along with the providers and purchasers of health care.

Briefly summarized, the *Statement* made the following points:

1. *The purchasers of care collectively should pay the total financial requirements of the health care institutions* (both current operating requirements and capital needs), which are listed below.

   a. Salaries, wages, employees' fringe benefits, services, supplies, normal maintenance, minor building modifications, and applicable taxes. (These expenses are normal, regular, and noncontroversial, with the possible exception of the interpretation of "minor building modifications.")

b. Interest on funds borrowed for capital needs and operating cash purposes. Interest on external loans for plant capital purposes would be reduced by income earned on investments of operating funds, endowments, gifts, and grants when such income was not assigned for specific purposes. The above offset would not apply to income on funds borrowed for current operating cash needs if the amount and application of the funds were "consistent with prudent fiscal management." (This is the net interest concept again, but with the added consideration of the interest earned on investment of borrowed current operating funds not being used to offset interest paid on borrowed funds. The AHA found difficulty in obtaining agreement on this exemption from the offset. This was a bargaining point which could be disallowed in exchange for some other advantage.)

c. Financial needs for approved educational programs above the amounts covered by tuition, grants, scholarships, and other sources. (This is the net educational cost discussed earlier.)

d. Financial needs for approved research projects related to patient care above the amounts covered by grants and other contributions. (This is the net research cost discussed earlier.)

e. All purchasers of care should be responsible for their appropriate share of the bad debts. (This is a little ambiguous in terms of what the appropriate share is, yet the point is important: that *all* purchasers should be responsible for a share of the bad debt. In the past, bad debts have not usually been considered an allowable cost.)

f. The cost of care of patients unable to pay—the medically indigent—should be appropriately shared by all purchasers of care. (The situation is directly parallel to the bad debts provision in the paragraph above—and is as important as that point.)

g. Capital needs are discussed generally under the headings:

   (1) Plant capital needs for preservation and replacement of plant and equipment; improvement of plant; expansion of plant; and amortization of plant capital indebtedness.

   (2) Operating cash needs to meet the fluctuating day-to-day obligations.

   (3) Return on investment for proprietary (for-profit) health care institutions. (The AHA *Statement* avoids the use of the words depreciation and plus factor and seems to be suggesting that a capital fund be established into which would be paid depreciation of buildings and equipment, gifts, grants and ap-

propriations, and some payment from patient services. From this seemingly suggested fund could be paid sums for: acquisition of land; replacement and major modernization of buildings; expansion of plant, equipment, and services; and amortization of capital indebtedness. Also, the need for operating funds demands a method for raising such monies. The purpose of AHA seemed to be to establish this need for capital funds and operating funds and the advisability of all purchasers of care paying their proportionate shares of these needs. Apparently it is assumed that these financial requirements could be negotiated by the large purchasers and the health care institution under suggested formulas. One point lightly touched upon was a recommendation that health care institutions being run for profit be allowed a fair return on their investment. If this is allowed, then it would seem that not-for-profit hospitals could rightfully ask for a plus factor for growth and to hedge against inflation in lieu of the return on investment.)

2. *The role and responsibilities of the health care institution*

   a. According to the *Statement,* the health care institution should maintain high quality of care, promote effective utilization of its patient care services, and inform and educate the community to the proper use of health care facilities. The institution should investigate the opportunities of sharing services, such as purchasing, laundry, and computers, with other facilities. Ongoing planning, both short- and long-term, should be the rule. Financial data should be available to the contracting parties and, when indicated, to the public.

   b. The contracting parties should strive to offer benefits as liberal as possible and should advise the public members covered by prepayment plans to contract for as wide a coverage as possible. The contracting parties should strive to improve the efficiency of their administration of the health care dollar while making retroactive appeal methods available for adjustment of charges. The parties should disclose information to the public on the utilization and financing of services.

   c. Areawide planning councils for health care should cooperate and assist both health care institutions and contracting parties and act as liaison with general community planning agencies. The councils should aid the community with respect to the "appropriateness, adequacy, priority, and location of health care services and facilities." The AHA would have the areawide planning council be an approving agency for new buildings and expansion plans as well as for purchase of major equipment. The capital spending fund the AHA would establish would be operative for new major spending under the advice of the areawide planning council.

d. The community is expected to support its health care institution with cash contributions and moral reinforcement.

FINANCIAL REQUIREMENTS OF HEALTH CARE INSTITUTIONS AND SERVICES, 1977 POLICY

The 1977 American Hospital Association policy is fundamentally a reaffirmation of the 1969 *Statement*. It does, however, differ from its predecessor in that it more firmly addresses the concept of operating margin, emphasizing that institutions must include in their financial requirements a factor that will enable them to assure that adequate resources will be available to finance necessary changes, that is, new technology, expansion, working capital requirements, and so forth. The 1977 policy also emphasizes that all purchasers must recognize and share fully in the institution's total financial requirements. In this regard, the point is made that "Any apportionment that permits a purchaser to assume a lesser responsibility is not appropriate and does not alter the total financial requirements of the health care institution. Rather, it requires other purchasers to make up the deficiency."

The 1977 policy statement is presented below.

INTRODUCTION

The delivery of health services requires a vast array of professional services, institutions, allied health organizations and educational programs, research activities, and community health projects. A high-quality health care delivery system is dependent upon the commitment of sufficient resources and their effective management. The system must ensure that necessary services are provided to the public in an effective, efficient, and economic manner. Coordination of the components of the health care delivery system and self-discipline of all participants within the system are necessary to meet this end. Three interrelated functions whereby such coordination and self-discipline can be achieved are effective planning, effective utilization, and effective management. These functions share the ultimate purpose of maintaining the highest standards of quality in the delivery of health care.

The health care delivery system has and should continue to have multiple sources of financing that must meet total financial requirements. These sources of financing should recognize that health care institutions must be financed at a level that supports the health objectives of the community, including uncompensated care costs as defined herein. The health care delivery system and its financing should be sufficiently flexible to change as needs of the community change and as new and effective technologies are developed so that the total financial requirements can continue to be met.

ELEMENTS OF FINANCIAL REQUIREMENTS

Institutional financial stability requires that there be a realistic appraisal of the two major financial components: (1) current operating requirements and (2) operating margin.

Meeting these financial requirements will enable the institutions to maintain and improve current programs and facilities and to initiate new programs and facilities consistent with community needs and advances in medical science.

Health care institutions differ in size, scope, and types of ownership and services, and therefore their operating and capital requirements differ. However, all elements of financial requirements must be reflected in the payments to health care institutions to provide adequately for demonstrated financial needs. The elements of financial requirements are described below.

CURRENT OPERATING REQUIREMENTS

Current operating requirements include the following costs:

1. *Patient care*
   These costs include, but are not limited to, salaries and wages, employee benefits, purchased services, interest expense, supplies, insurance, maintenance, minor building modification, leases, applicable taxes, depreciation, and the monetary value assigned to services provided by members of religious orders and other organized religious groups.

2. *Patients who do not pay*
   It must be recognized that a portion of the total financial requirements will not be met by certain patients who:

   a. Fail fully to meet their incurred obligation for services rendered;

   b. Are relieved wholly or in part of their responsibilities because of their inability to pay for services rendered. Therefore, these unrecovered financial requirements must be included as a current operating requirement for those who pay.

3. *Education*
   Where financial needs for educational programs having appropriate approval have not been met through tuition, scholarships, grants, or

other sources, all purchasers of care must assume their appropriate share of the financial requirements to meet these needs.

4. *Research*
   Appropriate health care services and patient-related clinical research programs are an element of the total financial requirements of an institution. The cost of these programs should be met primarily from endowment income, gifts, grants, or other sources.

OPERATING MARGIN

In order to meet the total financial requirements of an institution, a margin of net patient care revenues in excess of current operating requirements must be maintained. This difference will provide necessary funds for working capital requirements, capital requirements, and return on equity.

1. *Working capital requirements*
   Financial stability is dependent on having sufficient cash to meet current fiscal obligations as they come due.

2. *Capital requirements*
   Health care institutions are expected to meet demands resulting from such factors as population shifts, discontinuance of other existing services, and changes in the public's demand for types of services delivered. In order to be in a position to respond to such changing community needs, health care institutions must anticipate and include such capital needs in their financial requirements. There must be assurances that adequate resources will be available to finance recognized necessary changes.

   The capital requirements of a health care institution must be evaluated and approved by its governing authority in the context of the institution's role and mission in the community's health care delivery system. Coordination among the health care institution's governing authority, administration, and medical staff and the cooperation among health organizations and the appropriate areawide health planning agency are essential to this evaluation.

   a. *Major renovations and repairs*
      Funds must be provided for necessary major repairs of plant and equipment to ensure compliance with changing regulatory standards and codes and to finance planned and approved renovation projects.

   b. *Replacement of plant and equipment*
      Because of deterioration and obsolescence, assets must be replaced and modernized based on community needs for health care services. Funds that reflect the changes in general price

levels must be available for the replacement and modernization of plant and equipment.

c. *Expansion*
Sufficient funds must be available for the acquisition of additional property, plant, and equipment when consonant with community needs.

d. *New technology*
Advances in medical science and advances in the technology of delivering health services often require additional expenditures. Sufficient financial resources must be available for continued additional investment in the improvement of plant and equipment, consonant with community needs, so that health care institutions can keep pace with changes in the health care delivery system.

3. *Return on equity*
Investor-owned institutions should receive a reasonable return on their owners' equity.

RESPONSIBILITIES OF PURCHASERS FOR MEETING FINANCIAL REQUIREMENTS

Each institution's total financial requirements should be apportioned among all purchasers of care in accordance with each purchaser's use of the institution and measurable impact on the operations of the institution. Any apportionment that permits a purchaser to assume a lesser responsibility is not appropriate and does not alter the total financial requirements of the health care institution. Rather, it requires other purchasers to make up the deficiency.

RESPONSIBLITIES OF PROVIDERS

Health care institutions have an obligation to disclose to the public evidence that their funds are being effectively utilized in accordance with their stated purpose of operation. Institutions also have a responsibility not only to the purchasers of care but also to their community to provide effective management. An institution's goals and the methods that it uses to achieve those goals should be consonant with community planning and the resources in that community.

FINANCIAL REQUIREMENTS OF HEALTH CARE INSTITUTIONS AND SERVICES, 1979 POLICY

In 1979 the AHA House of Delegates approved a new definition of financial requirement and rephrased and reworked some of the 1977 policy statement.

The definition statement was:

> Financial requirements, as differentiated from accounting costs, are defined as those resources that are not only necessary to meet current operating needs, but also sufficient to permit replacement of the physical plant when appropriate and to allow for changing community health and patient needs, education and research needs, and all other needs necessary to the institutional provision of health care services that must be recognized and supported by all purchasers of care.

The 1979 statement stressed the community–health institution relationship, saying that if the health institution makes its role and mission consonant with community needs that as a corollary the institution should be assured that its financial requirements will be met. It seems the community is being reminded that it, through philanthropy or otherwise, must bear responsibility for the proper financing of its health care system.

Another suggestion in the 1979 statement seems to say that if investor-owned institutions receive a reasonable after-tax return on their owners' equity that the not-for-profit hospitals should also receive a reasonable return above cost. This would allow the not-for-profit institution to adjust to the community's changing needs for health services and to keep up with advancing technology.

AUTHORS' PLAN OF STUDY OF PROBLEMS IN PART II

The authors have taken what may appear to be an unusual approach to discussing hospital financial management by electing to discuss the subject of hospital revenues. In the preceding pages, it has been implied that the problems related to the sources of revenue are vital to the operation of a solvent hospital. It has been shown that third parties, or contracting parties as AHA states it, buy at wholesale rates on a cost or cost-plus basis where cost is not uniform due to the differing interpretations of cost. Furthermore, the self-pay patient has been pictured as one who pays a higher rate than Blue Cross or the government because his bill must absorb costs disallowed by the big purchasers.

New elements have been added to the reimbursement patterns in that health maintenance organizations (HMOs), preferred provider organizations (PPOs), and independent practice associations (IPAs), as well as diagnosis-related groups (DRGs), have altered approaches to reimbursement in many ways: from costs per day to costs per stay, to capitation rates, to contract rates, and actually to a modified all-inclusive rate. (See Chapters 6 and 7.)

Nevertheless, change is not as great as might be expected on the provider's side, for basically cost is the bottom line. The provider must at least recover costs for the services provided. So, if the provider operates under contract with third parties, costs cannot be denied in maintaining viability.

The purchaser of the provider's services is trying to widen his options to obtain the broadest and least expensive coverage for his subscribers, while the provider, as mentioned, is trying to recover costs or more.

Cost analysis will be described in the next chapter. Methods of allotting costs to centers of the hospital that produce revenue will be outlined. The methods will entail apportioning the salaries, supplies, and overhead expenses of the service departments that do not produce revenue to the departments that do. The total expense of the revenue departments (determined by adding the costs apportioned from the nonrevenue departments) then can be used as a basis for determining reimbursable costs and for setting rates and charges.

The chapter on cost analysis will be followed by one on Blue Cross and one on Medicare. In both of these chapters the philosophies of providing care of these two large purchasers will be examined, along with their methods of payment.

A later chapter will examine the relation of costs to charges and some methods of setting rates based upon that relationship.

SUGGESTED READINGS

American Hospital Association. "Equity in Financing" from *Report of the Task Force on Principles of Payment for Hospital Care,* pp. 27–44.

American Hospital Association. "Principles of Payment for Hospital Care."

American Hospital Association. *Statement on the Financial Requirements of Health Care Institutions and Services.*

Bower, James B.; Connors, Edward J.; Mosher, John E.; and Rowley, Clyde S. *Hospital Income Flow: A Study of the Effects of Source of Pay on Hospital Income.*

Fox, Peter D.; Goldbeck, Willis B.; and Spies, Jacob J. *Health Care Cost Management: Private Sector Initiatives.*

Foyle, William R. "Debatable Elements of Hospital Cost" in McNerney, Walter et al. *Hospital and Medical Economics,* pp. 935–56.

Mannix, John R. "Blue Cross Reimbursement of Hospitals."

Topics in Health Care Financing. "Financial Management Under Third Party Reimbursement," Fall 1976.

5

Cost Analysis

In Chapter 4 the importance of the sources of revenue to the financial status and position of hospitals was emphasized. It was pointed out that the great majority of the hospital's revenue comes from Blue Cross and Medicare, which base their reimbursements on costs. Certain costs are considered debatable; in fact, some seemingly legitimate costs are not even allowed in the reimbursement formulas. Hence, management necessarily must put great stress on cost finding or analysis, must formulate reasonable guidelines for the definition of cost, and must establish a firm base for all cost claims through cost analysis.

Thus, cost finding has become a resource tool for financial management in hospitals, particularly in recent years. On the one hand, cost finding has become a necessary procedure in apportioning costs to the patient care areas in order to comply with the reimbursement formulas of Medicare, Medicaid, and some Blue Cross plans.

On the other hand, any successful business, hospital or other, has to have a management team that is cost-informed, that plans with cost information at hand, that invests the business's capital with solid knowledge of the company's cost situation, and that sets prices and wages on the basis of real costs. That cost information comes from accurate cost finding.

The hospital's administrator, controller, and finance committee need accurate cost finding more than the executives of many other businesses because they operate on as little or less net profit than a giant supermarket or a chain of discount department stores. Also, they have less flexibility and less control of their financial environment.

A hospital cannot set rates and charges that are realistically related to costs unless the cost finding system accurately allocates both direct and indirect costs to the patient unit or patient service. Staffing of the nursing units, maintenance department, or an ancillary service should be done only with knowledge of the real costs as well as the real needs. Routine personnel problems involving financial questions (let alone union negotiations) should be approached only with sound cost information. Certainly, budgeting or any other projections of the financial future need solid grounding in the cost analysis of past performance.[1]

The hospital's purchasing department has worries of cost and inventory control, the dietary department has needs for cost controls down to the pennies per meal, laundry and housekeeping must consider their costs compared to contracted services—all these needs demand good cost information which comes with accurate cost finding methods.

Hospital administration handles millions of dollars of the community's money each year while walking a precarious path between rising costs and inadequate revenue. Hospitals cannot survive without the best possible cost information—the best possible cost finding or analysis.

It has been said, with some truth, that the need to develop cost figures for government and insurance claims has made for better financial management and administration in hospitals.

Cost finding, as it will be discussed in the following pages, will be considered the process of allocating all costs of operating the hospital to cost centers or departments that produce revenue.[2] Cost finding or cost analysis has also been defined as "the process of manipulating or rearranging the data or information in the existing accounts to obtain the costs of the services rendered by the hospital."[3] In other words, cost finding is a means of spreading the costs of plant maintenance, plant operations, and other general service departments or cost centers in a reasonable way to nursing care, operating room, emergency room, pharmacy, and other departments or revenue centers that enter charges for services provided for patients. An equitable cost determination for filing claims with the government or Blue Cross is a necessity; likewise, rates and charges for services

---

[1]The value of cost finding in budgeting and internal control of operations in the hospital is great. The budgeting process is discussed in Part IV.

[2]"All costs" include salaries, supplies, and other expenses of doing business, including depreciation.

[3]Three terms (cost finding, cost analysis, and cost accounting) will be used frequently in this text, which may cause some confusion because they have a common end product arrived at by two different techniques. *Cost finding* and *cost analysis* are used synonymously to refer to the technique of allocating direct and indirect hospital costs as explained in this chapter. They refer to an after-the-fact procedure in which data are taken from completed general accounting forms and then distributed to cost centers. *Cost accounting* is a procedure that is a part of the ongoing general accounting system and in which the cost allocations are done as the accounting forms are being prepared.

billed to other payers should be related to costs determined by some equitable method.

There seems to be a reasonable basis for relating charges patients are asked to pay to the costs of the hospital services they receive. The costs of the services are not only those expenses (salaries, supplies, food, medication) directly connected with the department providing the service, but also include such overhead items as maintenance, administration, depreciation, housekeeping, laundry, plant operation, and medical records. If the total costs of operating the hospital are to be recovered from the patients who receive service, an accurate assignment of all costs must be made to the departments providing services for which patients pay.

Some rational process of analyzing costs and assigning them appropriately to the proper patient service departments is patently necessary.

PREREQUISITES

There are five prerequisites a cost analysis system should meet if its function is to be fulfilled and if it is to operate efficiently.

1. There should be an organization chart and a chart of accounts relating to it.
2. There should be an identification of all cost centers as either general service cost centers or as final cost centers to which all costs are ultimately assigned.
3. There should be an accurate accounting system capable of accumulating financial data by cost center.
4. There should be a comprehensive information system capable of collecting nonfinancial data by cost center and by the total hospital providing: (a) the basis for distribution of costs from general service centers to final cost centers; and (b) the basis for calculating unit cost by final cost center.
5. A methodology for cost analysis should be chosen that is most practicable for the hospital situation.

THE ORGANIZATION CHART AND THE RELATED CHART OF ACCOUNTS

These have been discussed in Part I. These two items provide the road map by which costs can be routed through cost finding to the final cost center and a framework for the distinct functions of each center.

IDENTIFICATION OF ALL COST CENTERS

In the chart of accounts, cost centers should be established for all centers of activity and responsibility in the hospital. Some of the cost centers represent patient-centered activities, while others are primarily for general services such as: providing heat, light, and food; keeping the floors and walls clean; washing the linen; shoveling the snow; and doing the many other tasks necessary to the satisfactory operation of a complex organization such as a hospital. The hospital charges the patient directly for services such as: room, board, and nursing (under a daily rate); drugs and dressings; X ray; laboratory; physical therapy; and other therapeutic treatments and diagnostic procedures. These charges are usually itemized on his bill. However, the costs of many services (such as maintenance, housekeeping, and laundry) are not entered on the bill as direct charges. Thus, the second prerequisite in a cost analysis system is to identify (a) cost centers that produce revenue (for example, room charge) and (b) the general service cost centers that do not produce revenue (for example, maintenance, housekeeping, laundry). This identification is necessary because all the expenses, direct or indirect, incurred by the general service centers (nonrevenue-producing centers) must be allocated to the revenue-producing centers which are the final cost centers in the cost analysis process.

ACCURATE ACCOUNTING SYSTEM

After cost centers have been designated either as general service centers or as final cost centers, the accounting system must be accurate enough to accumulate and assign appropriately all financial data to the various cost centers. This is a necessary prerequisite not only if the direct costs of each cost center are to be accurately determined, but also if accurate total cost data are to be obtained.

COMPREHENSIVE INFORMATION SYSTEM
ON NONFINANCIAL DATA

As suggested in the paragraph above, much of the expense is not incurred by the cost centers independently, but is expense shared by many cost centers. It, therefore, must be prorated among the cost centers if accurate total cost data are to be obtained. To prorate equitably, it is necessary to have several kinds of nonfinancial data which can be used in dividing the cost among all centers. This nonfinancial information may include such statistics as square footage of each center, gross payrolls per center, number of employees per center, number of meals served, pounds of laundry washed, number of records processed, or number of patients cared for.

METHODS OF COST ANALYSIS

Several methods are commonly used in cost analysis, including

1. Direct apportionment
2. The step-down method
3. Double apportionment
4. Algebraic or multiple apportionment

DIRECT APPORTIONMENT

Allotting the cost incurred by nonrevenue-producing departments to revenue departments by direct apportionment can be done by any one of several methods. The simplest and least logical way is for administration to determine arbitrarily the percentage of the nonrevenue-connected expense each revenue center is to bear. Other yardsticks can be based on the percentage each revenue department represents of the total square footage of the hospital's buildings, or of the number of employees, payroll, pounds of laundry, patient days, or number of purchase requisitions. The reader can probably expand the list of possibilities even further. For instance, a person trained in the retail business might suggest: "Why not allot costs of the nonrevenue cost centers or departments to revenue departments in ratio to the revenue generated by each of those departments?"

Direct allocation, though administratively and clerically simple, is an inappropriate cost finding methodology, for it: (1) ignores the exchanges of services between nonrevenue-producing departments; and (2) does not compensate for the different demands for services by revenue departments on nonrevenue departments. For an example of the first point, the maintenance department might be called upon to do a large amount of work for the laundry. Since both departments are nonrevenue departments, there would be no means under direct allocation of charging any of the cost of the maintenance department to the laundry. To illustrate the second point: the intensive care unit may need more housekeeping service proportionately than any other nursing unit. For exchange of services between nonrevenue and revenue departments, the allocation of costs may not be in relation to the service provided. Consequently, direct allocation is neither a method of cost analysis recommended by the authors nor one accepted by most third parties.

THE STEP-DOWN METHOD

The step-down method is a more advanced cost finding technique than direct allocation, for it involves the distribution of the costs of nonrevenue-producing departments to other nonrevenue departments and, in turn, finally to revenue departments. The term "step-down" is used because of the format in which distributions of nonrevenue department costs are made. The costs of the nonrevenue department serving the most departments (both revenue and nonrevenue) are distributed first; the nonrevenue department serving the second largest number of departments is distributed next; the one serving the third largest number next, and so on. This technique results in a work paper that resembles a staircase or steps. Hence, the name of the method is obtained.

To explain the step-down distribution graphically, a ten-month cost apportionment of Community Hospital (Table 5.1) is used. The order of departments for apportionment was determined as first plant operations, then maintenance and repairs, and so on horizontally to the last department, superintendence and house orderlies.

Column 1 lists all the departments; Column 2 gives the square footage of each department; Column 3, the total operating and professional services expenses to be distributed. For example, the expense to be distributed for plant operations is $64,115.90.

Look across horizontal Row A to the third heading, plant operations, and note beneath the heading that the basis of allocation of this expense is square footage.

Column 4 shows how the total expenses of plant operations ($64,115.90) are distributed among the other departments, both nonrevenue and revenue, on the basis of the percentage of the total square footage of the hospital excluding that allotted for plant operations.

In Column 5 the $23,047.55 expense total of maintenance and repairs ($21,176.88 from Column 3 and $1,870.67 from Column 4, which was charged by plant operations to maintenance and repairs) is distributed to all remaining departments in ratio to the square footage of those departments.

The laundry department total of $22,311.74 shown in Column 7 was derived from the original department total of $18,287.18 in Column 3 plus $2,937.06 from plant operations in Column 4 and $1,087.50 from maintenance and repairs in Column 5. The laundry expense is prorated according to the total pounds of laundry issued as expressed in percentages in Column 6.[4]

The step-down process is continued through Column 18 until the six nursing care units have absorbed their proportionate share of costs of the nonrevenue service departments plus their own operating costs which are

---

[4]Besides square footage and pounds of laundry, it should be noted that other yardsticks are listed in horizontal Row B for use in cost allotment: patient days (Col. 10, 11); percentage of record keeping (Col. 11); departmental payroll (Col. 13, 16, 17); and priced requisitions (Col. 14, 15).

TABLE 5.1 Step-Down Method, Community Hospital

A. Department			Plant Operations	Maintenance and Repairs
	Departmental Square Footage	Total Operating and Professional Services Expenses		
B. Basis of Allocation			Sq. Footage	Sq. Footage
(1)	(2)	(3)	(4)	(5)
Plant operations	3,564	$ 64,115.90	$64,115.90	
Maintenance	1,349	21,176.88	1,870.67	$23,047.55
Laundry	2,118	18,287.18	2,937.06	1,087.50
Housekeeping	1,245	49,409.75	1,726.46	639.26
Purchasing and stores	1,228	6,144.34	1,702.88	630.53
Dietary—less revenue	3,592	62,173.72	4,981.06	1,844.34
Medical records	1,225	19,831.70	1,698.72	628.99
Administrative	1,703	100,216.17	2,361.56	874.42
Central supply	1,007	8,684.57	1,396.42	517.05
Medical and surgical	118	2,846.33	163.63	60.59
Nursing service		232,808.70		
Superintendence and house orderlies	209		289.82	107.31
Nursing centers				
Intensive care	1,380		$ 1,913.67	$ 708.57
Intermediate care	3,744		5,191.84	1,922.38
Continuing care	4,148		5,752.07	2,129.82
Self care	4,919		6,821.24	2,525.69
Pediatrics	2,445		3,390.50	1,255.40
Obstetrical	3,117		4,322.37	1,600.44
Subtotals	19,753		$27,391.69	$10,142.30
Emergency room	712	5,504.79	$ 987.33	$ 365.58
Operating room	3,903	30,213.87	5,412.33	2,004.02
Delivery room	3,313	21,475.76	4,594.17	1,701.08
Nursery	1,325	14,008.18	1,837.39	680.33
Pharmacy	343	39,225.89	475.64	176.11
Radiology	1,384	53,093.20	1,919.20	710.63
Laboratory	603	29,417.44	836.18	309.62
Anesthesia		2,897.98		
Oxygen		4,314.22		
Physical therapy	886	9,555.02	1,228.62	454.93
Occupational therapy	220	4,832.93	305.07	112.96
Total	49,800	$800,234.52	$64,115.90	$23,047.55

Laundry		Housekeeping	Purchasing and Stores	Dietary—less Revenue	Medical Records
	Amount				
Percentage of Total Pounds Issued		Sq. Footage	Sq. Footage	Patient Days	Estm'd Percentage of Record Keeping and Patient Days
(6)	(7)	(8)	(9)	(10)	(11)
	$22,311.74				
		$51,775.47			
		1,531.17	$10,008.92		
2.8%	624.73	4,478.79	892.18	$74,994.82	
		1,527.43	304.28		
		2,123.44	423.00		
10.5%	2,342.73	1,255.61	250.13		
		147.13	29.31		
		260.60	51.91		
5.3%	$ 1,182.52	$ 1,720.69	$ 342.76	$ 4,207.21	4.10%
14.0	3,123.65	4,668.32	929.95	16,986.33	17.72
14.9	3,324.45	5,172.06	1,030.30	19,371.16	19.22
15.0	3,346.76	6,133.41	1,221.81	18,898.69	19.12
4.3	959.40	3,048.62	607.31	7,079.51	6.17
18.5	4,127.67	3,886.52	774.22	8,451.92	8.67
72.0%	$16,064.45	$24,629.62	$ 4,906.35	$74,994.82	75.00%
2.1%	$ 468.55	$ 887.78	$ 176.85		5.00%
3.9	870.16	4,866.57	969.46		
		4,130.92	822.90		
		1,652.12	329.11		
		427.68	85.19		
1.0	223.12	1,725.68	343.77		
0.3	66.93	751.87	149.77		15.00
					5.00
7.4	1,651.07	1,104.74	220.07		
		274.32	54.64		
100.0%	$22,311.74	$51,775.47	$10,008.92	$74,994.82	100.0%

Continued

TABLE 5.1   Continued

A. Department	Medical Records	Administrative— less Telephone	Central Supply	Medical and Surgical
B. Basis of Allocation	Amount	Departmental Payroll	Priced Requisitions	Priced Requisitions
(1)	(12)	(13)	(14)	(15)
Plant operations				
Maintenance				
Laundry				
Housekeeping				
Purchasing and stores				
Dietary—less revenue				
Medical records	$23,991.12			
Administrative		$105,998.59		
Central supply		2,840.76	$17,287.27	
Medical and surgical				$3,246.99
Nursing service				
Superintendence and house orderlies				
Nursing centers				
Intensive care	$ 1,009.43	$ 11,055.65	$ 1,822.08	$ 586.73
Intermediate care	4,075.49	16,005.79	2,160.91	695.18
Continuing care	4,647.68	19,291.75	1,777.13	571.79
Self care	4,534.32	12,825.83	2,207.59	710.44
Pediatrics	1,698.57	6,815.71	565.29	181.84
Obstetrical	2,027.85	3,953.75	1,557.59	501.01
Subtotals	$ 7,993.34	$ 69,948.48	$10,090.59	$3,246.99
Emergency room	$ 1,199.56	$ 1,187.18	$ 409.71	
Operating room		7,123.11		
Delivery room		4,568.54		
Nursery		4,685.14	4,254.39	
Pharmacy		2,437.97	2,359.71	
Radiology		3,285.96	172.87	
Laboratory	3,598.66	4,971.33		
Anesthesia	1,199.56			
Oxygen				
Physical therapy		3,370.75		
Occupational therapy		1,579.37		
Total	$23,991.12	$105,998.59	$17,287.27	$3,246.99

Nursing Service	Superintend. & House Orderlies				Total Expense of Revenue-Producing Departments
		Total Nursing Cost	Patient Days	Nursing Cost per Pat. Day	
Departmental Payroll	Departmental Payroll				
(16)	(17)	(18)	(19)	(20)	(21)
$232,808.70					
$ 44,279.43	$44,989.07				
$ 29,806.47	$ 7,112.77	$ 61,468.55	1,230	$49.97	
43,135.50	10,293.50	109,188.84	4,971	21.97	
51,996.38	12,407.99	127,472.58	5,670	22.48	
34,557.42	8,246.50	102,029.70	5,531	18.45	
18,381.60	4,386.43	48,370.18	2,072	23.34	
10,651.90	2,541.88	44,397.12	2,473	17.95	
$188,529.27	$44,989.07	$492,926.97	21,947	$22.46	
					$ 11,187.33
					51,459.52
					41,547.76
					25,551.98
					43,001.35
					61,301.56
					40,101.80
					4,097.54
					4,314.22
					17,585.20
					7,159.29
$232,808.70	$44,989.07				$307,307.55

totaled in Column 18. Finally, in Column 21, the revenue departments other than nursing are shown as having absorbed their allotted shares of the costs of nonrevenue departments of the hospital. The sum of nursing costs in Column 18 ($492,926.97) and the total expense of the other revenue-producing departments ($307,307.55 in Column 21) equal the total operating and professional service expenses of the hospital ($800,234.52 as shown in Column 3). This completes the distribution of all expenses to revenue-producing departments.

It should be noted that the step-down method has been criticized as not allowing fully for interdepartmental charges between the different non-revenue departments. As an example, the housekeeping department was the fourth nonrevenue department to have its cost distributed in Table 5.1 of the step-down method. None of the housekeeping costs could be distributed to plant operations, maintenance, or laundry because those departments had already been closed out. Likewise, laundry charges could not be charged to plant operations or maintenance because both of those departments were closed out before laundry. The step-down method does finally allot all charges to the cost centers represented by the various revenue-producing departments. At present, step-down is a method approved by AHA and by many of the third parties. However, some accountants, due to the inaccuracies inherent in the step-down process, advocate different methods. Among the other methods is the double apportionment method, which uses two rounds of distribution in charging the nonrevenue costs to the revenue departments. An explanation of this method follows.

DOUBLE APPORTIONMENT[5]

Double apportionment, or double distribution, was designed to correct one of the major weaknesses of the step-down method. This weakness was shown above to be the failure to allow fully for interdepartmental charges between nonrevenue-producing departments. In double apportionment, two separate cost distributions are used (see Figure 5.1). In the first distribution all direct and indirect costs of all departments are distributed to the various cost centers according to the agreed upon basis of allocation. For example, costs of plant operations, maintenance, housekeeping, and purchasing are allotted to all departments (revenue and nonrevenue) in ratio to the square footage of the departments. Laundry costs are allocated to the departments served according to pounds of laundry each used, inpatient dietary costs are distributed to units served according to the patient days

---

[5]One weakness of double distribution is that it does not charge a department for its own services. Note in Table 5.2, Column 4, that plant operations expense ($64,115.90) is distributed to every department but its own.

FIGURE 5.1   Cost Finding Double Distribution Method

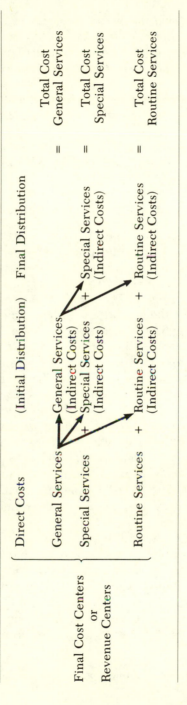

formula, and so on down the list of department costs to be distributed.[6]
*After the first distribution is completed, the costs that have been allocated
to the nonrevenue departments are then redistributed to the revenue-producing departments using the same bases of allocations as before (for example, square footage).*

In the double distribution method there is a more equitable allowance
for exchange of services between nonrevenue departments than in the step-
down method.

The following pages contain an explanation of the double apportionment method with an illustration in Tables 5.2 and 5.3.

THE FIRST DISTRIBUTION

By using Table 5.1 the step-down cost analysis sheet of Community
Hospital, and Table 5.2 for double apportionment, the differences and similarities in step-down and double apportionment can be shown. Basically,
double apportionment is two distributions of costs to reflect as accurately
as possible the interchange of services between nonrevenue departments
before costs are finally allotted to the revenue-producing departments. The
information in Column 3, which shows the total operating and professional
services expenses, is the same in both methods. Column 4 is the same in
both methods, with the total expense for plant operations distributed among
all other departments on a square footage basis. The difference between
the two methods begins in Column 5. Under double apportionment the
total expenses under maintenance and repair would be the figure shown
in Table 5.2, Column 3 ($21,176.88). This amount would be distributed in
Column 5 to all departments for which square footage is shown. Note that
the expenses were not accumulated (it was *not* $21,176.88 plus $1,870.67
to make $23,047.55); the amount distributed was the original expense total
in Column 3, or $21,176.88. Throughout the first distribution under the
double apportionment method the original expense total in Column 3 is
used for each department.

The distribution of the laundry costs to users of laundry will be in the
same proportion under both methods, but the amount of expense will differ
because under double apportionment just the original cost (not the accumulated cost) is distributed. The dietary department is also a special case
of distribution of the original expense of $62,173.72 (Column 3) to the nurs-
ing units according to the patient days. The original expense of medical
records ($19,831.70) is distributed under the formula shown in both ex-

---

[6]Other dietary costs (employees' cafeteria, for example) should be allocated to cost centers according to utilization.

hibits: 75% to nursing units on the basis of patient days; and 25% among emergency room, radiology, and laboratory on the basis of estimated usage.

The administrative expense ($100,216.17) would be distributed under double apportionment to all departments other than administration in ratio to departmental payrolls. The original expense total for central supply (Column 14) and medical and surgical supplies (Column 15) under double apportionment would be distributed to the same departments that received the accumulated allotments under the step-down method. After the nursing service payroll and the superintendence and house orderlies payroll (Columns 16 and 17) are distributed to the nursing units, the final computation of the first distribution of the double apportionment method can be undertaken. In Column 22 (not used in Table 5.1), totals of the expenses allocated to the various departments are made horizontally across the page. Column 22 will then contain the totals of all the allocated expenses of all nonrevenue departments, reflecting the interrelations of services provided by one department for another. A second distribution will now be needed to allot the nonrevenue expenses to the revenue departments. (See Table 5.3.)

THE SECOND DISTRIBUTION

When the horizontal totals (Column 22) have been determined for all of the nonrevenue departments, the second distribution, that of nonrevenue expenses to revenue departments, can be made. For example, the total for plant operations in Column 22, Table 5.2, is distributed to all the nursing units and other revenue-producing departments according to the ratio of the square footage of each revenue department to the total square footage of all revenue departments (see Table 5.3). The same bases of allocation are used in the second distribution as were used in step-down and in the first distribution of the double apportionment: square footage is used for plant operations, maintenance and repairs, housekeeping, and purchasing and stores; laundry usage ratio of the revenue departments would be used to distribute laundry expense; patient days for dietary; and so on. Once the second distribution is completed, and all of the expenses of the nonrevenue departments resulting from the first distribution have been allocated to revenue departments and totaled, the totals for each revenue department can be brought forward from Column 21 of Table 5.2 and a grand total made for each department as shown in Table 5.3.

Table 5.4 shows the double apportionment system; it is a more accurate method of distributing hospital costs than either the direct allocation or the step-down method. Even though it does entail more clerical work, it is the most desirable of the manual systems discussed.

TABLE 5.2 First Distribution, Double Apportionment Method,
Community Hospital

A. Department			Plant Operations	Maintenance and Repairs
	Departmental Square Footage	Total Operating and Professional Services Expenses		
B. Basis of Allocation			Sq. Footage	Sq. Footage
(1)	(2)	(3)	(4)	(5)
Plant operations	3,564	$ 64,115.90	($64,115.90)	$ 1,557.74
Maintenance	1,349	21,176.88	1,870.67	($21,176.88)
Laundry	2,118	18,287.18	2,937.06	925.74
Housekeeping	1,245	49,409.75	1,726.46	544.16
Purchasing and stores	1,228	6,144.34	1,702.88	536.74
Dietary—less revenue	3,592	62,173.72	4,981.06	1,569.98
Medical records	1,225	19,831.70	1,698.72	535.42
Administrative	1,703	100,216.17	2,361.56	744.34
Central supply	1,007	8,684.57	1,396.42	440.14
Medical and surgical	118	2,846.33	163.63	51.58
Superintendence and house orderlies	209	44,279.43	289.82	91.35
Nursing service		188,529.27		
Nursing centers				
Intensive care	1,380		1,913.67	603.16
Intermediate care	3,744		5,191.84	1,636.43
Continuing care	4,148		5,752.07	1,813.00
Self care	4,919		6,821.24	2,149.98
Pediatrics	2,445		3,390.50	1,068.66
Obstetrical	3,117		4,322.37	1,362.38
Subtotals	19,753		$27,391.69	$ 8,633.60
Emergency room	712	5,504.79	$ 987.33	$ 311.20
Operating room	3,903	30,213.87	5,475.33	1,705.90
Delivery room	3,313	21,475.76	4,594.17	1,448.04
Nursery	1,325	14,008.18	1,837.39	579.12
Pharmacy	343	39,225.89	475.64	149.92
Radiology	1,384	53,093.20	1,919.20	604.92
Laboratory	603	29,417.44	836.18	263.56
Anesthesia		2,897.98		
Oxygen		4,314.22		
Physical therapy	886	9,555.02	1,228.62	387.26
Occupational therapy	220	4,832.93	305.07	96.16
Total	49,800	$800,234.52	$64,115.90	$21,176.88

Laundry		Housekeeping	Purchasing and Stores	Dietary—less Revenue	Medical Records	
	Amount					
Percentage of Total Pounds Issued		Sq. Footage	Sq. Footage	Patient Days	Estimated Percentage of Record Keeping and Patient Days	
(6)	(7)	(8)	(9)	(10)	(11)	(12)
		$ 3,625.74	$ 450.84			
		1,372.75	170.65			
	($18,287.18)	2,155.29	267.93			
		($49,409.75)	157.50			
		1,249.52	($6,144.34)			
2.8%	512.05	3,652.94	454.38	($62,173.72)		
		1,246.47	154.97			($19,831.70)
		1,732.84	215.43			
10.5%	1,920.16	1,024.65	127.39			
		120.07	14.93			
		212.67	26.44			
5.3%	969.22	1,402.18	174.57	3,484.47	4.10%	813.10
14.0%	2,560.21	3,808.60	473.60	14,082.36	17.72%	3,514.14
14.9%	2,724.79	4,220.68	524.70	16,062.55	19.22%	3,811.66
15.0%	2,743.08	5,000.19	622.26	15,668.79	19.12%	3,791.83
4.3%	786.35	2,487.84	309.30	5,869.78	6.17%	1,223.62
18.5%	3,383.13	3,171.62	394.30	7,005.77	8.67%	1,719.41
72.0%	$13,166.78	$20,091.11	$2,498.73	$62,173.72	75.00%	$14,873.76
2.1%	$ 384.03	$ 724.48	$ 90.07		5.00%	$ 991.59
3.9%	713.20	3,988.73	493.70			
		3,371.05	419.10			
		1,348.22	167.62			
		349.01	43.39			
1.0%	182.87	1,406.25	175.08		15.00%	2,974.76
.3%	54.83	613.57	76.28		5.00%	991.59
7.4%	1,353.26	900.53	112.08			
		223.86	27.83			
100.0%	$18,287.18	$49,409.75	$6,144.34	$62,173.72	100%	$19,831.70

Continued

TABLE 5.2   Continued

A. *Department*	Administrative—less Telephone	Central Supply	Medical and Surgical	Nursing Service
B. *Basis of Allocation*	Departmental Payroll	Priced Requisitions	Priced Requisitions	Departmental Payroll
(1)	(13)	(14)	(15)	(16)
Plant operations	2,004.32			
Maintenance	2,004.32			
Laundry	2,004.32			
Housekeeping	7,516.20			
Purchasing and stores	501.08			
Dietary—less revenue	7,516.20			
Medical records	2,004.33			
Administrative	($100,216.17)			
Central supply	1,002.17	($8,684.57)		
Medical and surgical			($2,846.33)	
Superintendence and house orderlies	6,012.97			($44,279.43)
Nursing service				
Nursing centers				
Intensive care	5,010.80	694.77	227.70	4,427.93
Intermediate care	24,051.86	3,473.80	1,138.53	21,254.17
Continuing care	11,023.77	1,563.21	512.34	9,741.46
Self care	2,505.41	347.39	113.86	2,213.97
Pediatrics	5,010.81	694.77	227.70	4,427.93
Obstetrical	2,505.40	347.39	113.86	2,213.97
Subtotals	$ 50,108.05	$7,121.33	$2,333.99	
Emergency room	$ 5,010.81	$ 434.23	$ 142.32	
Operating room	4,008.65	694.77	227.70	
Delivery room	2,004.33	260.54	85.39	
Nursery	1,002.17	173.70	56.93	
Pharmacy	2,004.33			
Radiology	1,002.17			
Laboratory	1,002.17			
Anesthesia				
Oxygen	1,002.17			
Physical therapy	2,004.33			
Occupational therapy	501.08			
Total	$100,216.17	$8,684.57	$2,846.33	$44,279.43

Superintendence and House Orderlies					Total Expense of Nonrevenue Departments, Accumulated Horizontally
	Total Nursing Cost	Patient Days	Nursing Cost Per Patient Day	Total Expense of Revenue Departments	
Departmental Payroll					
(17)	(18)	(19)	(20)	(21)	(22)
	(stated in column 21)	(omitted for clarity)	(omitted for clarity)		(a) $ 7,638.64
					(b) 5,355.39
					(c) 8,290.34
					(d) 9,944.32
					(e) 3,990.22
					(f) 18,686.61
					(g) 5,639.91
					(h) 5,054.17
					(i) 5,910.93
					(j) 350.21
($188,529.27)					(k) 6,633.25
18,852.93				(l) $ 38,574.50	
90,494.03				(m) 171,679.57	
41,476.44				(n) 99,226.67	
9,426.47				(o) 51,404.47	
18,852.93				(p) 44,350.19	
9,426.47				(q) 35,966.07	
				(r) 14,580.85	
				(s) 47,521.85	
				(t) 33,658.38	
				(u) 19,173.33	
				(v) 42,248.18	
				(w) 61,358.45	
				(x) 33,255.62	
				(y) 2,897.98	
				(z) 5,316.39	
				(zz) 15,541.10	
				(zzz) 5,986.93	
$188,529.27				$722,740.53	$ 77,493.99

TABLE 5.3   Second Distribution, Double Apportionment Method, Community Hospital

		ICU	Intermed. Care	Cont. Care	Self-Care	Ped.	OB	ER	OR
(a)	Plant operations	$ 305.56	$ 907.10	$ 1,003.07	$ 1,105.85	$ 534.73	$ 763.86	$ 114.59	$ 946.20
(b)	Maintenance	214.20	642.60	696.15	803.25	374.85	535.54	80.45	642.65
(c)	Laundry	580.30	1,243.50	1,326.40	1,409.30	497.40	1,658.00	248.04	415.50
(d)	Housekeeping	397.76	1,293.28	1,292.72	1,491.60	696.08	994.43	99.14	1,193.28
(e)	Purchasing	159.60	438.72	518.70	598.50	279.30	399.02	79.98	478.80
(f)	Dietary	934.34	4,671.65	4,671.65	4,671.65	1,868.66	1,868.66		
(g)	Medical records	231.24	999.11	1,084.01	1,078.37	348.20	488.98	282.00	
(h)	Administrative	404.32	1,415.12	859.35	202.16	404.32	202.16	404.32	303.24
(i)	Central supply	472.10	2,367.13	1,063.18	236.05	472.10	236.05	295.55	472.10
(j)	Medical and surgical	28.02	140.07	63.04	14.01	28.02	14.01	17.51	28.02
(k)	Superintendence and orderlies	663.33	3,183.95	1,459.32	331.66	663.33	331.66		
	Dept. totals	$4,390.77	$17,302.23	$14,037.59	$11,942.40	$6,166.99	$7,492.37	$1,621.58	$4,479.79

TABLE 5.3 Continued

	Delivery	Nursery	Phcy.	Radiology	Lab.	Anesth.	O₂	PT	OT	Totals
(a) Plant operations	$ 763.86	$ 229.14	$ 315.56	$ 267.33	$152.70			$ 152.70	$ 76.39	$ 7,638.64
(b) Maintenance	535.54	160.65	214.20	187.56	107.10			107.10	53.55	5,355.39
(c) Laundry				165.80				746.10		8,290.34
(d) Housekeeping	994.43	298.32	397.76	298.32	198.88			198.88	99.44	9,944.32
(e) Purchasing	399.02	119.70	159.60	159.78	79.80			79.80	39.80	3,990.22
(f) Dietary										18,686.61
(g) Medical records				846.00	282.00					5,639.91
(h) Administrative	202.16	75.81	151.62	75.81	75.81		$75.81	151.62	50.54	5,054.17
(i) Central supply	177.41	119.26								5,910.93
(j) Medical and surgical	10.51	7.00								350.21
(k) Superintendence and orderlies										6,633.25
Dept. totals	$3,082.93	$1,009.88	$1,238.74	$2,000.60	$896.29		$75.81	$1,436.20	$319.82	$77,493.99

TABLE 5.4   Comparison of Cost Distribution Methods, Community
              Hospital

Unit	Step-Down Method	Double Apportionment Method
Intensive care	$ 61,468.55	$ 42,965.27
Intermediate care	109,188.84	188,981.80
Continuing care	127,472.58	113,264.26
Self care	102,029.70	63,346.87
Pediatrics	48,370.18	50,517.18
Obstetrics	44,397.12	43,458.44
Emergency room	11,187.33	16,202.43
Operating room	51,459.52	52,001.64
Delivery room	41,547.76	36,741.31
Nursery	25,551.98	20,183.21
Pharmacy	43,001.35	43,486.92
Radiology	61,301.56	63,359.05
Laboratory	40,101.80	34,151.91
Anesthesiology	4,097.54	2,897.98
Oxygen	4,314.22	5,392.20
Physical therapy	17,585.20	16,977.30
Occupational therapy	7,159.29	6,306.75
Total	$800,234.52	$800,234.52

MULTIPLE APPORTIONMENTS
(THE ALGEBRAIC METHODS)

Some accountants have developed methods of multiple distributions of costs which are sometimes referred to as algebraic methods. Conceivably, these distributions could be done manually, but from a practical standpoint double distribution remains the most feasible manual method.

Algebraic multiple distributions are made of expenses between non-revenue departments and then, finally, to revenue departments in an attempt to refine the cost analysis to the greatest possible degree of exactness. Although 10 or 12 distributions are made in some methods, it is most generally agreed that after 4 distributions there is little change in the ultimate cost figures.

To use multiple distributions to best advantage, a hospital should use a computer. In fact, a method of distributing interrelated costs has been devised in which simultaneous equations are programmed on a computer to take into consideration all cost interrelations between departments: nonrevenue departments to nonrevenue departments to revenue departments. The resulting cost analysis system is the most exact method yet devised, but it is beyond the capabilities of the average hospital accountant. The cost of programming and computer service time makes this type of cost analysis most practicable only when performed by a central service.[7]

HOW THE SYSTEMS COMPARE

At one time, William R. Foyle, a C.P.A. interested in hospital cost analysis, made a comparison of cost apportionment for three hospitals under each of the first four methods described in this chapter: direct allocation; step-down; double apportionment; and algebraic (multiple apportionment). Mr. Foyle's thesis was that the algebraic method using multiple apportionment would not only give a more accurate reckoning of the costs of the interchange of services among nonrevenue departments, but would also give a more accurate distribution of costs to general care departments in relation to ancillary services. The proper distribution of costs to general care departments is particularly important when the patient mix (high Medicare admission rate, for example) especially stresses the demand for general care over that of laboratory, radiology, and other ancillary departments. Mr. Foyle could demonstrate the difference in apportionment by the various methods of cost analysis, but concluded that the mathematical method was not the only factor to be considered in cost distribution. Certain management decisions made in the beginning, such as the basis of allocation (square footage, payroll allocation, accumulated costs, pounds of laundry), might widen differences more than mathematical methodologies.[8]

CONCLUSIONS

The most accurate method of cost analysis in terms of apportioning all allowable hospital costs to revenue-producing departments is a form of multiple apportionment.

To adjust for interdepartmental services, the simultaneous equation method programmed for a computer is the most exact. The double apportionment method is the most accurate of the feasible manual methods. Step-down, although acceptable to most third party payers, is less accurate because of the closing of a department for receipt of charges from other departments once its original and accumulated charges have been distributed.

A study of three hospitals showed a 1% or 2% variation by department

---

[7]One method widely used was devised by the MICAH Corporation, Ann Arbor, Michigan. The Hospital Administrative Services of the American Hospital Association also offers computerized cost analysis in its Cost Allocation Program (CAP). Dr. David Penn developed an algebra-equivalent method for Laventhol Krekstein Horwath & Horwath called a "successive iteration" method for practical use by accounting staffs.

[8]Foyle, William R., "Evaluation of Methods of Cost Analysis," an unpublished paper, c. 1964.

between the algebraic method (multiple apportionment) and the step-down, with double apportionment coming somewhere between. Consequently, on the basis of accuracy alone, the order of preference is: (1) algebraic (multiple apportionment); (2) double apportionment; (3) step-down; and (4) direct apportionment. From a practical standpoint of time and cost of the analysis, however, it would be better to consider the selection of manual methods as: (1) double apportionment; and (2) step-down.

SUGGESTED READINGS

American Hospital Association. *Cost Finding and Rate Setting for Hospitals.*
Bulletin of the Operations Research Society, Spring 1974.
Cleverley, William O. "An Input-Output Model for Hospital Costing."
MICAH Corporation. *The MICAH System for Hospital Cost Analysis.*
Perlman, Mark; Adams, Jeffrey; Wolfe, Harvey; and Shuman, Larry, *Methods for Distributing the Costs on Non–Revenue Producing Centers.*
Seawell, L. Vann. *Hospital Financial Accounting: Theory and Practice.*

6

Blue Cross

HISTORY AND PHILOSOPHY

The story of Blue Cross is said to have begun in 1929 when Dr. Justin Ford Kimball, the new executive vice president of Baylor University, found that the University Hospital in Dallas, Texas was in serious financial trouble because of the large amount of outstanding accounts receivable. The problem struck home to Dr. Kimball as an educator because many schoolteachers were prominent among the delinquent debtors.

The solution that was found for the problem in Dallas proved to be a prototype followed by many other communities. A prepayment plan for hospital care was developed under which teachers who joined the plan could pay six dollars a year and be assured of up to 21 days of hospital care in a semiprivate room at Baylor University Hospital. The prepayment plan worked: it solved the cash shortage dilemma facing the hospital and at the same time relieved the pressure of hospital bills for the teachers. By the end of 1929, 1,000 teachers were enrolled. This represented about 75% of the total. After a time, other groups in the community joined the teachers in the prepayment plan.

The Baylor prepayment idea caught on in other parts of the country where hospitals faced the problems of collecting unpaid bills and where workers worried about how to pay for unexpected hospitalization during times of increasing unemployment and decreasing wages. The workers liked the security of knowing that there was a definite period of care in a definite type of accommodation paid for in advance, if they needed it. The hospitals liked having the payment for the hospital care of a whole group of persons assured—and insured.

Shortly afterward other groups made contracts with hospitals in the Dallas area, but the contracts were between a certain group and a certain hospital. Multihospital prepayment contracts came later.

By 1932 plans were being developed in several communities of the country with contractual relations between each plan and more than one hospital.

In 1933, C. Rufus Rorem, Ph.D., a medical economist, joined the small staff of the American Hospital Association as associate director and brought with him a $100,000 grant from the Julius Rosenwald Fund for the development of group hospitalization plans. Under Rorem's guidance the Association developed criteria for acceptable group hospitalization plans. Among the features the Association recommended were

1. The plan should be founded as a public service not-for-profit agency.
2. The coverage should be for hospital care, not for physicians' services.
3. The plan should operate with the advice of physicians, hospital trustees, and others interested in public service.
4. There should be a free choice of hospital.
5. All recognized hospitals should participate in offering services under the plan.
6. The hospitals should be responsible for providing satisfactory care.
7. The plan should be financially sound.

In practice at least, the role of the American Hospital Association grew to that of being an accrediting agent of Blue Cross plans. The group plan idea began appearing in other states: New Jersey and Minnesota, among the first. (E.A. van Steenwyk of the Minnesota plan was the originator of the Blue Cross name and symbol.) In the various states the legislatures addressed themselves to the problems of the mushrooming hospital care plans and passed enabling acts that allowed the groups to solicit members without having financial reserves as large as required of commercial insurance firms. The enabling acts provided for state regulation of subscription rates (premiums) charged by the plans, usually by the office of the state insurance commissioner.

The question is often asked, does Blue Cross represent the hospital or the patient? This question cannot be answered simply, for the role of Blue Cross has been changing since the founding of the first plan. As has been indicated, Blue Cross was founded to save hospitals from financial ruin by reducing outstanding accounts receivable through a plan of prepayment of hospital care. The subscribers to the prepayment plan benefited by being relieved of hospital expenses that they probably would not have been prepared to pay. Originally the prepayment plan was fostered by hospitals with the American Hospital Association in the forefront as adviser. The public was included in a minority role on Blue Cross advisory boards. To this point, Blue Cross has been hospital- as opposed to patient-oriented.

However, as Blue Cross became more widespread, as hospital costs rose, and as premium rates rose in consequence, the public became more interested in the operation of the plans. The states that set Blue Cross premium rates resisted the requests for higher rates and demanded cost containment where possible. Blue Cross was forced by circumstances to begin controls by demanding better accounting methods in hospitals, by taking a firmer attitude on certain debatable costs, by fostering utilization review, and by experimenting with various methods of rate setting.[1]

At the time when Blue Cross became more conscious of the need for hospital cost containment and began to invite more public members to advisory boards, it can be said that Blue Cross became more subscriber-related.

It is difficult to generalize about Blue Cross, about its philosophy; its role; its benefits; its contracts; its membership; its reimbursement methods; or the direction in which it is going. It is difficult, if for no other reason than that in 1984 there were 68 separate plans in the United States, 4 in Canada, 1 in Puerto Rico, and 1 in Jamaica.

But people do generalize about Blue Cross in spite of the 74 separate corporations. Some persons say Blue Cross is social insurance. Without enumerating the pros and cons of Blue Cross as social insurance, it can be safely said that the Blue Cross concept calls for nongovernmental prepayment plans for hospital expenses—and there is a social overtone, to say the least. Blue Cross moves in the direction of one aspect of social insurance (comprehensive hospital care) in the "first day, first dollar" ideal goal of covering the whole hospital stay from the first day of admission and the first dollar of expense. Commercial insurance usually has a different base. It generally pays definite dollar indemnities for certain accommodations and for certain services.

Some of the Blue Cross contracts around the country limit benefits, or list hospital benefits with certain dollar or percentage deductions. Although it cannot be said that Blue Cross covers 100% of the hospital charges of its subscribers, the percentage of coverage is high. It might be easy to speculate that practically 100% of the bills would be paid by Blue Cross, except for special accommodations or extraordinary services some patients needed or demanded.

---

[1]Previously terms for methods of rate setting of Blue Cross–Blue Shield were "experience rating" of large groups or "community rating" of communities or areas. Both methods were ultimately based on the utilization of health services by categories of subscribers. Today the trend is for large purchasers to contract for specific benefits under a multioption choice of delivery based on utilization of services desired.

MEMBERSHIP

The growth of Blue Cross in number of plans and in number of members was particularly rapid from the 1930s up to 1958. In 1937 there were 37 plans with 1 million members; 10 years later (1947) the total membership had grown to 27 million, or 19% of the U.S. population. The growth spurted on until 1958 when 79 U.S. plans had 52 million members, equivalent to 30% of the U.S. population. Then, for the first time in over 20 years, Blue Cross membership did not increase. Unemployment in the automobile industry directly affected one of the largest groups of members.

After a time, increase in membership began again, both in gross numbers and in percentage of the U.S. population. By the end of 1973 the membership in the 74 U.S. Blue Cross plans had reached a total of over 80 million or 37.7% of the population of the areas served. This figure included nearly 5.4 million federal employees and dependents enrolled under the Federal Employees Health Benefits Program (FEP).

The implementation of Medicare on July 1, 1966 was responsible for Blue Cross's redesigning coverage for subscribers over 65. Subscribers thus were removed from regular membership and enrolled for complementary coverage. In 1980, 8.6 million Blue Cross members had coverage complementary to Medicare. This Blue Cross coverage in effect was designed to pay for the deductibles that the individual was expected to pay under Medicare provisions.[2]

The number of Blue Cross plans had been reduced from 79 to 68 through mergers by the end of 1980. In addition to the 68 U.S. plans, there was 1 in Puerto Rico and there were 4 in Canada and 1 in Jamaica, as previously mentioned. Canadian enrollment totaled about 5 million in 1980; the Canadian coverage was supplemental to that furnished under the various provincial health care plans.

The final report of 1984 as to the number of Blue Cross–Blue Shield subscribers was not available at the time of this writing. The regular membership plus federal employees, complementary Medicare enrollees, and military subscribers, along with those signed up in the associate plans should total over 80 million, of which 70% to 75% would be members of groups.

Generally, groups as small as 4 or 5 members are eligible for group Blue Cross rates if 100% of each group enrolls. When the group is larger (15 or more), the required percentage is about 70%. Arrangements are made to transfer from group to group with change of employment or to a conversion policy when a subscriber leaves a group but does not join another covered under Blue Cross. In the conversion, the subscriber may be charged a higher rate and receive fewer benefits.

---

[2]See Chapter 7.

Other fractions in membership besides the group, nongroup division are the regular and complementary membership classifications, which in turn are subdivided into individual and family enrollment.

With group enrollments there usually is not withholding of benefits for a period of time because of preexisting conditions (pregnancy being the most likely exception), but with nongroup enrollments there may be a waiting period for some preexisting conditions.

Enrollments can be for an individual or for a family. Under the family contract, dependent children are usually covered up to 19 years of age, unless married before that time. In some instances a totally disabled child will be covered after the age of 19.

BLUE CROSS AND BLUE SHIELD PLANS

The Blue Cross and Blue Shield plans combined are the largest health care insurer in the United States. Despite some slippage in numbers of subscribers due to competition from self-insurance plans and other optional and competitive plans, the Blues still command nearly 50% of the market. While some insurance companies are showing losses instead of profits in the health insurance business, the Blue plans are in good financial shape, with the majority of plans showing gains in reserves. (See Tables 6.1, 6.2, 6.3.) Furthermore the Blues' financial position is buttressed by the income derived from acting as the largest fiscal intermediary for Medicare.

Blue Cross and Blue Shield plans were classified in three categories in late 1984:

—*Category A*
   22 Blue Cross plans giving hospital coverage
   16 Blue Shield plans giving medical coverage

—*Category B*
   6 Blue Cross plans giving both hospital and medical coverage
   11 Blue Shield plans giving both hospital and medical coverage

—*Category C*
   40 Blue Cross–Blue Shield combined plans

This makes a total of 95 plans representing 68 Blue Cross and 67 Blue Shield units. The numbers will change because of forthcoming mergers.

The 68 Blue Cross units and the 67 Blue Shield units, in the first nine months of 1984, showed positive activities with revenues from subscribers at over $30 billion. Out of this claims of more than 27 billion (90.5%) were paid out, with an administrative cost of 7.5%. Reserves stood at over $6 billion.

TABLE 6.1 Blue Cross–Blue Shield Plans' (95) Financial Summary of Nine Months Ending September 30, 1984

Subscription revenue (net)	$30,142,271,000
Claims expense	27,282,485,000
Administrative expenses	2,255,211,000
Underwriting gain or (loss)	604,575,000
Investments and other income	789,557,000
Transferred to reserves	1,394,132,000

Source: Blue Cross and Blue Shield Association.

TABLE 6.2 Blue Cross–Blue Shield Plans' (95) Financial Summary, September 30, 1984

Current assets	$ 9,258,194,000
Total assets	$18,582,071,000
Current liabilities	$12,159,057,000
Long-term liabilities	$ 196,213,000

Source: Blue Cross and Blue Shield Association.

TABLE 6.3 Blue Cross–Blue Shield Plans' (95) Gains to Reserves for Nine Months Ending September 30, 1984

	Gains to Reserves
Category A	
22 Blue Cross Plans (hospital coverage only)	$417,705,000
16 Blue Shield Plans (medical coverage only)	92,127,000
Category B	
6 Blue Cross Plans (both hospital and medical-surgical)	81,559,000
11 Blue Shield Plans (both hospital and medical-surgical)	102,546,000
Category C	
40 Blue Cross and Blue Shield combined plans (both hospital and medical-surgical)	700,195,000
Total to reserves	$1,394,132,000

Source: Blue Cross and Blue Shield Association.

Blue Cross claims for the third quarter of 1984 showed evidence of the decline in hospital utilization that was common to the country in general.[3] Hospital patient admissions per 1,000 subscribers in 1984 declined compared to the same quarter of 1983—from 107 per 1,000 to 94 per 1,000. Inpatient days declined per 1,000 subscribers per year from 655 to 562. Average length of stay for hospital inpatients declined from 6.19 to 5.96 days per admission.

During the third quarter of 1984, however, benefit payments from Blue Cross increased over the preceding year. The average payment per inpatient admission increased 7.2%, from $2,331 to $2,499. The average benefit per inpatient day rose 9.7%, from $382 to $419. The average benefit payment per outpatient visit increased 10%, from $104.45 to $114.91.

ADMINISTRATION

One should always bear in mind when speaking of Blue Cross–Blue Shield that there are 95 autonomous plans in the United States plus Puerto Rico, Canada, and Jamaica. However, there is a national organization, the Blue Cross and Blue Shield Association (BCBSA), which is often the spokesman for the collective whole and which also acts as a clearinghouse of research information, a coordinator of national Blue Cross contracts, and a fiscal agent for a majority of the Medicare claims.[4]

There is no standard Blue Cross–subscriber contract for the U.S. plans, although there may be a slow movement in this direction because nationwide corporations, or large industrial unions, want uniform benefits for all the employees enrolled. In many instances the contracts negotiated by widespread companies call for benefits superior to those offered in some of the plans. Consequently, it has become necessary for BCBSA to form a subsidiary corporation to handle claims made under national contracts.[5] The largest of the national contracts, the Federal Employees Health Benefits Program, has over five million members, as already noted.

---

[3]Blue Cross plans in Puerto Rico, associate plans in Canada and Jamaica, and Medicare complementary coverage are not included.

[4]There were two national Blue Cross organizations until they merged in 1960: the Blue Cross Association and the Blue Cross Commission (a child of the American Hospital Association). The purposes of the current Blue Cross and Blue Shield Association are broadly: to coordinate the activities of the separate plans; to represent and speak for the plans on a national basis; to act as a clearinghouse for claims to be paid under contracts that cover employees of organizations that are spread over the territories of more than one plan, or for claims of members who were treated outside their own plan district. Since the merger, the national association has grown stronger. The association was strengthened again when it became the claims agent for Medicare for much of the country.

[5]Subsidiary corporations have also been formed to market life insurance and other types of insurance, as well as HMOs and PPOs.

The administrative officers of the plans are paid employees, but the governing boards are composed of voluntary members representing hospitals, medicine, and the public. Originally, the average ratio of the hospital members of the boards was over half and the public members about one-third. The trend has been for the hospital percentage to decrease and the public percentage to increase so that hospital members are no longer predominant in numbers.

The cost of administration of the plans has been impressively modest. Usually the plans report administrative costs of about 7.5%. The low cost can be accounted for partially because: Blue Cross plans do their own "selling" through salaried employees rather than through agents working on commission; they process their own claims; and they are not profit-oriented.

BLUE CROSS BENEFITS

Blue Cross and other health insurance policies are no longer simple contracts providing coverage for hospital care for subscribers. In the early days of prepaid group hospitalization, a subscriber for a rate as low as 50¢ a month might be insured for up to 21 days of hospital care. This was an inclusive rate that provided room and board, nursing care, ancillary services, and the use of the facilities—complete hospital care of the day.

Later, additional charges were added for family members, for maternity care, and for other special conditions. In the beginning commercial insurance varied somewhat in that premium rates were set on providing dollar benefits, an indemnity style of payment which was based on a certain number of dollars a day for hospital care, and which might or might not cover the hospital bill completely.

Early in the history of Blue Cross, complications in terms of coverage arose. The complications were national accounts. The insurer was asked to provide contracts for employees of companies with work places in many parts of the country. Problems such as this led to the national association of Blue Cross plans—first the Blue Cross Commission then the Blue Cross Association—setting up subsidiaries to handle national accounts across Blue Cross boundaries. Commercial insurance companies were able to adjust, first with their indemnity benefits and later with contracts tailored to large account specifications.

In the beginning Blue Cross premiums usually were paid by the employee. In fact, some labor unions were said to have refused an employer's wish to pay for his employees' insurance. Some unions were suspicious of any benefit from the hands of the employer that did not come as the result of collective bargaining.

A big change in the attitude of labor unions toward the employer paying all or part of health insurance costs came during World War II. There had been a wartime freeze on wages imposed in the war industries. War industries in general were working on a cost plus percentage of profit plan (for example, cost plus 10%). The federal government responded to pressure from labor unions for increased wages to offset inflation, particularly health care costs, by allowing employers to pay some of the health insurance costs of employees, and to charge that expense to the cost of doing business. Thus the employee received some benefits in lieu of wages and the employer was able to charge it off as cost on which he made his allowable percentage of profit. After the war, "fringe benefits" became a part of most union contracts.

Since fringe benefits became negotiable items in union contracts and were nontaxable to employees, they were viewed as preferred contract demands. In time, benefits increased and new items were added to the list. Time limits on days of hospital care were extended from a fairly limited number to 365 or 730 days per episode of illness. Other benefits were added such as dental care and inpatient days for mental illness. As the benefits increased, the premiums had to rise. This continued as long as the premiums were acceptable to the employers and the state rate-setting agencies.

However, the day came when employers began to protest that the high cost of fringe benefits made them unable to compete with foreign manufacturers. Employers began to speak of the fringe benefits as a high percentage of the cost of their products. General Motors and Chrysler talked about fringe benefits adding $500 to $600 to the price of every automobile they manufactured. This built-in cost factor added a dollar amount that exceeded the cost of steel in the vehicle. The weight of the cost of fringe benefits was felt especially during the recessions of the 1970s.

At the same time HMOs and other alternative methods of care were developing, and some employers were trying to find means of self-insurance. Copayments and deductibles became negotiable items. Options was a word used more and more frequently. The employee was offered inducements to use health services less often. (For example, a bonus might be given at the end of the year if no health services were used.)

PAYMENT OF PREMIUMS

A subtle influence on hospital utilization and on the cost of Blue Cross may be inherent in who pays the insurance premium.

In the early days of prepayment schemes for hospital care, the concern was to assure subscribers that they could have a reasonable number of days of hospital care as a benefit for monthly payments they could afford to pay. The premiums were paid to a hospital which, in consequence, was able to remain solvent during the Depression and provide needed services to the subscribers. It was a fairly simple one-to-one situation: a contract between a person and a hospital.

During the 1930s and later, complexities began to appear in the relationship between the subscriber and the provider: multihospital coverage became possible; a definition and refinement of the list of benefits developed; and the Blue Cross image emerged to make protection regional and even national in scope. Insurance coverage for hospital care became a desired goal of most American families. Linked with these changes was the development of large industrial labor unions with great power at the bargaining table. One of the fringe benefits sought by the labor unions was for the employer to share in the cost of hospital insurance as he did in the cost of social security. The trend developed for the employer to pay a share of the worker's insurance, or a share of the worker's and dependents' insurance or other combinations of payment—all moving toward the employer paying the total premium for worker and dependents.

Many thoughtful persons, while not disagreeing with payment of health insurance as a fringe benefit, have raised some questions. Do persons whose insurance is paid as a fringe benefit exercise the same prudence in requesting services as do persons who pay their own insurance premiums and know there is a direct relationship between services used and the cost of insurance? If employers pay most or all of the premiums for health insurance, does this contribute to more frequent admissions to hospital, higher costs, and higher premiums? These questions are unanswerable at present, but are worth pondering.

BLUE CROSS–BLUE SHIELD STANDARD OPTION PLAN

A good illustration of the use of an HMO plan calling for a sharing of premium costs and for one flat deductible of $100 for a hospital stay of up to 180 days[6] is the Blue Cross–Blue Shield Standard Option Plan for federal employees. In 1985 the rates charged the employees were

	Federal Employees (biweekly)	Postal Employees (biweekly)	Retired Employees (monthly)
Individual	$ 7.55	$1.89	$16.35
Family	$18.67	$5.33	$40.45

---

[6]After 180 days of hospital care the policy pays 75% of the bill.

HOSPITAL BENEFITS

All hospital costs after the initial $100 deductible are paid under the Blue Cross–Blue Shield Standard Option Plan and include

1. Semiprivate room and board
2. General nursing care
3. Operating room, recovery room, and treatment room services
4. Intensive care service
5. Labor and delivery room service
6. Drugs, X ray, EKG, EEG
7. Dressings, splints, plaster casts
8. Oxygen, anesthetics, laboratory service
9. Blood administration

The beneficiary has choice of physician and hospital.

OUTPATIENT CARE BENEFITS

After an annual deduction of $250 the Standard Option Plan pays 100% of

1. Outpatient treatment of accidental injury, in the emergency room or a doctor's office within 72 hours
2. Hospital charges for outpatient surgery

MEDICAL BENEFITS

Standard Option pays 75% of the customary, usual, and reasonable (CUR) charges for

1. Maternity care
2. Physicians' home and office visits (unlimited number)
3. Surgery, oral surgery, anesthesia
4. Diagnostic X-ray and laboratory service by a physician, independent laboratory, or hospital outpatient department
5. Doctors' hospital visits
6. Inpatient mental illness care up to 30 days
7. Inpatient consultation
8. Dental care related to accidental injury
9. Allergy tests and injections
10. Outpatient sessions for mental illness (up to 25 sessions)

11. Prescription drugs and insulin
12. Ambulance
13. Crutches and wheelchairs
14. Home nursing (25 visits)

MAJOR MEDICAL

Once any hospital deductible and the 25% major medical coinsurance total $2,500, the Standard Option Plan pays 100% of all covered expenses for all members of the family (on a family policy) for the remainder of the year.

DENTAL CARE

The Standard Option Plan helps pay for routine and preventive dental care including

1. Cleaning
2. Examinations
3. Extractions
4. Space maintainers
5. Fillings
6. Fluoride treatments

SUMMARY

The Standard Option Plan for federal employees is a comprehensive coverage scheme that offers nationwide hospital and medical service with choice of physician and hospital. The subscriber pays a reasonable share of the premiums and assumes responsibility for a $100 deductible on the hospital bill; assumes the balance of the medical bill after the Standard Option Plan pays 75% of the CUR charge. There is a 100% major medical coverage after deductibles and the 25% coinsurance reach $2,500 in a year. Dental care is covered partially according to a schedule of fees.

BLUE CROSS–BLUE SHIELD AND HMOS, IPAS, AND PPOS

Until about ten years ago Blue Cross–Blue Shield wrote contracts that insured subscribers for periods of up to a year or more of hospital and nursing care and for medical care within the hospital. There was some variation among contracts, especially among those written for large groups. Some contracts called for added benefits or for such control mechanisms as second opinions for surgery, utilization review, and preadmission procedures.

On the whole, Blue Cross–Blue Shield procedures developed in an orderly fashion until the early 1970s, when the federal government began asking for more than one option for health insurance contracts for federal employees. This was the time when certain prepaid group hospitalization plans took on the new name of health maintenance organization (HMO). The federal government passed legislation and issued regulations (rather tardily) that enabled entrepreneurs to start and operate HMOs.

The HMO was not a new idea although the name was. Existing HMOs as exemplified by Kaiser-Permanente and the Ross-Loos Clinic, both in California, offered medical care in the doctor's office and in the hospital, as well as hospital care and services, for a capitation fee. Physicians worked either for salaries or in a partnership arrangement. Kaiser-Permanente owns and operates hospitals and clinics in some of its areas of concentration; in others it contracts for space and service. The largest HMO, with over 4.6 million subscribers, Kaiser-Permanente is nonprofit, sells coverage on a capitation basis, and takes the financial risk of furnishing comprehensive health care services.

Kaiser cannot be taken as a prototype for many of the HMOs. In fact, there are so many kinds of HMO that it would be best at this point to consider a definition of HMO. Since many HMOs do not meet the description used by the federal government approval process, it is the generic definition Blue Cross–Blue Shield uses in its literature that we can adopt in the beginning, considering later some of the variations in structure and operation. The generic definition reads:

> A health maintenance organization (HMO) is an organized system which provides an agreed upon set of comprehensive inpatient and outpatient health services to a voluntary enrolled population in exchange for a predetermined, fixed, and periodic prepayment.

Most of the HMOs founded in recent years contract for hospital beds and services, rather than build them or buy facilities. In most cases the medical services have been contracted for from individual physicians or through IPAs (independent practice associations of physicians).

HMOs sell insurance and take the risk of furnishing medical, hospital, and related services, as well as administering the plans. By February 1985, there were in the United States over 16 million subscribers in more than 330 HMOs.

Most of the early HMOs were not-for-profit, but the trend now seems to be for-profit organizations, with not-for-profit HMOs changing to for-profit. Big investors are getting into the HMO business: Prudential, Metropolitan, and Aetna life insurance companies have separately entered the for-profit field as have Health America, Maxicare, U.S. Health Care, and others. A question in the minds of many is whether the trend toward for-profit will raise the cost of health care.

Another factor to consider is the development of HMO management companies. The effect of management companies on cost and efficiency remains to be seen.

The next logical step in HMO development is for HMOs to unite in networks or to arrange for service interchange so that national accounts can be accommodated. Kaiser-Permanente in the past few years has moved toward a national structure. It has expanded from its original territory on the West Coast into Colorado, Texas, Ohio, Connecticut, and the District of Columbia, among other places. Reports in early 1985 were that Kaiser-Permanente would like to merge with the Health Insurance Plan (HIP) of New York City. This would add over 900,000 subscribers to Kaiser.

Over the past decade, since HMOs have been an option to the traditional Blue Cross–Blue Shield contracts, the Blues have been losing some members. To protect their market where optional plans were being offered in addition to their own, the Blue plans have developed HMOs and an HMO network, HMO-USA. Its title describes its goal: to have a national network of Blue Cross–Blue Shield HMOs. Early 1985 figures showed an HMO-USA network of 62 HMOs in 31 states, established by 44 Blue Cross–Blue Shield plans, with an enrollment in excess of two million members.

There are several varieties in structure of Blue Cross–Blue Shield HMOs, which have been classified under two broad headings: the Group category and the IPA category.

The Group category is divided into Staff and Group subcategories. Staff HMOs furnish medical services through physicians who are salaried employees. Group HMOs contract with a medical group practice to purvey medical care services, usually on a capitation basis.

In the IPA category there are several subcategories. In a Group Practice Network, an HMO contracts with more than one group practice. An IPA type of HMO is one that contracts with an association of physicians in individual practice. An IPA Network is one in which an HMO contracts with more than one individual practice association (IPA). Mixed Networks are HMOs that contract both with medical groups and with IPAs. (See Table 6.4.)

HMO-USA is already making some headway in enrolling national accounts. United Airlines and Goodyear are two well-known companies that have signed up. During 1984, HMO-USA increased its number of subscribers by 37% while the HMO industry as a whole showed only a 22% increase. This enabled Blue Cross–Blue Shield HMOs to increase their share of the national market from 11% to 12%.

The Blues established 10 new HMOs in 1984, bringing their total to

TABLE 6.4   Blue Cross–Blue Shield HMO Enrollment by Models, December 31, 1984

	HMOs	Membership	
Group Category			
Staff	7	210,745	
Group	13	260,794	
Total			471,539
IPA Category			
Group practice network	10	662,750	
Mixed network	9	596,017	
IPA	16	187,115	
IPA network	7	133,779	
Total			1,579,661
Grand total	62		2,051,200

Source: Blue Cross and Blue Shield Association.

62. The range of enrollment in the 62 plans was from 309,000 persons in the Health Maintenance Network in Southern California to a few hundred in the plans in the process of formation. The median of the top 40 fully operative plans was about 33,000 subscribers.

It would seem that there will be a period of shakedown and merger among existing HMOs and the formation of a few national chains or networks. (Maxicare is reported to be absorbing Health America.) Certainly Kaiser-Permanente, HMO-USA, an organization sponsored by a commercial insurance company or two, an investor-owned hospital chain, and possibly an investor-owned HMO corporation will survive at least the first general adjustment.

Another option in health insurance is that sold and administered by preferred provider organizations (PPOs). The PPOs contract with providers: hospitals, physicians, visiting nurses, clinics, and other professionals. The contracted fees are usually lower than customary rates, and are given by the providers because they expect that PPOs will steer business into the empty beds or into the open appointment times. Conditions are attractive for many providers to sign such contracts because of overbedded hospitals, the coming glut of medical graduates, the decline of length of stay in hospitals, and the growing ratio of use of outpatient services over inpatient care when possible.

SELF-INSURANCE

Another option is self-insurance by the employer. Sometimes the employer assumes the cost of health care of his employees but has an insurance company or a third party administrator (TPA) process the claims. Another plan is for the employer to pay claims up to a certain dollar amount and then have the insurance company take over claims beyond that amount— a stop-loss arrangement.

Self-insurance and all the optional plans have cut into the writing of traditional policies to the extent that Blue Cross–Blue Shield and commercial insurance companies also have had to offer optional plans to stay competitive. However, self-insurance may be a shortsighted way to go unless enrollees are young; older people offer greater risk.

In 1984 surveys by Coopers & Lybrand and by the Wyatt Company showed respectively that 60.9% and 57% of the companies surveyed were self-funding in some degree in health insurance plans. The 1984 figures were about three times as large as those of surveys in 1980.

COSTS OF HEALTH CARE

Mention has been made of the costs of health insurance and other benefits expressed in terms of the average cost per automobile manufactured in the United States. Health cost totals given by officials of various national organizations varied from $362 billion to $600 billion as the health care costs including insurance for the nation in 1984. One computation had the U.S. population spending an average of $12,000 per second in 1984 for health care. Another estimate had fringe benefits totaling $138 per week per worker. Obviously the estimates are based on several different definitions of costs and of benefits, but, whatever the standards, costs are tremendous and are a sizable and growing percentage of the GNP.

COST CONTAINMENT

Blue Cross–Blue Shield and other insurers have attempted to contain costs while maintaining good health protection for subscribers. Some of the efforts have been through

1. Certain copayments and deductibles
2. Reducing inpatient length of stay
3. Adoption of a DRG reimbursement plan for all inpatients
4. Requiring a second opinion on all nonemergency surgery
5. Preadmission procedures for nonemergencies
6. Conducting health education and fitness programs
7. Encouraging outpatient care
8. Setting up one-day surgical centers

9. Early discharges under home health care service
10. Establishing hospice service for the terminally ill
11. Promoting early discharge after normal maternity

COSTS IN RELATION TO REIMBURSEMENTS

The basic issue in reimbursement is allowable costs. No matter whether reimbursement is based on cost, cost plus, contracts on costs, prospective cost agreement, DRGs, or per capita costs, the bottom line for purchaser, provider, or beneficiary is cost—the word of the day.

(The chapter on cost analysis in this book describes various definitions of costs and different methods of computing costs, while DRGs are discussed in an appendix to Chapter 7 on Medicare and Medicaid.)

From the early days of Blue Cross there has been much discussion on what costs were allowable. In fact, in the beginning many Blue Cross plans did not base their payments on cost but paid the actual charges the hospital billed the patient, or paid an agreed upon fixed per diem rate. In 1947 only about 10% of the Blue Cross plans paid on the basis of an average per diem cost. In the 1960s and 1970s the movement was toward paying hospital charges or actual cost of the hospital stay plus 2%—whichever was the lower.

Reimbursement from Blue Cross is changing now from either a cost plus 2% or a charges base. The Blue Cross plans are now moving toward discounted contract day rates and, in a few cases, toward a DRG-type reimbursement. The situation is in flux, with the many options mentioned elsewhere (HMOs, PPOs, IPAs) becoming more and more popular with insurance purchasers, which in turn causes pressure for more creative financing.

A CHANGE IN BLUE CROSS REIMBURSEMENT

In June 1984 the Ohio Insurance Commission approved the merger of Blue Cross of Northeast Ohio and Medical Mutual of Cleveland (Blue Shield). In August 1984 the merged Blue Cross and Blue Shield Mutual of Northern Ohio announced that hospitals in the area would have to bid competitively for a share of the $500 million spent annually by Blue Cross in the region. This was a departure from the cost-plus reimbursement arrangement of the past. In fact, there is question whether the contractual method will survive the courts.

Blue Cross undoubtedly has found a pressure point because the northern Ohio region is overbedded, possibly by as much as 25%. It was estimated that fixed costs to pay for those surplus beds might amount to $130 million a year. Furthermore, not only was the area overbedded, but also in

1983 the average cost of hospital stay in the Cleveland area was $3,811, which compared unfavorably with the national average of $2,875.

With the hospitals in a vulnerable position because of surplus beds, some of them might be tempted to reduce drastically their charges to Blue Cross to help fill empty beds and pay fixed costs. (So the thinking went.)

The annual bidding was instituted originally for three northern Ohio counties with 34 hospitals. At a later date hospitals in eight more counties were to be affected. The bid criteria were drawn up by the Center for Health Policy Studies and made allowances for hospitals serving a large percentage of indigents. Allowances were made also for "medical teaching institutions." The DRG principle was used in determining costs, thus making provision for case mix by diagnosis.

Under the contract terms, all emergency care for Blue Cross–Blue Shield subscribers will be reimbursed no matter where the care takes place. Subscribers who choose to go to a hospital not under contract will be reimbursed 70% of the hospital bill.

In the original bidding in the three Ohio counties with 34 hospitals, the bids of 9 hospitals were rejected—4 of them in Cleveland. The 9 rejected hospitals were further irritated by a Blue Cross advertising campaign that listed the accepted and the rejected hospitals. Two of the rejected hospitals secured a court order to stop the advertising until the Ohio Insurance Commission could review the incident.

At this writing in mid-1985 the matter is in the courts. At least three of the nine rejected hospitals are suing Blue Cross. Lakewood Hospital in April 1985 was awarded $4.5 million in County Common Pleas Court on the basis of an Ohio law that states that the not-for-profit health insurance organization must furnish equal benefits at institutions of the subscriber's choice. Blue Cross stated its intention to appeal. In the meantime the rejected hospitals are laying off some employees and tightening operations in face of possible loss of patients.

NEW SITUATIONS FOR BLUE CROSS–BLUE SHIELD TO MEET

Blue Cross and Blue Shield are affected directly or indirectly by many problems extant or rising. Some of the more evident are as follows.

COVERAGE FOR SENIORS BEYOND MEDIGAP

Medicare beneficiaries are finding that the federal government is paying less than 50% of their health bill, with out-of-pocket expenses still rising.

Some of the Blue Cross plans have signed contracts with the Health Care Financing Administration (HCFA) allowing them to offer to Medicare beneficiaries HMO-IPA plans giving comprehensive coverage at reasonable rates (in some cases about $15 a month more than medigap policies) and with no balance billing or other added costs. HCFA pays the Blue Cross–Blue Shield plan about 95% of the Medicare benefits due in the case, and the monthly senior premium covers the remainder.

There is a free choice of physician (who often works through a contract with an IPA). The doctor accepts full payment from the Blue Cross–Blue Shield plan under a fee schedule with no balance billing. There is no need for the beneficiary to file claim papers or otherwise arrange payment.

In a recent move, the Kansas City Blue Cross–Blue Shield announced a senior plan, Total Health Care 65, which, under contract with HCFA, offers Medicare benefits plus additional coverage for comprehensive care. For Missouri subscribers the premium ranges from $19.96 a month for a female aged 65 to $27.40 a month for a 74-year-old male to $39.40 a month for an 85-year-old or older female or male. Other Blue Cross plans have similar arrangements with comparable rates.

COALITIONS

Coalition is a word being widely used in the health care vocabulary to describe groups of employers and other businessmen who are talking together about methods of joint effort or counsel in combating the rising costs of employer-paid health insurance and other fringe benefits.

This move, brought on by the pressure of rising costs, has had an impact on Blue Cross and other carriers.

PROBLEMS FOR PHYSICIANS

Two problems affecting the physician and, indirectly, Blue Cross–Blue Shield are the large number of medical school students being graduated, and the terrific increase in malpractice insurance premiums, particularly for medical and surgical specialists.

In the 1950s many persons believed there was a growing shortage of physicians in the United States, which would cause a crisis in health care by the 1980s or 1990s. This prompted federal assistance to the medical schools to correct the situation.[7] Existing schools were enlarged and new schools were started, particularly after 1960. Many of the new schools offered clinical experience through community hospitals rather than through university medical centers. The effects of the larger medical student enrollment began to show in the number of graduates in the 1970s. According to the American Medical Association in 1960 there were 7,081 graduates of American medical schools; in 1983 there were 15,728 graduates. This increase does not include the thousands of graduates of foreign medical schools

---

[7]Financial aid came in many forms: research and training grants to teachers, student loans, construction aids, Hill-Burton aid to hospitals affiliated with medical schools.

who came to the United States for clinical education and to open offices and practice medicine. The ratio of doctors of medicine to population in the United States rose from approximately 145 per 100,000 in 1960 to 205 in 1980. Now in the mid-1980s it appears that instead of a crisis in health care due to a shortage of doctors, the country may face a crisis of oversupply, or glut as it is being described by some, in the 1990s.

The AMA Masterfile listed 501,958 physicians in the United States in December 1982, with 408,663 (81.5%) in direct patient care. Female physicians made up 12.8% of the total, foreign medical school graduates 21.4%.

The U.S. Department of Health and Human Services (DHHS) in early 1985 estimated that there were 502,000 physicians in the United States, 26% of whom were linked to hospitals—52% of them on salary, 33% in fee-for-service arrangements.

The oversupply of physicians by the 1990s raises the question of how this will affect physicians' practices and thus affect the third party payers. Will the physician see each patient more often to fill up the appointment schedule? Will he prescribe more treatments in his office than before? Will he increase his fees? Will he be more competitive and cut his fees to benefit from a larger volume of patients?

The second problem affecting physicians and, indirectly, the third parties is the high cost of malpractice insurance. With attorneys offering their services for fees on a contingency basis, malpractice litigation has blossomed. The "injured" patient may think of himself as suing a rich doctor protected by a rich insurance company in front of a sympathetic jury willing to hand down seven-figure damages.

Some insurance companies have increased premiums for malpractice protection 50% or more. In fact, some companies have gone out of the malpractice business. The *New York Times* recently reported premium rates of doctors on Long Island, N.Y. Obstetrics-gynecology specialists had their annual premium rates raised from $54,282 to $82,500; neurosurgeons from $66,468 to $101,100; pediatricians from $10,689 to $16,200. There seems to be a great difference in the premiums in a metropolitan area compared to some of the smaller cities: obstetrics-gynecology rates in Albany, N.Y. were quoted as being $23,394 while in Brooklyn they were $45,000.

Some hospital associations and group practices have established independent insurance companies to try to bring the situation under control. Rising premium rates add to the total costs of health care and affect all parties concerned.

BALANCE BILLING

A physician practice that is costly and irritating to patients and which can be detrimental to the image of the doctors, is balance billing.

Balance billing refers to the charges some physicians make above and beyond the fee schedules set up as customary, usual, and reasonable (CUR) by Blue Shield, insurance companies, and other third parties.

In Massachusetts in the past, Blue Shield paid 95% of CUR fees to physicians. (The other 5% was for administrative costs.) Blue Shield tried to adjust for the percentage of inflation each year but was restrained by a ruling of the Massachusetts insurance commission in 1976.

The result of this restraint was a feeling on the part of physicians that they were being misused, and the ruling led to extended court action by physicians. The legal action seemed favorable until the physicians were stymied by 1984 legislation, signed by Governor Michael S. Dukakis, which allowed Blue Shield to set CUR fee schedules and disallowed balance billing. At this writing, the state medical society is petitioning the U.S. Supreme Court for a hearing on the situation, which the Court so far has refused to review.

Balance billing is not a new practice. Physicians, particularly surgeons, have long felt justified in charging a sum above the amount allowed by insurance companies or other third parties. The practice has seemed arbitrary and greedy to many patients, particularly the poor and elderly. The physician may feel justified in his action, but he is likely to find himself characterized unpleasantly.

PROBLEMS OF INSURANCE

There is a sizable mass of individuals and families who are not properly insured. They include the underinsured, the uninsured, and the uninsurable.

Blue Cross–Blue Shield and commercial insurance companies have tried to correct these conditions whenever possible. To correct one phase of underinsurance, they have issued special policies as previously mentioned to the seniors through contracts with HCFA so that seniors can have comprehensive coverage from HMOs. Comprehensive coverage has become an option for working age persons also.

Unemployed and laid off workers often have lacked insurance. Carriers have lowered rates for the unemployed in some cases. However, if the employer can carry the employee's insurance for only a limited time, the employee is faced with not being able to pay even a lowered premium. In joining the uninsured, the out-of-work have to turn to welfare medicine—Medicaid—for help in time of illness.

The uninsurables often can be covered through a pool of insurance companies.

Under the present system there are unpaid hospital bills. Fortunately most of the unpaid bills are small, under $25,000. Unpaid bills often occur in cases of care of accident victims.

EXTENDED INSURANCE COVERAGE

In the past few years Blue Cross–Blue Shield and other insurance carriers have broadened coverage in several areas. Some of these areas have proved to be more widely used than anticipated, and some have been more expensive than expected. Among treatments newly covered or for which benefits have increased are

1. Drug abuse
2. Alcohol abuse
3. Mental illness
4. Fertilization (in vitro)
5. Organ transplants (full or partial payment—see following pages)

Some insurers have offered lower rates for nonsmokers, people who are not overweight, and persons with blood pressure within the normal range. There may be a problem of monitoring such special classes of insurees.

Some insurers have included coverage of the services of professionals such as psychologists, nurse midwives, and chiropractors. There has been some move to extend maternity benefits to all women enrolled in either family or individual coverage.

TRANSPLANT INSURANCE COVERAGE

Blue Cross–Blue Shield and other insurance carriers are faced with many unknowns in trying to arrange for surgical transplantations of organs in human beings. Although there has been a cautious approach to the situation and some carriers have covered transplants of some organs, it still seems that there are more questions than answers.

The success of some organ transplants is difficult to demonstrate (particularly hearts and artificial hearts). The prospect of a normal life after a transplant operation, especially a heart transplant, does not seem to be predictable.

The range of transplants attempted is wide: kidney, heart, heart and lung, artificial heart, bone marrow, small intestine, skin, liver, pancreas, cornea, and others. The line between experimental surgery and established procedures is sometimes very thin. The question of how to distinguish and authorize capable and experienced surgical teams in the various transplant procedures is arousing ire in the medical world. The need for approving institutions for conducting transplant surgery has offended some large medical centers that have not established a reputation for this kind of surgery. A general Blue Cross–Blue Shield practice seems to be to cover procedures in transplants approved by the FDA.

Other problems in organ transplantation are how to procure organs; how to select patients to receive transplants (age, physical condition, projected life span, and ability to pay); how to encourage potential donors to register for future donations; how to keep the system as fair as possible; and how to keep procurement of organs on a not-for-profit basis.

One aspect of organ transplants is how to meet the costs. Who will pay the $50,000 to $200,000 bill? Some of the insurance carriers, including some Blue Cross–Blue Shield plans, are writing benefits to cover some of these operations for a few dollars a month. Some of the coverage is on a selective basis, covering "established" procedures and not covering experimental procedures, as may be defined by the carrier. This can include preauthorization of the surgery and of the surgery team or institution.

In line with insurance coverage of organ transplants, other problems appear likely. Assume that insurance coverage on most transplant surgery comes within the financial reach of everyone who has health insurance and that certain subscribers do not choose to take transplant coverage. What happens when need arises for transplant surgery for the uninsured person and money for the surgery is not available? This may be the case of an unfortunate person whose life could depend on an operation costing $100,000. On a rare occasion the money might be raised by public subscription, but what if this situation becomes common? Will it be necessary to make mandatory the coverage of organ transplants? Will transplants be covered for Medicaid recipients? Will Medicare beneficiaries be omitted because of age? Will the government have to take a hand to regulate the procedures?

HOSPICE CARE

Many of the Blue Cross plans are offering hospice services for the terminally ill (persons whose life expectancy is six months or less). Much of the care can be performed in the subscriber's home by visiting nurses and hospital-based or community-based home care helpers. Medical supplies and physical therapy, as well as bereavement counseling, are included in the coverage. On some occasions readmissions to hospital for short periods for special procedures are required. Patients seem to prefer being cared for at home whenever possible.

Costs for hospice care have been much lower than hospital inpatient costs. A pilot study in Vermont, reported by Blue Cross–Blue Shield in February 1985, showed an average length of patient participation of 36 days at an average cost of $1,307. This cost figure is probably lower than found in many hospice programs, but it seems safe to say that hospice care is much cheaper than inpatient care in the same community, while being more satisfying to the terminal patient.

WALK-IN HEALTH CARE CENTERS

Walk-in clinics are becoming a new option for emergency care for complaints that might be handled in a physician's office or, in some cases, the emergency room of a hospital. A patient can walk in without an appointment, at any hour of the day or night in many situations, receive treatment, pay a reasonable fee, and be on his way.

It was estimated that there were about 2,300 of these freestanding urgent care centers operating in the United States in 1984, and they grossed about $880 million dollars in revenue. Since the clinics usually operate on a cash or insurance basis, the founders of such centers tend to stay out of the poorer sections.

Since the freestanding clinics have demonstrated their success, the for-profit hospital chains have been attracted to the field. Humana was operating 80 Medfirst clinics in 13 states in 1984 and was planning to expand. National Medical Enterprises, another chain, was operating 18 clinics in early 1985 and expected to have 35 clinics in operation by summer of that year.

All freestanding clinics do not prove to be successful, and some close. However, it would seem likely the total number will grow, with many solvent clinics remaining after the shakedown.

IMAGING, CLINICAL LABORATORY, AND COST CONTAINMENT

Blue Cross–Blue Shield, commercial insurance companies, hospitals and other service providers, physicians, employers supporting group hospitalization, self-insurers, optional delivery systems (HMOs, PPOs, IPAs), outpatient departments and freestanding clinics, the federal government (prospective payment systems, DRGs, tightening of Medicare and Medicaid regulations), hospices, home care, second opinions on nonemergent surgery, and members of the public—these have all contributed to the slowdown of the rise in health care costs in the United States. In spite of all the efforts, the rise is a greater percentage than the rate of inflation.

One of the areas that might offer a field for cost reduction is that of ancillary services, particularly clinical laboratory and radiology services. The clinical laboratory workload has been affected by the practice of so-called defensive medicine. Defensive medicine has come about primarily because of the constant threat of malpractice suits against physicians. The physician is likely to order more tests, more X rays, more images than necessary to demonstrate that he has taken every means of giving his patient the highest quality of care. Defensive medicine is expensive medicine. Proper monitoring is needed to bring utilization into an acceptable and prudent range.

In recent years more sophisticated techniques and equipment are being used by radiologists in addition to X ray, fluoroscopy, sonar, and other more traditional devices. New words and new diagnostic machines have entered the radiology department, such as computerized axial tomography (CAT or CT) and magnetic resonance imaging system (MRIS) or nuclear magnetic resonance (NMR). This equipment is expensive, and the fees for use are high. The first step used in control is to limit the purchase of the expensive technological equipment until sufficient need can be shown. The second control, after the purchase, is to limit use of the equipment until diagnostic need can be demonstrated. (No need for a $600 procedure for a simple headache.)

In June 1984 Blue Cross and Blue Shield Association published "Medical Necessity Guidelines," a pamphlet outlining actions not indicated in several imaging modalities—mostly routine chest X rays. Guidelines for the use of the new, sophisticated imaging devices are no doubt being written now. The need is great to specify "not indicated" when use is superfluous.

TAX ON FRINGE BENEFITS

At the present time Congress is trying to reform the tax structure of the United States. Among the many possible reforms suggested is the need to be fair about fringe benefits. The argument used has been that if a worker makes $1,000 in wages he pays income tax on that amount. If a worker receives $1,000 in fringe benefits, including health insurance, he pays nothing. The call is to be fair. If wages are taxed, fringe benefits should be also, say the advocates of fairness in taxing.

Some in Congress are trying to find a middle road that will recognize the principle but temper the tax. For example, a compromise might be reached whereby amounts of premiums for health care insurance paid by the employer which exceed $175 per month per family or $70 a month for the individual would be taxable as income of the employee.

Another more likely tax would be on any return of employer-paid premiums or bonuses to employees for nonuse of health services during a period. This money paid the employee for nonuse could be considered income for the employee and subject to tax.

The insurance industry is likely to oppose strongly a tax on any kind of insurance premium paid by the employer. There seems to be little chance that fringe benefits will be taxed.

THE FUTURE

The future of Blue Cross–Blue Shield and health care delivery is discussed in the final chapter of this book. Needless to say, the authors look for a great influx of change and restructuring in the years ahead.

SUGGESTED READINGS

Anderson, Odin W. *Blue Cross Since 1929: Accountability and Public Trust.*

Anderson, Odin W. *Health Services in the United States: A Growth Enterprise Since 1875.*

Blue Cross Association–American Hospital Association. *Financing Health Care of the Aged.*

Rorem, C. Rufus. *Origins of Blue Cross.*

Rorem, C. Rufus. *Private Group Clinics.*

Rorem, C. Rufus. *A Quest for Certainty: Essays on Health Care Economics, 1930–1970.*

Somers, Herman M. and Somers, Anne R. *Doctors, Patients and Health Insurance.*

Weeks, Lewis E. (ed.). *Odin W. Anderson: In First Person, An Oral History.*

Weeks, Lewis E. (ed.). *George Bugbee: In First Person, An Oral History.*

Weeks, Lewis E. (ed.). *Robert M. Cunningham, Jr.: In First Person, An Oral History.*

Weeks, Lewis E. (ed.). *James Hague: In First Person, An Oral History.*

Weeks, Lewis E. (ed.). *Walter J. McNerney: In First Person, An Oral History.*

Weeks, Lewis E. (ed.). *John R. Mannix: In First Person, An Oral History.*

Weeks, Lewis E. (ed.). *Maurice J. Norby: In First Person, An Oral History.*

Weeks, Lewis E. (ed.). *James R. Neely: In First Person, An Oral History.*

Weeks, Lewis E. (ed.). *Daniel Pettengill: In First Person, An Oral History.*

Weeks, Lewis E. (ed.). *C. Rufus Rorem: In First Person, An Oral History.*

Weeks, Lewis E. (ed.). *Robert Sigmond: In First Person, An Oral History.*

Weeks, Lewis E. (ed.). *Kenneth Williamson: In First Person, An Oral History.*

Weeks, Lewis E. and Berman, Howard J. *Shapers of American Health Care Policy: An Oral History.*

Wirick, Grover. *Hospital Use and Characteristics of Michigan Blue Cross Subscribers: An Analytical Interview Survey.*

7

Medicare and Medicaid

M Day was July 1, 1966. This was a day of great social adjustment in the United States. It was the day that health service benefits were initiated by the federal government under Medicare and Medicaid, otherwise known as Title XVIII and Title XIX of the Social Security Act.

Medicare and Medicaid together made more impact on the way we live in the United States than any other piece of social legislation since the original Social Security Act passed in the mid-1930s during the administration of Franklin D. Roosevelt. In fact, Medicare and Medicaid have direct ties to the Roosevelt administration and every administration since then. Some kind of plan for a national health insurance or service has been conceptualized, introduced as a bill into Congress, or at least stated as a goal in some politician's campaign during every administration since the thirties. President Lyndon B. Johnson chose to honor the efforts of former President Harry S. Truman to have health insurance legislation passed in Congress by flying to Independence, Missouri, so that he could sign the bill that made Medicare and Medicaid into law in the presence of Mr. Truman.

Medicare and Medicaid are compromises between several divergent views of what the benefits under such plans should be, and how the plans should be financed and administered. The compromises have made administration difficult, but it is better to have compromises than no plan, or no benefits. It would seem that U.S. Representative Wilbur D. Mills (D., Ark.), chairman of the House Ways and Means Committee in 1965, thought this way also, for he is credited with bringing about a meeting of minds through compromise. A stalemate over health legislation had existed for years, caused by the differing positions of various Congressmen, the American Medical

Association, the American Hospital Association, the Blue Cross Association, trade unions, business associations, and other special interest groups.

Medicare helps pay for two kinds of service for persons 65 years of age or over: Part A (HI) is insurance for hospital care and related services; and Part B is insurance to help pay doctors' bills for service in or out of the hospital, and for other related services. This Part B insurance is also known as the Supplementary Medical Insurance Program (SMI).

Medicaid provides help at the state level for the medically indigent (persons unable to pay for medical care even though they may be able to defray other ordinary living expenses). There is no age limit for Medicaid recipients; the only test is need. Many of the so-called welfare medical cases, including the blind, the disabled, and crippled children, come under Medicaid.

Although Medicaid has been the source of help for the medically indigent at the state level since the SSA Amendments went into effect in 1966, there were other changes made under the SSA Amendments of 1972 (Public Law 92–603) which further affected certain of those persons:

1. Persons under 65 who have been receiving disability benefits under Social Security for at least 24 consecutive months are now eligible for hospital insurance under Medicare Part A and also may enroll in the medical insurance program, Part B.

2. Widows, 50 or over, who were eligible for disability benefits for two years or more but did not file a disability claim because they were getting Social Security checks as mothers caring for young or disabled children, are eligible for Part A hospital insurance and may enroll in the Part B medical insurance program.

3. Persons under 65 who need hemodialysis or renal transplantation for chronic renal disease are eligible for hospital insurance under Medicare Part A and may enroll for Part B medical insurance, if they meet certain work requirements under Social Security, or are receiving Social Security benefits, or are the spouses or dependent minor children of such individuals. Eligibility for coverage begins with the first day of the third month after the month in which a course of renal dialysis begins and continues through the twelfth month after the month in which dialysis terminates, or 36 months following the month of a kidney transplant. If the transplant fails, or if after the 36 months the person needs maintenance dialysis or a new transplant, Medicare coverage can be reinstated without a waiting period.

MEDICARE (PART A) HOSPITAL INSURANCE

The fact that Medicare is structured in two parts illustrates the compromise effected by Congress. Part A helps pay for hospital care, extended care, and home health service for persons 65 years of age or older who are registered under Medicare. Part A is financed by a special percentage assessment added to the Social Security payroll deduction of employees, and to the SSA contributions of employers and the self-employed. The general fund of the federal government makes up any deficit.[1] However, there is an annual review of costs so that adjustments can be made in coinsurance ratios, if needed. The coinsurance arrangements call for the beneficiary to pay a part of the cost and for Medicare to pay the remainder. Claims are handled through an intermediary or fiscal agent for the government. This agent usually is the local Blue Cross plan acting under a subcontract with the Blue Cross Association, or an insurance company.

The structure of Part A of Medicare satisfied the exponents of financing by payroll deduction through the Social Security Administration with supplements from the federal government when needed. Part A was also designed to meet the demands of those who favored coinsurance. The extensive claims facilities of Blue Cross and major commercial insurance companies were also needed.

The SSA Amendments of 1972 made provision for persons aged 65 and over who previously were not eligible for Medicare hospital insurance to secure such coverage on a voluntary basis by agreeing to pay a monthly hospital insurance premium and also by agreeing to enroll for Part B Medicare medical insurance. The basic premium as of July 1, 1973 for hospital insurance under this voluntary provision was $33 a month. By January 1, 1986 the basic premium for a person 65 years of age had risen to $214 a month.

MEDICARE (PART A) BENEFITS

Three kinds of facility are the major sources of service benefits for Medicare Part A recipients: care in the hospital; care in a skilled nursing facility after a hospital stay; or services from a home health care agency to bed patients who are at home after a stay in a hospital or a skilled nursing facility[2] (see Table 7.2). For changes in hospital insurance copayments see

---

[1]Table 7.1 gives a profile of the increase in contributions since 1966. Both percentage of contribution rate and annual earnings base are likely to be increased in the future.

[2]A change in title was made by using "skilled nursing facility" to replace "extended care facility" under the SSA amendments of 1972. See section on skilled nursing facilities, pages 172–73.

TABLE 7.1   Contribution Ratio for Medicare Hospital Insurance
                 (HI) Part A

Beginning	Annual Earnings Base	Contribution Rate (%) Employee and Employer, each	Maximum Contribution each
1966	$ 6,600	0.35	$ 23.10
1967	6,600	0.5	33.00
1968	7,800	0.6	46.80
1969	7,800	0.6	46.80
1970	7,800	0.6	46.80
1971	7,800	0.6	46.80
1972	9,000	0.6	54.00
1973	10,800	1.0	108.00
1974	12,000	1.0	120.00
1975	14,100	1.0	141.00
1976	15,300	1.0	153.00
1977	16,500	1.0	165.00
1978	17,700	1.0	177.00
1979	22,900	1.05	240.45
1980	25,900	1.05	271.95
1981	29,700	1.30	386.10
1982	32,400	1.30	421.20
1983	35,700	1.30	464.10
1984	37,800	1.30	491.40
1985	39,600	1.35	534.60
1986	42,000	1.45	609.00

Source: Social Security Administration.

Table 7.3; for changes in supplementary medical insurance premiums see
Table 7.4.

Benefits are governed by benefit periods. A Medicare benefit period
begins the first time that a person registered under Medicare enters a hospital as a bed patient and ends whenever he has not been in a hospital or
in a facility offering skilled nursing care for 60 days in a row. The key to
understanding the benefit period is the 60-day interval necessary between
the end of one benefit period and the beginning of another.

TABLE 7.2 Medicare and Medicaid: Benefits, Financing, and Coinsurance

	Persons Covered	Benefits (Services)	Benefits (Length)	Methods of Financing	Coinsurance Costs
MEDICARE A	Aged 65 or older who are registered with SSA. Also exceptions for certain disabled.	Certain services from hospitals, SNFs, and home health agencies.	Hospitals: 90 days in each benefit period. SNFs: 100 days of care in each benefit period. Home health nurse or therapist: 100 visits within one year after hospital or SNF stay.	Primarily by Social Security tax of 1.45% of first $42,000 annual earnings (1986) each by employee and employer.	Hospital: recipient pays first $492, and from 61st to 90th days pays $123 a day. Lifetime reserve: recipient pays $246 a day. SNF: recipient pays $61.50 a day from 21st through 100th day. Home health care: if recipient qualifies under Medicare A, 100 home visits, after discharge from hospital or participating SNF are fully paid by Medicare.
MEDICARE B	Aged 65 or older who are registered with SSA for Supplementary Medical Insurance.	Certain services from physicians, hospital outpatient departments, and home health agencies.	Services during a calendar year.	By a monthly premium paid by the recipient and an equal amount by the federal government. Premiums can be raised as SSA benefits are raised. Premium in 1986 was $15.50 per month per person.	Recipient pays first $75 cost of a calendar year.
MEDICAID	Medically indigent, as needed.	Hospital services as inpatient or outpatient, laboratory tests, X rays, physicians' services, home health care visits.	Year	Shared federal and state program.	None

TABLE 7.3   Hospital Insurance (HI) Copayments for First
                 Amounts and for 61st through 90th day of
                 Hospitalization per Benefit Period

		Pay First	From 61st to 90th Day Pay per Day	Lifetime Reserve Days Pay per Day
Prior to 1969		$ 40	$ 10	$ 20
Beginning January	1969	44	11	22
	1970	52	13	26
	1971	60	15	30
	1972	68	17	34
	1973	72	18	36
	1974	84	21	42
	1975	92	23	46
	1976	104	26	52
	1977	124	31	62
	1978	144	36	72
	1979	160	40	80
	1980	180	45	90
	1981	204	51	102
	1982	260	65	130
	1983	304	76	152
	1984	356	89	178
	1985	400	100	200
	1986	492	123	246

Source: Social Security Administration.

PART A HOSPITAL BENEFITS

These benefits provide for care in a semiprivate room (two to four beds in a room) with all meals, including special diets, for up to 90 days in a benefit period. Other hospital care expenses included under coinsurance are

1. Drugs furnished by the hospital

2. Laboratory tests

3. Nursing services (regular but including special care units)[3]

4. Medical supplies such as splints and casts

---

[3]Items not paid for under Part A coinsurance include private duty nurses, extra charge for a private room unless patient needs it for a medical reason, telephone, radio, television, or physicians' services (covered under Part B).

TABLE 7.4   Supplementary Medical
                       Insurance (SMI) Premiums

Prior to April 1, 1968	$ 3.00	a month
Beginning April 1, 1968	4.00	
July 1, 1970	5.30	
July 1, 1971	5.60	
July 1, 1972	5.80	
July 1, 1973	6.30	
July 1, 1974	6.70	
July 1, 1976	7.20	
July 1, 1977	7.70	
July 1, 1978	8.20	
July 1, 1979	8.70	
July 1, 1980	9.60	
July 1, 1981	11.00*	
July 1, 1982	12.20	
January 1, 1984	14.60	
January 1, 1985	15.50	
January 1, 1986	15.50	

Source: Social Security Administration.

*Future increases in premiums will be possible only in per-
centage ratio to general increases of Social Security benefits.

5. Operating room and recovery room costs

6. X-ray and other radiological services including radiation therapy,
   billed by the hospital

7. Use of appliances and equipment furnished by the hospital, such
   as wheelchair, crutches, and braces

8. Rehabilitation services, such as physical therapy, occupational
   therapy, and speech pathology services

9. Care in a participating psychiatric hospital for not more than 190
   days in a lifetime

10. Blood (except for nonreplacement fees for the first three pints)

PART A HOSPITAL COINSURANCE PAYMENT

Coinsurance requirements in force January 1986[4] were the following:
For the first 60 days in the hospital a bed patient registered under Medicare
Part A pays the first $492 of the hospital bill, and for the 61st through the

[4]Periodic adjustments have been necessary in the coinsurance percentages and dollar
amounts because of rising costs.

90th days pays $123 a day.[5] Medicare pays all other covered charges. The initial $492 is paid only once in a benefit period, even if the patient is in the hospital several times.[6]

PART A SKILLED NURSING FACILITY (SNF) BENEFITS

These benefits apply to beneficiaries who become bed patients in the SNF (after leaving a hospital) for up to 100 days in each benefit period. The benefits include care in a semiprivate room (two to four beds in a room) with all meals and, if needed, special diets. Other expenses covered with coinsurance provisions include

1. Drugs furnished by the SNF
2. Regular nursing service
3. Physical, occupational, and speech therapy
4. Medical supplies such as splints and casts
5. Medical social services
6. Use of appliances and equipment furnished by the SNF, such as wheelchair, crutches, and braces[7]

CONDITIONS NECESSARY FOR A PATIENT TO QUALIFY FOR PART A SNF CARE BENEFITS

These conditions include

1. Medical needs requiring continuing nursing care
2. A physician determining that a patient needs SNF care, ordering such care, and certifying that patient receives that care
3. The patient having been in a participating or qualified hospital for at least three days in a row before admission to SNF
4. Patient being admitted to the SNF within 30 days of leaving the hospital
5. Patient being admitted to SNF for further treatment of condition treated in hospital

---

[5]Besides the 90 days of hospital care allowed per benefit period, there is also a "lifetime reserve" of 60 days available to Medicare patients. If a Medicare patient needs to use more than 90 hospital days during one benefit period he may use some of his lifetime reserve days. Medicare pays all covered charges, except $246 per day for lifetime reserve days used. There is another special rule that limits benefits: a beneficiary has a lifetime limit of 190 hospital days in a psychiatric hospital.

[6]The Social Security Administration keeps a record of benefit days for the beneficiary.

[7]Expenses not covered in the SNF include private duty nursing, extra charge for a private room unless the patient needs it for a medical reason, telephone, radio, television, and physicians' services (covered under Part B).

6. Utilization review organization or PRO of the facility not disapproving the stay

Two new qualifying factors under the 1972 SSA Amendments affected extended care benefits: advance approval of extended care and home health benefits; and modification of the transfer requirement for extended care benefits.

As of January 1, 1973 the secretary of HEW was authorized to establish minimum periods during which beneficiaries would be presumed to be eligible and payment could be made for extended care or home health benefits after hospitalization. Medical conditions, length of stay, or number of visits are the basis for the regulations. The attending physician is required to certify that the condition is one designated in the regulations and to furnish a plan of treatment prior to or at the time of the admission or the first visit under home health service. Certifications and patient stays are subject to review.

A waiver in the requirement that a patient is entitled to extended care benefits only if he is transferred to an SNF within 30 days of discharge from a hospital is possible

1. If appropriate bed space is unavailable in the geographic area during the 30-day period.

2. In cases where skilled nursing care or rehabilitative services cannot be utilized within the 30-day period due to the patient's medical condition. For example, after a fracture, physical therapy or restorative nursing might not be indicated within the regular period after hospital discharge. Therefore, transfer to an SNF should be made at a medically appropriate time.

COINSURANCE PROVISIONS FOR CARE IN A SKILLED NURSING FACILITY

These provisions call for the beneficiary to pay $61.50 per day for care from the 21st day through the 100th day.

PART A HOME HEALTH BENEFITS

These benefits can include certain services furnished to the patient in his home by a participating home health agency.[8]

1. Part-time nursing care

2. Physical therapy and speech therapy

---

[8]Medicare does not pay as a home health benefit the expenses of full-time nursing care, drugs and biologicals, blood transfusions, personal comfort or convenience items, or meals delivered to the home.

If the patient needs part-time skilled nursing care, physical therapy, or speech therapy, Medicare can also pay for

3. Part-time services of home aides
4. Medical social work
5. Medical supplies furnished by the agency
6. Durable medical equipment (80% of approved cost)

Up to 100 visits by the nurse, therapist, or other persons supplying service are allowed within a year after the most recent discharge from a hospital or a participating SNF.

CONDITIONS NECESSARY TO QUALIFY FOR PART A HOME HEALTH BENEFITS

The following four conditions must all be met before Medicare can pay for home health visits:

1. Needed care includes part-time skilled nursing care, physical therapy, or speech therapy.
2. The patient is confined to his home.
3. A doctor determines the patient's home health care needs and sets up a home health care plan.
4. The home health agency providing services is participating in Medicare.

HOSPICE CARE

Hospice care is a mode of care for terminally ill patients which has been effective in bringing comfort and relief to patients whose expected life is six months or less. The care generally is given in the home surroundings by the hospice provider, which can be connected with a hospital or can be a separate agency.

Medicare defines a hospice as "a public agency or private organization that is primarily engaged in providing pain relief, symptom management, and supportive services to terminally ill people and their families."

Exceptions to home care are made when inpatient hospital care is medically necessary or when respite care is needed. Respite care has been described by Medicare as a short-term inpatient stay which may be necessary to give temporary relief to the person who regularly assists with the home care. Inpatient respite care is limited each time to stays of not more than five days in a row. Medicare hospital insurance can help pay for hospice care if all of the following conditions are met:

1. A doctor certifies that a patient is terminally ill.
2. A patient chooses to receive care from a hospice instead of standard Medicare benefits for the terminal illness.
3. Care is provided by a Medicare-certified hospice program.

PART A HOSPICE BENEFITS

Medicare hospital insurance can pay for the following hospice services:

1. Nursing services
2. Doctors' services
3. Drugs, including outpatient drugs for pain relief and symptom management
4. Physical therapy, occupational therapy, and speech-language pathology services
5. Home health aide and homemaker services
6. Medical social work
7. Medical supplies and appliances
8. Short-term inpatient care, including respite care
9. Counseling

There are no deductibles or copayments in hospice care except for part of the cost of outpatient drugs and inpatient respite care as described below.

Medicare hospital insurance cannot pay for the following services:

1. Treatment other than for pain relief and symptom management of the terminal illness
2. Five percent of the cost of outpatients drugs or $5.00 per prescription, whichever is less
3. Five percent of the cost of respite care, up to a total of $400 (1985 figure)

MEDICARE (PART B) MEDICAL INSURANCE

Part B is the medical insurance section of Medicare designed to help pay for doctors' services, outpatient services, medical services and supplies outside the hospital coverage, and those home health services not covered in Part A. Part B is financed by a monthly insurance premium, $15.50 per month per person during 1986,[9] paid by the Medicare beneficiary and an

---

[9]Higher rates must be paid by those beneficiaries who did not enroll within the first year of eligibility after becoming 65 years of age. The rate is about 10% higher after the first year, about 20% higher after the second, and about 30% higher after the third.

amount contributed by the federal government.[10] The premium rate has been reviewed each year in December or before, and a new rate has been set to become effective in January of the following year. This system was established to ensure that costs could be met by contributions of the beneficiaries and the government. Under the SSA Amendments of 1972, however, beneficiary premiums for medical insurance cannot be increased unless there has been a general Social Security benefit increase since the current premium rate was established, and the percentage of premium increase cannot exceed the percentage of the general Social Security increase.

The contribution method of financing for Part B Medicare illustrates another of the compromises effected between differing views in health insurance proposals to the Congress. Part B also has provisions for coinsurance and for a nongovernment fiscal agent to act as the "carrier" or intermediary agent. Usually, the carrier is a Blue Shield plan or an insurance company handling claims for a state or a large area of a state. Both the coinsurance and nongovernment carrier provisions could be called compromises.

The SSA Amendments of 1972 made provision to avoid levying penalties due to neglect of eligible persons to enroll in Part B (SMI) insurance. Beneficiaries receiving monthly SSA or Railroad Retirement benefits prior to age 65 are now deemed to have enrolled in SMI the month before the month they are entitled to Part A hospital insurance (HI). Those who have not previously received benefits will be deemed to have enrolled likewise before the HI entitlement. Disability beneficiaries will be deemed to have enrolled in the 24th consecutive month of receiving benefits. However, an individual can decline SMI if he wishes. The requirement that beneficiaries enroll within three years of initial eligibility or reenroll within three years of termination has been eliminated. There was no change made in the provision that only one reenrollment is permitted after a termination, or in the approximately 10% increase in the basic premium for each 12 months one could have been, but was not, enrolled.

PART B COINSURANCE

Part B requires the beneficiary to pay the first $75[11] (1985 rate) in rea-

---

[10]The Part B insurance premium is deducted from the monthly checks of those who receive Social Security benefits, Railroad Retirement benefits, or Civil Service annuities. Those who do not receive such checks pay their premiums directly to Social Security, or their premiums are paid by a state social agency (Medicaid).

[11]The provision that the first $75 Part B expense in a calendar year is deducted from benefits is modified by a special carry-over rule that covers the last three months of the year. Any Part B expenses incurred in the last three months of the calendar year that can be counted toward the $75 deductible for that year can also be counted toward the $75 annual deductible for the next calendar year.

sonable charges[12] in a calendar year. After the first $75 expense, Medicare Part B insurance will pay 80% of all reasonable charges for the rest of the year.

MEDICARE (PART B) BENEFITS

Benefits for Part B expenses are paid in either of two ways: (1) payment can be made to the doctor or supplier, or (2) the payment can be made directly to the beneficiary.

Under method (1) the doctor or supplier agrees to apply for the medical insurance payment at a rate not to exceed the reasonable charge set by the carrier. The beneficiary is responsible for any of the $75 deductible not met that year and for the 20% coinsurance of the amount above the $75 deductible. (This is called the assignment method.)

Under method (2), after the proper forms have been signed by the doctor or supplier, the beneficiary can apply for direct payment. In turn, he can pay his doctor or supplier for services rendered.

There is a time limit for filing claims for Part B Medicare benefits: services received in the fourth quarter of year 1 and services received in the first three quarters of year 2 must be filed before the end of year 3. For example, claims for services received between October 1, 1984 and September 30, 1985 must be filed by December 31, 1986.

PART B—DOCTORS' SERVICES COVERED[13]

Medicare Part B benefits cover

1. Medical and surgical services including anesthesia by a doctor of medicine or osteopathy.
2. Certain medical and surgical services by a dentist (see following section).
3. Chiropractic by licensed and Medicare-certified chiropractors, limited to manual manipulation of the spine to correct a subluxation.

---

[12]"Reasonable charges" for covered services are set by the carrier after taking into account the customary charges of the doctor or other supplier of services and after considering, as well, the customary charges made by other doctors or suppliers for that service in the community.

[13]Services not covered include routine physical check-ups; routine foot care, eye refraction and examinations for prescribing, fitting, or changing eyeglasses; hearing examinations for prescribing, fitting, or changing hearing aids; immunizations (except pneumococcal vaccinations); those of certain practitioners such as Christian Science practitioners and naturopaths. Some health care services and supplies are not generally accepted by the health community as being reasonable or necessary for diagnosis of treatment. These include acupuncture, histamine therapy, and various kinds of medical equipment.

4. Services of a licensed podiatrist including the removal of plantar warts. Treatment of mycotic toenails is limited to once every 60 days unless more frequent care is ordered by the patient's physician. Routine foot care (hygienic care, flat feet and other structural misalignment, removal of corns, calluses, and most warts) is not covered unless a medical condition affecting the lower limbs (such as severe diabetes) requires such care to be performed by a podiatrist or a doctor of medicine or osteopathy.

5. Other services ordinarily furnished by the doctor's office and included in his bill, such as: diagnostic tests and procedures; medical supplies; services of the office nurse; drugs and biologicals that cannot be self-administered; transfusions of blood and blood components; and physical therapy and speech pathology services.

6. Services by radiologists and pathologists to hospital inpatients will be paid 100% of reasonable charges.

7. Doctors' services for outpatient treatment of a mental illness will be paid to the extent of no more than $250 in any one year.

PART B—DENTAL SERVICES COVERED[14]

The medical insurance of Part B covers services of dentists only when surgery of the jaw or related structures, or setting of fractures of the jaw or facial bones is involved.

PART B—LABORATORY AND RADIOLOGY SERVICES BY DOCTORS FOR HOSPITAL INPATIENTS

Medicare Part B insurance pays 100% of all reasonable charges by doctors for radiology and pathology services for Part B inpatient beneficiaries in a participating or otherwise qualified hospital. Since these fully paid expenses for the services of radiologists and pathologists are an exception to the coinsurance feature of Part B insurance, these expenses cannot be counted toward the $75 deductible.

PART B—INDEPENDENT LABORATORY SERVICES

Medicare medical insurance can pay the full approved fee for covered diagnostic tests provided by independent laboratories that accept Medicare assignment. The laboratory must be certified by Medicare for the services received.

---

[14]Medical insurance of Medicare Part B does not pay for dental services such as filling, removal, replacement, or other care of the teeth, or for the treatment of gum areas, or surgery or other services related to these kinds of dental care.

PART B—AMBULANCE SERVICE COVERED

Medicare medical insurance will help pay for ambulance transportation of a Part B beneficiary by an approved ambulance to a hospital or a skilled nursing facility only when

1. The ambulance and its equipment and personnel meet Medicare requirements.
2. Transportation by other means would endanger the patient's health.
3. The patient is taken to a facility serving the locality or the nearest facility equipped to take care of the patient.

PART B—OUTPATIENT HOSPITAL BENEFITS

The following are outpatient hospital services that Part B medical insurance helps pay for:[15]

1. Laboratory and other diagnostic services billed by the hospital
2. X-ray and other radiology services billed by the hospital
3. Emergency room or outpatient clinic services
4. Medical supplies, such as splints and casts
5. Drugs and biologicals that cannot be self-administered
6. Blood (except for the first three pints)

Under the 1972 SSA Amendments, covered speech therapy services may now be provided to inpatients of hospitals and SNFs under Part B Medicare medical insurance as outpatient services if the patients have exhausted their inpatient days or are otherwise not entitled to hospital insurance Part A.

PART B—OUTPATIENT PHYSICAL THERAPY AND SPEECH PATHOLOGY SERVICES

Physical therapy services are covered when they are furnished by a qualified hospital, SNF, home health agency, clinic, rehabilitation agency, or public health agency, and they are furnished under a plan established and periodically reviewed by a physician. One may receive physical therapy or speech pathology services as part of treatment in a doctor's office. Services may also be received directly from a Medicare-certified physical therapist in the office or in the patient's home if the treatment is prescribed

---

[15]Part B medical insurance does not help pay for tests given in a routine check-up, eye refractions and examinations, immunizations (except pneumococcal vaccinations or immunizations required because of an injury or immediate risk of infection), routine foot care, or hearing examinations for hearing aids.

by a doctor (the maximum amount medical insurance can pay is $80 in a year).

A hospital or an SNF may now provide covered outpatient physical therapy or speech pathology services under Medicare Part B medical insurance to its own inpatients if they have exhausted their inpatient days under Medicare Part A or are otherwise not entitled to Part A coverage of these services.

PART B—HOME HEALTH BENEFITS

Under Part A the Medicare hospital insurance helps pay for home health benefits after a stay in a hospital and/or a skilled nursing facility. Part B covers home health care without the necessity of the beneficiary previously having been a bed patient of a hospital or an SNF in the same benefit period.[16]

PART B—OTHER MEDICAL SERVICES AND SUPPLIES

When any of the services listed below are furnished by a participating hospital, a skilled nursing facility, or a home health agency, that institution will file a claim with the carrier and will also bill the patient for his share under the coinsurance arrangement. Among the services Part B medical insurance helps pay for are[17]

1. Diagnostic X-ray and laboratory tests furnished by approved independent laboratories
2. Radiation therapy[18]
3. Portable diagnostic X-ray services in the home under a physician's supervision
4. Surgical dressings, splints, casts, and similar devices
5. Rental or purchase of durable medical equipment prescribed by a physician for use in the home (wheelchair, hospital bed, oxygen equipment
6. Services (other than dental) to replace all or part of an internal body organ (included are corrective lenses after a cataract operation)
7. Certain ambulance services

---

[16]Home health services not paid for under Part B include full-time nursing, drugs and biologicals, personal comfort or convenience items, noncovered levels of care, and meals delivered to the home.

[17]Part B insurance does not pay for prescription drugs and drugs that are self-administered (insulin, for example), for hearing aids, eyeglasses, false teeth, orthopedic shoes, or other supportive devices for the feet.

[18]Medical insurance will help pay for these items in cases where Part A hospital insurance cannot pay.

MEDICARE (PART A) AND THE HOSPITAL

For the Medicare program the federal government sets standards of certification and conditions for participation for the suppliers of institutional services, established procedures for reimbursement of the suppliers, specified that fiscal intermediaries[19] be selected for processing Part A Medicare claims, and set up a nongovernment council of health and financial experts to act in an advisory capacity.[20]

Under the law it is required that state or local health agencies (or other appropriate agencies) be used to certify that institutional providers of care and independent laboratories meet conditions for participation set by the federal government. The costs for this initial survey and for periodic rechecking are paid by Medicare. The details of the certification process and the conditions for participation are discussed in a section that follows.

Reimbursements for covered services provided by hospitals, skilled nursing facilities, and home health agencies under Part A are based on reasonable costs. Acceptable cost-finding methods, allowable costs, and reporting methods for this reimbursement are discussed later in the chapter.

The intermediaries for Part A providers (hospitals, skilled nursing facilities, and home health agencies) were originally nominated by groups of those institutions for consideration and judged for approval by the Social Security Administration. The intermediaries were chosen by SSA for the ability to act as a claims agent and payer of claims and also on the ability to furnish consultative services on cost-finding and accounting procedures so that the Part A providers will receive equitable payments for services rendered. However, if the provider chooses it may deal directly with SSA.

At the beginning of the Medicare program, the American Hospital Association nominated the Blue Cross Association as fiscal intermediary of its member hospitals. (A few of the member hospitals, however, chose other intermediaries.) Blue Cross was chosen by about 91% of the hospitals, 54% of the SNFs, and 78% of the home health agencies.[21] The next largest group

---

[19]The fiscal agents for medical insurance claims under Part B, called carriers, have somewhat wider responsibility than fiscal intermediaries of Part A. Carriers must be experienced in the health field to the degree that they are competent not only to accept and pay claims, but also that they can determine whether a provider's charge is reasonable, whether it is his customary charge for the service, and how it compares with customary charges in the community for like services. The carriers at the beginning of Medicare consisted of 33 Blue Shield plans, 15 commercial insurance companies, and 1 independent health insurer. These carriers served the 64 geographic regions into which the country was divided. Group prepayment plans are reimbursed on a reasonable cost basis directly by the Social Security Administration.

[20]The advisory body was called the Health Insurance Benefits Advisory Council (HIBAC). It was composed of nongovernment health and financial experts who advised the SSA on general policy for both Medicare and Medicaid.

[21]Myers, Robert J., *Medicare*, p. 179.

of intermediaries was of commercial insurance companies. A few other health organizations were chosen as intermediaries; a small percentage of providers chose to deal directly with SSA.

CERTIFICATION OF HOSPITALS (PART A)

The requirements of the Joint Commission on Accreditation of Hospitals (JCAH) or of the American Osteopathic Association (AOA) for approval of hospitals are generally accepted as satisfying conditions for participating hospitals under Title XVIII unless a state or region imposes higher restrictions for purchases of services. In practice, a state agency determines eligibility or ineligibility of an institution to participate in the Medicare program. The state agency certifies that the hospital

1. Is accredited by JCAH or AOA
2. Has established a utilization review plan meeting the requirements of the act and that the plan is in effect, or will be in effect, the first day of the hospital's participation
3. Has met the statutory requirements of the act, or if certain deficiencies with respect to one or more conditions of participation have been found, that reasonable plans have been made to correct the deficiencies; and, despite the deficiencies, adequate care is being given, without hazard to the health and safety of the patients

Certification of a hospital by the state agency (acting under agreement with the secretary of HEW, now HHS) as being in substantial compliance will be for a period of two years. A list of deficiencies of standards will be noted, and whether the deficiencies create a serious hazard to health and safety, and whether the hospital is making reasonable plans and efforts to correct the deficiencies within a reasonable period. Notice of eligibility or ineligibility for participation made by the secretary on the basis of the state agency certification will be sent to the institution being considered by the SSA.

In like manner, the state agency will certify that an institution is not in compliance or is no longer in compliance. If on the basis of the state agency's certification of noncompliance or no longer in compliance the participation agreement is terminated, the hospital can request that the determination be reviewed.

Special certification can be allowed in isolated regions where the denial of certification would seriously limit the accessibility of beneficiaries to hospitals. The special certification can be allowed only if the deficiencies noted do not place the health and safety of patients in jeopardy. Resurveys are required annually for specially certified institutions.

Another exception to general rules allows payments to be made for emergency services in nonparticipating hospitals under special conditions.

Under the SSA Amendments of 1972, a new mechanism for continued validation of the voluntary accreditation process was set up. The secretary of HEW was authorized to enter into an agreement with any state to have the state certification agency survey hospitals accredited by JCAH on a selective sample basis, or a specific hospital on the basis of substantial allegations and evidence of a condition adverse to health and safety. If a survey institution is found to have significant deficiencies relative to Medicare health and safety standards, the institution may be terminated from participation in the program. An institution certified on the basis of JCAH accreditation must agree to authorize JCAH to release to the secretary of HHS a copy of the most current JCAH accreditation survey if the institution is included in a certification survey.

CONDITIONS FOR PARTICIPATION OF HOSPITALS, PART A

The conditions outlined for participation of the providers of services under Part A represent good organization and good practice. The conditions for participation of hospitals have been chosen for detailed description and discussion, but the same careful controls seem to have been used for all providers. An administrator could use Medicare conditions of participation guidelines as rules of practice.

The conditions for participation of hospitals under Title XVIII include

Compliance with State and Local Laws. The participating hospital must meet all laws of licensure and standards; staff must be registered and licensed in conformity to laws; the hospital must operate in compliance with laws relating to fire and safety, to communicable and reportable diseases, to post-mortems, and to other relevant matters.

The Governing Body of the Hospital. This body (or the legal body responsible for the conduct of the hospital) must be operated generally as follows:

1. Under a set of written bylaws which stipulate the selection, term of office, and duties and requirements of the members and which specify to whom responsibilities for the operation and maintenance of the hospital are delegated.

2. The governing body shall have regular meetings to plan for and evaluate the operation of the hospital and the care of patients.

3. There shall be a committee structure consistent with the size and scope of the hospital. Principal among these committees should be: an executive committee to coordinate the activities and the general policies of the various hospital departments and of the special committees established by the governing board; a finance committee;

a joint conference committee to act as a liaison with the medical staff; and a building and maintenance committee.

4. The governing body appoints members of the medical staff. This staff in turn works under written bylaws, rules, and regulations that outline procedures for submission and processing of staff applications and definitions of physicians' privileges.

5. The governing body appoints a qualified hospital administrator or executive officer, preferably one with formal training in a graduate program of hospital administration approved by the Association of University Programs in Health Administration. The administrator is to act as executive officer of the governing body in the management of the hospital and in providing liaison among the governing body, medical staff, nursing staff, and other departments of the hospital.

6. The governing body must establish a policy requiring: every patient to be under care of a physician; a patient to be admitted to the hospital only on the recommendation of a physician; that a physician is on duty or on call at all times and available within 15 or 20 minutes at the most.

7. The governing body is responsible for providing a physical plant staffed and equipped to provide services needed for patients.

The Physical Environment. Buildings should be constructed and maintained to assure safety and well-being of the patients as required by state laws and codes. Factors to be considered are facilities for the physical separation of isolation patients and for handling contaminated linens; at least 100 square feet floor space for a private room and 80 square feet area per patient in multiple rooms; facilities for emergency power, lighting, gas, and water; regular inspection and cleaning of all intake sources; proper waste disposal facilities; and generally good housekeeping. Fire control standards should be rigid and enforced. A sanitary environment should be maintained by an infection committee and by infection control procedures. Also, the hospital should provide adequate diagnostic and therapeutic facilities to permit an acceptable level of patient care.

The Medical Staff. The staff, organized under bylaws approved by the governing body, should be responsible to that body for the quality of medical care provided patients of the hospital. The staff should work through a committee structure to carry out the policies of both the medical staff and the hospital. There should be enforced disciplinary procedures for infractions of hospital and medical policies.

The medical staff should attempt to secure autopsies in all cases of unusual deaths and of medico-legal interest and education. A minimum of 20% of all terminal cases should be autopsied.

Standards should be set for consultations with qualified physicians under conditions where: the patient is not a good medical or surgical risk; the diagnosis is obscure; there is doubt as to the best therapeutic measures; or there is question of criminal action. The consultation should include an examination of the patient and a written and signed opinion to be included in the patient's medical record.

Medical staff appointments should be made by the governing board, with reappointments made periodically after reappraisal of the members' competence and character.[22] The staff membership or professional privileges should not be granted solely on certification, fellowship, or membership of a specialty body or society.

The active medical staff of the hospital performs the organizational duties of the medical staff: maintains proper quality of medical care in the hospital; adopts rules and regulations for governing the medical staff (with the approval of the governing body); elects its officers (or recommends appointments to the governing body if called for in bylaws); makes recommendations to the governing body about appointments to the staff and grants of medical staff privileges; and makes recommendations to the governing body about matters of concern to the medical staff.

Other staff categories, which may be supplemental to the active staff but which in no way reduce the responsibility of the active staff, include

1. The honorary staff is usually composed of former active staff members, retired or emeritus, or other distinguished physicians the hospital desires to honor.

2. The consulting staff is usually composed of recognized specialists serving in consulting capacity rather than as admitting or attending physicians.

3. The associate staff category usually includes the members who use the hospital infrequently or who are less experienced or who are going through a period of probation before an appointment to the active staff.

4. The courtesy staff members are usually those who want to attend patients in the hospital, but, for some reason, not disqualifying, are ineligible for appointment in another category of the staff.

The medical staff officers are usually elected by and from the active staff members (unless in rare situations, the officers are appointed by the governing board or by some other means).

The chief of staff as chief executive officer of the staff has the following responsibilities:

---

[22]Appointments are made after consideration of recommendations of the credentials committee and of the medical staff voting membership.

1. To organize and administer the medical staff in accordance with terms of the staff bylaws and the rules and regulations
2. To act in coordination and cooperation with the hospital administrator in all medico-administrative matters to carry out the policies adopted by the governing body
3. To be responsible for the careful supervision over all clinical work in all departments of the hospital

Medical Staff Bylaws and Rules and Regulations. These regulations which have been adopted to enable the medical staff to carry out its responsibilities include

1. A descriptive outline of the medical staff organization
2. A statement of qualifications of physicians necessary for staff membership, and the duties and privileges of each category of membership
3. A procedure for granting and withdrawing privileges of physicians
4. A method of appeal from decisions affecting staff membership or privileges
5. A specific statement forbidding the splitting of fees
6. A provision for regular meeting of the medical staff
7. Provisions for the keeping of complete and accurate clinical records
8. A provision making the physician in charge of a surgical patient responsible for seeing that all tissue removed at an operation is delivered to the hospital pathologist, and that a routine examination and report are made at that time
9. A rule permitting a surgical operation only on the consent of the patient or a legal representative, except in emergencies
10. A statement providing that consultations be required except in emergencies
11. A regulation requiring all physicians' orders to be recorded and signed
12. If dentists and oral surgeons are to be accorded staff membership, necessary qualifications, privileges, and rights of this group must be stated in the bylaws

Medical Staff Committees. Certain committee functions are required. In a small hospital the medical staff might work as a committee of the whole, but an organization structure with at least two or three major committees would be preferred. Those major committees would probably include

1. An executive committee to coordinate the activities of the medical staff, receive and act upon reports of other committees of the staff, and represent the staff as a whole where this is indicated

2. A credentials committee to review applications for appointments and reappointments to the medical staff and make recommendations to the executive committee on those applications and on the staff privileges connected with them

3. A joint conference committee composed of members of the governing body and medical and administrative staffs (the committee acts as a liaison among those groups)

4. A medical records committee composed of staff members representative of a cross section of the clinical services of the hospital to supervise the maintenance of the medical records system

5. A tissue committee to review and evaluate all surgery done in the hospital on the basis of agreement or disagreement among the preoperative, postoperative, and pathological diagnoses and on the acceptability of the procedures followed

6. A utilization review committee composed of staff members representative of the clinical services to evaluate the quality of patient care under a regular utilization review plan

Medical staff meetings should be held at frequent and regular intervals to "review, analyze, and evaluate" the work of the medical staff members. In addition, where the size of the hospital makes it feasible (all except the small general hospital of 75 beds or less), the medical staff should be organized in clinical services headed by a chief of service. The chief should be responsible for the administration of the clinical service and the quality of care given patients there.

The Nursing Department. The hospital must have an organized nursing department with a licensed registered professional nurse on duty at all times and with professional nursing service available for all patients at all times. Standards are given for supervisory personnel and for working relationships with physicians and with other departments of the hospital. Written nursing care procedures and written nursing care plans for patients are required as are constant review and evaluation of nursing care provided patients.

The Dietary Department. An organized dietary department under the direction of a qualified dietitian is required. Standards are set for written procedures, facilities, food storage, and therapeutic diets. Provision is made for contract food service from an outside management company as long as standards of trained personnel and other requirements are met.

Medical Records Department.   A medical record must be maintained for every patient admitted for care in the hospital. Standards are given for the necessary contents of the record, its completion, its indexing and filing, and its preservation.

Pharmacy or Drug Room.   The hospital must have a pharmacy under the direction of a registered pharmacist or a drug room under proper supervision. Standards are given for facilities, personnel, records to be kept, control of dangerous and toxic drugs, and a pharmacy and therapeutic committee to set standards and controls for drugs dispensed.

Laboratories.   The hospital should have a well-organized and adequately supervised clinical laboratory to perform those services commensurate with the hospital's needs. Anatomical pathology services and blood bank services should be available in the hospital or by arrangement with other facilities.

Medical Library.   The library should contain modern textbooks and current periodicals relative to the clinical services offered by the hospital. The library should be easily accessible and available at all times to the medical and nursing staff.

Complementary Departments.   Standards are listed for departments or services of surgery, anesthesia, dentistry, and rehabilitation as to effective policies and procedures relating to the staff and the functions of the services to assure health and safety of the patients.

Outpatient Department.   For hospitals that have outpatient departments there are stated effective policies and procedures relating to the staff, the functions of the service, the facilities, and outpatient medical records.

Emergency Service or Department.   The hospital must at least be prepared to take care of an occasional emergency case even though the hospital does not have an organized emergency service. For the hospital with an organized service, there are effective policies and procedures relating to the staff, the functions of the service, the medical records kept for the emergency room, and the facilities deemed adequate.

Social Work Department.   This department is not a requisite for participation in Medicare Part A. If such a department is in a participating hospital, standards are given for its organization, direction, personnel, and necessary records.

Utilization Review Plan.   The participating hospital is to have a plan for utilization review which applies at least to services furnished by the hospital to inpatients who are beneficiaries under Title XVIII. An acceptable plan would review utilization on a sample basis (or another plan) of admissions, duration of stays, and professional services furnished. Also under the plan there must be provisions for a review of each case of continuous extended duration. Under section 238 of the 1972 SSA Amendments, if the utilization review committee of a hospital or skilled nursing facility in its sample or other review of admissions finds a case in which inpatient care is no longer medically necessary, Medicare payment will be cut off three days after notice of the committee finding.

REIMBURSEMENT TO HOSPITAL PROVIDERS — PART A

Historically, the reimbursement to hospitals for services provided Medicare Part A beneficiaries is based on reasonable costs. The formula for reimbursement based on reasonable costs was established after extended consultations and on the advice of leading health organizations and individuals such as: American Hospital Association; American Nursing Home Association; American Association of Hospital Accountants (now Healthcare Financial Management Association); Blue Cross Association and local plans; Health Insurance Association of America and private insurance firms; the former Health Insurance Benefits Advisory Council (HIBAC); and many hospital administrators and comptrollers.

The experience of third party payers such as the Blue Cross plans and various state and federal agencies was studied. The cost-based programs particularly were examined, and the AHA's "Principles of Payment for Hospital Care" was used as a guideline in considering allowable costs.

The objective of the reasonable cost reimbursement formula to providers of hospital care under Medicare Part A included

1. To make the payments to providers as current as possible

2. To make retroactive adjustments to cover increases in costs as they occur

3. In making reimbursements, to take into account the percentage of total patients who are 65 years of age or older, to account also for the difference in rate of utilization and in length of stay in hospital for patients 65 and over

4. To have flexibility at the beginning of participation to allow for the differences in record keeping among hospitals

5. To attempt to accord equitable treatment to profit and nonprofit providers

6. To recognize the needs of institutions to keep abreast of developments in the health sciences and the healing arts[23]

---

[23]At the beginning of Medicare a 2% "plus factor" was allowed for keeping abreast of developments and for other contingencies. This was dropped a year or two later.

Two methods of apportioning costs have been used in the past. One was based on Medicare beneficiaries' share of total charges figured by individual departments; the second was a combination based on average cost per day for room, board, and routine nursing charges plus the beneficiaries' share of the total charges of nonroutine and ancillary services. The methods will be discussed more fully in later paragraphs.

Payments, as stated, were to be kept as current as possible. A system was established of making interim payments at intervals of no less than once a month, with the payments based on estimates of costs. (This voluntary payment plan is sometimes referred to as "periodic interim payment" or PIP.) In most cases experience with other third party payers had given an accounting basis for estimates of cost. A retroactive adjustment was scheduled for the end of each accounting period.

Annual costs reports and other financial data are required of hospital providers under Part A. Definitions, statistics, and reporting and accounting practices are those standard for the hospital field.

Authority to place a limitation on provider costs to be recognized as reasonable under Medicare was given to the secretary of HEW under the 1972 SSA Amendments. The limitation is based on comparisons of the costs of covered services by various classes of provider in the same geographic area. Providers of services are allowed to charge beneficiaries for the unreimbursed costs of services in excess of, or more expensive than, services necessary for the efficient delivery of needed health services. (The exception to this rule would be cases in which the physician who admitted the patient had a financial interest in the facility.) The provider would be required to notify the beneficiary of the charges for expensive or luxury services prior to admission. One overriding provision was that SSA would always pay the lesser of costs or charges.

PRINCIPLES FOR SPECIFIC REIMBURSABLE COSTS

One of the key points stressed in Chapter 4 was that the debatable areas of cost were areas critical to the operation of a solvent hospital. Considerable space was given to consideration of items such as depreciation, bad debts, education, and research. The position of the AHA, both early and current attitudes, was examined in detail. The same critical area must be considered again, this time from the standpoint of health insurance for the aged as it affects providers of hospital care. The federal government also has a set of principles on this gray area of debatable costs. Each of them will be considered briefly.

Depreciation. An allowance for depreciation as a cost is given when it is based on historical cost or on market value at time of donation for donated items. The method of computation can be: straight line; double declining balance; or sum-of-years digits. However, accelerated depreciation is no longer allowed on new assets, is limited to 150% of straight line when allowed, and is allowed only when it is proved necessary to supply the capital account. Medicare allows depreciation and interest expense on capital planning for amounts over $100,000 only when approved by an area planning agency. One favorable ruling is the allowance of depreciation on assets being used by the provider at the time it enters the program, even if already wholly or partially depreciated on the provider's books.

Interest Expense. The Medicare principle is that necessary and proper interest on current indebtedness is an allowable cost. Interest on loans that result in surplus funds or on loans not reasonably related to patient care would not be considered allowable cost. Interest expense to be an allowable cost would first be reduced by the amount of interest earned on investments, except for interest earned on gifts and grants, restricted or not restricted, but held separate and not commingled with other funds. Although depreciation funding is not required, it is encouraged by the provision that interest earned on the invested depreciation fund is not deducted from the interest that is considered an allowable cost.

Bad Debts, Charity, and Courtesy Allowances. All three of these items are considered deductions from revenue and cannot be included in allowable costs. One exception is made regarding bad debts. If beneficiaries under Medicare fail to pay the deductible and coinsurance amounts they have incurred, those amounts can be included by the provider in the Medicare program's share of costs after reasonable collection efforts have been made.

Educational Costs. An appropriate part of the net cost of educational activities is an allowable cost. The appropriate part, of course, is the Medicare program's share according to the reimbursement formula chosen. The educational activities include medical, osteopathic, dental, and podiatric internships and residency programs, other recognized professional and para-medical educational training programs either licensed by the state or conducted by professional and technical societies and associations, and approved by the Social Security Administration. The "net" educational cost refers to the stipends of trainees, teacher salaries, and other costs less any reimbursements from grants, tuition, or directed donations.

Research Costs. Costs incurred for research purposes "over and above usual patient care" are not considered allowable costs. This ruling is based on the fact that federal research grants and funds from foundations and private donors are sufficient to finance most research. However, the provider is allowed to include expenses of studies, surveys, and analyses necessary to the provider's administrative and program needs.

Grants, Gifts, and Income from Endowments. Unrestricted grants, gifts, and income from endowments should not be deducted from operating costs in computing costs under the reimbursement formula. However, if the grants, gifts, or income from endowments have been designated by the donor for paying specific operating costs, then those amounts should be deducted from the specific costs or category of costs.

Value of Voluntary Services. The principle covering voluntary services is similar to that of other third party cost reimbursement plans. The provider that has sisters or other members of a religious order working in the hospital in positions necessary to normal patient care can include as an allowable cost for each of these volunteers an amount equal to that a lay employee of like training would earn in the community. The donated services of other individual volunteer workers cannot be included.

Purchase Discounts, Allowances, and Refunds of Expenses. All discounts, allowances, and refunds of expenses are reductions in the cost of goods or services purchased and are not income.

Compensation of Owners. In proprietary institutions the owner can be compensated for necessary duties at a rate comparable to that paid by comparable institutions. In addition, Medicare allows the owners of an institution a reasonable return on their investment.

Cost to Related Organizations. The principle relating to this point is stated: "Costs applicable to services, facilities, and supplies furnished to the provider by organizations related to the provider by common ownership or control are includable in the allowable cost of the provider at the cost to the related organization. However, such cost must not exceed the price of comparable services, facilities, or supplies that could be purchased elsewhere."

Plus Factor. As mentioned previously, a plus factor of 2% originally was allowed to cover contingencies, but later was dropped.

Differential on Nursing Wages. Formerly an 8.5% differential in nursing costs was allowed to compensate for the added care needed by Medicare patients. This has been discontinued.

THE SKILLED NURSING FACILITY

The SSA Amendments of 1972 made provisions for using the term "skilled nursing facility" to replace the terms "extended care facility" used previously under Medicare (Title XVIII) and "skilled nursing home" used under Medicaid (Title XIX).

Care requirements of a skilled nursing facility were defined in a U.S. government announcement of the 1972 SSA Amendments as:

> A single common definition of care requirements for extended care services under Medicare and skilled nursing services under Medicaid is established as follows: Skilled nursing care provided directly by or requiring the supervision of skilled nursing personnel, or other skilled rehabilitation services, which the patient needs on a daily basis, and which as a practical matter can be provided only in a skilled nursing facility on an inpatient basis. The Medicare requirement that extended care services must be a continuation of treatment for a condition treated in a hospital is retained.

For Medicare patients this covers two classes of patient who may not have been covered before:

1. The patient who needs a variety of unskilled services on a regular daily basis, if the planning and overseeing of the aggregate of the unskilled services requires regular daily involvement of skilled personnel.

2. The patient who is in regular need of skilled rehabilitation services (other than nursing) which are essential to his recovery after a hospital stay or to prevent his condition from worsening, and which as a practical matter should be provided in a skilled nursing facility.

A facility meeting the definition of skilled nursing facility (SNF) can participate in both Medicare and Medicaid provided it agrees to terms of participation. The definition of a skilled nursing facility is basically the former Medicare definition plus new provisions for submission of information on ownership, for adherence to certain fire and safety codes, for independent medical evaluation and audit of patients and patients' need for skilled nursing care, and for certain institutional planning requirements. The secretary of HHS under present Medicare arrangements with state agencies will certify SNFs requesting participation in both Medicare and Medicaid. State agencies will continue to certify SNFs requesting participation in Medicaid only.

The secretary is authorized also to waive the requirement for a registered nurse on one full shift seven days a week in certain rural areas where RNs are in short supply. Those rural institutions caught in shortage of help situations may be allowed to operate on a 40-hour-per-week five-day coverage if the physician certifies patients can be without registered nurses for 48 hours, or if physicians or other nurses can cover the institution when patients need skilled help during the regular nurse's days away. Furthermore, the 1972 SSA Amendments say that SNFs cannot be required to provide medical social services as a condition of participation in either Medicaid or Medicare.

A further ruling affecting SNFs is one that authorizes state certifying agencies, subject to the approval of the secretary of HHS to provide such specialized consultative services to a skilled nursing facility as the facility may request and need to meet one or more conditions of participation.

MEDICARE CHANGES UNDER THE TAX EQUITY AND FISCAL RESPONSIBILITY ACT OF 1982 (TEFRA), PL 97–248

The Tax Equity and Fiscal Responsibility Act of 1982 (PL 97–248) will have some of the most far-reaching effects on the Medicare program of any legislation since the original act passed in 1965. One could point to the 1972 Social Security Amendments as having an important effect on Medicare but must note that they affected benefits and services, while PL 97–248 has a notable impact on providers, particularly on hospital payment.

There were predictions for several years that something would have to be done about Medicare costs and utilization. By as early as mid-1967 observers knew that Medicare was on a troubled course. In the beginning the best actuaries and analysts had underestimated the cost and utilization of Medicare—by at least 50%. However, that original underestimate was only part of the problem. Medicare was in what is popularly called a cost spiral, a whirlwind of runaway costs and utilization. Many experts could explain it, but could not explain it away. Medicare demands continued to grow in an absolute sense and as an increasing proportion of the total service load provided by hospitals. For example, Medicare patients accounted for 20% of the total inpatient hospital care in 1970, and 29% in 1980—a 45% increase in proportion.

This increased use of hospital services by the aged population can be partially explained away by the steady increase in the ratio of the aged in our population. There may have also been an increased or growing expectation for health services among the aged which would be difficult to estimate.

The increase in the number of aged and their higher utilization rate do not account for the entire increase in Medicare costs. There are many other causes, which are discussed below.

Labor costs in hospitals are up sharply. This is partly due to the fact that for years hospital employees were paid much less than similar workers outside hospitals. Hospital employees have been catching up. As a special case, nurses have benefited from a competetive labor market because they have been in short supply. Concurrently (and possibly because of the nurse shortage), the technician sector of the hospital labor force has increased in ratio to others. Another factor in higher labor costs is that the ratio of full-time equivalent employees to patients has grown 4% or 5% a year, thus doubling in the past decade. Unionization, which usually brings higher labor costs, has been growing among hospital service employees. As a whole, increasing wages, labor shortages, personnel upgrading, and higher ratio of employees to patients have had a significant effect on labor costs for hospital care, including that of Medicare patients.

Inflation in the cost of all kinds of wages, services, and supplies has affected costs in the hospital field.

Growth in technology has added to overall costs involving expensive equipment and the specialized personnel needed to operate it.

Any manager could itemize a long list of other cost factors that have been a part of the cost spiral in his institution.

The above helps explain that the 1982 legislation was an attempt to slow down rising health care costs, which have surged above the inflation rate of the national economy and are representing a larger percentage of the GNP each year.

In fact, it has been remarked that in the past 15 years there have been only two periods when the rate of increase in health care costs declined. One was under the stopgap Economic Stabilization Program of the Nixon years. The other was the Voluntary Effort fostered by the American Hospital Association and the American Medical Association. The Economic Stabilization Program could have no permanent effect because it was an artificial barrier designed to give a temporary respite. The Voluntary Effort was a valiant attempt but, because it was voluntary, it had limited long-term control that could be wielded from the top. It had to depend on the goodwill of managers who were working against overwhelming forces.

The 1982 legislation is a new approach to reimbursement in which payment is on the basis of cost of hospital stay (operating cost per stay) rather than cost per day or total annual cost. There may be enough of a difference between cost per case and cost per day to alert the manager to the better possibilities of sharing in any savings on costs in the cost per case method over the cost per day method. The incentives have been changed by focusing on the case and allowing a sharing of the savings. With these new incentives, will hospitals respond?

PAYMENT PLANS

Two methods are presented in the 1982 legislation for computing operating costs per case: the individual hospital's target method and the average cost of groups of hospitals under Section 223 rules. Under the plan a hospital would be paid a maximum of either its individual target or the Section 223 limit, whichever had the lower operating cost per case—which translates into the observation that never would the payment for reimbursement ever be more than the Section 223 group hospital payment formula.

The individual hospital target method is based on the hospital's his-

torical operating cost for routine and special units and for ancillary services
(excluding capital and teaching costs) per Medicare case for the last fiscal
year ending before October 1, 1982. Each year any increase due to inflation
is adjusted by using the HCFA market basket index as a base and by adding
a 1% factor to adjust for possible expenses due to technological advances.
(The adjustment for inflation for FY 1983 is estimated at 6.9% plus 1% for
technology.)

The formula used to compute the individual hospital base limit cost
per case is to take the total of allowable inpatient Medicare costs for the
last base year and divide that total by the number of Medicare discharges
for that base year. This gives an average cost per case for Medicare patients
for the last base year. To that average cost per case then add any HCFA
market basket index adjustment for the new base year.

The group hospital method is used to compute the average cost per
case of all hospitals in standard metropolitan statistical areas (SMSAs) and
all rural hospitals over 50 beds for inpatient Medicare care under Section
223 limits. The average Medicare cost per case is determined by dividing
total allowable costs by the number of Medicare discharges in the group of
hospitals for the past fiscal year (in the beginning, FY 1982). Under the
group hospital method the average cost per case for FY 1983 was considered 120% of the FY 1982 average; 115% for FY 1984; and 110% for FY 1985.
Thereafter the average base rate (110% of FY 1982) will be used. Under the
group hospital method some adjustments may be made for differences in
hospital case mix (disproportionate numbers of Medicare and Medicaid
patients, for example), for regional variations in wage rates, for psychiatric
hospitals, or for unusual educational costs.

Calculation of payments is made under the following format:

Step one. The first step is to compare the hospital's actual average cost
per case to the average cost per case limits set in the group hospital method.
If the hospital's actual average cost per case equals or exceeds the limit set
under the group method, then the group method will apply. If the hospital's
actual average cost per case *does not* equal or exceed the limit set under
the group hospital method, then the individual hospital target method applies, as set forth in step two.

Step two. To repeat, if the actual average hospital cost per case does
not equal or exceed the limits set under the group hospital method, then
payment is calculated against the limits of the individual hospital target
method.

Rewards and penalties. If the hospital is reimbursed under the group
hospital method, it is paid a maximum of only the group hospital cost per
case (mentioned again for emphasis), regardless of what the actual costs are.
Any cost in excess of the limit must be absorbed by the hospital.

If the hospital is reimbursed under the individual hospital target limit and is able to hold its costs below the target limit, it shares 50% in the savings, as long as the hospital's share of savings is not over 5% of the target amount. If the hospital's average cost per case exceeded the target limit under the individual hospital method in fiscal years 1983 and 1984, the hospital had to absorb 75% of any cost above the target limit. Since FY 1985, the hospital must absorb all costs in excess of the target limit.

OTHER CHANGES IN MEDICARE

Several other important changes were made in the 1982 legislation. These are summarized below.

Assistants in surgery are not paid under the act if the hospital has an approved medical training program or if a qualified member of the house staff is available. Assistants in surgery are paid if an assistant's services are required because of exceptional medical circumstances or because the assistant is part of a team performing a complex procedure (Sec. 113).

Audits and medical claims. In addition to any other funds that were appropriated, $45 million per year was provided for the fiscal years 1983 through 1985 to intermediaries and carriers for provider cost audits and reviews of medical necessity. The monies came from the Medicare Part A trust fund (Federal Hospital Insurance Trust Fund) and the Part B trust fund (Federal Supplementary Medical Insurance Trust Fund) (Sec. 118).

Contracted services. Providers are not to be paid for the cost of services contracts that are based on a percentage of charges, revenues, or claims. Contracts for physician services to patients are not affected generally. (Also see *Radiologists and pathologists* below.) Likewise, customary commercial business contracts are not affected if they are reasonable or provide incentives for providers to be efficient and economical.

It would seem that this disallowance would apply to monies paid to management contracts, employees, consultants, or others unless it could be shown that the contract was a standard business contract. (An example would be paying a standard percentage commission in a real estate transaction) (Sec. 109).

Diagnosis-related groups (DRGs). One of the measurements for hospital case mix that probably will be a regular method of adjustment (by indexing hospitals) in the new Medicare payment plans is the DRG concept. The Health Care Financing Administration (HCFA) has already made an extensive study of the DRG classification of Medicare patients, although critics have said that severity of illness has not been factored into the classification. On the basis of the HCFA study the DRG classification has been proposed to Congress as a formula accommodating the difference in the kinds of patients in hospitals, the different conditions in hospitals in various regions of the country—metropolitan versus rural, small hospitals versus tertiary care hospitals. Special consideration will be given long-term, pediatric, and psychiatric hospitals.

Elderly workers, aged 65 to 69 years, may choose between Medicare coverage and employer-furnished health insurance coverage. There is some question about how employers will react in hiring practices (Sec. 116).

Health maintenance organizations. Medicare beneficiaries may enroll in HMOs, with the federal government paying a premium on the basis of a formula involving per capita cost of health care in the area. This is a refinement of an existing condition (Sec. 114).

Hill-Burton charity cases. Hospitals that have received grants under Hill-Burton in the past have been expected to do some charity work as part of their program. Medicare has taken the position that this Hill-Burton charity work was not an allowable cost. It stated this position in PL 97–248, but whether or not that position will prove tenable will depend on the outcome of several suits in which hospitals are trying to justify this charitable work as an allowable cost based on arguments that there is a financing cost or a capital cost that is beyond the generally considered "charitable" cost (Sec. 106).

Home health agencies. A slight change in wording in the Social Security Act establishes a single payment limit—based on cost experience of freestanding home health agencies—for hospital-based and freestanding home health agencies alike. (In the past the hospital-based cost was higher (Sec. 105).)

Hospice service is available to terminally ill Medicare patients with expected life of six months or less, for two 90-day periods and an additional 30-day period as needed. This experimental program provides physical therapy, occupational therapy, speech therapy, medical social services, home health aide services, medical supplies, physician services, short-term inpatient care, and counseling for the terminal individual. Copayments for respite services and prescription drugs have been set at 5% (Sec. 122).

Ineffective drugs. In the 1982 law Congress prohibited payments under Medicare and Medicaid for "less than effective" prescription drugs. These are drugs that the Food and Drug Administration declares to be ineffective in limiting the problems related to them (Sec. 115).

Interest charges on overpayments and underpayments. Often in the Medicare cost settlement process, after the cost report is audited, the provider pays or receives a difference between the amount of payment received and the final settlement amount after audit. Any payment due either to the provider or to Medicare is subject to interest after 30 days, according to a rate of interest paid under a Federal Hospital Insurance Trust Fund formula (Sec. 117).

Medicare coverage of federal employees is a part of the new law and made them subject to Social Security Hospital Insurance Tax effective January 1, 1983. This changed the situation in which federal employees in the past could work for a short time in the private sector after being retired from a federal job and become fully eligible for Medicare coverage (Sec. 121).

Medicare Part B premiums cannot annually be increased more than the percentage of increase in Social Security benefits for that year. The premium rate for January 1, 1986 was $15.50 a month in contrast to the original rate of $3.00 in 1966 (Sec. 124).

Merchant seamen had free health care under the Public Health Service until that care was discontinued in 1981. Some of the seamen were qualified to enroll under Medicare Part B but failed to do so before a penalty period. PL 97–248 provided an open enrollment period from October 1, 1982 through December 31, 1982 with a period of coverage retroactive to October 31, 1981 (Sec. 125).

Nursing differential. The nursing salary cost differential (5% to hospitals, 8.5% to nursing homes) has been eliminated by Congress (Sec. 103).

Overhead payments in outpatient clinics. An amendment has been made in the wording of the Social Security Act in an attempt to eliminate a double charge for overhead when a physician serves a patient on hospital premises for which overhead has already been charged (Sec. 104).

Periodic interim payments (PIP) to hospitals in FY 1983 and FY 1984 were delayed three weeks to shift, for federal fiscal accounting and reporting, some of the expense to the following year (Sec. 120).

Private room subsidy. In the past the Medicare program has reimbursed hospitals and skilled nursing facilities for routine care on the basis of average cost of all rooms (private or semiprivate), including depreciation, interest, and other greater costs of private rooms. This private room subsidy was eliminated effective October 31, 1982 (Sec. 111).

Provider-based physician services in hospitals and skilled nursing facilities will be reimbursed on the basis of reasonable charges under Medicare Part B only if the services are professional medical services personally rendered by the physician for an individual patient and contribute to the diagnosis or treatment of an individual patient. (This is meant to differentiate services rendered to an individual patient from services rendered to the general benefit of patients in a hospital or an SNF.)

Professional standards review organizations (PSROs). This program has been repealed, but a similar but smaller organization for utilization review will replace it. (See *Utilization and quality control peer review organizations* below.)

Radiologists and pathologists. Their reimbursement rate under Medicare will be reduced from 100% of reasonable cost to 80%, the same percentage as other physicians are paid. The 20% portion of Medicare not paid cannot be charged off to bad debts (Sec. 112).

Skilled nursing facilities (SNFs). The new law removes the requirement for three days of prior hospitalization of the beneficiary before admission to an SNF (Sec. 123).

Union organizing activities. According to the new legislation, the expense of opposition to unionization on the part of hospitals will not be considered a reimbursable cost under Medicare (Sec. 107).

Utilization and quality control peer review organizations (PROs). The 1982 law, PL 97–248, effectively ended PSROs as they had existed since the 1972 Amendments. However, existing PSROs continued until the secretary of HHS could organize the new PROs based preferably in state areas, although some regional and local organizations proved possible also.

HHS negotiates two-year performance contracts with not-for-profit and for-profit PROs. No contracts are made with hospitals or hospital affiliates, although subcontracts may be permitted. There were no contracts with intermediaries or insurance companies for the first 12 months.

If more than one group is available for contract, preference is given to groups of physicians.

MEDICAID CHANGES

Under the new law states are allowed to charge Medicaid patients for almost any services, as of FY 1983. This can include charges for routine services and laboratory tests. Family planning services will be exempt from charges as will be care for children under 18 and for pregnant women.

States will be allowed to place liens on the homes of poor nursing home residents receiving Medicaid. Such a lien cannot be collected until after the death of the recipient. If there is a surviving spouse or a minor child living at home, the lien cannot be collected while that spouse or minor child is there. Also, the state will be allowed to deny Medicaid services to those who transfer ownership of a home for less than market value.

Medicaid will pay for home care for children if it is not more expensive than institutional care.

POSSIBLE MANAGEMENT ADJUSTMENTS

Managers of hospitals are faced with a test of skill in adjusting to meet the financial restraints of the new Medicare/Medicaid legislation. This in many cases will undoubtedly lead to

1. Tighter control of staffing schedules
2. Reexamining services offered and the scheduling of those services
3. A hard look at the diagnostic and treatment procedures
4. A critical review of admission and discharge practices

5. Revamping reporting and data systems
6. Developing better management and performance measurements
7. Reexamining shared and contract services in place or in potential
8. A full use of the new utilization review program

Of great importance is the need to involve physicians of the medical staff and the hospital trustees in meeting the challenge of the new legislation. Physicians order admissions, care, ancillary services, and patient discharges. Thus physicians have great control over the financial condition of the hospital. Physicians should be made aware of the legislation and the problems it has caused—and of their need to participate in solving or mitigating those problems. The members of the board of trustees should also be drawn into meeting the challenge by assessing in a realistic way the health care needs of the community and the possible options the hospital has for meeting those needs.

TRENDS

It appears that the new law, PL 97–248, is the first step in what may become a series of revisions in Medicare and Medicaid. The secretary of the Department of Health and Human Services sent a plan for prospective payment for consideration by Congress in 1983. There were also some hints from HHS and from Congress that following 1982, the year of the hospital, would be 1983, the year of the physician. The year 1983 was not the year of the physician in terms of increased regulation. Many expect the physician to come under stricter regulation in the near future.

Greater copayments for Medicare A have been suggested because the federal contribution to Medicare A far exceeds the 50% planned originally.

The new legislation provided for the group hospital base rate to reach a plateau in FY 1985 of 110% as far as allowing an overrun of the current base rate without penalty. The individual hospital target rate and the sharing of savings expired in 1985, so only the group hospital 110% formula remained.

The unanswered question: can hospitals generally operate efficiently enough to remain viable under the cost-of-stay formula?

MEDICARE PROSPECTIVE PRICING, PL 98–21

The costs for providing inpatient hospital care to Medicare beneficiaries have risen explosively with little or no control since the Medicare program began in 1966. In fact, the trust fund for Part A hospital care is in danger of being depleted within a few years.

The first year of Medicare ended in mid-1967 with a cost of about

$3 billion; in 1982 it was $33 billion. In the period 1979 to 1982 the average cost of a day of hospital care increased annually almost 18%; Medicare expenditures for hospital care rose at an annual rate of 19%. In 1982 hospital costs increased by 15.5%, or three times the rate of the inflation in the economy as a whole (*Federal Register,* January 3, 1984). Not only was there an increase in hospital costs generally but there was also a percentage increase of Medicare patients among the hospital inpatient total.

Several methods have been used to try to find an equitable means of paying for provider services. One of the principal methods used was retrospective reimbursement based on reasonable costs. Then the Tax Equity and Fiscal Responsibility Act of 1982 (TEFRA) PL 97–248 was enacted.

Basically TEFRA called for reimbursement based on an average cost per case for Medicare inpatients. The plan is described in foregoing pages of this chapter. In the legislation there was a requirement that the secretary of Health and Human Services develop, in consultation with the Senate Finance Committee and the House Ways and Means Committee, a legislative proposal for Medicare payments to hospitals, skilled nursing facilities, and other providers on a prospective basis, thus offering a predictable payment for services.

As required under 1972 legislation, the Health Care Financing Administration, a division of the Department of Health and Human Services, did conduct research and demonstrations of methods of payment to providers of care for those enrolled under Medicare. One of the purposes was to constrain costs.

One of the methods of payment investigated was what is now called the diagnosis-related groups method. This DRG approach was a product of extensive research by a team at Yale University. The researchers studied patients in a national sample of 332 hospitals. Records of over 1.4 million patients were classified by diagnosis and related clinical information including principal diagnosis, secondary diagnosis, surgical procedures carried out, age, sex, and discharge status. The diagnoses were first classified in 23 major diagnostic categories (MDC). Later these were more broadly classified.

The information developed at Yale University was used during a demonstration with New Jersey hospitals. There, 356 categories of DRGs were used. The New Jersey demonstration was not labeled successful or unsuccessful, but it did furnish needed experience for the Medicare DRG prospective payment plan.

The Yale University and New Jersey research was the experiential basis for PL 98–21 which was enacted and became commonly known as the prospective payment system (PPS).

PPS calls for a change from the cost per case method of reimbursement of allowable costs for Medicare Part A hospital services retrospectively, to one of payment computed prospectively under a formula of payment adjusted for diagnostic groups, for certain clinical characteristics of the patient, for hospital, region, wage levels, and other pertinent factors.

The Medicare PPS is based on 470 diagnostic classes coded according to the 1979 *International Classification of Diseases, 9th Revision, Clinical Modification (ICD–9–CM)* developed by the Commission on Professional and Hospital Activities.

There has been a three-year transition period for PPS in which the adjustment from a more or less local or regional view of reimbursement to a national or federal perspective has taken place. During the three years there were adjustments to problems that arose. In fact, even the matter of the beginning date of the program in individual hospitals was tied to their fiscal year. The PPS program went into effect October 1, 1983. Hospital participation started with those institutions whose fiscal year began on that date. Other hospitals began participating on the beginning of their fiscal years which began after October 1. This gradual phasing in lessened the impact of the new program nationally and made the experience of the earlier participants possibly helpful to programs starting later.

Pricing of payments to providers of inpatient care (excluding hospitals such as long-term, children's, psychiatric, and rehabilitative) under PPS is determined by applying the weight of the proper DRG category to a base Medicare rate (plus other adjustments to be explained later). This applies to DRG categories 001 to 468. Categories 469 and 470 are used temporarily for improperly matched or invalid data that require special attention. Cases in these two DRG categories must finally be assigned to one of the 468 categories that have cost weights.

The DRG weight, simply defined, is the relative cost of treating the average Medicare patient for a particular DRG as compared to the cost of treating the average Medicare patient. The relative weights were determined by HCFA using a 20% sample of all Medicare bills in 1980, giving attention to routine care, special care, ancillary services, length of stay, area wages, and teaching activities. Those cases not falling within three standard deviations of the mean in costs were dropped from the computation of the DRG weight. This reduced the risk of a few extreme cases unduly affecting the average costs.

PRICING METHOD

The PPS pricing method is rather complicated and slightly overwhelming because of all the adjustments that have to be made. Basically, however, the concept is relatively simple. For the first three years of the PPS (October 1, 1983 through September 30, 1986), the payment to a hospital for a

Medicare patient under the DRG concept was made by combining a hospital rate and a federal rate on a stated proportionate basis for each year. The method for determining each is described.

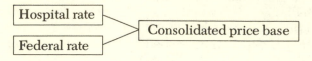

HOSPITAL RATE

The hospital factor in the standard Medicare price was obtained from the hospital's average operating inpatient cost per case of the cost reporting year prior to TEFRA.[24] Under the PPS hospital inpatient operating costs include all costs *except:* depreciation; interest; capitalized lease costs; return on equity for investor-owned hospitals; and direct costs of medical, nursing, and allied health professions education programs operated by the hospital.

Many of the items listed as exceptions to inclusion as operating costs are passed through and added to the hospital's total Medicare payments as reasonable cost items (depreciation, interest, capitalized lease costs, return on equity, and educational costs). (One change from the TEFRA design is that malpractice insurance costs to the hospital are included in the hospital rate.)

Other adjustments have to be made to the hospital rate besides exclusion of items from operating costs.

Hospital case mix index adjustment is one. This is the amount by which a hospital's average cost per case would differ from the national average given the mix of patients it admits.

Updating factor. As an updating factor, an adjustment rate is set based on three items: a consumer price index market basket of costs related to inpatient health services; a technology allowance of 1%, and a budget neutralizer to prevent the actual PPS payments from becoming higher or lower than those that would have been paid in the same period had TEFRA continued. The updating factor for the year ending September 30, 1984 was set at 1.13242. This factor served as a stabilizing force during the transition period.

The hospital rate is thus computed:

Hospital's base year average per case operating expense amount	÷	Hospital's case mix index	×	Updating factor	=	Hospital rate

---

[24]The hospital's fiscal intermediary computed the hospital factor via an audit.

FEDERAL RATE

Federal base rates (with urban and rural variations) were set by HCFA for federal fiscal year 1984 for nine census regions, determined for labor-related items (DRG portion) and non–labor-related items.

The urban rate applies to all hospitals in metropolitan statistical areas (MSAs); the rural rate applies to all hospitals outside MSAs. So, the Medicare PPS uses MSAs to define the boundaries of urban and rural areas, while TEFRA used standard metropolitan statistical areas (SMSAs). Some SMASAs have been split, or redrafted, into two or more MSAs and may include larger gross territory than before. Consequently, some hospitals classified as rural under TEFRA may now be considered urban or vice versa.

To compute the federal rate component several adjustments have to be made. *The labor portion of the proper regional standard base rate* (urban or rural) is stated first (Table 7.5).

The area wage index adjustment is made to the labor portion of the regional standard base rate for area wage variations. The index of area wage adjustments is set forth in the *Federal Register* (September 1, 1983, Table 4b).

Nonlabor portion. The applicable urban or rural nonlabor portion of the regional standard base (Table 7.5) must be added to the adjusted labor portion.

Cost of living adjustment. The states of Alaska and Hawaii only are allowed a cost of living adjustment for the nonlabor portion of their regional standard base rate because of higher material costs due to greater shipping costs.

Outlier patients must be adjusted for. Payments in addition to the DRG price are made for outlier patients, those who exceed either the length of stay or the cost of stay limits. (The outlier adjustment applies only to the federal component.)

Length of stay outliers are those patients who exceed the DRG stay by the lesser of 20 days or 1.94 standard deviations from the mean stay for that diagnosis. Payment will be made for approved outlier days at the rate of 60% of the average per diem federal rate for the DRG.

Cost outliers are patients whose cost of treatment adjusted by multiplying the total billed charges by the national cost-to-charge ratio (.72) exceeds the DRG price by the greater of $12,000 or 150%. Payment for patients who qualify as cost outliers will be 60% of the difference between the outlier cost cutoff and the estimated actual costs. (The billed charges will be reduced by the hospital's indirect medical education adjustment.)

Length of stay outliers are identified automatically by the hospital's fiscal intermediary. Cost outliers must be identified by the hospital. Before

TABLE 7.5   Regional Standard Base Rates

| | Urban | | Rural | |
Region	Labor	Nonlabor	Labor	Nonlabor
Region 1 New England	$2,332.56	$635.51	$1,994.31	$482.14
Region 2 Middle Atlantic	$2,096.87	$628.04	$1,984.97	$488.97
Region 3 South Atlantic	$2,183.42	$581.98	$1,796.04	$406.30
Region 4 East North Central	$2,330.77	$677.44	$1,950.90	$455.12
Region 5 East South Central	$1,962.32	$517.99	$1,811.73	$380.17
Region 6 West North Central	$2,273.55	$602.65	$1,820.63	$390.59
Region 7 West South Central	$2,137.03	$570.02	$1,754.37	$378.77
Region 8 Mountain	$2,099.73	$605.05	$1,818.61	$425.10
Region 9 Pacific	$2,210.17	$708.49	$1,900.63	$495.70

Source: *Federal Register.* Vol. 49, No. 1, January 3, 1984.

outlier payments are made, length of stay or costs must be approved by a PSRO or a PRO.

The federal rate is computed thus:

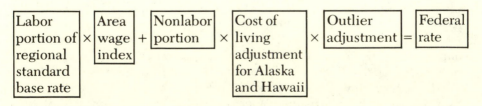

Labor portion of regional standard base rate × Area wage index + Nonlabor portion × Cost of living adjustment for Alaska and Hawaii × Outlier adjustment = Federal rate

CONSOLIDATED PRICE BASE

The consolidated price base is computed by adding the hospital rate and the federal rate while making an adjustment for blend factors the first three years.

Blend factors used in the consolidation of hospital and federal rates the first three years were as follows: the first year (fiscal year 1984) the consolidated rate was 75% of the hospital rate for that year and 25% of the federal rate,[25] the second year (FY 1985) the blend was 50% each of the hospital and federal rates; the third year (FY 1986) the blend was hospital rate 25% and federal rate 75%. The fourth year (FY 1987) the rate will be 100% of the federal rate.

The consolidated price base/Medicare patient DRG charge is compiled as follows:

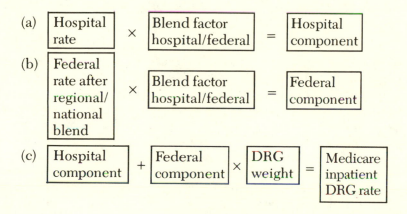

MISCELLANY

In any exposition of a concept or system it is likely that there are comments or definitions related to factors of the system that have not been included in the general text. Below there are listed alphabetically a number of comments and definitions related to this DRG discussion.

Bad debts due to unpaid deductibles and coinsurance owed by Medicare beneficiaries will be reimbursed fully under PPS.

Blue Cross and other payers. Some Blue Cross plans (seven in practice or in process of setting up) have adopted the PPS payment plan (DRGs).

---

[25]The federal rate also has a blend factor. The federal rate will blend annually, the first three years between regional and national, urban or rural. The first year (FY 1984) the blend was 100% regional, urban or rural; the second year (FY 1985) the blend was 75% regional, 25% national, urban or rural; the third year (FY 1986) 50% regional, 50% national, urban or rural; the fourth year (FY 1987) the federal rate will be 100% national, urban or rural.

The Department of Health and Human Services is working on a PPS for skilled nursing facilities.

Budget neutrality. This is a provision of PPS that stipulates that for the first two years of the PPS plan the cost to the federal government will be no more and no less than what would have been paid if TEFRA had remained in place.

Case mix changes. TEFRA case mix index (not PPS case mix) may be recomputed due to changes in the hospital's circumstances. Some examples of change are

—Change in hospital's organization such as a merger with another hospital

—Change in range of services such as establishment of a new and added service unit

—Change in the medical staff due to granting staff privileges to doctors of added specialties and subspecialties

A hospital, to request a change of case mix status, must be able to demonstrate a change in case mix, the factors responsible for the change, and the effect of the change on costs. It is necessary to compare the case mix indices of the base year with those of the year in question, to assess the factors causing change, and to establish the effect of changes on costs.

Complication and comorbidity[26] *factor.* The DRG Grouper computer program automatically searches the list of any secondary diagnoses on a patient's bill for a complication or a comorbidity. If such a condition is found, the patient will be classified in a DRG on the basis of having that complication. A substantial complication or comorbidity is defined as a condition that increases the length of stay by at least one day in 75% of all patients.

Copayments and deductibles. Patients under Medicare PPS are affected very little as to copayments, deductibles, and uncovered charges (for example, telephone, TV, and added charge for a private room when requested by the patient for nonmedical reason). Patients are billed for those items as before.

One new regulation is helpful to certain patients: Medicare PPS will pay full DRG rate even if a patient had only one day of benefits left on day of admission. If there are outlier days involved, payments are made for the outlier days covered; the patient is billed for outlier days not covered.

Disproportionate share. Under the statute HCFA has been authorized to give special treatment to hospitals having a disproportionate share of Medicare and low income patients. However, HCFA has not exercised this

---

[26]Comorbidity is an illness, usually a chronic illness, present at the time of the illness evidenced by the principal diagnosis.

authority because its internal studies have failed to show any significant relationship between disproportionate Medicare patient load and average cost per case. (The validity of these internal studies has been questioned by many hospitals.)

DRG Grouper. This title signifies a computer program that assigns DRGs by using the principal diagnosis and other information from the patient's bill or medical record. Two features of the DRG Grouper program (the surgical procedure hierarchy and the complication and comorbidity factor—which see) eliminate the need to consider the order in which surgical procedures and secondary diagnoses are listed on the medical record or patient's bill.

DRGs, relative occurrence. Although the principle of the DRG concept is to assign one of the 468 regular DRGs to the patient's record, it should not be inferred that there is anywhere near an even distribution of DRGs. In the 1980 study of Medicare cases by HCFA it was found that 100 DRGs accounted for 80% of the cases, 27 DRGs accounted for 50% of the cases, and 8 DRGs accounted for 25% of the cases. Furthermore, it was found that 114 DRGs were not used for the Medicare patients studied, and that many hospitals used only 30 or 40 DRGs.

Exempt hospitals. Certain hospitals are exempt or otherwise excluded under the Medicare prospective payment system as described below:

—Long-term hospitals—characterized as those with lengths of stay greater than 25 days

—Children's hospitals—with patients predominantly under 18 years of age

—Psychiatric hospitals—having a Medicare certificate of participation

—Rehabilitation hospitals—offering intensive services meeting additional organizational and staffing requirements

—Cancer hospitals—meeting guidelines of the National Institutes of Health under which 80% or more of the patients discharged have a diagnosis of cancer

Hospitals exempt under PPS are reimbursed on the basis of reasonable costs under a target rate increase established under TEFRA.

Certain other hospitals have special conditions of participation:

—Rural referral centers (see also *Referral centers*) of acute care with 500 beds or more classified at the same rate as urban

—Sole community provider

—Hospitals covered under state-controlled reimbursement systems have a special exclusion. The states called waiver states include New York, New Jersey, Massachusetts, and Maryland.

Exempt hospital units. Rehabilitation and psychiatric units in general hospitals are exempt from Medicare PPS if the units are physically distinct and the hospital

—Has separate admission and discharge policies for rehabilitation and psychiatric units (transfers from regular nursing care units to rehabilitation or psychiatric units must go through discharge and new admitting procedures and have separate bills for stays in regular nursing units and in special psychiatric and rehabilitation units)

—Can identify direct and indirect costs for routine and ancillary services for patients admitted to the special rehabilitation and psychiatric units

—Can meet special criteria for type of patient admitted, and for organization and staffing of the unit

Kidneys for transplants. The costs for the acquisition of kidneys are passed through the Medicare PPS and are paid for on a reasonable cost basis to hospitals qualifying as renal transplant centers.

Medical education. Direct educational costs for both undergraduate and graduate medical education, nursing education, and allied health professions programs are pass-through costs which are paid as a reasonable cost separate from the DRG cost.

Indirect medical costs will be arranged for in a lump sum payment according to a formula based on full-time equivalent interns and residents per bed ratio. The lump sum allowance "will be equal to 11.59 percent of the federal component payments in proportion to the federal component blend factor for each full-time equivalent intern and resident per bed employed by the hospital" (American Hospital Association, Special Report #6).

Nursing salary differential. A few years ago a percentage was added to Medicare reimbursements, called a nursing salary differential, for the purpose of an allowance for the extra nursing care needed by Medicare patients. This differential was removed under TEFRA. It was *not* restored under Medicare PPS.

Part A. Medicare PPS payments are for Part A nonphysician services. In a few cases there may have been in effect a practice whereby some charges normally under Part A have been charged under Part B. A waiver of termination of the practice is available up to three years where the termination might be considered to threaten the stability of patient care. An example is a situation where the hospital and the physical therapist are unable to agree on a contractual relationship wherein the hospital would pay the therapist, and no substitute provider is available. In this instance the hospital could receive a waiver to obtain time to find alternative providers. The hospital would receive the DRG payments less an offset equal to the amount of Part B billings rendered by the therapist.

Periodic interim payments (PIP) are available to qualifying hospitals on a biweekly basis according to a percentage of estimated total annual prospective payments due them.

Principal diagnosis. The principal diagnosis is determined at discharge as being that condition chiefly responsible for the patient's admission to the hospital. All principal diagnoses are verified by the fiscal intermediary, PSRO, or PRO that reviews the bill. The principal diagnosis is used rather than the admitting or primary diagnosis, which often proves to be different from the principal or final diagnosis.

Referral centers. A referral center is a rural hospital with 500 or more beds, or a hospital that obtains at least 50% of its patients from other hospitals or from physicians *not* on the staff of the hospital. Under the latter criteria, at least 60% of the Medicare patients must live more than 25 miles from the hospital, and at least 60% of all services the hospital furnishes to beneficiaries must be furnished to patients who live more than 25 miles from the hospital. The *Federal Register* (January 3, 1984) states that referral centers located in rural areas and having 500 or more beds must use the rural wage index applicable to that hospital.

Research. Under the research and demonstration section of the Social Security Amendments of 1983, research will be carried on about the effect of incorporating capital costs into the PPS rate; reimbursement for physician inpatient services on a DRG basis; prospective payment for hospitals not presently covered under PPS; and payments to all providers under PPS. (At least 18 such research projects were under way in early 1984.)

Reviews and appeals. Budget neutrality adjustments and the weights and definitions of DRGs, by statute, are not reviewable judicially or administratively. With other items, appeal procedures are the same as under the reasonable cost plan.

Sole community providers. A hospital designated as a sole community provider continues to have its DRG price schedule based on a blend of 75% hospital and 25% federal rate rather than undergoing the changes during the transition years to heavier weighting toward the federal rate each year. Also the sole community provider remained eligible for additional payments during the three-year transition period to ensure recovery of fixed costs should admissions decline by more than 5%.

These providers are defined as hospitals in rural areas meeting one of these conditions:

—There is no acute hospital within 50 miles.

—There is no acute hospital within 25 miles *and* either (1) the hospital provides services to 75% of its service area, or (2) other hospitals are inaccessible for at least a month (30 full consecutive days) during the year.

—There is no acute care hospital within 15 miles and, because of travel conditions, other hospitals are inaccessible for at least a month (30 full consecutive days) during the year.

—The provider is an under-50 bed hospital located between 25 and 50 miles of neighboring hospitals and a PRO or fiscal intermediary certifies that the hospital would have met the utilization criteria were it not for the fact that patients in the service area were forced to utilize alternative hospital services due to the unavailability of certain services at the requesting hospital.

Surgical procedure hierarchy. A surgical patient is first classified in a major diagnostic category (MDC) according to the principal diagnosis. Next the patient is classified in a DRG using a surgical procedure from all the procedures that might have been performed on the patient. A computer program automatically classifies the patient according to the most resource-intensive surgical procedure related to the principal diagnosis. The order of the listing of the procedures has no significance; the accurate coding of the principal diagnosis is the key. If the surgical procedures listed are not related to the principal diagnosis, the record is coded DRG 468 (a surgical procedure unrelated to the principal diagnosis) for special attention and review.

Transfers. When a Medicare patient is treated by more than one hospital, each hospital used will be separately paid. Medicare PPS automatically pays the DRG charges including any outlier payments to the hospital that discharges the patient to his home, to a skilled nursing facility, or to other non-PPS facilities. The transferring hospital is paid the DRG (of the national average length of stay) per diem for the days the patient is in the hospital.

COMMENT

The early data show that PPS is working: the length of stay is falling and the number of hospital personnel is growing at the slowest rate in a decade.

MEDICARE HMO AND CMP CONTRACTING REGULATIONS

The Health Care Financing Administration published final regulations implementing Section 114 of the Tax Equity and Fiscal Responsibility Act of 1982 on January 10, 1985. Section 114 established many of the details for the determination of Medicare payment to prepaid health plans (PHPs) categorized as either health maintenance organizations (HMOs) or competitive medical plans (CMPs).

Details of the regulations include

1. Eligibility criteria for a qualified organization
2. Eligibility criteria for risk basis contracting
3. Level of payment for risk basis contracts

The regulations restate the legislated criteria and establish the administrative process for contracting between eligible organizations and the Medicare program. The regulations became effective February 1, 1985.

PRIOR HMO PARTICIPATION IN MEDICARE

HCFA previously contracted with federally qualified HMOs through reasonable cost contracts, risk contracts, or demonstration programs.

Under *reasonable cost contracts* interim payments are made to the HMO during the year based on an estimate of the HMO's annual operating costs. Payment is adjusted at year-end to reflect the actual costs incurred by the HMO. Actual cost is determined through allocation and apportionment of direct patient care and overhead costs.

Under the *risk contract* the HMO's actual costs and an adjusted average per capita cost (AAPCC) are determined. The AAPCC is an actuarial estimate of what HCFA would have paid for care provided to the Medicare subscriber group by the HMO if that care had been provided in a non-HMO setting in the same, or a similar, geographic area. AAPCC estimates are made for several different subscriber groups which are defined by variables such as age and sex. Based on the HMO's Medicare enrollment, an aggregate AAPCC payment is computed for the HMO. The HMO's actual costs are compared to the aggregate AAPCC. If actual costs are less than the aggregate AAPCC, the HMO retains half the difference, not to exceed 10% of the AAPCC. If the reverse occurs, the HMO absorbs the entire difference as an operating loss.

Demonstration projects are paid at 95% of a prospectively set AAPCC amount. There is no retrospective year-end adjustment. The demonstration HMOs assume full financial risk at the 95% AAPCC payment level.

The major changes brought about by the legislation and the regulations are to

1. Expand the use of the existing demonstration contracts as risk contracts without retrospective adjustment. (Eligible organizations may continue to contract as cost basis contracts if they wish to.)
2. Expand the number of eligible organizations to include some previously nonqualified organizations.

CONTRACTING PROCESS

There are two steps to the contracting process. First, an entity must be certified as a federally qualified HMO or CMP. Second, the entity must meet Medicare's contracting criteria.

ELIGIBLE ORGANIZATIONS

In these regulations an eligible organization is defined as a prepaid health plan that is organized under state laws and meets the provisions of the federal HMO act as defined in section 1301(d) of the Public Health Service Act, or complies with all of the following:

1. Provides physician, laboratory, X-ray, preventive, and emergency services directly or under contract
2. Provides out-of-area coverage to its subscribers
3. Provides contracts for inpatient hospital services
4. Assumes full financial risk for the care of its subscribers on a prospective fixed price basis or shares financial risk with the actual providers of the services delivered
5. Has adequate provision against insolvency

Once an entity has been deemed eligible for participation as an HMO or a CMP, it may seek to contract with HCFA on either a prospective risk basis or a cost basis.

CONTRACTING CONDITIONS

To qualify for a risk contract, an HMO or a CMP must

1. Provide evidence to HCFA that it is capable of bearing the risk of potential financial losses
2. Have at least 5,000 total enrollees, or 1,500 enrollees if it serves a primarily rural area
3. Have at least 75 Medicare enrollees, or an acceptable plan to achieve this in two years
4. Agree to enroll Medicare beneficiaries on a first-come-first-serve basis up to its predetermined limit (With certain exceptions which are not discussed in the regulations, Medicare and Medicaid enrollment may not exceed 50% of the total enrollment.)
5. Have an open enrollment period of at least 30 days each year
6. Be capable of direct delivery of a complete range of medically covered services with the exception of hospice care

7. Furnish the required services through providers and suppliers that meet applicable Medicare statutory definitions and implementing regulations

8. Have an operating and verifiable quality assurance program

To qualify as a reasonable cost contract, the HMO or CMP must

1. Meet all the criteria of risk contract eligibility, but choose cost basis payments, *or*

2. Meet all the criteria of risk contract eligibility, but fail to provide adequate assurances to HCFA of ability to bear the potential financial losses, *and*

3. Have at least 250 Medicare enrollees by the beginning of its fourth contract period

BASIS OF PAYMENT UNDER RISK CONTRACT

Under the risk basis contract HCFA will make capitated payments to the HMO or CMP on behalf of the enrolled Medicare subscriber population based on a prospectively determined monthly rate. Minimally, those services normally covered under Medicare Parts A and B must be provided in the HMO or CMP benefits package. The actual payment and benefit level contracted for between HCFA and the HMO or CMP is a function of the HCFA-promulgated rate schedule of AAPCC and a provider-developed estimate of the organization's adjusted community rate (ACR).

The AAPCC is HCFA's prospective estimate of the average per capita costs for full Part A and Part B services for a class of Medicare subscribers if services were provided by non-HMO organizations in the same or a similar geographic area. AAPCCs are calculated currently for 120 different beneficiary groups based on beneficiary age, sex, disability, Medicaid, and institutional status. A complete list of the applicable rates is in the February 10, 1985 *Federal Register*. The maximum HMO or CMP payment per enrollee is a per subscriber rate equal to 95% of the appropriate AAPCC amount. HCFA will make monthly payments in accordance with the HMO or CMP's actual enrollment in each AAPCC group.

A weighted average of the AAPCC subscriber rates is then projected based upon an estimate of Medicare enrollment in the HMO or CMP. A comparison is made between the weighted average rate and the organization's ACR. In the event that the weighted average per subscriber rate exceeds the ACR, the HMO or CMP must choose from the following options:

1. Forego payment of all or part of the difference by accepting a lower payment percentage

2. Offer additional benefits to the Medicare subscribers beyond those required at current Part A and Part B benefits levels

3. Have a portion of its current payments withheld by HCFA for use in subsequent years to prevent excessive fluctuation in the level of the additional benefits

4. Offset the difference against the beneficiary obligation to pay Medicare deductibles and copayments

Where an organization has insufficient data to make the ACR calculation, HCFA will make the calculation based on all available information including, if necessary, the experience of the other HMO organizations. A retrospective reconciliation of total payments and a weighted average AAPCC based on actual enrollment will be made to correct for errors in original enrollment projections.

HCFA will also determine an actuarial equivalent to the average Medicare deductible or copayment amount. This amount is deducted from the Medicare payments and will be paid by the Medicare enrollee in the form of a premium to the HMO or CMP.

Should a cost basis HMO or CMP wish to provide services to Medicare subscribers on a risk basis, the law requires that two new risk basis Medicare subscribers be enrolled by the HMO for each cost basis enrollee that changes to a risk basis. The conversion from cost to risk must be at the election of the enrollee and must occur in an unbiased fashion.

BASIS OF PAYMENT UNDER COST CONTRACTS

The costs incurred by an HMO or a CMP under a cost contract are reimbursed if they are found to be proper and necessary, are reasonable in amount, and are arrived at in accordance with established Medicare payment principles. The services of physicians and other Part B suppliers must be priced competitively within the HMO or CMP service area. If these services are purchased on a fee-for-service basis, the costs are considered reasonable only if they do not exceed the reasonable charge criteria mandated for non-HMO and non-CMP providers by existing Medicare regulations. If the services are supplied by the HMO or CMP, Medicare costs are derived through Medicare's cost apportionment and cost allocation principles.

In addition to the determination of the individual reasonability of the costs of providing services, HCFA also will supply an absolute limitation on the total amount paid to the HMO or CMP based on a weighted average of the AAPCC for each class of Medicare enrollee in the HMO or CMP.

IMPLICATIONS FOR HOSPITALS

A hospital may participate in the Medicare prepaid health plan in three alternate ways: (1) as a noncontracting hospital, (2) as a contracting hospital, or (3) as an HMO or CMP. Hospitals that do not contract with HMOs or CMPs will not be unaffected by the regulations. If a local HMO or CMP does achieve Medicare eligibility, total Medicare admissions within the community may decline if the HMO or CMP tightly controls the level of Medicare inpatient utilization for its subscribers.

The magnitude of the potential impact on Medicare inpatient admissions depends on the number of Medicare beneficiaries that enroll in the program, the current Medicare inpatient utilization patterns, and the selective contract pattern used by the HMO or CMP. For example, if the HMO or CMP contracts with those hospitals that are already treating the majority of the Medicare beneficiaries, then there may be little, if any, redistribution in Medicare utilization patterns. However, all hospitals may experience a reduction of inpatient admissions for the HMO or CMP Medicare subscriber group.

A noncontracting hospital may also receive HMO subscribers for emergency services and urgently needed services. The regulations define emergency situations as covered inpatient or outpatient services that are furnished by an appropriate source other than the HMO or CMP, that are immediately needed, and where the time to reach a contracting supplier would risk permanent damage to the patient's health. Urgently needed services are defined as covered services required to prevent serious deterioration of an enrollee's health resulting from an unforeseen illness or injury while the enrollee is absent from the HMO or CMP's geographic area and where receipt cannot be delayed until this enrollee returns. According to the procedures utilized during the demonstration projects, final responsibility for determining if the services provided qualify as emergency or urgent care rests with the fiscal intermediary.

Where such services are provided, the ultimate financial risk is assumed by the HMO or CMP. The HMO or CMP may choose from two payment options: having the fiscal intermediary pay the hospital or paying the hospital directly. A hospital should, whenever possible, contact the HMO for specific billing instructions before submitting a bill to the fiscal intermediary.

If payment is made through the fiscal intermediary, it will be in accordance with existing Medicare payment principles for the services rendered. Generally, prospective DRG payments for inpatient services and cost payments for outpatient services will take place. In states with Medicare waivers, payment would be made in accordance with the state program. Medicare will adjust the aggregate payments made to the HMO or CMP by the exact dollar amount paid out to noncontracting hospitals on behalf of the risk basis provider. To receive full payment, it will be necessary for the hospital also to receive payment for those costs paid as "pass throughs." This should mean that Medicare HMO charges and statistics will be included in the total Medicare data on the provider's cost report. HCFA has been asked to specify how the applicable statistics for Medicare HMO payments received under the fiscal intermediary option are to be treated in the hospital's cost report.

If the HMO chooses to make payment directly, its incentive is to pay at a rate no higher than the Medicare direct payment amount. Hospitals should be careful to collect full payment from the HMO, including applicable adjustments for capital costs, direct medical education, and indirect medical education adjustments.

Noncontracting hospitals should take care not to provide services other than emergency or urgent care to an HMO or CMP Medicare enrollee. Nonemergency or nonurgent services do not have to be paid for by the HMO or CMP or by the Medicare program.

EMERGENCY AND URGENT SERVICES

If the hospital is presented with a patient and it is unclear as to whether the circumstances represent either emergency or urgent care, and time permits, the hospital should contact the HMO or CMP. If the HMO or CMP advises the hospital that the proposed treatment is not of an urgent or emergency nature, the hospital should advise the patient in writing of the HMO or CMP's decision. The letter should indicate that the HMO or CMP has been contacted and the beneficiary is responsible for payment if services are still rendered. If the hospital believes the care to be of an urgent or emergency nature, it is in a difficult position. The hospital may continue to treat the care as an emergency, bill the fiscal intermediary, and await final determination. In submitting the bill for payment, the hospital should advise the fiscal intermediary of the HMO or CMP's determination. If the fiscal intermediary rules against the hospital, no payment will be made.

In the event that the HMO or CMP agrees that the care is of an urgent or emergency nature, then the hospital should request billing instructions from the HMO or CMP. If the fiscal intermediary is billed directly, the hospital should advise the intermediary of the HMO or CMP's decision. If the fiscal intermediary denies payment, then the bill should be directed to the HMO or CMP for payment.

In many potential emergency and urgent situations, however, the hospital cannot risk the time to make contact with the HMO or CMP. Therefore, the final determination of the emergency or urgent situation must be based on the facts at the time the patient presents himself and on the judgment of the medical personnel present on the site. The regulations were written to provide such latitude. The American Hospital Association has taken the position that all emergency and urgent care services provided in good faith should be paid for. The Association is awaiting clarification from HCFA. In the meantime, the medical needs of all patients based on the judgment of on-site personnel must remain the primary bench mark of the level of care and services provided.

NONEMERGENCY SERVICES

The HMO and CMP regulations state that the HMO or CMP is required to assume the risk for all nonemergency and nonurgent care provided solely at HMO or CMP contracting facilities. With proper beneficiary education and identification, noncontracting hospitals should be able to avoid inappropriate risk.

It is essential in all instances where an individual presents himself that the noncontracting hospital be able to determine if a Medicare beneficiary is an HMO or CMP enrollee or a regular Medicare beneficiary. At this time HCFA has not issued a uniform rule on HMO and CMP subscriber identification. Where the hospital provides treatment of a nonemergency or nonurgent nature under the belief that the individual is a regular beneficiary, neither HCFA nor the HMO or CMP is required to make payment. Until a method of identification is established locally, hospitals must be on guard. Speific questions aimed at determining HMO or CMP benefits should be instituted into admitting procedures. Local hospital groups may wish to monitor HMO and CMP development and to work subsequently with local HMO and CMP organizations to share information on local identification procedures. The American Hospital Association has petitioned HCFA for a national identification procedure.

CONTRACTING FACILITIES

The HMO or CMP also has the option of negotiating its own contract outside the Medicare prospective pricing system with local hospitals. This contract between the hospital and the HMO or CMP is completely independent of current Medicare regulations.

The actual experience of those hospitals that do contract with a Medicare-certified HMO or CMP will be a function of the HMO or CMP's enrollment and the HMO or CMP's utilization controls. Ideally the hospital would realize increased inpatient admissions from both the Medicare and non-Medicare enrollment population. The hospital should be aware that the reductions in utilization by the HMO or CMP in general can offset a part of any potential increases in potential patient population for a contracting facility. HMO or CMP contracting hospitals may also experience a change in the average severity of their patients. Just as in the case of overall admissions, the HMO or CMP utilization review methods may eliminate potential low severity admissions, leading to an overall increase of the severely ill in the case mix. Finally it is critical that the contracting hospital negotiate a payment that reflects its direct patient operating costs, its costs of capital, and applicable adjustments for medical education, as well as for indigent care.

HOSPITALS AS HMOS OR CMPS

Any organization that can meet the requirements of the HMO act or the CMP requirements delineated in the regulations may seek to qualify as a Medicare HMO or CMP. This includes existing hospital prepaid health plans. Hospitals with high Medicare utilization may be interested in developing an HMO or a CMP. Such facilities are already treating significant numbers of Medicare beneficiaries. With the hospital as an HMO or a CMP, these beneficiaries could continue to receive service at the hospital. Financial benefits from the management of a full range of services under a prepaid plan are just as available to hospitals as they are to nonhospital organizations. The regulations, however, do not allow for the development of a Medicare-only HMO or CMP. With certain exceptions, a maximum of no more than 50% of the HMO or CMP's enrollees can be Medicare or Medicaid eligible.

The ability of hospitals to compete on the open market with larger, already organized HMOs may be the primary deterrent to hospitals' achieving HMO or CMP designation. It appears that many established HMOs are ready to move quickly toward attaining eligibility and enrolling Medicare subscribers. A hospital's ability to establish the necessary organizational functions and to market itself to the Medicare beneficiary may be hindered by

1. Its geographic limitations with respect to fixed plant and facility
2. Its historical relationship with its medical staff as an independent provider
3. Its inability to shed the high costs perceptions of the non-Medicare purchasers necessary to spread financial risk and meet the regulatory enrollment limitations

MEDICARE HMO OR CMP: CONCLUSIONS

The promulgation of the Medicare HMO and CMP regulations presents both options and challenges for hospital providers. Initially many short-term issues exist that relate to the interaction between the Medicare HMO or CMP and hospitals. These issues relate to the proper assignment of the financial risks intended in a capitated services arrangement. Many operating questions remain unanswered. Until answers are available hospitals must be guarded in providing nonemergency services to potential HMO or CMP subscribers once a Medicare HMO or CMP begins to operate in their service area. Many questions may need resolution at the local level until national clarification and instructions are issued.

In the longer term, the issues are related to market entry. Depending on their geographic situation, market share, and prior HMO activities, some hospitals may be able to obtain HMO or CMP eligibility on their own. Others may find that they can achieve eligible status and compete locally through partnerships with other hospitals and providers, and with third party payers. Finally, many more hospitals may enter into contracts with Medicare eligible HMOs and CMPs as preferred providers. Even in this latter situation, hospitals must proceed cautiously. The management of the hospital should have full knowledge and understanding of the terms of the arrangement including the relationship of the payment of the HMO or CMP to the cost anticipated in treating the subscriber population, the impact on current hospital operating resources, and the anticipated effect of the HMO or CMP's utilization review criteria.

Finally, as continued pressure on the Medicare trust funds and annual federal budgets continues, pressures to control utilization of benefits by subscribers will grow. Therefore, in the longer term, it will become important that hospital participation be made more viable. This may only be achieved, however, through future legislative changes in the eligibility and compliance criteria coupled with changes in the methods of hospital health care delivery.

MEDICAID

Medicaid is the stepchild of political expediency, in fact, a kind of afterthought of Medicare. When the Social Security Amendments of 1965 were written, one of the pressing needs addressed was that of establishing a health care program for the elderly—Title XVIII, or, more commonly called, Medicare.

Persons under 65 needing help were receiving some aid under a variety of federal, state, and county programs. It is likely someone in Washington thought it would be an excellent idea to lump together the blind, the disabled, the families of dependent children, and others at the poverty level of all ages in one large federal-state program supported in great measure by federal funds. That became Medicaid, otherwise known as Title XIX.

The revenues from Medicaid (and Medicare) are important to hospitals, nursing homes, laboratories, physicians, pharmacies, home care services, therapists, and other providers, because the number of recipients of benefits from federal and state funds is growing in percentage of revenue of those providers year by year.

Some people felt that Medicaid was a stopgap program that would aid the poor and medically indigent until Hubert H. Humphrey was elected President of the United States in 1968 and persuaded Congress to pass a national health insurance act. Of course, this did not come to pass.

In the years preceding Medicaid, the elderly, the blind, the disabled, and sick children had been aided through the Kerr-Mills Act and related legislation, but there was still a great need to be addressed.

Medicare was designed for those persons over 65 who might need hospital and medical care. It was an insurance plan that included many compromises: employee-employer financing as well as federal general funds; hospital care and skilled nursing facility care with deductibles paid by the patient; and a separate insurance plan (Medicare B) with costs shared by the beneficiaries and the federal government to pay, at least partially, the fees charged by physicians for their services—to mention a few.

Medicaid may have been an afterthought to help the categorically needy previously mentioned (the blind, the disabled, children, the aged who needed assistance, the poor). Certainly there were many poor who were not receiving needed medical care, and there were many aged who could not pay the deductibles charged by hospitals and skilled nursing facilities. Also many aged persons needed financial assistance to stay in intermediary care homes (commonly called nursing homes) after their discharge from a hospital or an SNF. So Medicaid was structured as a means of taking care of this undetermined number of needy Americans.

Medicaid, or Title XIX, as it came out of Congress, was *not* a law which was put into action uniformly in all parts of the country. Again, Medicaid was a compromise. Possibly only a compromise could pass Congress. The Hill-Burton Act of the 1940s may have been an example Congress followed. Hill-Burton provided for building hospitals in the postwar period and was heavily weighted in funding to the South and to rural areas. In administration, the states operated in true states' rights tradition. Medicaid was and is heavily weighted to the poor states.

FINANCING

Medicaid is a program to provide health care to the needy, with the financing shared by the federal government and the individual participating states. A state pays from 17% to 50% of the costs depending on the per capita income of the state in relation to the country as a whole. The federal government pays the remaining costs, after the the state's share, on an open-ended basis.

BASIC AND OPTIONAL BENEFITS

Under Title XIX each state wishing to participate in Medicaid could enter into an agreement with the secretary of Health, Education, and Welfare (HHS now) to furnish at least certain basic mandated health services to a group of individuals in need of financial assistance and others considered categorically needy.[27] The state income level below which individuals were considered to be in need of financial assistance was set by the state.

The mandated services presently are

1. Inpatient hospital care
2. Outpatient hospital care
3. Physicians' care
4. Laboratory and X-ray diagnostic services
5. Skilled nursing facility care
6. Home health care
7. Early and periodic screening, diagnosis, and treatment for needy children under 21 years of age

States were allowed also to include certain optional benefits, with the state paying its contracted share of costs. Optional services could include any of the following at a level and amount set at the discretion of the state:

1. Medical care by practitioners other than medical doctors
2. Private duty nurses
3. Clinic services
4. Dental services
5. Physical therapy and related services
6. Prosthetics and eyeglasses
7. Other diagnostic, screening, preventive, and rehabilitative services
8. Inpatient hospital, skilled nursing facility, intermediary care facility care for persons over 65 for tuberculosis or mental illness
9. Intermediary care facility care
10. Other medical care

ADMINISTRATION OF MEDICAID

Medicaid may be a financially shared program between the individual state and the federal government, but the administration is primarily by the state (with a few basic guidelines set in Washington). From state to state the administrative body differs. Administration may be under the aegis of the state welfare department, the state health department, a combined

---

[27]All states did not immediately apply for a Medicaid program. Nearly a decade passed before the last two states, Alaska and Arizona, began programs. The Arizona program was soon challenged in the courts and was withdrawn, but was later revived.

health and welfare body, or, in at least one case (Mississippi), under a separate department. Whatever the administrative leadership, the Medicaid program retains aspects of a welfare program. In fact, welfare departments in most states determine eligibility of persons for Medicaid benefits.

The few basic guidelines set in Washington, as mentioned above, came through Medical Services Administration (MSA) of DHHS which has federal oversight of the state programs. From the start of Medicaid, this body has been trying to coordinate the effort. MSA was given only six months lead time at the beginning of Medicaid to negotiate and approve all the varied programs entered into with the states.

In the early 1970s Howard Newman became commissioner and brought some order to MSA activities, but it would seem that the inherent weaknesses of Medicaid make an equitable program impossible.

MEDICAID ELIGIBILITY

Certain persons are eligible for assistance in any Medicaid program. Basically these include anyone previously helped under assistance to the blind (AB), to the aged (OAA), to families of dependent children (AFDC), and to the partially or totally disabled (APTD)—the Kerr-Mills recipients, whose program was phased out in 1969 whether or not a state established a Medicaid program.

In addition, certain other individuals became eligible who formerly had been ineligible because of state laws with restrictive residence and age requirements. Under Medicaid these restrictions were removed.

Another large group became eligible because their family income was below the poverty level set in their state for a means test. The income level for qualification varies widely from state to state, more than 100% from lowest to highest. For example, when Medicaid became operative in New York State, an income of $6,000 for a family of four was set as a level below which Medicaid would apply. This figure for 1966 was a relatively good income. In fact, this $6,000 income for a family of four, and related levels for other sized families, affected nearly 45% of the state's population. Since New York is a comparatively high per capita income state, the state's portion of the Medicaid cost was 50%. The program was such a drain on the state treasury that a downward adjustment in the income level to qualify had to be made. MediCal (California Medicaid), which began with an eligibility level of $4,092 for a family of four, also found the program to be a tremendous financial burden.

Each state set its own level of income below which persons living anywhere in the state could qualify for Medicaid benefits. This often had a built-in inequity, particularly in states with extremes of metropolitan and rural areas. In New York State a $6,000 eligibility level had a much greater impact in upstate New York than in metropolitan and rural areas. A great number of upstate residents were eligible for Medicaid who probably did not consider themselves victims of poverty.

Besides including the so-called categorically needy—AB, AFDC, OOA, APTD, and the low-income people—the states have the option of also including others who are sometimes called medically indigent. Medically indigent persons can be described as those who have incomes over the means test level but who have incurred medical expenses which, if deducted from their incomes, would place them at the public assistance level. Usually in a case of this sort, the person would spend for medical expenses down to the eligibility level and would then qualify for assistance. This spending down has sometimes been called the "notch effect."

MEDICAID COSTS

In the first years the states were attracted to Medicaid, particularly in regard to clients on public assistance, because some of the load that the states may have been bearing alone could now be shifted to federal sharing of 50% to 83% of the expense.[28] Hospitals began getting paid on the basis of reasonable costs for welfare and former charity patients, and this was a much better payment pattern. Nursing homes which had tried to negotiate rates that would cover costs for state- or county-supported patients now found a better payment climate both in rates and in promptness. Physicians and other providers began to collect for their services according to negotiated rates based on usual and customary fees. Outside of the mass of paper work it seemed a good situation for the states and most providers, not to mention the people who were assisted.

What was not anticipated was the tremendous growth of the program both in numbers of recipients and in dollars spent. The actuarial figures used in projecting the cost of Medicaid were woefully under actual costs. What had been estimated as a $2 billion program became, within a decade, a $20 billion cost with about 24 million recipients.

To be fair, the program was hardly started before the effects of Vietnam and the attending inflation were felt. Many workers in the health field, particularly nurses and other hospital workers, were underpaid in comparison to workers in industry. The wage adjustments that had to be made were costly to the providers and therefore to Medicaid. Also, the rapid rise of technology in health care increased costs through added capital expenditures and new patterns of utilization of the "machines."

MEDICAID AND QUALITY OF CARE

The states are responsible for the quality of care under the Medicaid program. Various devices have been used to oversee tbe programs: utili-

---

[28]Under Reagan budget cutting, the federal percentage allowed the states could be reduced.

zation committees, PSROs, and other types of peer review. Measurement of quality of care has always been a difficult task except for the most gross measurements. Researchers have always searched for but never found the perfect method. Some progress has been made, particularly through utilization studies, but there is still a long way to go.

MEDICAID FRAUD AND ABUSE

Any agency or program that has a cash flow of $20 billion a year is going to attract the covetous. Unfortunately there are the covetous in all the strata and in all the professions of the health care arena, as there are in any cross section or sample of the American population. The federal government has uncovered fraud and abuse among all kinds of providers and among recipients. There has been false billing, Medicaid "mills" where a patient gets a few seconds of attention, storefront laboratories working in collusion to defraud with those who refer work to them, and many other ingenious schemes to get a piece of the $20 billion. Unofficial estimates say that 5% of Medicaid expenditures is being drained off illegally. This figure may be optimistically low. Whatever the figure, vigilance is called for.

MEDICAID AND HMOS

Some states are experimenting by enrolling persons eligible for Medicaid assistance in local HMO programs. Originally it was believed that economies could be effected at the same time that quality medical care could be ensured. The HMO enrollment has not been in practice long enough to generalize about results.

MEDICAID UTILIZATION

The use of Medicaid services has risen much faster and to a much greater extent than expected, with more than 10% of the population currently being recipients. According to DHEW, the trend in the decade 1967 through 1976 showed some decrease in the use of inpatient hospital facilities and an increase in outpatient care. There seems to be a greater demand for services by the elderly, particularly in intermediary care. Medicaid services are likely to change. This is discussed in the last chapter of the book.

SCOPE OF MEDICAID SERVICE

Medicaid programs differ greatly in the 50 states as has been mentioned previously—differing in the range of services, in qualifying factors for beneficiaries, in payment methods, in length of stay limitations, and in accommodation limitations for inpatients as well as different handling of outpatients and rural health care.

On the plus side, 30 of the 50 states now recognize the principle of medical indigence and include the medically needy among those eligible for benefits. Of course there is a great difference in income levels in the various states as a base for considering a person or family in need.

On the minus side, economic conditions have made it more and more difficult for many states to finance the state portion of the Medicaid cost. With budget reduction at the federal level, Medicaid expenditures are likely to be restricted as well as at the state level.

A profile of the operation of the Medicaid programs is seen as follows:

Method of Payment.   Thirty-one states were on a cost basis, 14 on a combination cost/charge, and 6 on prospective methods of payment. Note that more than one mode of payment in a state makes for double counting.

Approval Requirement.   Seven states required prior approval or preauthorization before payment was made, five required PRO certification, three states required utilization review, four a physician's certificate, and one professional review.

Length of Stay Limitation.   Nineteen states had LOS limitation. These limitations ranged from a number of days per calendar or fiscal year to a number of days per admission or per diagnostic code.

Accommodation Limitations.   There were accommodation limitations by seven states. One of the states limited patients to semiprivate rooms, another to multibed rooms, another allowed private rooms for isolation necessary to protect other patients, another allowed reimbursement for semiprivate and private rooms only when medically necessary, while others had restrictions against weekend admissions.

Methods of Payment: Outpatient Hospital Services.   The methods of payment for outpatient services were somewhat similar to those for inpatient services: 25 were cost-related; 10 charge-related; 9 by fee schedules; 3 prospective; and 3 combination cost/charge basis.

Methods of Payment: Rural Health/Ambulatory Services.   Here the distribution of methods of payments was different: 30 were charge-related; 14 by fee schedules; and 6 cost-related.

The years ahead are uncertain for Medicaid. Many adjustments may be necessary to keep the state programs solvent and within their present (often inadequate) scopes.

MEDICARE AND MEDICAID INTERRELATIONSHIPS

There has to be an interrelationship between the two programs because the insurance program which is Medicare cannot operate with deductibles to cover a population that cannot pay deductibles. There has to be a supplement to help those people who are medically indigent. If a person over 65 cannot pay the Medicare B premium, then Medicaid has to be the assisting arm. There are many critics of Medicaid who complain about inadequate health care, inefficiency, fraud, and many other things. On balance, however, progress has been made.

1972 Social Security Amendments

Listed alphabetically below under key words are items touched upon in the 1972 amendments to the Social Security Act which affect the Medicare and Medicaid programs. Many other changes under the 1972 amendments have already been discussed in the text of this chapter.

BENEFIT CLAIMS-REASSIGNMENT (SEC. 236)

Payment for claims under Medicare can be made only to the patient, the physician, or the supplier who provided a covered service and accepted assignment except: (1) the payment may be made to the employer of the physician or supplier if the physician or supplier is required as a condition of his employment to turn over such fees to his employer; or (2) the payment may be made to the facility where the services are provided if the facility has a contractual arrangement with the physician or supplier giving it the sole right to bill Medicare for the services. Also, direct payment can be made to an organization administering a health care delivery system such as a prepaid group practice.

CAPITAL EXPENDITURES LIMITATIONS (SEC. 221)

Certain amounts of reimbursement based on capital expenditures may be withheld or reduced to providers of health services and to health maintenance organizations under Medicare, Medicaid, and child and maternal health programs by the secretary of HEW when those expenditures are deemed inconsistent with health service or facility decisions made by designated state planning agencies. Procedures will be set up for the facility or organization proposing a capital expenditure to appeal an adverse decision.

CHIROPRACTIC SERVICES IN TREATING A SUBLUXATION OF THE SPINE BY MANUAL MANIPULATION (SEC. 273)

The subluxation must have been demonstrated by X ray. The practitioner must be licensed and meet certain educational requirements.

COLOSTOMY SUPPLIES (SEC. 252)

Colostomy bags and necessary accessories are no longer classed as surgical dressings but as prosthetic devices. Coverage was extended to irrigation and flushing equipment and other items directly related to colostomy care, whether or not attachment of a bag is required.

DISCLOSURE OF INFORMATION UNDER MEDICARE AND MEDICAID (SEC. 249C)

The secretary of HEW will make available for public inspection: formal evaluations of carriers, intermediaries, and state agencies; comparative evaluations of the performance of contractors; and formal evaluations of the performance of providers of services. Such reports will not be made public until the contractor has had the opportunity (60 days maximum) to review the report and offer comments.

Also (in Section 299D) the secretary is required to make available to the public information from surveys of providers relating to the presence or absence of deficiencies in areas such as staffing, fire safety, and sanitation.

DURABLE MEDICAL EQUIPMENT (SEC. 245)

The secretary of HEW is authorized to experiment in various geographic areas with reimbursement approaches intended to prevent unreasonable expenditures for prolonged rentals of durable medical equipment. Among methods to be considered were: lend-purchase arrangements; lump-sum payment when outright purchase would be cheaper for estimated period of use; and waiver of 20% coinsurance if beneficiary purchased used equipment at price at least 25% less than reasonable charge to purchase new equipment.

HEALTH MAINTENANCE ORGANIZATION (SEC. 249F)

An HMO is defined as an organization that provides comprehensive health care on a per capita prepayment basis. Under the 1972 amendments, established HMOs can qualify for an incentive reimbursement plan under Medicare by entering into a contract with the secretary of HEW. The contract would specify the per capita amount the HMO would be paid in advance each month. The HMO would submit financial statements at the end of the fiscal year from which the secretary would determine the average per capita cost for Medicare patients had the services been provided the beneficiaries under other health care arrangements. If the HMO's incurred costs were less than the other arrangements, the difference (savings) would be shared by the HMO and the Medicare Trust Fund under a stated formula.

LABORATORY-DIRECT BILLING (SEC. 279)

The secretary is authorized to negotiate a payment rate with independent diagnostic laboratories for covered laboratory services which, if the laboratory accepts assignment, would be paid in full by Medicare. No coinsurance would be collectible from the beneficiary because the rate accepted would be the full charge for the procedure.

MEDICAL INSURANCE HEARING (SEC. 262)

Enrollees, physicians, or suppliers who are dissatisfied with the determination or the promptness of action on a Medicare Part B medical insurance claim may file for a fair hearing if $100 or more is at issue.

PENALTIES FOR FRAUD AND FALSE REPORTING (SEC. 242)

Certain acts, statements, or representations in connection with furnishing items or services, with program payments, or with certification of providers have been defined as subject to penalties under the Medicare program.

PHYSICAL THERAPISTS (SEC. 251)

Services of a licensed independently practicing physical therapist furnished in his office or the patient's home under a physician's plan, and meeting health and safety conditions specified by the secretary, have been covered under Medicare medical insurance since July 1, 1973 up to $100 of incurred expenses in a calendar year (subject to medical insurance deductible and coinsurance).

PHYSICIANS' CHARGES (SEC. 224)

Provisions have been made to set limits for physicians' charges in the Medicare, Medicaid, and maternal and child health programs by a formula relating to the charges of the previous fiscal year.

PLANNING (SEC. 234)

Hospitals, skilled nursing facilities, and home health agencies are required under Medicare to have a written plan reflecting an annual operating budget and at least a three-year projected capital expenditures plan.

PROFESSIONAL STANDARDS REVIEW (SEC. 249F)

The 1972 SSA Amendments authorized the establishment of independent professional standards review organizations (PSROs) under which practicing physicians would assume certain responsibility for reviewing the quality and appropriateness of care provided under Medicare, Medicaid, and maternal and child health programs. PSRO areas were established throughout the country by geographic or medical service areas, each area generally containing a minimum of 300 practicing physicians. The PSROs assumed responsibility in their areas for assuring that services were medically necessary and provided in accordance with professional standards. PSROs were not involved with reasonable charge determinations.

There was a review mechanism provided for reconsideration of a PSRO determination. PSROs have been replaced by PROs.

PROFICIENCY DETERMINATION FOR CERTAIN HEALTH PERSONNEL (SEC. 241)

The amendment made provision for the secretary of HEW (in conjunction with professional organizations and state health and licensure agencies) to determine the proficiency of certain health personnel (experienced practical nurses, therapists, laboratory technicians) now excluded, or limited in responsibility, under Medicare regulations through December 31, 1977. Since that date these health personnel have had to meet specific formal education, professional membership, or other requirements established by regulations.

PROSPECTIVE REIMBURSEMENT DEMONSTRATIONS (SEC. 222)

Under the 1972 amendments the secretary of HEW was directed to develop and carry out experiments and demonstrations in prospective reimbursement in Medicare. Experiments were authorized in testing changes in methods of reimbursement with performance incentives for intermediaries and carriers. Experiments can be tried with new types of provider (such as organizations providing comprehensive, mental, or ambulatory services, including ambulatory surgical centers), with the use of intermediate care or homemaker services by beneficiaries who could leave the hospital but are unable to maintain themselves at home unassisted. Also, experiments can be tried for improving rehabilitation treatments of patients in long-term facilities and to determine if clinical psychologists should be more available under Medicare.

PROVIDER CHARGES (SEC. 233)

Payment for provider charges is made at the lesser of reasonable cost or customary charge. Where there is a public provider of service at no charge or at only a nominal fee, payment is made on the basis of reasonable cost.

REIMBURSEMENT APPEALS BY PROVIDERS (SEC. 243)

A five-member Provider Reimbursement Review Board reviews appeals by providers when the intermediary makes a final cost determination with which the provider is dissatisfied. At least $10,000 must be involved, and the provider must appeal within 180 days of the determination. Groups of providers may file an appeal on common issues when the aggregate amount is at least $50,000. The secretary may, within 60 days, reverse or modify a board decision favorable to the provider. In this event the provider has recourse to judicial review.

SERVICES OUTSIDE THE UNITED STATES (SEC. 211)

Inpatient hospital services furnished by a foreign hospital are covered for U.S. citizens under Medicare under certain conditions:

1. If the foreign hospital is closer to, or substantially more accessible from, the beneficiary's residence than the nearest hospital in the United States that is suitable and available for his treatments
2. If the foreign hospital has been accredited by JCAH or a hospital approval program essentially comparable

Coverage is extended in these cases to any ambulance or physicians' service furnished. Benefits for these U.S. citizens are payable regardless of where the illness or accident occurred or whether an emergency existed. Present provisions covering emergency inpatient hospital services outside the United States when the emergency arises in the United States are retained. Emergency coverage is extended to include beneficiaries who incur an emergency in Canada while traveling without delay on the most direct route between Alaska and another state. The reimbursement methods are essentially the same as for nonparticipating hospitals in the United States.

TEACHING PHYSICIANS (SEC. 227)

The payment of teaching physicians under Medicare is made on the basis of reasonable costs rather than fee-for-service, unless

1. A bona fide patient relationship exists between the physician and the patients for whom a fee-for-service charge is made; or
2. The hospital had, in the two-year period ending in 1967 and every year thereafter, regularly billed all inpatients for such physicians' services, and reasonable charges had been collected from at least 50% of patients in these periods.

Medicare payments will be authorized on a cost basis for services provided to hospitals by the staff of certain medical schools, but only in respect to services that would be eligible for cost reimbursement, if they were furnished by the hospital.

Payments for services donated by volunteer physicians can be paid into a fund designated by those physicians if the fund is to be used for educational and charitable purposes.

TERMINATE MEDICARE PAYMENTS TO SUPPLIERS (SEC. 229)

Under the 1972 amendments the secretary was given authority to terminate payment, with public notice, for service rendered by an institutional provider of services, a physician, or any other supplier of health and medical services determined by the secretary to be engaged in overcharging, furnishing excessive, inferior, or harmful services, or making a false statement to obtain payment.

THERAPY SERVICES (SEC. 251)

A definition of reasonable cost under Medicare for covered physical, occupational, speech, or other therapy services or services of other health-related personnel (except physicians) is that the cost cannot exceed an amount equivalent to the salary that reasonably would have been paid, and any other costs that would have been payable, had the services been performed in an employment relationship. Any other reasonable expenses related to the service which an individual not actually working as an employee might have been paid could be recognized. These other expenses might include such items as travel expense, office expense, and similar costs.

WITHHOLDING MEDICAID PAYMENTS TO TERMINATED MEDICARE PROVIDERS (SEC. 290)

The secretary has been authorized since October 30, 1972 to withhold future federal financial participation in state Medicaid payments to institutions that have withdrawn from Medicare without refunding Medicare overpayments or without accounting for Medicare payments to them.

SUGGESTED READINGS

GENERAL

Myers, Robert J. *Medicare*, Selections.
Somers, Herman M. and Somers, Anne R. *Medicare and the Hospitals: Issues and Prospects*, Selections.
Stevens, Robert and Stevens, Rosemary. *Welfare Medicine in America: A Case Study of Medicaid*, Selections.
Stuart, Bruce C. and Spitz, Bruce. *Rising Medical Costs in Michigan*, Selections.
Topics in Health Care Financing, Spring 1979.

MEDICARE CHANGES UNDER TEFRA

American Hospital Association. Special Report #1, Special Report #2, Medicare Payment: Cost Per Case Management.

American Hospital Association. Office of Public Policy Analysis. Hospital Economic Performance: 1981. Policy Brief #42.

Ernst & Whinney. *The Tax Equity and Fiscal Responsibility Act of 1982: Provisions Affecting Medicare and Medicaid Programs,* 1982.

Hospital Week. September 24, 1982 to January 14, 1983.

Hospitals. October 1, 1982 to January 1, 1983.

MEDICARE PROSPECTIVE PRICING

American Hospital Association. *Managing Under Medicare Prospective Pricing.*

American Hospital Association. Special Report #4, The Medicare Case Mix Index.

American Hospital Association. Special Report #6, Medicare Prospective Pricing. Summary of Regulations.

American Hospital Association. Special Report #7, Diagnosis Related Groups.

Commission on Professional and Hospital Activities. *International Classification of Diseases, 9th Revision, Clinical Modification (ICD–9–CM).*

Federal Register. September 1, 1983, p. 39,871.

Federal Register. January 3, 1984, pp. 234–340.

Price Waterhouse. *The Challenge of Prospective Payment.*

8

Charges and Rate Setting

The previous chapters have considered the two major sources of hospital revenues—Blue Cross and Medicare. However, a discussion of the sources of operating revenues would be incomplete without an examination of the matter of charges and rate setting. Admittedly, charges or revenues from self-responsible (self-pay) patients generally represent a relatively small segment of a hospital's total revenues. Nevertheless, it is a segment that, as will become clear, is critical to the total financial well-being of a hospital. Therefore, it is important for a complete understanding of hospital financial management that the reader be familiar with the techniques, mechanics, and philosophical issues related to the setting of rates for hospital services.

BACKGROUND—THE PROBLEM

In Chapter 1 the objective of the manager of a commercial enterprise was stated as being that of maximizing owner's wealth, that is, $W = E/R$. To achieve this objective, assuming that the capitalization rate (R) is constant and that earnings (E) are the difference between revenues and costs, the manager must not only minimize cost, but also set price at a level that will allow production to proceed to that point wherein marginal revenue equals marginal cost. Thus, the commercial manager is confronted with a two-sided problem.

In contrast, the hospital manager, though confronted with a substantial array of financial and economic problems, has not been forced to pay particular attention to the pricing problem. Due to the dominance of cost-based reimbursement agreements, concern has been focused, in the main, on cost as opposed to price. The hospital manager, therefore, primarily has concentrated his talents and abilities on controlling costs and assuring quality services.

For the most part, hospital managers have traditionally viewed revenues from self-responsible patients as the balancing factor in their revenue structure. That is, they have known, at least approximately, the hospital's financial needs and the amount of revenues that could be expected from third party and philanthropic sources. Given this information, the amount of additional revenues necessary to meet or balance any deficit occurring between financial needs and expected revenues becomes obvious. Knowing this amount, charges to self-responsible patients have then been set at levels that will generate revenues sufficient to balance financial needs and income. Thus, charges historically have been established not on the basis of cost, but rather on the basis of financial expediency. Table 8.1 illustrates this situation.

This approach to establishing charges has resulted in the hospital industry participating in what can perhaps be best described as overt price discrimination. As should be clear by this point, hospital prices discriminate in favor of patients covered by third party payers. These patients, in effect, pay for care at cost, while self-responsible patients pay for care on the basis of charges that are dictated by financial expediency and need; that is, charges are established at levels designed to generate revenues equal to cost plus whatever additional funds are needed to meet the hospital's financial requirements.

TABLE 8.1   Charges Based on Financial Expediency

Step 1

           Revenues from third parties*
  + Revenues from philanthropy
  + Revenues from other sources

           Expected revenues

Step 2

           Financial needs*
  − Expected revenues (from Step 1)

           Revenue deficit (Revenue needed from
           self-responsible patients)

Step 3

$$\frac{\text{Revenue deficit}}{\substack{\text{Expected units of service provided} \\ \text{to self-responsible patients*}}} = \substack{\text{Charges to self-} \\ \text{responsible patients}}$$

*Assume that the values for these items are at least approximately known by management.

In the case of commercial firms, such a pricing practice would likely violate antitrust laws and would be illegal. However, for whatever the reasons, the legality of this practice has not been questioned in the hospital industry until recently.[1]

It should be realized that there is nothing inherently or implicitly wrong with third party payers purchasing hospital services at cost. Third party payers argue, with some validity, that they are not only volume purchasers of care, but that they are also reliable and faithful purchasers. Therefore, they maintain that they should pay for care at a price that is less than that paid by an individual payer.

The first part of the above argument is basically the contention that all large volume purchasers put forth as justification for quantity discounts. This justification, while valid in some commercial and industrial instances, is not valid in the hospital setting. An industrial firm, due to the operational economies inherent in volume production, can offer a purchaser a quantity discount on large volume sales because its operating costs are less. Costs are reduced, for the firm can "tool up" for and run, in a single batch, a large quantity that it has neither to store nor to market. Unfortunately, these same conditions do not exist in the case of the third party purchaser of hospital services.

Admittedly, Blue Cross or the government purchases in total a large quantity of hospital services. However, these services are not purchased either all at the same time or all from the same hospital. Instead, the situation is one in which a large number of piecework purchases are made from various hospitals. Under these conditions, an individual hospital cannot reduce its production costs simply due to the fact that payment is derived from a single source. Thus, on pragmatic financial grounds the argument that third party payers should receive a quantity discount is neither justified nor valid.

In contrast, the notion that third party payers should receive a price discount because they are reliable and faithful payers can, to some extent, be justified. Historically, third party payers have not defaulted on their obligations, and hospitals generally can be assured of receiving payment. Thus, a hospital, when dealing with third party payers, incurs less of a business risk, for it can be confident of receiving payment and, hence, does

---

[1]The basic issues in question were tested in court (U.S. Dist. Ct. Western Dist. Pa.; Civil No. 68–69, January 6, 1972). In the case, the Travelers Insurance Company contended that Blue Cross of Western Pennsylvania violated the provisions of the Sherman Act. The court dismissed the suit, finding that Blue Cross's competitive status was not acquired by boycott or intimidation; it is not a monopolist, for it cannot control rate making or establish its own rates, has not violated the Sherman Act, and is entitled to McCarran Act exemption. In essence, the court concluded that Blue Cross has not established artificial restraint-of-trade practices.

not have to concern itself with the problems and costs of bad debts. The implication of this situation is that the economic costs, that is, out-of-pocket plus intangible operating costs, of providing services to patients covered by third party payers are relatively less (by the bad debt cost element) than the cost of providing the same services to self-responsible patients (see Figure 8.1). Given this fact, it is reasonable for third party payers to pay less for services than individual payers, for their costs are less.

It is important to note that the foregoing does not imply that third party payers should not pay full costs. Due to reduced business risk, the full costs of providing services may be somewhat less for third party payer patients than for self-responsible patients. Third parties may thus pay somewhat less for services. However, if a hospital is to maintain a sound financial position, third party payers must pay at least their appropriate share of these costs. This approach to charging or billing for services is consistent with the common business practice of offering price discounts to reliable purchasers.

As was discussed in Chapter 4, third parties are not entirely satisfied with paying for services at their appropriate share of full costs. They want to exclude, by definition, several real operational cost elements from the items included in determining their share of cost. Thus, third parties, in effect, want more than just the price discount that should be available to any reliable purchaser. They want to pay for services on the basis of an adjusted cost, which obviously would be less than full cost.

FIGURE 8.1   Rate Setting—Theory

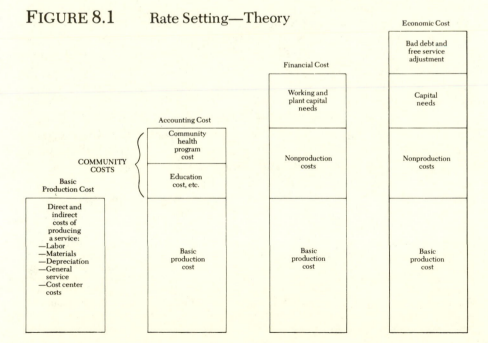

Due primarily to both their bargaining power and the precarious financial position of most hospitals, third parties have been able to impose this adjusted basis of reimbursement on hospitals. The result of this has been that hospitals have had to look at other revenue sources to obtain the funds necessary to meet the costs excluded by third parties. Self-responsible patients have traditionally been the source to which hospitals have turned for these additional revenues.[2] The effect of this has been that self-responsible patients—by paying more than their economic costs—have been subsidizing the care of third party beneficiaries.

At a time when hospital costs are increasing at a rapid if not explosive rate, it is inequitable to charge any category of patients more than its just costs. This situation of self-responsible patients subsidizing other patients must be corrected. To accomplish this, two things must be done. First, third party cost-based reimbursement agreements must be renegotiated to include all economic costs of operation so that reimbursement will equal full economic cost. Second, hospital charges must be established on the basis of economic costs, not financial expediency.

If all payers for care are to be treated equitably, the need for the above actions is obvious. The matter of substantially changing the philosophy behind third party payment contracts is basically a political problem, which is beyond both the scope of this book and the power of an individual hospital. However, the problem of setting charges on the basis of economic costs is germane to this text.

CURRENT PRACTICE

As indicated earlier, charges or rates have historically been established on the basis of financial expediency. However, perhaps it would be more appropriate to describe the current practice of most hospitals as that of setting charges on a consensus basis which is then modified by financial expediency and need.[3]

The technique commonly used, except in those few states that have rigorous rate-setting legislation,[4] can be defined as a consensus approach, for a hospital—to avoid public scrutiny of its rates and to be able to claim that its rates are reasonable—sets its rates based upon the rates of similar hospitals. That is, an urban hospital would consider the rates of other urban hospitals and establish its charges at corresponding levels. Thus, to the

---

[2]Hospitals could also look to philanthropy and the government for these additional funds. However, neither of these sources is as easy to turn to as self-responsible patients. Philanthropy cannot be relied upon as a regular source of funds. Also, government is often unwilling or unable to provide funds to nongovernmental hospitals.

[3]Kaitz, Edward M., *Pricing Policy and Cost Behavior in the Hospital Industry*, Chapters 3 and 4.

[4]In these states, rates are based on cost or economic cost as is suggested in this chapter.

extent that hospitals follow the patterns established by similar hospitals, rate setting is done by consensus. However, to the extent that revenues from charges are used as a balancing factor in a hospital's revenue structure, the consensus is modified; that is, rates are adjusted to meet financial needs. Thus, the approach that hospitals actually use can be most aptly described as a modified consensus approach.

This technique for establishing charges, along with the custom of setting the rates for routine services (room, board, and nursing services) at less than cost—so that they would be more comparable to hotel and restaurant charges—was probably initially adopted by hospitals as a defense mechanism against public opinion and pressure. Hospitals, however, are beginning to change their approach to setting charges.

The cost finding data that Medicare requires are providing hospitals with the basic quantitative information necessary to determine charges equitably. The impact of this increased knowledge is already apparent, as charges are now more closely corresponding to cost.[5] Additionally, the American Hospital Association's *Statement on the Financial Requirements of Health Care Institutions and Services* will, if and when operationally adopted, force third parties to pay for services on a cost basis that includes all economic costs in the reimbursement formula. If this is done, there will no longer be a need for hospitals either to view or to use charges as the balancing factor in their revenue structures. Instead, hospitals will be financially able to establish charges on the basis of economic costs.

How, though, does one set rates so that the charges for services will correspond to the economic costs of providing those services? To answer this question, it is necessary first to identify those cost elements that constitute economic cost.

RATE SETTING

THEORY

The American Hospital Association, in its publication "Factors to Evaluate in the Establishment of Hospital Charges," states that

the rates charged for each individual service should reflect properly the operating expenses of the service rendered, plus an equitable share of the other financial needs for which the patient is responsible.[6]

The Association thus provides a reasonable and financially realistic philosophical guideline for establishing charges. However, it does not spe-

---

[5]Feldstein, Paul J. and Waldman, Saul, "The Financial Position of Hospitals in the First Two Years of Medicare," *Inquiry*, Volume VI, No. 1, pp. 19–27.

[6]American Hospital Association, "Factors to Evaluate in the Establishment of Hospital Charges," p. 10.

cifically indicate the cost elements that must be considered if charges are properly to reflect operating expenses and other financial needs, that is, reflect economic costs.[7]

Perhaps the simplest approach to identifying and conceptualizing the costs that constitute total economic cost, and that should be included in setting rates, is to view a charge as comprising a stack of premiums or cost elements. Figure 8.1 illustrates this concept.

As can be seen from the figure, the first cost element that should be included is the basic cost of producing the service. This cost is really nothing more than the sum of the actual direct and indirect costs of production.

In addition to basic production costs, the hospital, if it is to maintain a sound financial position, must also include premiums for community costs. That is, it should include cost premiums for services it provides to the community that are neither directly nor indirectly related to the actual production of any particular unit of patient service. Examples of costs of this nature are education, research, and community health program costs. The sum of these two categories of cost—basic production plus community costs—can be defined as accounting cost. This cost is the total cost of a revenue or final cost center as determined through cost finding.

Economic costs, such as additional working and plant capital needs, should also be included as part of the stack of premiums. The inclusion of these cost elements is necessary to maintain both the quantity and quality of the hospital's capital stock. The total of these cost factors, plus accounting cost, can be identified as financial cost. This cost accurately reflects the financial requirements of the hospital, for not only are operating expenses considered, but other financial needs also are taken into account. Thus, if charges are to be equitable to both the payer and the hospital, they should be equal to the financial cost of producing a unit of service.

If a hospital were to set charges at the above rate, and if it were to receive payment on all its bills, it would generate revenues equal to its financial requirements. Unfortunately, hospitals do not always receive payment on all their patient billings. Therefore, financial cost must be adjusted for bad debts and free services. That is, an additional premium or cost element must be included in the charge structure. The inclusion of this last element sets the charge structure equal to economic cost. If a hospital were to charge for services at this rate, it would both receive revenues—billings less bad debts and free services—equal to its financial requirements and establish an equitable charge structure.

---

[7]It is interesting to note that the concept of economic cost, first introduced in this text in 1971, is becoming increasingly accepted. The Blue Cross Association has recognized it in its policy on "Payment to Health Care Institutions." The federal government has recognized it in PL 93–641 (the Health Services Resources and Development Act of 1974), and state governments, as in the state of Maryland, have recognized it in their rate review laws. See Appendix 8 for a further discussion of legislated rate setting.

The foregoing reflects an implicit assumption that the institution is a nonprofit (Section 501(c)(3)) hospital. As a result, a cost element to reflect a rate of return on invested equity has not been included in the model. If the hospital were investor-owned (proprietary), a rate of return on equity would be a real operating cost and charges would have to be set at a level sufficient to generate revenue to meet this financial requirement. This would be accomplished by adding another premium or cost element to the financial cost stack in Figure 8.1.

The question of whether hospitals should be organized for profit, and have the added cost of a rate of return, is a complex ethical, economic, and public policy issue. It must be recognized that investor-owned institutions are a significant and growing force in the hospital industry, with over 1,060 hospitals and 105,657 beds. Moreover, the profit motive has proven in many phases of the economy to be a beneficial driving force requiring no apology. However, as a countervailing point, one must appreciate that, unless the profit motive produces compensating improvements in operating efficiency, the rate of return is an added cost—due to organizational form—that increases the price of hospital care.

Viewing the charge for a service as a stack of premiums is fine in theory. However, this theory, though fostering an understanding of how charges should be established, does not explain how actually to establish charges. Therefore, let us turn now and examine the mechanics of rate setting.

MECHANICS

The American Hospital Association has suggested three basic methodologies or techniques for determining the rates applicable to the products or services of the various revenue centers within a hospital. Each of these methodologies utilizes the notion of economic cost as the basis for establishing charges and attempts to apportion this cost—as reasonably as possible—to the particular units of service produced by the revenue center in question. The mechanics of each technique and the type of revenue center for which it is most appropriate are discussed below.

Weighted Procedure Rate Method. Those revenue centers, such as laboratory, radiology, and inpatient units, that produce various but relatively standardized services or products should determine their service charge in terms of average cost per weighted procedure or service. This technique requires that each different product that is produced by the revenue center be assigned a unit weight or value based upon the relative time, resources, and skill required to produce that product. That is, the unit value should represent the cost of performing a service relative to some other service which is used as a base, that is, has a unit value of one. Table 8.2 presents the example relative value units suggested at one time by the Connecticut Hospital Association for laboratory services.

Given a listing of unit values, the next step in calculating the service charge is to multiply the unit value for each service by the expected number of services that will be produced in order to determine the total number of weighted units.[8] Total economic cost should then be divided by total weight units to determine charge per weighted unit. Based upon these calculations, the charge per service is determined simply by multiplying the charge per weighted unit by the predetermined value of each service. Tables 8.3 and 8.4 illustrate this technique for inpatient and laboratory revenue centers.

Admittedly, this technique for computing rates is relatively complex. However, if the unit values assigned to each service are appropriate, the resulting charge structure will be equitable to all parties. Thus, the critical and, obviously, the most difficult factor in this process is the selection of unit values. Various sources, such as the American College of Pathology and the American College of Radiology, have developed listings of unit values which may be appropriate to a particular hospital's needs.[9] However, a hospital, before completely accepting any of these unit values, should first review them in terms of its own physical plant layout, processing tech-

---

[8]It should be noted that it is difficult, if not impossible, to establish equitable charges without first developing accurate demand forecasts and expense budgets. The basic principles underlying budgeting are discussed in Part IV. However, readers desiring additional information on these subjects should see H. Berman and P. Bash, *Operational Budgeting Systems;* M. Lash, *The Development of an Expense Budgeting Procedure;* or J. R. Griffith, *Quantitative Techniques for Hospital Planning and Control.*

[9]Remarks of Owen M. Johnson, Jr., Director, Bureau of Competition, Federal Trade Commission. Mr. Johnson's remarks were made in April 1977 to the National Health Lawyers Association.

"Another area of Commission concern is the promulgation and use of relative value scales by professional groups. For those of you who are not familiar with the relative value scale (or RVS), it is a listing of procedures or services with assigned comparative values. Where the comparative values are expressed in dollar terms, the publication and circulation of these schedules may constitute direct price-fixing. Even where these procedures or services are ranked by some other numerical index (for example, the recommended time for a procedure), physicians may, by agreeing on a monetary conversion factor (for example, $75 per hour), produce a price-fixing schedule.

"Promulgation of RVSs by members of a professional group can diminish price competition in a number of ways. First, the scale, by its very nature, eliminates a degree of independent choice for those who use it. Variation in overhead, direct costs, and desired profits—the components of pricing in a competitive marketplace—are ignored by RVSs. More importantly, these scales make it difficult, if not impossible, for the conscientious health care shopper to derive any benefits from comparative pricing.

"In a series of cases the Commission has obtained consent orders from three professional associations, the American College of Obstetricians and Gynecologists, the American College of Radiology, and the American Academy of Orthopaedic Surgeons; and a proposed consent settlement with a fourth association, the Minnesota State Medical Association, is currently on file for public comment. These orders require the organizations to withdraw all copies of RVSs and to refrain from publishing or participating in the development of any such scales in the future. *Continued on p. 248.*

TABLE 8.2 Example Relative Value Units

	Suggested Values		Suggested Values

I. CHEMISTRY EXAMINATIONS
Acetone (serum) 20
ACTH response test with
  administration 300
Aldosterone 750
Albumin 30
Albumin & globulin with total
  protein 60
Alcohol, blood 100
Aldolase 100
Amino acids, blood or urine 100
Amino nitrogen 100
Aminotransfases (see transaminase) . 50
Ammonia 00
Amylase 40
Ascorbic acid (Vit. C) 80
Barbiturates, quantitative 50
Barbiturates, specific identification .. 120
Bilirubin, direct & total 35
Bilirubin, micro or amniotic 50
Blood gases-complete
Blood gases, Ph PCO$_2$ Cal. HCO$_3$ ... 80
Blood gases, PO$_2$ alone 50
Blood gases, O$_2$ Sat. calculated extra 10
Blood gases with pH, PGO$_2$ and PO$_2$ 100
Bromide 50
BSP 50
Blood urea nitrogen (BUN) ....
Blood urea nitrogen, manual 25
Blood urea nitrogen,
  large batch volumes 20
Blood volume dye 100
Calcium, manual 50
Calcium, large volumes 40
Catecholamines 200
Carbon dioxide, manual 35
Carbon dioxide, large volumes 25
Carbon monoxide, qual, sean 50
Carotenes 50
Cephalin cholest. flocculation 20
Chlorides, manual 30
Chlorides, large volumes 25
Cholesterol, total 50
Cholesterol, free and esters 100
Cholinesterase, typical 50
Cholinesterase, debucane atypical .. 75
Copper 100
Cortisol, plasma 100
Creatine 50
Creatine phosphokinase 50
Creatinine, serum manual 40
Creatinine, large volumes 30

Clearance calculation 10
Cryoglobulins with collection at
  37°C 40
Doriden 120
Electrophoresis, serum protein 80
Electrophoresis, large batch 60
Electrophoresis, immuno 200
Electrophoresis, lipoproteins 100
Electrophoresis, urine, CSF, protein 100
Electrophoresis, haptoglobin ....

II. HEMATOLOGY
Anticoagulants, circulating 50
Bleeding time, Ivy 35
Blood counts
  Eosinophils 30
  Platelets, smear estimate 20
  Platelets, quantitative 50
RBC 15
RBC, manual 15
Reticulocytes 30
WBC, semi, large volume 10
WBC, manual 15
WBC, differential, smear 20
Blood indices (math only) 5
Blood volume-Evans dye 100
Bone marrow (aspiration, H & E, Fe
  on clot and/or interpretation) 300
Clot retraction, qualitative 10
Coagulation time ....
Coagulation time, Lee White 60
Fibrinogen, quantitative 75
Fibrinolysins, qualitative 10
Fragility of crythrocytes 150
G-6-P-D, screen qualitative 50
G-6-P-D, semiquantitative
  histochem 100
Hematocrit 10
Hemoglobin, manual 15
Hemoglobin, large volume 10
Hemoglobin, plasma 50
Hemoglobin, type F (Fetal) 60
Hemoglobin, electrophoresis 80
Hemoglobin, A2 ....
Hemolysins, acid or cold screen 20
Hemolysins, quant acid-Ham T 100
Hemolysins, auto 50
L-E preparation 100
Leukocyte alkaline phosphatase 100
Malaria smear 50
Methemoglobin 50
Electrophoresis, hemoglobin 80

TABLE 8.2   Continued

	Suggested Values		Suggested Values
Electrophoresis, A2	100	Uric acid, manual	40
Placental estriols		Uric acid, large volumes	30
Fatty acid, total		VMA	
FSH		VMA, quantitative	100
Galactose tolerance,		Xylose, urine, no dose	100
see glucose per spec	30	17 Ketosteroids, total	75
Gamma globulin salting out	30	17 Ketogenic, steroids	125
Glucose, manual	25	ABO immune antibody screen & titer	
Glucose, large volume	20	of infant	75
Haptoglobin		RB cells washed	150
Hemoglobin, plasma free	50	Platelets concentrate	225
Hydroxyindolacetic acid (5HIAA)	30	Leukocyte poor blood preparation	50
17 Hydroxysteroids (Porter-Siller)		Open head workup-simple	375
Iodine, PBI alone	75	Open head workup-complex	625
Iodine, PBI large batch	50	Packed cells preparation	25
Iodine, BEI	150	Plasmaphoresis per event	600
T3 by column		Phlebotomy	50
T4		Platelet concentrate preparation	150
Iron, serum	50	Cryoprecipitate	225
Iron, binding capacity	100	Antibody technique fluorescence	100
LDH, manual	40	Antistreptolysin O titers	65
LDH, large volumes	30	Agglutinations (slide) febrile each	30
LDH, fractionation isoenzymes	80	Agglutinations (tube) brucella only	60
Lipase	50	Agglutinations (tube) coccydiomyces	60
Lipids, total	100	Agglutinations leptosera, rubella,	
Lipids, triglycerides	100	tularemia, typhoid O silicosis	60
Lipids, phospholipids	60	Antibiotic sensitivity disc	30
Lithium	50	Antibiotic sensitivity tube	125
Macroglobulin, sia H2O test	20	Autogenous vaccine	300
Macroglobulin, electrophoresis		Cold agglutinins with titer	65
Macroglobulin,		C-reactive protein	40
immunoelectrophoresis		Culture, general bact.	50
Magnesium, manual	50	Culture, general bact. with	
Methemoglobin	50	sensitivity	75
NPN	50	Culture, blood with sensitivity	125
Osmolarity	25	Culture, stool or urine with	
Phosphatase, acid (total only)	40	sensitivity	75
Phosphatase, prostatic & total	60	Culture, fungi	75
Phosphatase, alkaline manual	40	Culture, fungus with definitive ID	100
Phosphatase, large volume	30	Culture, Tbc with smear	125
Phosphorous, manual	30	Dark field	75
Phosphorous, large volumes	25	Direct smear clinical material	
Potassium, manual	25	including tbc	40
Proteins, total, chemical	30	Heterophile, screen	30
Proteins, refractometer	20	Heterophile with absorption titer	65
Salicylates, quantitative	30	Immunoglobulins by diffusion	
Sodium, manual	25	Ig G, Ig A, Ig M (all three)	100
Sodium, large batches	20	Latex fixation for slide R.A.F. with	
Sulfonamides	50	one dilution	40
Thymol turbity	25	Peripheral smear for parasites	50
Transaminases, manual	40	Plasma clotting factors	
Transaminases, large volumes	30	Factor V	125

Continued

TABLE 8.2   Continued

	Suggested Values		Suggested Values
Factor VIII	125	Sugar, quantitative	25
Factor IX	125	Sulkowitch	10
Factor X	125	Urinalysis, routine, complete	30
Factor XIII	25	Urobilinogen	25
Platelet aggregation	10		
Prothrombin time	25	**VI. MISCELLANEOUS**	
Prothrombin consumption	50	Gastric analysis per specimen by pH	
Partial thromboplastin time (PTT)	25	meter specimens fasting and max	
Peroxidase stain	40	stim, pH and total acid output	30
RBC morphology Only	20	Diagnex	30
Sedimentation Rate	15	Occult blood	10
Sickle cell preparation	20	Sweat tests, plate	25
Siderocyte stain (Fe)	30	Sweat tests, complete	
Thrombin time, alone	30	Sweat tests, Na or Cl	
Thromboplastin generation test		Sweat tests, nails	
(TGT complete)	50		
Tourniquet test	50	**VII. ADMINISTRATIVE**	
		Stat collection only	40
III. TRANSFUSION SERVICE		Night performance	20
ABO, cell grouping	20	Routine collection	20
ABO, grouping & Rh typing (routine)	35	Drawing separating and added	
Rh cell typing (anti D, anti CD) slide	15	packaging, transportation, and	
Rh subgrouping (anti C, D, E, c, e)	50	record costs	
Subgrouping other than common		a. Simple, 1st class	25
Rh & ABO antigens	25	b. Complex (dry ice) also special	100
Crossmatch-routine (saline, albumin,		Local reduction (in a specific test)	
antiglobulin)	40	units	
Direct antiglobulin (Coombs) test	30	Because another institution as-	
Indirect antiglobulin (Coombs) test	35	sumed drawing, sending, and bill-	
		ing costs	10
IV. SEROLOGY-BACTERIOLOGY		Local reduction of a specific test unit	
Antibody titer (i.e., anti-Rh)	65	as above but billing	5
Antibody screen (simple)	40		
Antibody identification	200	**VIII. ISOTOPES**	
Rhogam workup with maternal		Au 198 microaggregate	340
& infant screen		Blood volume, dye	100
ABO immune antibody screen		Blood volume, RISA first	25
& titer of mother	75	Blood volume, RISA with repeats	
Osmolarity	15	Bloodvolume, Cr51 RBC's	140
pH	10	Blood volume, Cr51 repeats with same	
Porphorins-screen	15	cells	100
Copro, Uro, porphobilinogen	100	Latex fixation for thyroid globulin	
Phenylketonuria-(fe C13)	10	antibodies	40
		Pregnancy-chorionic gonadotrophins	
V. CLINICAL MICROSCOPY		Pregnancy-chorionic full titer	150
Phenolsulphonthalein (PSP)	20	Pregnancy-serologic slide test	40
Porphobilinogen	35	Pregnancy-titers (3 tubes)	80
Protein, qualitative	10	Rubella hemagglutination inhibition	80
Salicylates, screen (fe C13)	30	Serologic test for syphilis, VDRL	15
Sediment see mx	10	Premarital VDRL	20
Specific gravity, alone	10	Treponema fluorescent antibodies	100
Sugar, qualitative	10	Thyroid antibodies tube test	65

TABLE 8.2   Continued

	Suggested Values		Suggested Values
C. S. F. tests		G-II 131 protein loss (PVP)	
Cell count with differential	50	G-I Cr51 RBC intestinal blood loss ..	
Fecal tests		Insulin binding index	100
Qualitative stool fat	20	Insulin immunoassay	100
Microscopic examination of stool	25	I 131 excretion, 48 hours	80
Occult blood	10	I 131 excretion, repeat 48 hours	40
Ova & parasites, complete	75	I 131 plasma descence	
Pin worm preparation	10	I 131 PBI	
Urobilin, qualitative	25	I 131 uptake, single determination .	
Trypsin by titer	30	I 131 uptake, multiple	150
Sperm analysis		I 131 uptake, with thyroid	
Sperm count & mobility	100	suppression	150
Urinalysis		I 131 uptake with TSH stimulation ..	440
Addis count	75	I 131 uptake with scintiscan	150
Routine & microscopic	30	Lung microaggregates	340
Acetone	0	Pancreas scan, Se 75	125
Bence-Jones protein heat	25	Placental scan	150
Bence-Jones protein-electrophoresis	100	Renal scan	380
Bile ictotest	10	Renogram, hippuranil I 131 or Hg	
Calculus chemical analysis	50	203	300
Cell count & differential	75	Rose Bengal, liver	220
Fat particles (free)	40	Rose Bengal, with scintiscan	
Hemoglobin (free)	10	Spleen scan with sequestration	190
Hemosiderin	40	T3 uptake with RBC	50
Hemogentisic acid	20	T3 uptake with resin sponge	60
Melanin	25	T4 Murphy-Pattee	100
Microscopic only (centrifuge)	15	Phatmologram	20
Myoglobin-screen	15	Ferrokinetics	400
Myoglobin-qualitative	100	RBC survival Cr51	200
Body scan, whole	400		
Bone, 1st section scan	260	IX. TISSUES & CYTOLOGY	
Bone, 2nd section scan	350	Gyn-cervical & vaginal	50
Brain, cisternograph with RISA	540	Sputum, urine and cavity fluids	75
Brain, technicium (te)	410	Gastric with collection	150
B12 Schilling, initial	140	Sex chromatin determination	50
B12 Schilling, with intrinsic factor ..	200	Tissues	
Cardiac output with ISHA		Gross only includes pathologist	30
Cardiac cisternograph with RISA	540	Gross & microscopic	300
Cardiac scan (peripheral effusion) ...	220	Frozen section consultation	300
Circulation time		Bone marrow	300
G-II 131 triolein study		Autopsy	5000
G-II 131 oleic acid study			

Source: Connecticut Hospital Association, Relative Value Schedule-Laboratory. Used by permission of the Connecticut Hospital Association.

TABLE 8.3   Laboratory Charges

I.   *Assumptions*
     A.   Accounting costs for the laboratory = $150,000.
     B.   Financial and economic costs for the laboratory = a 20% addition or
          $30,000.*
     C.   Total economic cost for the laboratory (financial requirements) =
          $180,000.
     D.   Weighted units computation (example represents only a sample of all tests
          performed).

Amylase, blood	2,000	2.5†	5,000
Bleeding time	2,500	1.9	4,750
Hematocrit	3,800	.8	3,040
Platelet count	3,900	1.0	3,900
Uric acid	1,500	1.5	2,250
Total weighted units (all tests)			120,000

II. *Calculation*
     Step A

$$\frac{\text{Total economic cost}}{\text{Total weighted units}} = \text{Charge/Weighted unit}$$

$$\$180,000 \div 120,000 = \$1.50$$

     Step B

(Charge/weighted unit) × (Unit value of test) = Charge/Test
$1.50 × 2.5 = $3.75 Charge/Amylase, blood test
$1.50 × 1.9 = $2.85 Charge/Bleeding time test
$1.50 × .8 = $1.20 Charge/Hematocrit test
$1.50 × 1   = $1.50 Charge/Platelet count test
$1.50 × 1.5 = $2.25 Charge/Uric acid test

*Premium for economic and financial costs should be based on historical accounting data
(bad debt and free service element), subjective estimates, and policy decisions.

†These weighting factors are used just for purposes of illustration. Individual hospitals
should select weighting factors on the basis of their unique physical plants, processing techniques, capital-labor mix, and so forth.

---

[9]*Continued from p. 243.*

   "One aspect of our RVS orders which has caused confusion has been the effect of the
Commission's actions on the value scales of third-party payers. It should be noted that these
consent orders in no way restrict health insurers—whether private or government—from
developing guidelines for assessing the reasonableness of charges. The Commission's concern has been confined to physicians' adoption of RVSs and efforts to ensure adherence to
these schedules. Use of similar scales by third-party payers does not make them participants
in price-affecting agreements of the type proscribed by the Commission's consent orders. In
short, it is one thing for consumers to develop guidelines for evaluating fees, but quite
another for competitors to publish and enforce pricing schedules. Despite this distinction,
it is interesting to note that the Social Security Administration has directed private insurers
who administer physician payments for Medicare to cease references to relative value scales
banned by the Commission."

TABLE 8.4   Inpatient Unit Charges

I. *Assumptions*
    A. Type of facility

	Private Room	Semiprivate Room	Ward	Total
Expected patient days	2,000	6,000	2,000	10,000
Facility unit value	2	1.5	1	
Total weighted units	4,000	9,000	2,000	15,000

    B. Costs
        Accounting, financial, and economic costs to be allocated on the basis of patient days = $350,000.
        Accounting, financial, and economic costs to be allocated on the basis of unit value = $150,000.

II. *Calculation*
    Step A

$$\frac{\text{Costs to be allocated on the basis of patient days}}{\text{Patient days}} = \frac{\text{Patient day}}{\text{charge factor}}$$

        $350,000 \div 10,000 = $35

    Step B

$$\frac{\text{Costs to be allocated on the basis of unit values}}{\text{Total weighted units}} = \frac{\text{Unit value}}{\text{charge factor}}$$

        $150,000 \div 15,000 = $10

    Step C

        (Unit value charge factor) × (Unit value of facility) = Unit value charge factor/facility
            $10 × 2   = $20 Unit value charge factor/Private room bed
            $10 × 1.5 = $15 Unit value charge factor/Semiprivate room bed
            $10 × 1   = $10 Unit value charge factor/Ward bed

    Step D

        (Patient day charge factor) + (Unit value charge factor/Facility) = Charge/Inpatient unit
            $35 + $20 = $55 Charge/Private room bed
            $35 + $15 = $50 Charge/Semiprivate room bed
            $35 + $10 = $45 Charge/Ward bed

III. *Explanation (Patient Days)*
    A. Certain cost elements, such as nursing, dietary, medical records, and working capital needs, are, for the most part, used or applied uniformly to all patients. Thus, they should be allocated on the basis of patient days. Therefore, based on accounting data (budgets), the hospital should determine the total amount of cost that should be allocated on a patient day basis. This cost should then be divided by total patient days to determine cost per patient day.
    B. Those cost elements that cannot be allocated appropriately on a uniform basis should be distributed on a weighted value basis. The mechanics of this distribution are basically the same as those depicted in Table 8.3. Cost elements that fall into this category are bad debts, plant capital needs, depreciation, housekeeping, plant operations, and so forth.
    C. As the final step, the charges, as determined in items A and B above, should be combined to produce charge per type of facility.

niques, capital and labor mix, and costs. If the proposed values are not suitable, the hospital should either subjectively modify them or, using industrial engineering techniques, develop its own value system. This latter alternative is quite costly and should only be used as a last resort when subjective modification does not provide workable results.

Hourly Rate Method. Those revenue centers, such as operating room, physical therapy, and anesthesia, whose patient service is hours of use, should determine their service charge in terms of rate per hour. An example of the mechanics of determining charge per hour of usage for the operating room is presented in Table 8.5.

It should be noted that the operating room rate is expressed in terms of both rate per manhour and rate per operating room hour. The calculation of both rates provides the hospital with the flexibility necessary to assure that rates are as equitable as is practically feasible. Thus, when a procedure is an average or typical procedure, that is, the average number of personnel participate, the rate per operating room hour is appropriate. However, if a procedure is atypical, that is, more or fewer than the typical number of personnel are involved, the rate per manhour should be used. In this way, the hospital can tailor its rates to fit the actual service provided.

The charge for operating room use also can be calculated on the basis of the average cost per weighted procedure. However, due to the wide range of possible variation in the time, resources, and skill required to

TABLE 8.5   Hourly Rates

I. *Assumptions*
    A. Accounting costs for the operating room = $100,000
    B. Financial and economic costs for the operating room = a 30% addition or $30,000
    C. Total economic costs for the operating room = $130,000
    D. Expected hours of use = 2,000
    E. Average number of personnel per operation = 4

II. *Calculation*
    A. (Total economic cost) ÷ (Hours of usage) = Rate/Hour
            $130,000 ÷ 2,000 = $65 Charge/Hour
        This rate should be used when a procedure utilizes the average number of personnel.
    B. (Hours of usage) × (Typical number of personnel) = Manhours of usage
            2,000 × 4 = 8,000 manhours
        1. (Total economic cost) ÷ (Manhours of usage) = Rate per manhour
                $130,000 ÷ 8,000 = $16.25 Charge/Manhour
        2. This rate should be used when a procedure involves more, or less, personnel than typical. For example, for a one-hour procedure that utilizes 5 persons, the charge should be 5 × $16.25, or $81.25.

perform any given procedure, this technique is more suited to revenue centers that provide reasonably standardized services, such as those discussed above, than it is to the operating room. Therefore, hourly rates are recommended as the preferred basis for charging for operating room services.[10]

Surcharge Rate Method. Those revenue centers, such as pharmacy and central supply, that serve primarily a merchandising function, should determine their rates in terms of a surcharge which should be "added on" to the cost of the goods they supply. That is, those revenue centers whose function is that of either handling or preparing goods for final distribution should establish charges on the basis of the cost plus a surcharge for handling and processing. An illustration of this method of determining charges is presented for pharmacy in Table 8.6.

RATE SETTING PRAGMATISM

The above methodologies, with some minor modifications such as that necessary for inpatient units, will provide the hospital with the techniques needed to establish charges equal to economic costs for each of its revenue centers. However, determining or knowing the theoretically ideal charge for each service is not enough. For example, if the charge for a particular service based on economic cost appears excessive, management may as a matter of policy reduce the charge for that service and subsidize it by increasing the charges for other services.

Perhaps the best illustration of this type of situation was referred to earlier in regard to routine service rates. As was pointed out, hospitals, to avoid or at least to minimize public pressure and scrutiny, as a matter of policy set routine service charges at less than cost so that they will compare more favorably with hotel and restaurant rates. The obvious result of this practice is that inpatient units operate at a loss, that is, costs exceed revenues. To recover this loss, profits, that is, revenues in excess of cost, must be generated by other revenue centers. Thus, it is common to find laboratory, radiology, and pharmacy producing profits, while operating room, delivery room, and inpatient units operate at a loss.

In addition to adjusting the rate structure for seemingly excessive charges, management may also be forced to alter rates due to third party payer attitudes and practices. As has been discussed, third party payers, in principle, should pay essentially the same rates as all other payers. However, as should be realized by this point, the simple fact is that they do not pay

---

[10]Hourly rates, while an improvement over the weighted procedure method, are still not ideal for they ignore the matter of personnel mix. Thus, to the extent that a rate can be adjusted for the actual mix of personnel used in any given procedure, it can be made more equitable.

TABLE 8.6   Pharmacy Charges

I. *Assumptions*
    A. Accounting cost for pharmacy = $50,000.
    B. Financial and economic cost for pharmacy = a 20% addition, or $10,000.
    C. Total economic cost for pharmacy = $60,000.
    D. Cost of drugs billed to patients = $45,000.

II. *Calculations*
    Step A

        (Total economic cost) − (Cost of drugs billed to patients) = Total
        surcharge
            $60,000 − $45,000 = $15,000
    Step B

$$\frac{\text{Total surcharge}}{\text{Cost of drugs billed to patients}} = \text{Percentage markup}$$

            $15,000 ÷ $45,000 = 33.3%
    Step C

        (Percentage markup) × (Cost of drugs*) = Surcharge
            33.3% × $12 = $4
    Step D

        (Surcharge) + (Cost of drugs) = Charge/Drugs
            $4 + $12 = $16 Charge

*Assumed drug cost for a particular prescription.

on the same basis. Accordingly, rate structures applicable to other payers must be adjusted if a hospital is to maintain a financially sound position.

The implications of these pragmatic factors, regardless of how distasteful, should be obvious. To maintain a financially viable position, management must adjust charges to meet financial realities. This fact, though philosophically repugnant, is a fiscal fact of life which intelligent management cannot ignore. The foregoing theory and techniques will provide management with the understanding and information necessary to determine the costs of these decisions and, one hopes, will enable better decisions to be made. However, neither theory nor technique will change the fact that rate adjustment decisions are necessary.

CONCLUSION

Based on both the previous chapters and the above material, the reader should now have an understanding of the sources of hospital operating revenues, their philosophies, and the financial problems and considerations related to these sources.

SUGGESTED READINGS

American Hospital Association. *Cost Finding and Rate Setting for Hospitals.*

Berman, Howard J. and Bash, Paul L. *Operational Budgeting Systems: Hackley Hospital, Muskegon, Michigan*

Dowling, William L. (ed.). "Prospective Rate Setting."

Dowling, William L. "Prospective Reimbursement of Hospitals."

Kaitz, Edward M. *Pricing Policy and Cost Behavior in the Hospital Industry.*

Lash, Myles P. "The Development of an Expense Budgeting Procedure."

Ruchlin, Hirsch S. and Roger, Harry M. "Short-Run Hospital Responses to Reimbursement Rate Changes."

Topics in Health Care Financing. "Rate Regulation."

APPENDIX 8[11]
LEGISLATED RATE SETTING

When the foregoing chapter was first written, the notion of economic cost was little more than a theoretical construct whose principal value lay in its usefulness in explaining desired management behavior. Similarly, the notion of third party cost-based reimbursement agreements being renegotiated to include all economic cost was little more than an idealistic goal. However, in 1969 the state of New York enacted legislation giving the commissioner of the Department of Health the responsibility for certifying that proposed hospital rates were reasonably related to the cost of delivering efficient health care services. The commissioner has implemented this responsibility through a formula approach to rate setting.

Since 1969, 16 states have enacted and one state (Colorado) has rescinded legislation that requires the disclosure, review, or regulation of hospital rates or budgets.[12] Table 8.A-1 summarizes, with the exception of Illinois where the program is not yet operational, the major characteristics of each of these state programs. Of the 14 operational programs, 4 states (Connecticut, Maryland, Massachusetts, and Washington) have rate-setting commissions with full authority to review and approve hospital budgets or rates. Two other states (New York and New Jersey) have given authority to state agencies to set Medicaid and Blue Cross rates.

The remaining 8 states, with the exception of Wisconsin and Rhode Island, use a variety of organizational mechanisms to review and comment on publicly or to disclose findings as to the reasonableness of hospital rates. The Rhode Island program is carried out by Blue Cross. Wisconsin uses a

---

[11]Material for this appendix has been drawn, in large part, from *Abstracts of State Legislated Hospital Cost Containment Programs,* HCFA Pub. No. 017 (5–78).

[12]In 1980 the American Hospital Association also rescinded its guidelines on "State Level Review and Approval of Budgets for Health Care Institutions."

joint committee of the Department of Health, Blue Cross, and the state hospital association. Both the Rhode Island and Wisconsin programs require hospital compliance with the findings of the review process.

Participation in each of the programs is mandatory for all nongovernmental hospitals. Compliance with the programs is mandatory in all the involved states except for Arizona, Maine, Minnesota, Oregon, and Virginia. It should be recognized, however, that states with voluntary compliance believe that public pressure and third party contractual payment processes will result in actual compliance.

It is interesting to note that though support for legislated rate-setting programs exists in many areas, the cost containment effectiveness of such programs is still an open question. To begin to provide answers, the Health Care Financing Administration has financed the evaluation of six rate-setting programs: that is, western Pennsylvania, upstate and downstate New York, New Jersey, Rhode Island, and Indiana.[13] Of the programs, four—western Pennsylvania, upstate New York, New Jersey, and Rhode Island[14]—were shown not to have had a statistically significant impact on hospital costs. In contrast, the other two programs—Indiana and downstate New York—both showed a statistically significant cost impact.

This latter evidence does not, however, make it easier to draw firm conclusions about the effectiveness of legislated programs.[15] While the New York program is legislated, the Indiana program is just the opposite—a voluntary effort, established in 1960 by the Indiana Blue Cross Plan and the Indiana Hospital Association.

The Federation of American Hospitals (FAH), the national association of investor-owned hospitals, also has attempted to examine the effects of hospital rate regulation. The FAH financed a study, conducted by ICF Corporation, to examine in 17 states the impact of rate regulation on hospital costs and revenues. The 17 states were grouped into three categories:

1. Mandatory rate regulation (Maryland, Connecticut, New York, New Jersey, Massachusetts)

2. Voluntary or private payer operated rate regulation (Arizona, Indiana, Ohio, Pennsylvania, Wisconsin)

---

[13]Hellinger, Fred J., "State Rate Review: A Critical Assessment." *Hospitals*, September 1, 1978.

[14]The New Jersey and New York programs are legislated programs. Indiana, Rhode Island, and western Pennsylvania are voluntary efforts.

[15]There is very little indication that hospital rate regulation has a more significant effect than other factors on controlling hospital expenditures per case and per capita and in limiting hospital revenues per case and per capita; to the extent that any effect could be discerned, the states with voluntary rate regulation programs exhibited 1% to 2% better performance than either of the other two groups on most measures over the period studied.

3. No rate regulation (Texas, Virginia, North Carolina, Florida, Illinois, Minnesota, California)

The findings of the study can be summarized as follows:

1. States with mandatory rate regulation exhibited performance similar to states with no rate regulation at all; however, two factors are relevant here:

   a. First, the only period in which mandatory rate regulation seemed to have a slight effect was in reducing hospital expenditures per case in the post-ESP period (1974–75). However, this effect was more than offset by an increase in hospital utilization that produced higher expenditures per capita; thus, effective utilization controls appear to be an essential component of mandatory rate regulation; more research and consideration should be focused upon whether PROs are capable of such reductions or whether other approaches are required;

   b. Second, it is possible that socioeconomic factors might have produced higher rates of increase in the absence of mandatory rate setting; however, examination of states from the two groups with similar socioeconomic characteristics (Illinois and New Jersey) and in the periods before and after the introduction of rate regulation in other states (Maryland) provided little support for this possibility.

2. States with voluntary programs might well form a good basis for further experimentation and research; despite the current emphasis on mandatory rate regulation programs, the study found evidence that voluntary programs hold as much or more promise; thus, further consideration should be given during research and experimentation to disclosure-oriented programs (such as Arizona) and other voluntary approaches (for example, the use of competitive bidding to establish reimbursement levels).

3. States considering development of rate regulation systems should consider the expected impact carefully; the researchers were unable to identify any significant initial impact of rate regulation, and the impact over time was greatly affected by other factors, such as socioeconomic conditions, changes in utilization, and the Economic Stabilization Program.

In considering the above findings it is important to bear in mind that these evaluations focused on so-called first generation programs. As rate-setting programs continue, it is likely that they will evolve into increasingly sophisticated and potentially potent cost containment programs. Whether such potency will accrue to the community good—or just fuel a regulatory

TABLE 8.A-1*   State Legislated Hospital Cost Containment Programs†

State	Responsible Agency	Type of System	Voluntary vs. Mandatory	Payers Covered
Arizona	Department of Health Services: Local HSAs	Budget/Rate review	Mandatory review Voluntary compliance	Charge-based including Blue Cross
California	Department of Health Facilities Commission	Disclosure	Mandatory disclosure	Not applicable
Connecticut	Commission on Hospitals and Health Care	Budget/Rate review and approval	Mandatory	Charge-based
Maine	Health Facilities Cost Review Board: voluntary budget review organization	Budget/Rate review voluntary compliance	Mandatory review Voluntary compliance	Charge-based
Maryland	Health Services Cost Review Commission	Budget/Rate review and approval	Mandatory	All payers
Massachusetts	Massachusetts Rate Setting Commission	Cost/Rate review and approval	Mandatory	Blue Cross
		Budget/Rate review and approval	Mandatory	Charge-based
		Rate setting	Mandatory	Medicaid
Minnesota	Department of Health Minnesota Hospital Association	Budget/Rate review	Mandatory review Voluntary compliance	Charge-based including Blue Cross
New Jersey	State Department of Health	Budget/Rate review and approval	Mandatory	Medicaid and Blue Cross
New York	State Department of Health	Rate setting	Mandatory	Medicaid and Blue Cross
Oregon	State Health Planning and Development Agency	Budget/Rate review	Mandatory review Voluntary compliance	Charge-based including Blue Cross
Rhode Island	State Budget Office: Blue Cross of Rhode Island	Negotiated budget/rate review and approval	Mandatory	Medicaid and Blue Cross
Virginia	Virginia Health Services Cost Review Commission: voluntary cost review organization	Cost/Charge review	Mandatory review Voluntary compliance	Not applicable
Washington	Washington State Hospital Commission	Budget/Rate review and approval	Mandatory	All payers Charge-based
Wisconsin	State Department of Health: Rate Review Committee	Budget/Rate review and approval	Mandatory	All payers except Medicare

Source: Health Care Financing Administration; Office of Policy, Planning, and Research; Office of Demonstrations and Evaluations.
*Abstracts of State Legislated Hospital Cost Containment Programs, HCFA Pub. No. 017 (5-78), May 1978.
†Illinois is not listed due to the initial development stage of the program.

Revenue Control Method	Unit of Payment	Frequency of Review	Adjustments	Appeals
Total revenue	Charges	Prior to any rate change	Not applicable	Not applicable
Not applicable	Not applicable	Annually	Not applicable	Not applicable
Total revenue	Charges	Annually	Retroactive volume: unforeseen and material change in expense	
Not applicable	Charges	Annually	Not applicable	Not applicable
Total revenue: departmental revenue or guaranteed revenue per case or maximum revenue per case	Rate-based charges	Annually and as necessary	Retroactive possible for volume and uncontrollable costs	Public hearing before Commission
Cost-based	Routine per diem, ancillary charges	Annually be denied	Excess costs may	Courts
Total revenue	Charges	Annually	None	Division of Hearing Officers
Cost-based	Per diem	Annually	Uncontrollable costs	Division of Hearing Officers
Total revenue	Charges	Annually and when requested during year	None	DOH-Public hearings before independent hearing examiner: MHA-hearing before appeals panel
Cost-based	Per diem	Annually	Retroactive: for volume, economic factors, pass-through items	Formal appeal before independent hearing officer
Cost-based	Per diem	Annually	Retroactive adjustment for actual economic factor: volume in downstate Blue Cross	Formal appeal before State hearing officer
Total revenue	Charges	Annually and when requested during year	Not applicable	Not applicable
Total revenue	Charges	Annually	Retroactive volume	Binding arbitration before independent mediation
Not applicable	Not applicable	Annual disclosure budgets as necessary	Not applicable	Not applicable
Total revenues rates per unit of service by revenue center	Rate-based charges	Annually	None	Formal hearing before commission or independent hearing officer
Total revenue	Charges	Prior to any rate change at most once a year	None	Hearing before independent appeals board

agency's need to demonstrate that it can be tough regardless of the community cost—is, at the moment, a moot point.

The only conclusion that can be drawn now is one of uncertainty.
Given the state of the art, there is nothing inherently wrong with reaching
this finding. Successive generations of legislated programs do, however,
merit careful monitoring so that more reasoned and knowledgeable judgments can be made as to their ultimate usefulness and role.

NOTE

As a related point it is interesting to note the results of the research
completed by Abt Associates for the Health Care Financing Administration
on the effects of prospective hospital financing programs on hospital
expenditures.[16]

The Abt Associates analysis yields four conclusions:

1. Prospective payment mechanisms are effective devices for controlling hospital costs.

2. Only in the most recent years have prospective payment systems
   shown a statistically and practically significant effect on hospital
   expenditures. (However, the fact that programs that were implemented in the mid-1970s produced an effect almost immediately
   does suggest that the payment system does not have to be in existence for four or five years before it influences hospital behavior.)

3. Both voluntary and mandatory prospective payment programs have
   been successful in reducing hospital expenditures.

4. Mandatory prospective payment programs appear to have a higher
   probability of being successful. (However, aside from suggesting
   that mandatory programs are more likely to be effective in controlling costs than are voluntary programs, the results provide relatively
   little indication of which other characteristics are likely to be important determinants of effectiveness.)

---

[16]Coelen, Craig and Sullivan, Daniel, "An Analysis of the Effects of Prospective Reimbursement Programs on Hospital Expenditures," *Health Care Financing Review*, Winter 1981.

PART

III

Working Capital Management

General Principles

The previous sections have attempted to aid the reader in developing a feeling for the financial environment of a hospital and an understanding of it. The inclusion of this background material was necessary to provide a foundation for the following discussion of the financial subsystems of hospitals. The emphasis of this section will be on developing an understanding of the tools and techniques needed to guide and control the operation of these systems. In this chapter and the next we shall examine the general principles of working capital management. In the subsequent chapters, the management and financing of specific systems (cash, marketable securities, inventories, and accounts receivable) will be discussed.

INTRODUCTION

The most appropriate way to begin a discussion of working capital management is to define what is meant by the term working capital. Historically, there has been substantial disagreement among financial managers, accountants, and economists as to the exact definition of working capital. Some authorities have gone so far as to argue that the term is both misleading and inaccurate and that, to avoid confusion, it should not be used at all. They prefer to focus attention on the individual elements of working capital—cash, accounts receivable, investments. To do so, however, fails to recognize properly that the changes within these elements merely reflect short-term management decisions as opposed to longer-term investment and operating strategies. As a result, the majority of authors and practitioners accept the concept of working capital and have defined it as being the total current assets of the hospital. Working capital, thus, refers to the sum of the hospital's investment in short-term or current assets—cash, marketable (short-term) securities, accounts receivable, and inventories.

Net working capital is also a commonly used term. It should be noted, however, that net working capital and working capital are not synonymous. Net working capital is defined as the excess of total current assets over total current liabilities—accounts payable, accrued wages, and any other short-term liabilities. Thus, working capital equals total current assets, and net working capital equals total current assets less total current liabilities.

The important matter, however, is not definitions. Certainly, it is necessary to start with an understanding of what is meant by the two terms. The critical question, though, is what is the importance of working capital management? Why is sound working capital management needed for efficient "least cost" hospital operations?

IMPORTANCE OF WORKING CAPITAL

To understand the importance of working capital management, it is necessary first to realize the significance of working capital to hospital operations. In the vocabulary of financial management, the word capital is a synonym for the term total tangible assets, that is, the capital of the hospital is equal to the sum of its assets. Total assets, in turn, can be classified into basically two categories—fixed or long-term assets, and liquid or current assets. Long-term (fixed) assets include such items as land, plant, equipment, and all other assets that the hospital expects to hold for more than one year. Conversely, current (liquid) assets consist of cash and those other assets that the hospital expects to convert into cash within one year, for example, accounts receivable, inventories, and short-term securities.

Fixed assets are obviously needed if patient care services are to be produced. However, fixed assets alone cannot be productive. A hospital building cannot produce patient care. It holds the productive capacity or the potential to produce care, but unless another element or ingredient is combined with fixed assets this potential cannot be realized. Thus, if fixed assets are to be productive they must be combined with another type of asset or capital. Current assets or working capital is the element that must be combined with fixed assets if their productive potential is to be achieved.

Working capital can be viewed as the catalyst that changes the productive potential of fixed assets into patient care services. Working capital, though it has no innate patient care potential of its own, is the means of converting buildings and equipment into patient care services. The obvious question, however, is how does working capital accomplish this? How is working capital able to make fixed assets productive?

Working Capital Management

To understand fully the importance of working capital and the methods for managing it, it is essential to obtain a firm understanding of the manner in which a hospital generates and uses working capital. Keep in mind that the definition of net working capital is simply the mathematical difference between the hospital's total current assets and total current liabilities. If the hospital has more current assets than current liabilities, it has a positive working capital reservoir; if there are more current liabilities than current assets, the hospital has a negative working capital reservoir. Any difference results from an accumulation of individual management actions in the hospital's accounting records.

In its simplest form, the principal sources of working capital are the funds derived from the payments for services rendered. To generate working capital, the hospital converts its assets into production capacity and hospital resources, which in turn generate patient service revenues. As payment is received for these services, management converts the revenues back into hospital assets through a choice between operational and investment decisions. Correspondingly, the principal use of working capital is the financing of the hospital's day-to-day operating expenses.

To simplify the understanding, it is helpful to view working capital as consisting solely of cash. In Figure 9.1, cash is converted first into inventory to be utilized in the delivery of patient care. As specific services are rendered, requiring the depletion of the inventory, a patient charge for the use of the inventory and the associated personnel costs is generated. Until paid, the charge exists as an account receivable. The liquidity and negotiability of the account receivable are a function of the hospital's collection history. Upon payment, the hospital realizes a return of its original cash invested. The hospital also realizes an increase in net worth, current assets, and working capital because of the element of profit margin included in its charges.

Viewing working capital as cash, it is relatively simple to see how working capital is able to activate and bring out the productive potential of other assets. Fixed assets, inventories, and other nonpersonnel assets must all be combined with cash that pays the hospital's operating expenses— labor, utilities—to generate the hospital services that result in the establishment of a patient charge. With working capital, the hospital exists as a dynamic, productive community resource. Without it, the hospital can never put its bricks, mortar, and supplies to work in the production of patient services.

The presence of sufficient amounts of working capital also provides hospital management with the necessary breathing room for making effective operational decisions. The most obvious advantage occurs in the area

FIGURE 9.1   Cash Cycle
(Steps 1 and 4)

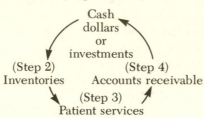

1. Assume that the hospital begins operations with cash holdings of $10,000. Its initial balance sheet would be as follows:

Step 1 Balance Sheet

Assets		*Liabilities & Net Worth*	
Cash	$10,000	Capital stock	$10,000
		Total liabilities	
Total assets	$10,000	& net worth	$10,000

2. Cash is needed to purchase merchandise which, in turn, will be used to produce services. Assuming that half the cash is used to purchase medical inventories for patient care, the balance sheet would be as follows:

Step 2 Balance Sheet

Assets		*Liabilities & Net Worth*	
Cash	$ 5,000	Capital stock	$10,000
Inventories	$ 5,000	Total liabilities	
Total assets	$10,000	& net worth	$10,000

3. If the remaining cash and the entire inventory are used at cost plus 20%, the position statement would be as follows:

Step 3 Balance Sheet

Assets		*Liabilities & Net Worth*	
Accounts receivable	$12,000	Capital stock	$10,000
		Retained earnings	2,000
		Total liabilities	
Total assets	$12,000	& net worth	$12,000

4. The accounts receivable are all paid, and the firm receives $12,000 in cash. However, management does not feel that it is necessary to hold all $12,000 in cash and, therefore, it invests $2,000 in short-term securities which readily can be converted back to cash. The balance sheet at the completion of these transactions would be as follows:

Step 4 Balance Sheet

Assets		*Liabilities & Net Worth*	
Cash	$10,000	Capital stock	$10,000
Short-term invest-		Retained earnings	2,000
ments	2,000	Total liabilities	
Total assets	$12,000	& net worth	$12,000

of accounts receivable and accounts payable management. The presence of a working capital reservoir relieves the pressure of constant cash shortfalls. Otherwise, temporary operational gains that do occur must be channeled instantly into operational contingencies to avert potential disruption in patient services. Another advantage is in the area of investment earnings. The existence of working capital permits management to take the most effective position with regard to the investment of available funds and to take advantage of longer-term investment opportunities. If working capital is predictable and available in sufficient amounts to finance operations in the near term, management is free to utilize its excess funds to establish long-range revenue streams, which in turn increase the hospital's production capacity and its future revenues. Increased revenues result in still more funds for more long-range expansion or increased future working capital reserves.

Finally, hospitals with the appropriate levels of working capital have an easier time availing themselves of the debt markets. Most creditors assess their risk in terms of the borrower's ability to continue operations and to experience sufficient excess revenue to repay the funds borrowed. The proper levels of working capital provide some assurance that additional short-term borrowing is unnecessary and that an interruption in operations is unlikely. Therefore, future revenue streams are not jeopardized, nor is the creditor's loan in any danger.

Hospitals that have either no or insufficient working capital reservoirs are in a continually poor operating position. They can be described as effectively stagnant. The absence of a sound financial position is characterized by an absence of sound financial planning, uncertainty in management decision making, and inefficient utilization of the hospital's assets. On the operating side, management addresses one short-term crisis after another. The hospital is plagued by poor outside relations with suppliers and creditors and an inability to expand its credit base. Current creditors become fearful of recouping current obligations, and future creditors see little opportunity for additional revenue. The hospital's financial position continues to deteriorate, operations suffer, plant deteriorates, medical and staff morale declines, and public confidence is jeopardized. Once the financial position is sufficiently weakened, the trend toward further spiraling declines is difficult to reverse.

Internal factors affecting working capital are largely within the scope of management control. The goal of managing working capital is to maximize operational cash inflows, manage operational cash outflows, and minimize the use of outside funds in the maintenance of continuing operations.

Management controls the efficiency of the production process. The more efficient the operation, the more operating margin that is generated by the operation, the more working capital available. Therefore, efficiency is one means available to management to maintain or improve a working capital position. Management can also control the level and availability of the working capital through its decisions on the allocation and mix of funds between short-term (current) and long-term (noncurrent) assets. Both the investment of funds and the shifting of funds should be fully analyzed to measure the return, the opportunity costs anticipated, and the residual effects on operations. Finally, the choice of credit and payment, billing, and collection policies will determine the velocity of working capital inflows and outflows.

External forces, such as third party payment practices and supplier credit restrictions, will also affect the level of the working capital required by affecting the terms of the hospital's accounts payable policies. General economic conditions will affect the level of consumer funds available and the level of third party payer funding and, therefore, the hospital's accounts receivable policies. Indirectly, consumer attitudes and third party payer policies directed at the level of health care expenditures in the community in general will also affect the respective payment attitudes.

Hospitals can control the impact of the external forces to some degree by availing themselves of advance payment programs or periodic interim payments. These can prevent elongated and fluctuating payment cycles during which the hospital must finance its accounts receivables. It is also important for the hospital to strive for a balanced payer mix. A balanced mix will assure that the payment policies of a single payer do not inappropriately affect hospital operations or adversely affect management decisions. Similarly, hospitals may want to enter into long-term arrangements with suppliers to insure price and credit stability.

SOURCES AND USES OF WORKING CAPITAL

The financial and accounting world of the hospital does not exist in the simplistic world of cash basis accounting. While it was useful to utilize cash to illustrate the production potential of working capital, it must also be clear that working capital arises from sources other than the production of services. Hospitals, just as most financial entities today, utilize the accrual basis of accounting for financial reporting. Accrual accounting is the means by which accounting gives rise to accounts such as accounts receivable, accounts payable, and accrued expenses. Accrual accounting recognizes revenues and other resource acquisitions when the hospital is legally entitled to receipt or title of the goods; expenses and liabilities are recognized when the hospital is legally obligated to make payment. As a result, accounting entries are made in both situations prior to any actual inflow or outflow of cash. Because the definitions of working capital and net working capital go beyond cash, the interaction among current assets, current liabilities, and noncurrent accounts also gives rise to sources and uses of working capital.

This matter of interdependence should be clarified further before proceeding. In Figure 9.1, cash is utilized to obtain the necessary inventory for the production of patient services. However, because both cash and inventory are current assets, the net effect on both working capital and net working capital is zero. Alternatively, the hospital's management could utilize trade credit to obtain the necessary goods. In these situations, cash is not reduced, yet inventories are increased. Under accrual accounting, a current liability for the amount of the trade credit received is recorded. For example, if the only transaction were the purchase of $5,000 of drugs through the use of credit, the hospital's simplified balance sheet would be as follows:

Current Assets	
Inventory—Drugs	$5,000
Total Current Assets	$5,000
Current Liabilities	
Accounts Payable	$5,000
Total Current Liabilities	$5,000

The hospital has obtained a current asset (inventory), but has also obligated itself to a current liability (an account payable) of the same amount. From the standpoint of net working capital, the use of a current liability to acquire a current asset is similar to the use of cash. However, from the standpoint of total working capital, the hospital is able to increase its working capital reservoir by $5,000 because the increase in inventory (a current asset) results in an increase in total current assets. The account payable has in effect substituted itself temporarily for cash and has financed the acquisition of items necessary for the operation of the institution. Obviously, at some point the account payable will need to be paid. At that time a decrease in total working capital will result because cash will necessarily be diminished. Ideally, this would not occur until sufficient funds become available from patient charges to maintain the higher working capital position.

Credit does not always behave in this manner. In another situation, the same hospital purchases some laboratory equipment with a short-term note of $50,000. In this example, the hospital obtains a noncurrent asset (laboratory equipment) by obligating itself to a current liability (a note payable). Although the dollar amounts are identical, the result is a loss of net working capital because the note represents a current item, included in the definition of net working capital, while the laboratory equipment is a fixed asset and is noncurrent.

The laboratory equipment is classified as a noncurrent asset because its full value will not be utilized to increase the production capacity of the

Current Assets

Inventory—Drugs	$ 5,000
Total Current Assets	$ 5,000

Fixed Assets

Laboratory Equipment	$50,000
Total Fixed Assets	$50,000
Total Assets	$55,000

Current Liabilities

Accounts Payable	$ 5,000
Notes Payable	$50,000
Total Current Liabilities	$55,000
Total Liabilities	$55,000

hospital in the current operating period. Although the total productive potential of the hospital increases immediately, that increase is not immediately reflected in the hospital's financial statements. The full effect of the increase in capacity is expected over the useful life of the equipment. This may span several accounting periods.

STATEMENT OF CHANGES IN FINANCIAL POSITION

Many operational and investment decisions have a direct impact on the level of working capital evident in the hospital's financial statements. The impact of some decisions is disguised, in that the actual current asset and liability accounts are affected only as a transaction passes through them. To fragment multipart transactions and to illustrate the actual sources and uses of working capital, accountants utilize the "Statement of Changes in Financial Position." By analyzing this statement, it is possible to identify the specific transactions that give rise to the working capital levels being maintained. The full list of accounting transactions that generate or use working capital is provided in Table 9.1. See also Figure 9.2 for statement of changes in a hospital financial position.

After net income from the production of patient services, the most prevalent source of hospital working capital is depreciation. Depreciation is the pro rata allocation of the cost of a piece of equipment or of the hospital plant over its useful life. Depreciation is a source of working capital because it reduces net income in the current period.

TABLE 9.1   Statement of Changes in Financial Position

Actions increasing working capital (Sources of working capital)
Net income from operations
Expenses not requiring the outlay of working capital in current period
    Depreciation expense
    Amortization of premium or discount on debt issuance
    Amortization of leasehold improvements
    Increases in the level of deferred income
    Amortization of good will
Other sources
    Proceeds from the sale of a fixed asset
    Proceeds from the sale of stock
    Proceeds from a mortgage or issuance of long-term bonds
    Proceeds from long-term investments
    Proceeds from the cash surrender value of employee life insurance
    Proceeds from the sale of good will

Actions decreasing working capital (Uses of working capital)
Credits not resulting in working capital
    Parents' share of undistributed subsidiary income
    Gains on the sale of a fixed asset
Other uses
    Dividends declared
    Increases in long-term investments
    Purchase price of fixed assets
    Purchase price of treasury stock
    Purchase price of good will
    Purchase price of subsidiary stock
    Increases in the cash surrender value of employee life insurance

QUANTITY OF WORKING CAPITAL

It is axiomatic that if the total cost to the community of patient care is to be minimized, then the cost of working capital must also be minimized. To accomplish this, management must control two interrelated factors. It must determine both the level or quantity of assets and the proper asset financing combination so that these two factors, when taken together, will result in working capital costs being held to a minimum. Since this is a two-part problem, let us consider in this chapter the quantity aspect and in the next chapter the matter of financing current assets.

Perhaps the simplest approach to understanding how the level of working capital is determined is to return to the notion of working capital being cash. With this notion in mind, consider Figure 9.3.

Figure 9.3 pictures, in a rather elementary manner, two cash flow streams—a cash inflow stream and a cash outflow stream. The cash inflow stream represents the flow of cash payments to the hospital in return for

FIGURE 9.2   Saint Anthony Hospital and Health Center—Statement
               of Changes in Financial Position of Unrestricted Funds,
               Years Ended December 31, 1984 and 1983

	1984	1983
Funds provided		
From operations		
Income (loss) from operations	$ 90,205	(28,085)
Add item that does not require an outlay of		
working capital in the current period—		
depreciation	570,671	561,327
Total funds provided from operations	660,876	533,242
Nonoperating revenue	217,975	119,789
Additions to long-term pension liability	—	184,985
Transfer from plant replacement and		
expansion fund	556,867	738,480
Additions to long-term debt	429,009	98,027
Decrease in cash—Board-designated fund	10,329	—
Decrease in deferred Medicare receivable	14,300	473,240
Donated equipment	—	4,350
Total funds provided	1,889,356	2,152,113
Funds applied		
Increase in cash—Board-designated	—	10,329
Increase in lease deposits	3,909	2,629
Increase in deferred charges	—	32,526
Additions to property, plant, and equipment	298,381	394,877
Funding of depreciation	570,671	560,530
Decrease in long-term debt and lease		
obligations	459,388	—
Decrease in long-term pension liability	240,015	370,828
Total funds applied	1,572,364	1,371,719
Increase in working capital	$ 316,992	780,394

Continued

services rendered. It can be viewed as consisting of two components: a
production cycle and an accounts receivable cycle. The timing of cash inflows, that is, the length of time between the initial production of a service
and receipt of payment for that service, is hence a function of (1) how long
it takes to produce the service (production cycle) and (2) how long it takes
to receive payment for the service after it is produced (accounts receivable
cycle). In this example, the cash inflow stream is assumed to consist of a
production cycle of 7 days and an accounts receivable cycle of 21 days. That
is, the average length of stay is assumed to be 7 days and the average delay
in payment from the time the bill for services is submitted to the time the

FIGURE 9.2   Continued

	1984	1983
Changes in components of working capital		
Increase (decrease) in current assets		
Cash	$ (60,878)	133,432
Accounts receivable and due from third party payers	42,142	1,641,381
Other receivables	237,940	(38,679)
Inventories	(4,610)	60,264
Prepaid expenses	83,189	(32,994)
Increase in current assets	297,783	1,763,404
Increase (decrease) in current liabilities		
Accounts payable	309,591	151,314
Accrued expenses	(93,731)	72,322
Accrued payroll and related withholdings	(139,862)	1,038,415
Accrued vacation pay	(53,951)	13,193
Refund due to patients	16,624	39,538
Current installments of pension liability	239,421	(166,500)
Current installments of long-term debt	(22,646)	18,026
Current installments of obligations under capital lease agreements	22,788	37,374
Notes payable	(59,000)	11,000
Due to third party payers	191,600	69,970
Due to specific purpose funds	(323,177)	(238,072)
Due to plant replacement and expansion fund	(106,866)	(63,570)
Increase (decrease) in current liabilities	(19,209)	983,010
Increase in working capital	$ 316,992	780,394

payment is received is assumed to be 21 days. Therefore, the timing of the cash inflow is 28 days.[1]

In addition to the cash inflow stream, the cash outflow stream must also be considered in determining the quantity of working capital. This is due to the fact that the minimum level of working capital that a hospital needs is equal to the difference between its initial cash inflow and outflow streams. The cash outflow stream represents the flow of payments that the hospital must make to obtain labor, supplies, and other items needed to produce services. It can be viewed as consisting of two basic components:

---

[1]Patient arrives on day 1 and stays until day 7. Therefore, the production cycle is 7 days. The bill for services is submitted on the day of discharge. Therefore, day 7 is the last day of the production cycle and day 8 is the first day of the accounts receivable cycle. If the accounts receivable cycle is assumed to be 21 days, then the sum of the two cycles is 28 days.

FIGURE 9.3   Quantity of Working Capital

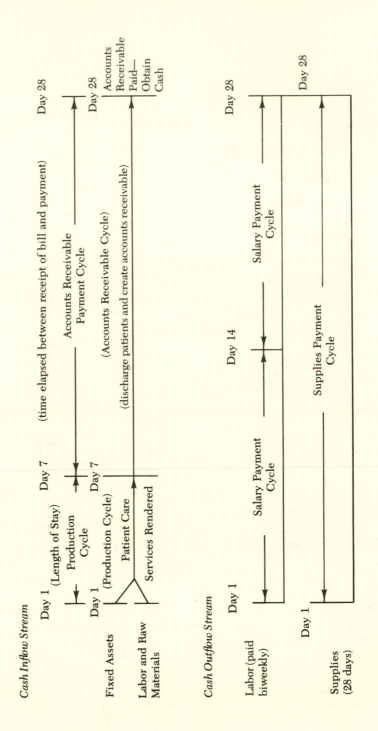

a salary payment cycle and a supplies payment cycle. The salary payment cycle represents the time period between salary payments. The supplies payment cycle represents the time elapsed between the receipt of supplies and the payment for those supplies. In this example, for the sake of simplicity, it is assumed that salaries are paid biweekly and that supplies are paid for 28 days after receipt. Therefore, in a single cash inflow cycle (28 days), salaries are paid twice and supply expenses are paid once.

In the initial 28-day period there will be three cash outflow items. Offsetting these outflows will be one cash inflow. Due to the length of the production and accounts receivable cycles, on day 28 the fees for the first 7 days of production, that is, for those patients entering the hospital on day 1 and discharged on day 7, will be received. Therefore, in the example 28-day period, the hospital (assuming charges are equal to costs) will receive payments equal to 7 days' costs, but must make payments equal to 28 days' costs.[2]

Obviously, there is an imbalance existing here. Revenues equal to 7 days' costs cannot possibly pay for the costs of 28 days of operation. Therefore, funds from some source other than revenues must be used to pay the costs that cannot be offset by the cash inflow stream. This other source of funds is the working capital or cash that must become available at the beginning of or during the period if the hospital is to be able to meet its obligations and continue to operate until it achieves a self-sustaining position.

The amount of cash, or the quantity of working capital, that must be held is a function of the timing and amount of cash inflows and outflows. At a minimum, it is equal to the difference between the cash inflows received and the cash outflows paid during the initial cash inflow or, if it is longer, outflow cycle. Expressed algebraically, the minimum quantity of working capital that must be held is equal to $CO_j - CI_j$ where CO_j equals the cash outflows in period j, CI_j equals the cash inflows in period j, and j equals the time period necessary to complete either a single cash inflow cycle or, if it is longer, a single cash outflow cycle, that is,[3]

$$CO_j - CI_j = \text{Minimum Quantity of Working Capital.}$$

[2]Again, for the sake of simplicity, assume that the term costs refers only to labor and supplies costs. Admittedly, there are other cost factors. However, inclusion of these other factors will not change the conclusions reached, but will greatly complicate the explanation. Therefore, it seems advantageous at this point to ignore these factors.

[3]At this point the matter of uncertainty has not been considered. However, if the minimum quantity of working capital is to be determined accurately and realistically, the problem of uncertainty in regard to the timing and amount of cash inflows cannot be ignored. In the following chapters this matter will be discussed further.

This same concept can be illustrated in a somewhat different manner through the use of Table 9.2 and Figure 9.4. Table 9.2 is based on the cycle timing assumption set out in Figure 9.3 and the following costs:

Cash Outflows
   Salary cycles (2 cycles at $10,000) each = $20,000
   Supplies cycle   = $ 2,000

$$CO_j = \$22,000$$

Cash Inflows
   Cash receipts on day 28   = $ 5,500 $CI_j = \$ 5,500$

Using the formula described above, the quantity of working capital or the initial cash reserve that the hospital needs to be able to meet its cash outflows and attain a self-sufficient financial position is $16,500, that is,

Quantity of Working Capital   = $CO_j - CI_j$
                               = $22,000 - $5,500
Quantity of Working Capital   = $16,500

As can be seen from Table 9.2, if the hospital has an initial working capital investment of $16,500, it is able to meet all of its obligations.[4] The initial working capital investment acts as a pool or reservoir of funds that can be drawn upon, along with the cash inflows, to pay cash outflows. Figure 9.5 illustrates the reservoir conceptualization of working capital. Cash inflows of $5,500 are combined with a $16,500 reservoir of working capital to enable the hospital to pay costs of $22,000.

Figure 9.5 also illustrates how the timing and amount of cash inflows and outflows determine the level of the reservoir, that is, the quantity of working capital needed. As can be seen from the figure, as cash inflows increase less working capital is needed. Conversely, as cash outflows increase more working capital is needed. Table 9.2 describes in numerical terms the effect that the timing of inflows and outflows can have on the quantity of working capital.

Table 9.3 and Figure 9.6 are based, with one exception, on the same cost and timing assumptions that were used in Table 9.2. The single exception is in regard to the timing of the accounts receivable cycle. In Table 9.2 the accounts receivable cycle was assumed to be 21 days. However, for purposes of Table 9.3, it is assumed that the cycle is accelerated from

---

[4]If volume or cost changes result in changes in the absolute amount of cash inflows and outflows, then the quantity of working capital needed to achieve a self-sufficient financial position will also change at a corresponding rate. For example, if volume were to double, causing labor expenses to increase to $40,000 and supplies expenses to increase to $4,000, then, all other factors being equal, the minimum quantity of working capital would also double to $33,000.

TABLE 9.2 Quantity of Working Capital

Day of Position Statement	Balance Sheet				Expenses
	Current Assets		**Current Liabilities**		
Day 0	Cash =	$16,500	Net worth =	$16,500	
Day 1	Cash =	$16,500	Accts. pay. =	$ 2,000	
	Inventory =	2,000	Net worth =	16,500	
	Total	$18,500	Total	$18,500	
Day 7	Cash =	$16,500	Accts. pay. =	$ 2,000	
	Inventory =	1,500	Accrued salaries =	5,000	
	Accts. rec. =	5,500	Net worth =	16,500	
	Total	$23,500	Total	$23,500	
Day 14	Cash =	$ 6,500	Accts. pay. =	$ 2,000	Salaries =
	Inventory =	1,000	Net worth =	16,500	$10,000
	Accts. rec. =	11,000			
	Total	$18,500	Total	$18,500	
Day 28	Cash =	$ 0	Accts. pay. =	$ 0	Salaries =
	Inventory =	0	Net worth =	16,500	$10,000
	Accts. rec. =	16,500			Supplies*=
	Total	$16,500	Total	$16,500	$ 2,000
Day 35	Cash =	$ 5,500	Accts. pay. =	$ 2,000	
	Inventory =	1,500	Accrued salaries =	5,000	
	Accts. rec. =	16,500	Net worth =	16,500	
	Total	$23,500	Total	$23,500	
Day 42	Cash =	$ 1,000	Accts. pay. =	$ 2,000	Salaries =
	Inventory =	1,000	Net worth =	16,500	$10,000
	Accts. rec. =	16,500			
	Total	$18,500	Total	$18,500	
Day 49	Cash =	$ 6,500	Accts. pay. =	$ 2,000	
	Inventory =	500	Accrued salaries =	5,000	
	Accts. rec. =	16,500	Net worth =	16,500	
	Total	$23,500	Total	$23,500	
Day 56	Cash =	$ 0	Accts. pay. =	$ 0	Salaries =
	Inventory =	0	Net worth =	16,500	$10,000
	Accts. rec. =	16,500			Supplies =
	Total	$16,500	Total	$16,500	$2,000
Day N	Cash =	$16,500	Net worth =	$16,500	

Cash Receipts and Working Capital		Cash Outflows	
Cash inflows, days 1–28 =	$ 5,500	Supplies	$ 2,000
Initial working capital =	$16,500	Salaries	20,000
Total	$22,500	Total	$22,000

*Attain financial self-sufficiency; that is, cash inflows will equal outflows for any given period of length j.

FIGURE 9.4   Quantity of Working Capital

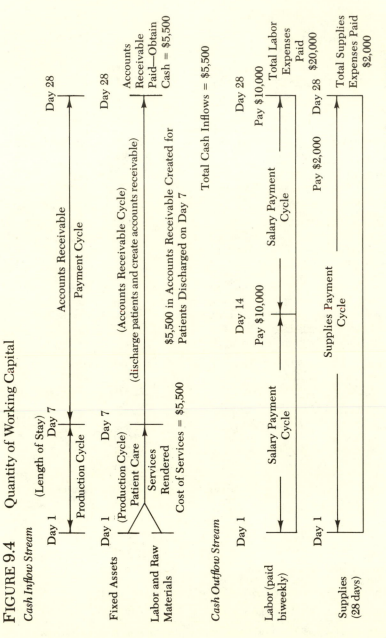

Cash Inflow Stream

Cash Outflow Stream

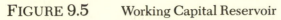

FIGURE 9.5   Working Capital Reservoir

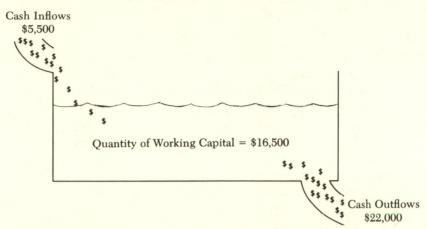

21 days to 7 days. That is, the time period between patient discharge and patient payment is accelerated or shortened from 21 days to only 7 days.

Based upon these assumptions, in a single (28-day) cash outflow cycle, expenses, as was the previous case, will be $22,000. However, cash receipts for the same period will be greater than the $5,500 of the previous example. Due to the acceleration of the accounts receivable cycle, three cash inflows instead of only one will be available to offset cash outflows. Cash receipts of $5,500 will be received on days 14, 21, and 28. Therefore, as is indicated in the table, receipts will be $16,500, payments will be $22,000, and $5,500 in initial working capital will be needed; that is, $CO_j = \$22,000$, $CI_j = \$16,500$, and $j = 28$ days:[5]

$$
\begin{aligned}
\text{Quantity of Working Capital} \quad &= \quad CO_j - CI_j \\
&= \quad \$22,000 - \$16,500 \\
\text{Quantity of Working Capital} \quad &= \quad \$5,500
\end{aligned}
$$

Accelerating the timing of the accounts receivable cycle thus results in a reduction in the amount of working capital needed to attain a self-sustaining financial position. This is a critical point that should be kept in mind, for it will be referred to again later in the text.

Note that at the end of each of the preceding examples, the total level of available working capital in the reservoir is zero. The obligations of the period have entirely utilized the cash available at the beginning of the period and all cash generated during the period. This requires management to locate funds from outside operations at the beginning of each period to

---

[5]It should be noted that since the cash outflow cycle is longer than the cash inflow cycle, that period *j* is equal to the length of the cash outflow cycle—28 days.

TABLE 9.3   Quantity of Working Capital—Timing Factors

Day of Position Statement	Balance Sheet				Expenses
	Current Assets		*Current Liabilities*		
Day 0	Cash =	$ 5,500	Net worth =	$ 5,500	
Day 1	Cash =	$ 5,500	Accts. pay. =	$ 2,000	
	Inventory =	2,000	Net worth =	5,500	
	Total	$ 7,500	Total	$ 7,500	
Day 7	Cash =	$ 5,500	Accts. pay. =	$ 2,000	
	Inventory =	1,500	Accrued salaries =	5,000	
	Accts. rec. =	5,500	Net worth =	5,500	
	Total	$12,500	Total	$12,500	
Day 14	Cash =	$ 1,000	Accts. pay. =	$ 2,000	Salaries =
	Inventory =	1,000	Net worth =	5,500	$10,000
	Accts. rec. =	5,500			
	Total	$ 7,500	Total	$ 7,500	
Day 21	Cash =	$ 6,500	Accts. pay. =	$ 2,000	
	Inventory =	500	Accrued salaries =	5,000	
	Accts. rec. =	5,500	Net worth =	5,500	
	Total	$12,500	Total	$12,500	
Day 28*	Cash =	$ 0	Accts. pay. =	$ 0	Salaries =
	Inventory =	0	Net worth =	$ 5,500	$10,000
	Accts. rec. =	5,500			
					Supplies =
	Total	$ 5,500	Total	$ 5,500	$ 2,000
Day 35	Cash =	$ 5,500	Accts. pay. =	$ 2,000	
	Inventory =	1,500	Accrued salaries =	5,000	
	Accts. rec. =	5,500	Net worth =	5,500	
	Total	$12,500	Total	$12,500	

Cash Receipts and Working Capital		*Cash Outflows*	
Cash inflows	= $16,500	Supplies	$ 2,000
Initial working capital =	$ 5,500	Salaries	20,000
Total	$22,000	Total	$22,000

*Attain financial self-sufficiency; that is, cash inflows will equal outflows for any given period of length *j*.

FIGURE 9.6   Quantity of Working Capital

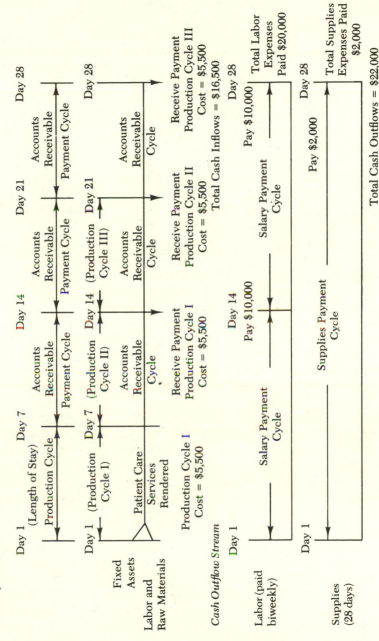

reestablish the working capital reservoir. Effective management of working capital requires an analysis that overlaps the billing and payment cycles of the hospital into a sufficiently long period for manipulation of cash flow factors and current versus noncurrent resource shifts.

Figure 9.7 illustrates a longer-term approach to analyzing and managing working capital. Assuming a payment cycle of 28 days, the billings from Production Cycle I are received at the end of Payment Cycle I (day 1), the billings from Production Cycle II are received on day 7, and so forth. The result is an even inflow of working capital, such that the inflows replenish the working capital reservoir by the end of the period. In a short-term planning period, it is important to insure that the ending working capital reservoir is of a sufficient level to fund the working capital needs of subsequent periods. Because the hospital's cash receipt and payment functions are slow to change, as a general rule, cash inflows during a period must be sufficient to meet the operating outflows of the period and replenish the initial working reservoir.

An analysis of working capital by month reveals the peaks and valleys in the cash inflows and outflows and allows management to anticipate significant shortfalls as well as the availability of excess funds for short-term investment. This type of analysis is shown in Table 9.4 and may be used for either working capital or cash analysis.

Note that each month has a positive working capital balance which is carried forward to the beginning balance of the next month. This occurs through May. During these months, the excess working capital should be invested in short-term interest-yielding securities to earn a return. In May, the beginning balance in the working capital reservoir plus the cash inflows for the period are not sufficient to cover the required cash outflows. To avoid a disruption in production, management must take steps to increase the total level of working capital by increasing the beginning balance, increasing the period's cash inflow, or decreasing the period's cash outflow. To increase the beginning balance of working capital, management may consider sources of funds from outside of operations including debt or the conversion of noncurrent assets to current assets. These actions must be analyzed to determine if they will have adverse operational effects in later periods. For example, debt will carry with it an interest obligation that will increase the cash outflows in future periods. If debt is utilized in the short term to effect a positive working capital position, then the repayment schedule must be structured so as not to create further negative positions at a later date. Management may also choose to defer creditor payments or to accelerate its own cash collections efforts. These, however, must be examined in relationship to longer-term credit and collection procedures. Whichever strategy is adopted, its effects must be felt beyond May or the hospital depicted in this example will break even for the six months shown but have similar difficulties in July due to the absence of an ingoing reservoir.

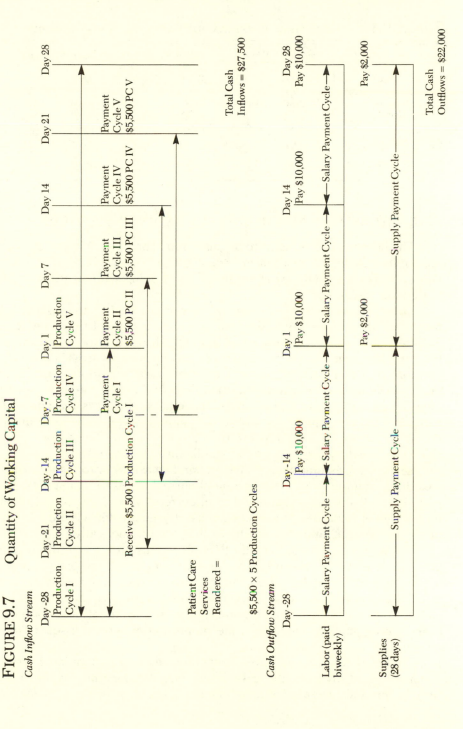

FIGURE 9.7   Quantity of Working Capital

Cash Inflow Stream

Day -28	Day -21	Day -14	Day -7	Day 1	Day 7	Day 14	Day 21	Day 28
Production Cycle I	Production Cycle II	Production Cycle III	Production Cycle IV	Production Cycle V				
			Payment Cycle I	Payment Cycle II $5,500 PC II	Payment Cycle III $5,500 PC III	Payment Cycle IV $5,500 PC IV	Payment Cycle V $5,500 PC V	

Receive $5,500 Production Cycle I

Patient Care Services Rendered =

$5,500 × 5 Production Cycles

Total Cash Inflows = $27,500

Cash Outflow Stream

| Day -28 | Day -14 | Day 1 | Day 14 | Day 28 |
| | Pay $10,000 | Pay $10,000 | Pay $10,000 | Pay $10,000 |

Labor (paid biweekly) — Salary Payment Cycle — Salary Payment Cycle — Salary Payment Cycle — Salary Payment Cycle — Salary Payment Cycle —

Pay $2,000   Pay $2,000

Supplies (28 days) — Supply Payment Cycle — Supply Payment Cycle —

Total Cash Outflows = $22,000

TABLE 9.4   Analysis of Working Capital Requirements by Month

	January	February	March	April	May	June
Beg. W. C. balance	$16,500	19,500	17,500	8,500	3,500	(1,500)
Budgeted Operations						
Oper. revenues	12,000	10,000	8,000	8,000	9,000	12,000
Oper. expenses	10,000	13,000	18,000	14,000	15,000	10,000
Oper. margin	2,000	(3,000)	(10,000)	(6,000)	(6,000)	2,000
Plus: Depr. expense	1,000	1,000	1,000	1,000	1,000	1,000
End W. C. balance	$19,500	17,500	8,500	3,500	(1,500)	1,500

WORKING CAPITAL AND OPERATIONAL RESULTS

The question that remains to be answered is how the quantity of working capital affects the level of operating costs. What is the cost of maintaining working capital? What are the costs of being without it? How are these costs measured?

The relationship between the cost of working capital and operational results can be seen clearly in the case of a manufacturing firm or any other commercial enterprise. Assume that both the absolute amount and the efficiency of managing accounts receivable and inventories are held constant and that the other current assets of the firm, cash and short-term investments, yield a lower return (profit) than that obtained on the firm's investment in fixed assets (land, buildings, and equipment). It is reasonable to make this last assumption, for cash earns nothing and if short-term investments earn more than fixed assets, then the firm should be in the marketable securities business instead of manufacturing.

Given these assumptions, management, to maximize profit and owner's wealth, must minimize the proportion of current assets to total assets. The more assets that can be channeled from current to fixed assets, with their higher rate of return relative to current assets, the greater will be the total profits of the firm. Table 9.5 illustrates this point numerically.

Investment in working capital thus represents an opportunity cost to the firm equal to the return lost by investing in current assets as opposed to fixed assets. The greater the quantity of working capital relative to total assets, the greater is this cost. Therefore, both to minimize the opportunity cost of working capital and to maximize profits, management should attempt to reduce, as much as is feasible, the proportion of current assets to total assets.

The relationship of the level of working capital to operational results is somewhat abstruse in the case of the hospital, for rates of return on various hospital investments are difficult, if not impossible, to calculate.

TABLE 9.5   Cost of Working Capital—Manufacturing Enterprise

Assume the following rates of return

Cash	=	0%
Short-term investments	=	8%
Fixed assets	=	12%

Case 1

Allocation of Assets		Returns
Cash	$ 100,000	$ 0
Short-term investments	$ 150,000	$ 12,000
Fixed assets	$ 750,000	$ 90,000
	$1,000,000	$102,000

Case 2. Assume that assets ($150,000) are channeled from current assets—short-term investments—to fixed assets.

Allocation of Assets		Returns
Cash	$ 100,000	$ 0
Short-term investments	$ 0	$ 0
Fixed assets	$ 900,000	$108,000
	$1,000,000	$108,000

Conclusion
The lower the proportion of current assets (working capital) to total assets, the greater is the firm's return on total investment.

Nevertheless, it can be argued, at least on a subjective basis, that the rate of return on a patient service program, on a lifesaving piece of equipment, or on a piece of equipment that makes a patient more comfortable, is greater than that which could be obtained from an investment in cash or short-term securities. If this is the case, management should attempt to minimize the relative proportion of assets invested in working capital (cash and short-term investments) in order to maximize the return to the owner, that is, the community.

The relationship of the quantity of working capital to operational results can also be viewed in another manner which may be somewhat easier to visualize. In this case, the matter of concern is the effect of the level of working capital on the costs borne by patients. To understand how the quantity of working capital affects the amount of costs that have to be borne by patients, it is necessary to view costs as net costs. That is, the costs borne by patients are equal to operating costs less nonoperating revenues. The costs of care borne by patients thus vary inversely with nonoperating revenues, that is, as the amount of nonoperating revenues increases, the amount of revenues to be obtained from patients—the cost of care borne by patients—decreases.

This view of costs is not entirely contrived. As was discussed in previous chapters, third party payers offset nonoperating revenues against operating costs to determine the basis for computing reimbursable costs. Also, hospitals generally base their charge structure on the difference between their total revenue needs and the sum of both nonoperating revenues and revenues obtained from third party payers. Thus, in reality, the cost of care borne by patients is determined, at least in part, by the nonoperating revenues of the hospital.

Given this view of costs, consider once again the example described in Tables 9.2 and 9.3. With these examples in mind, assume that a hospital originally had $16,000 invested in working capital, but that it changed its credit and collection policies so that only $5,500 is now needed. If this were the case, there would be a cash surplus of $11,000. This cash would no longer be needed for day-to-day operations and therefore could be invested in revenue-generating securities. Assuming that it were invested in long-term corporate bonds earning 8%, this cash surplus would return an annual nonoperating revenue of $880.

Admittedly, $880 is not a great deal of money. However, it is sufficient to illustrate the point. A reduction in the quantity of working capital has enabled management to invest former working capital funds in revenue-gathering securities. These securities yield a nonoperating revenue that can be used to reduce the cost of care borne by patients. Eight hundred eighty dollars is now available to meet operating costs that previously had to be met through funds provided by patients. Thus, by reducing the quantity of working capital, management is able to reduce the cost of care borne by patients.[6] Table 9.6 numerically illustrates this process.

As was the case with the commercial enterprise, investment in working capital represents an opportunity cost to the hospital. This cost is equal to the rate of return that could have been achieved if the hospital's working capital investment were reduced and the excess funds were invested in other assets. The greater the quantity of unnecessary or excessive working capital, the greater is this opportunity cost. Thus, to reduce the cost of care borne by patients, management must minimize the working capital investment of the hospital.

As has been seen in the above example, the quantity of working capital can be reduced if cash inflows are accelerated. Also, as will be discussed later, the quantity of working capital can be reduced by decelerating cash outflows. Therefore, if management is to reduce the cost of care borne by patients, it must minimize the quantity of working capital by accelerating cash inflows and/or decelerating cash outflows.

---

[6]It should be noted that if the $11,000 had been invested in capital equipment instead of securities, the cost of care borne by patients would still be reduced. In this instance, the hospital would not have to build as much of a premium into the patient's bill for capital equipment. Thus, the patient's bill would be less.

TABLE 9.6   Working Capital and Cost of Care Borne by Patients

Assumptions

1. Operating costs = $100,000/year
2. Working capital investment
   - Original .... = $16,500
   - Improved management .... = $ 5,500
3. Assets for investment
   - Original .... = $ 0
   - Improved management (surplus funds created due to the decrease in working capital investment) .... = $11,000
4. Nonoperating revenue
   - Original .... = $ 0
   - Improved management ($11,000 invested at 8%) .. = $ 880

	Original Example	*Improved Management Example*
Operating costs	$100,000	$100,000
Nonoperating revenue	0	– 880
Cost of care borne by patients	$100,000	$ 99,120

Conclusion

A reduction in the cost of care borne by patients can be achieved by reducing the necessary quantity of working capital and investing the surplus funds in revenue-generating securities.

CONCLUSION

A word of caution should be expressed at this point. It should be clear now that the cost of care cannot be minimized if the hospital has an excessive amount of working capital. The operational rule or guideline is that management should attempt to minimize the hospital's investment in working capital. However, this does not mean that the hospital should have a zero working capital investment. Just as too much working capital prohibits least cost operation, too little not only can result in additional costs from such factors as having to borrow at inopportune times or having to forego purchase discounts, but also may result in insolvency and even—in the extreme—failure. Thus, management should strive not for the minimal, but rather for the optimal quantity of working capital, that is, that quantity that is sufficient but not excessive.

The following chapters will discuss the techniques for determining the optimal investment for each of the components of working capital. Given these techniques, the reader will be familiar with the tools needed to optimize the total quantity of working capital and minimize costs.

SUGGESTED READINGS

Anthony, Robert N. and Reese, James S. *Management Accounting*, Chapter 12.

Archer, Stephen H. and D'Ambrosio, Charles A. *The Theory of Business Finance*, Chapter 17.

Beranek, William. *Working Capital Management*, Chapters 1 and 2.

Cleverley, William O. *Financial Management of Health Care Facilities*, Chapter 8.

Dewing, Arthur S. *The Financial Policy of Corporations*, Chapter 23.

Knight, W.D. "Working Capital Management—Satisficing Versus Optimization," pp. 33–40.

Lindsay, J. Robert and Sametz, Arnold W. *Financial Management: An Analytical Approach*, Chapter 3.

Weston, J. Fred and Brigham, Eugene F. *Managerial Finance*, pp. 439–45.

Financing Working Capital

As has been discussed in the previous chapter, working capital management, by definition, is a two-part problem. To minimize the cost of working capital, management must determine not only the proper level or quantity of assets, but also the proper asset financing combination. The foregoing chapter has examined the quantity aspect of the problem, or the relationship between the quantity of working capital and the cost of working capital. Therefore, this chapter will be addressed to the matter of financing working capital.

SOURCE OF FUNDS

Working capital can be financed from two basic sources of funds— equity and debt. Equity is the owner's investment in the hospital. It is the funds provided or contributed by the community both to obtain the hospital's physical plant and facilities and also to prime its operational pump, that is, provide the initial working capital needed to sustain operations until the hospital reaches a self-sustaining position. Table 10.1 illustrates the manner in which equity can be used to finance working capital. The specific role of equity as a source of financing will be discussed below. For the moment, it should just be noted that equity is the owner's permanent investment in the hospital and can only be repaid or returned if the assets of the hospital are liquidated (see Table 10.1).

In addition to or in place of equity, debt can be used to finance working capital. Debt can be viewed as a temporary investment in, or loan to, the hospital which must be repaid. If the loan matures or must be repaid within a year, the debt is considered to be short-term. If the period until payment

TABLE 10.1   Working Capital Financing—Equity

Assumptions
1. The community donates $18,500,000 to be used for the creation of
   Philanthrophy Memorial Hospital.
2. A 100-bed hospital is constructed at a cost of $18,000,000.

Balance Sheet 1
As of End of Construction*

Assets		*Liabilities and Net Worth*	
Current assets		Current liabilities	$ 0
Cash	$ 500,000		
Fixed assets		Net worth	
Building & equipment	$18,000,000	Owner's equity	$18,500,000
Total	$18,500,000	Total	$18,500,000

Balance Sheet 2
As of Several Months of Operation†

Assets		*Liabilities and Net Worth*	
Current assets		Current liabilities	
Cash	$ 100,000	Accounts payable $ 100,000	
Accounts receivable	$ 400,000	Net worth	
Inventories	$ 100,000	Owner's equity	$18,500,000
Fixed assets			
Building & equipment	$18,000,000		
Total	$18,600,000	Total	$18,600,000

*The $18,500,000 investment has been used to build and equip the building and provide working capital of $500,000. This $500,000 is needed to pay for wages, supplies, and other expenses until that time when cash inflows become sufficient to meet cash outflows. Thus, the balance sheet after several months of operation may be as follows.

†As is illustrated by balance sheet 2, the $500,000 in cash that was financed through owner's equity has been used to pay operating expenses and is represented by the cash of $100,000, and the accounts receivable of $400,000. As these accounts receivable are paid, the hospital should achieve a self-sustaining position. For the sake of simplicity, no profit margin has been assumed in the services offered by the hospital. In reality, owner's equity should increase as services are provided, because profits are earned by the provider. The profits, in turn, also increase the hospital's cash and accounts receivable and its working capital reservoir.

is greater than one year, the debt is generally categorized as long-term. The significance of the timing of debt maturity and its relationship to the cost of working capital will be discussed at a later point. Table 10.2 illustrates the manner in which debt can be used to finance working capital.

EQUITY FINANCING

A hospital acquires its initial base of equity from public contributions or from the sale of ownership rights to individual stockholders. Philanthropic contributions provide the primary basis of equity financing to vol-

TABLE 10.2   Working Capital Financing—Debt

Assume the same situation as was described in Table 10.1 with the only difference being that $18,000,000 instead of $18,500,000 was contributed. Given these assumptions, balance sheet 1 would appear as follows:

Balance Sheet 1
As of End of Construction*

Assets			Liabilities and Net Worth		
Current assets	$	0	Current liabilities	$	0
Fixed assets			Net worth		
Building & equipment	$18,000,000		Owner's equity	$18,000,000	
Total	$18,000,000		Total	$18,000,000	

Balance Sheet 2
As of First Day of Operation†

Assets			Liabilities and Net Worth		
Current assets			Current liabilities	$	0
Cash	$	500,000	Long-term liabilities		500,000
Fixed assets			Net worth		
Building & equipment	$18,000,000		Owner's equity	$18,000,000	
Total	$18,500,000		Total	$18,500,000	

Balance Sheet 3
As of Several Months of Operation‡

Assets			Liabilities and Net Worth		
Current assets			Current liabilities		
Cash	$	100,000	Accounts payable	$	100,000
Accounts receivable		400,000			
Inventories		100,000	Long-term liabilities		500,000
Fixed assets			Net worth		
Building & equipment	$18,000,000		Owner's equity	$18,000,000	
Total	$18,600,000		Total	$18,600,000	

*The $18,000,000 has been used to build and equip the hospital. However, no funds are available to finance the working capital that is needed if the hospital is actually to operate. Therefore, assume that $500,000 is borrowed to finance working capital. The balance sheet, as of the first day of operations, would be as follows.

†The $500,000 is needed to pay wages, supplies, and other expenses until that time when cash inflows become sufficient to meet cash outflows. Thus, the position after several months of operation may be as follows.

‡As is illustrated by balance sheet 3, the $500,000 in cash, which was financed through long-term debt, has been used to pay operating expenses and is represented by the cash of $100,000 and accounts receivable of $400,000. As these accounts receivable are paid, the hospital should achieve a self-sustaining position.

untary, nonprofit hospitals. Funds are donated by private individuals, hospital auxiliaries, or organized hospital fund-raising subsidiaries. Once the funds are given, the donor relinquishes all rights to the funds. There is no residual control or return provided to the donor. Donated funds may be unrestricted by the donor, such that management is free to utilize the funds as it wishes, or may be restricted, such that management must utilize the funds for a purpose identified by either management or the donor at the time of transfer.

For-profit or investor-owned hospitals utilize the issuance of negotiable stocks to acquire equity capital. The process used by the investor-owned hospital is similar to the process utilized by non–health care, for-profit corporations to raise funds through the sale of public stocks. In purchasing the stock of the propriety hospital, the stockholder establishes a pro rata claim to the assets of the corporation and the expectation that a distribution of the annual earnings will occur.

Some argue that the availability of capital through the stock markets provides management with a great deal of flexibility, both in raising the funds and in ultimately utilizing them. The flexibility available from stock transactions is a function of the increased control and maneuverability management can attach to the sale. In a stock sale, management may analyze the market and choose the timing of the sale and the volume necessary to achieve the desired equity return and to protect the rights of current stockholders. Most important, the sale is a cash transaction. The equity is received as the stock is purchased. Philanthrophy is much less certain. Timing is elongated because of planning, solicitation, and collection periods. Because nothing, with the exception of a personal income tax deduction is available in return, management may have to be very explicit in its plans for the use of the funds to gain donor confidence. Finally, a pledge is not always fully collectible. Pledges in excess of necessary funds may be needed to achieve the desired level of funding.

The most consistent and direct source of working capital after the operations of the institution commence is the net margin generated through the provision of services to the hospital's patients. The operating margin that results from the generation of aggregate revenues in excess of aggregate expenses increases the funds available to the hospital. These funds either become a part of the working capital reservoir or are utilized to establish contingencies for expansion of the hospital's production capacity. Table 10.3 expands on the position illustrated in Table 10.2. In this case, however, a profit margin of 20% on all services is assumed. If gross revenues for the period are $1,000,000, the operating margin (profit) to the hospital is $200,000. The $200,000 increases the hospital operating fund balance and unless dispersed to the owner to repay a portion of the initial contributions, it increases the total equity available to management.

The transactions for the period include $800,000 for operating supplies and $200,000 in operating margin. The operating margin is recorded as fund balance in the net worth section of the balance sheet. In turn, a current asset of $1,000,000 (some combination of cash and accounts receivable) results from the billings generated.

TABLE 10.3   Working Capital Financing—Operational Margins

Assume the same situation as described in Table 10.2, Balance Sheet 3. In this case, the hospital incurs $800,000 of expense which depletes the hospital's cash and accounts receivable balance and increases the accounts payable balance by $300,000. With the supplies obtained from the expenditures, the hospital generates gross revenues of $1,000,000.

Balance Sheet 3
As of Several Months of Operations

Assets		*Liabilities and Net Worth*	
Current assets		Current liabilities	
Cash	$ 0	Accounts payable	$ 400,000
Accounts receivable	1,000,000	Total	$ 400,000
Inventories	100,000		
Total	$ 1,100,000	Long-term liabilities	$ 500,000
Fixed assets		Net worth	
Building & equipment	$18,000,000	Fund balance	$ 200,000
		Owner's equity	18,000,000
		Total	$18,200,000
Total	$19,100,000	Total	$19,100,000

The definition of working capital from Chapter 9 can now be related to the situations described here to illustrate the effects of an operating margin on working capital.

Working Capital = Current Assets − Current Liabilities
(Table 10.2) WC = $ 600,000   − $100,000
           = $ 500,000
(Table 10.3) WC = $1,100,000   − $400,000
           = $ 700,000
△ WC = $ 700,000   − $500,000
           $ 200,000

DEBT FINANCING

When sufficient cash levels are not present, such that operations may not be maintained at acceptable levels, debt provides the hospital with another source of immediate cash for the necessary working capital reservoir. Ultimately, however, whether the debt is short-term or long-term, the operating margin must be sufficient to provide funds to cover the full amount of the debt undertaken. Therefore, while debt initially increases the hospital's working capital, it also establishes a drain on the funds generated by operations in future periods. Growth in the hospital's operating margin must be sufficient to cover the increased demand for cash at a level that equals both the loan principal and the loan interest.

Debt comes in several forms. It can be long-term or short-term. It may also be obtained as an explicit loan action by management or it may be obtained as a byproduct of the hospital's trade accounts.

TRADE CREDIT

It is possible to finance working capital through the use of accounts payable or "trade credit." Technically, an account payable is a form of short-term debt. Accounts payable are debt obligations that arise out of the regular course of operational transactions—as opposed to being financial transactions such as the negotiation of a loan. Normally, a buyer receives and uses goods before he is required to pay for them. This procedure represents the extension of trade credit by the seller and is reflected in the records of the buyer as an account payable.

Recall, for a moment, the example that was described in Table 9.2 of the previous chapter. In that example, it was assumed that in a single cash inflow cycle of 28 days, salaries of $20,000 were paid, supplies expense of $2,000 was paid, and $16,500 in initial working capital and $5,500 in cash inflows were needed in order to pay these expenses. However, if the timing of the supplies cycle changes, so that the payment for supplies is due in 56 days instead of 28, the initial working capital needs of the hospital also change. This situation is illustrated in Tables 10.4 and 10.5.

As is obvious from the tables, the extension of the due date for paying for supplies resulted in initial working capital needs decreasing by $2,000. However, under either set of assumptions, $22,000 in labor and supplies was needed during the 28-day period. Thus, if less initial working capital was needed under the second set of assumptions, financing or support from some other source, equal to $2,000, must have been obtained. As should be apparent from the example, the other source of support was the supplier who extended the payment period from 28 to 56 days, that is, extended trade credit of 56 days. The extension of the payment period, therefore, is in effect a 56-day, $2,000 loan to the hospital.

The 56-day loan is a monetary obligation or liability of the hospital and is reflected in the current liabilities section of the hospital's position statement as an account payable for the purchase price of the goods in question. Thus, through the use of accounts payable the hospital was able to reduce its cash outflows and to use less of its own cash. Accounts payable, therefore, have financed or supplied part of the hospital's working capital needs.

At first glance, this approach to financing working capital appears to be ideal. Through the use of accounts payable, the example hospital has been able to finance its working capital requirements with less of its own funds. It would thus seem reasonable that the hospital should take advantage of trade credit whenever it is offered, that is, incur an account payable whenever possible, for it provides the mechanism by which the hospital can reduce its investment in working capital and thereby free assets for investment in other areas. The decision rule, however, is not as clear-cut as the foregoing statement would lead one to believe.

COST OF TRADE CREDIT

Suppliers of goods realize that when they offer trade credit they are actually offering a loan. Additionally, they are aware of the fact that the granting of such a loan involves a cost to them, either in terms of an opportunity cost equal to the earnings that could have been obtained by using the loaned funds in some other manner, or an out-of-pocket cost equal to the interest expenses that have to be paid to some other source in order to obtain the funds required by the suppliers for their operational needs. Thus, suppliers are neither able nor inclined to provide trade credit for free. They also realize that it is inconvenient, if not impossible, both for themselves and for purchasers, to require cash payments. Therefore, they have adopted

TABLE 10.4   Effect of Timing of the Supplies Cycle on Initial Working Capital Needs

Original Assumptions (see Table 9.2)

Salaries expense of $10,000 due 14th and 28th days	= $20,000
Supplies expense of $2,000 due 28th day	= $ 2,000
Cash outflows	= $22,000 = CO_j
Cash receipts on the 28th day	= $ 5,500
Cash inflows	= $ 5,500 = CI_j
Quantity of working capital	= $CO_j–CI_j$
	= $22,000–$5,500
	= $16,500

Chapter 10 Assumptions

Salaries expense of $10,000 due 14th, 28th, 42nd, and 56th days	= $40,000
Supplies expense of $2,000 due 56th day	= $ 2,000
Cash outflow	= $42,000 = CO_j
Cash receipts on the 28th, 35th, 42nd, 49th, and 56th days	= $27,500
Cash inflows	= $27,500 = CI_j
Quantity of working capital	= $CO_j–CI_j$
	= $42,000–$27,500
	= $14,500

TABLE 10.5   Quantity of Working Capital

Day of Position Statement	*Balance Sheet*				*Expenses*
	Current Assets		**Current Liabilities**		
Day 0	Cash =	$14,500	Net worth =	$14,500	
Day 1	Cash =	$14,500	Accts. pay. =	$ 2,000	
	Inventory =	2,000	Net worth =	14,500	
	Total	$16,500	Total	$16,500	
Day 14	Cash =	$ 4,500	Accts. pay. =	$ 2,000	Salaries =
	Inventory =	1,000	Net worth =	14,500	$10,000
	Accts. rec. =	11,000			
	Total	$16,500	Total	$16,500	
Day 28	Cash =	$ 0	Accts. pay. =	$ 2,000	Salaries =
	Inventory =	0	Net worth =	14,500	$10,000
	Accts. rec. =	16,500			
	Total	$16,500	Total	$16,500	
Day 35	Cash =	$ 5,500	Accts. pay. =	$ 4,000	
	Inventory =	1,500	Accrued salaries =	5,000	
	Accts. rec. =	16,500	Net worth =	14,500	
	Total	$23,500	Total	$23,500	
Day 42	Cash =	$ 1,000	Accts. pay. =	$ 4,000	Salaries =
	Inventory =	1,000	Net worth =	14,500	$10,000
	Accts. rec. =	16,500			
	Total	$18,500	Total	$18,500	
Day 49	Cash =	$ 6,500	Accts. pay. =	$ 4,000	
	Inventory =	500	Accrued salaries =	5,000	
	Accts. rec. =	16,500	Net worth =	14,500	
	Total	$23,500	Total	$23,500	
Day 56	Cash =	$ 0	Accts. pay. =	$ 2,000	Salaries =
	Inventory =	0	Net worth =	14,500	$10,000
	Accts. rec. =	16,500			
					Supplies =
	Total	$16,500	Total	$16,500	$2,000 *
Day N	Cash =	$14,500	Net worth =	$14,500	

Cash Receipts and Working Capital		*Cash Outflows*	
Cash inflows, days 1–56 =	$27,500	Supplies	$ 2,000
Initial working capital =	$14,500	Salaries	40,000
Total	$42,000	Total	$42,000

*Attain financial self-sufficiency; that is, cash inflows will equal outflows for any given period j.

a compromise approach that allows for a variable cost of credit arrangement with the purchaser. For the sake of convenience and business practicality, trade credit is offered for a limited period at no explicit cost.[1] Beyond the grace period, an explicit charge is made to the purchaser for the use of the credit.

The mechanism that is used to affect this variable price arrangement is one of selling on terms that allow for a purchase discount if payment is made within a specified time period. The exact nature of the sales terms that are offered varies with industry convention and the financial needs of the seller. Generally, terms are set at 2-10, net 30.

Terms of 2-10, net 30 mean that if a hospital pays for a purchase within 10 days of the date of invoice (the discount period) then the price of the purchased goods can be discounted or reduced by 2%. Thus, if a $100 purchase is made and paid for within 10 days, the hospital only has to pay $98 for the purchased goods. If the purchase is not paid for within 10 days, then the hospital has to pay $100 by the 30th day—the due date or the end of the net period.

The use of the foregoing sales arrangement means that the hospital is actually being offered the opportunity to purchase two different items. Obviously, it is purchasing goods. Additionally, if it does not exercise its option of paying within the discount period, it is purchasing credit. The purchase of credit, however, has a cost. If a hospital is to minimize its costs, it should not incur the cost of trade credit unless it is the least cost credit financing alternative.[2]

Assuming that a $100 purchase is made and terms of 2-10, net 30 are offered, the cost of trade credit is $2.00 for the use of $98.00 for a 20-day period. On an annual basis, since there are approximately 18 20-day periods in a year, the cost of credit in percentage terms is 18 times $2.00 over the amount of money ($98.00) that is being borrowed. The cost of trade credit, therefore, is 18 times 2 over 98 or about 37%. Trade credit is thus a relatively costly source of financing. Table 10.6 illustrates the mechanics of calculating the cost of trade credit.

The nature of the cost of accounts payable can be more clearly understood through the use of Figure 10.1. The vertical axis of the diagram measures the cost of credit in terms of an annual rate of interest. The horizontal axis represents time elapsed after the receipt of goods by the purchaser.

---

[1]As has been indicated, trade credit has a cost to the supplier. However, offering credit for at least a limited period is a necessary part of business and, therefore, represents a normal business cost which is included in establishing the purchase price, as opposed to being set out as an additional explicit factor.

[2]In actual practice, hospital management typically makes a determination of its least cost financing alternative and establishes an accounts payable policy that is applied uniformly to bills containing discount terms. This policy should be reviewed routinely to determine if any of the assumptions of the cost of the various sources of credit have changed.

During the discount period—day 1 to day 10—the cost of credit is not explicitly set out, and the credit can be viewed as being virtually an interest-free loan. This is the case due to the fact that the purchase price remains the same whether the goods are paid for on day 1, day 10, or any day in between. Thus, while admittedly there is a cost for the use of credit during the discount period, the cost is buried or hidden in the purchase price and cannot be avoided.

After the expiration of the discount period—day 11—the hospital incurs an explicit cost for the use of the credit for the next 20 days, that is, until the end of the net period—day 30. Whether the goods are paid for on day 11 or day 30, the cost is still the same. Thus, if a $100 purchase were made on terms of 2-10, net 30 and paid for on the 11th day, the purchaser would pay $2.00 for the use of $98.00 for just one day. Since there are 365 one-day periods in the year, the cost in dollars of using trade credit would be $2.00 times 365, or $730. In terms of an annual rate of interest, the cost of using trade credit would be 2 times 365 over 98, or 744.89%. As the graph indicates, as payment is delayed the cost of credit declines. The annual rate of interest is approximately 37% if the purchase is paid for by the due date, i.e., the 30th day. As payment is delayed beyond the due date,

TABLE 10.6   Cost of Credit

Cost of credit is a function of
1. The rate of discount
2. The discount period
3. The net period

Assumption
Hospital makes a $100 purchase and terms of 2-10, net 30 are offered:
    Rate of discount = 2%
    Discount period = 10 days
    Net period = 20 days
    Cost of goods = quoted price ($100) minus the discount.
              = $98 (This is the amount being borrowed.)*

Cost of credit on annual basis

1. $2 for every 20-day period, or $\dfrac{365}{20}$ = 18.25 × $2 = $36.50

2. amount borrowed = $98

3. interest rate = $\dfrac{\text{interest expenses}}{\text{amount borrowed}}$ = $\dfrac{\$36.50}{\$98.00}$ = 37.2%

*Under the above assumption, the hospital can obtain the goods for $98 by paying within 10 days. However, if it chooses not to pay until the end of the 30-day period, this decision will cost it an additional $2. Therefore, if the goods are not paid for until the end of the 30-day period, the hospital has borrowed $98 for 20 days at a cost of $2. It should be noted that the loan is considered to be for 20 days because no explicit charge is made if payment is made before day 10.

FIGURE 10.1   Cost of Credit

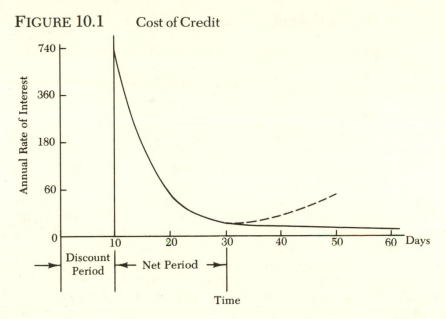

the annual interest rate will continue to fall. In fact, the annual rate can decline indefinitely.

Suppliers will attempt to prevent the cost curve from falling indefinitely by mailing past due notices, placing follow-up telephone calls, and taking stronger action, if necessary. These measures obviously increase the cost to the seller of offering trade credit. However, they do not raise the cost of credit to the purchaser for the invoice already outstanding. Failure to pay its obligation on time will raise questions about the hospital's ability to pay, the acumen of its management and, perhaps, even the trustworthiness of its management and governing board. These questions and doubt not only will make suppliers and other potential lenders less willing to offer credit to the hospital, but also will probably increase the cost of future purchases; that is, the hospital may have to pay cash in the future or may have to use vendors who charge more in order to compensate for the added costs of dealing with slow payers.

The nature of this future cost is illustrated by the dotted line in Figure 10.1. The line represents the indirect cost that is incurred by the hospital if payment is past due on the current bill, that is, it represents the future costs that will be levied against the hospital if it defaults on its present obligation. Thus, if trade credit is used, the due date (the end of the net period) is the long-run low point of the cost curve.

Given the nature of both the trade credit purchase arrangement and the foregoing cost curve, the use of accounts payable or trade credit as a means of financing working capital has some interesting managerial implications. In terms of financial management rules of thumb, the following guideline can be set out:

The potential user of trade credit should choose one of two points at which to pay—

1. Either the *end* of the discount period, or

2. The *end* of the net period

It should be noted that in both instances emphasis is placed on paying at the end of the period. This is the case because, if the hospital is going to take the discount, the cost of goods is the same regardless of whether the payment is made on day 1, or the day on which the discount expires. If the hospital elects not to take the discount, then the cost of credit is incurred, but this cost is constant throughout the entire net period. Therefore, there is no financial incentive to force payment prior to the last day of the net period. Actually, the financial incentive lies in the direction of delaying payment to maximize cash availability as long as possible. By delaying payment until the end of either the discount period or the net period, the hospital can more productively use its assets, for instead of committing funds to inventories, it can invest in revenue-generating securities which will provide a return.

Based upon the above guideline, the matter of when to pay under either alternative is clear. However, the critical question is how does one determine which alternative to select? In general terms, the answer to this question is simply that the best choice between the two is determined by the cost of credit from other available sources. If credit is needed, whether or not the discount is taken should depend on the costs of the various alternative sources of credit. Thus, if an alternative source of credit is less costly than trade credit, the discount should be taken and the alternative source should be used as the means of financing working capital. Conversely, if trade credit is the least cost alternative, the discount should not be taken. It is only through this type of financing strategy that management can minimize the total cost of working capital.

The decision as to whether or not the discount should be taken may also depend on the alternative uses to which funds can be put. If funds are immediately available to pay a bill, then before they are used in this manner, management should compare the return that could be earned by investing the funds in some other manner versus the cost of trade credit. Thus, if the revenues that can be earned through investment exceed the cost of the trade credit, it would be financially imprudent to take the discount and forgo the revenue.

Additionally, if the revenues are less than the cost of trade credit but exceed the cost of the least cost credit alternative, then the discount should be taken and the least cost source of credit should be used as the source of financing. Thus, the decision as to whether or not trade credit should be used depends, in the case where credit is needed, upon the cost of alternative sources of credit and, in the case where credit is not absolutely needed, on the revenues that could be earned from alternative uses of funds and the cost of alternative sources of credit.

One further point should be noted in regard to the cost of credit. Management, in determining the least cost credit alternative, should examine cost not only in terms of a percentage annual interest rate, but also in terms of absolute dollar costs. In the previous example, $98.00 could be borrowed for 20 days at a cost of $2.00. Thus, the cost of credit in absolute dollars would be $2.00, and in terms of annual interest rate, about 37%. As an alternative, however, assume that the hospital could also borrow $98 from its bank at an annual interest rate of 10%, but that it must hold the loan for at least six months.

At first glance, the bank loan appears to be the least cost source of credit—10% versus 37%. When absolute dollar costs are considered, however, trade credit is the least cost alternative—$2.00 versus $4.90. Thus, to minimize the total cost of operations in this instance, trade credit should be used as the means of financing working capital, for its full cost is less than the cost of the short-term bank loan (less any interest that may have been earned on the unused loan balances). Tables 10.7 and 10.8 contain numerical examples of the foregoing decision rules.

COMMERCIAL DEBT

As has been indicated, commercial debt can also be used as a means of financing purchases and, therefore, it can be viewed as a source of financing for working capital. In addition, commercial debt can play a primary role in the financing of working capital needs. In order to understand the nature of this primary role, it is necessary first to consider the exact character of the hospital's working capital needs.

As is illustrated in Figure 10.2, the working capital needs of a hospital can be viewed as consisting of two components—a permanent segment and a temporary segment. Permanent working capital can be defined as the minimum working capital investment that the hospital must have if it is to be able to maintain the factors of production necessary for operations; that is, it is the level of assets that is needed to finance the lowest expected level of operations. This quantity is represented by segment AB in Figure 10.2.

As is apparent from the diagram, the hospital's working capital needs fluctuate over time, but at no time do they fall below point B. Thus, if the hospital is to be able to operate, it must have available on a continual basis a working capital investment equal to line segment AB.

Working capital investment (volume and costs remaining constant) will

TABLE 10.7 Decision Rule—Use of Trade Credit when Additional Financing Is Necessary

Basic Rule

Whether the discount is taken or not depends on the cost of credit from the cheapest alternative source. If the alternative rate lies below the low point of the trade credit cost curve, the financially prudent decision would be to take the discount, borrow from the alternative source, and pay the invoice prior to the expiration of the discount period. If the alternative source of credit has a rate higher than the low point on the trade curve, then trade credit should be used.

Example I
A. Assumptions
    1. $100 purchase on terms of 1-10, net 30.
    2. Alternative source—factor or sell accounts receivable at a discount rate of 7%.
B. Costs
    1. Dollar = $1; interest rate about 18%
    2. Dollar = $7; interest rate = none—have sold property
C. Decision
    Trade credit is the least cost alternative. Therefore, the discount should not be taken.

Example II
A. Assumptions
    1. $100 purchase on terms of 1-10, net 30.
    2. Alternative source A—factor accounts receivable at a discount of 7%.
    3. Alternative source B—obtain a 30-day, 8% bank loan for $150 (note the added $50 is for the required compensatory balance).
B. Costs
    1. Dollar = $1; interest rate = about 18%
    2. Dollar = $7; interest rate = none
    3. Dollar = $1; interest rate = 8%
C. Decision
    On a cost basis it is a matter of indifference between trade credit and bank loan. Subjective factors should determine the choice.

Example III
A. Assumptions
    Same as in II, except terms of sale are 2-10, net 30.
B. Costs
    1. Dollar = $2; interest rate = about 37%
    2. Dollar = $7; interest rate = none
    3. Dollar = $1; interest rate = 8%
C. Decision
    The bank loan is the least cost alternative. Therefore, the discount should be taken.

TABLE 10.8   Decision Rule—Use of Trade Credit When Additional Financing Is Not Necessary

Basic Rule

Whether or not the discount is taken depends on both the cost of credit from the cheapest alternative source and the return that can be earned by investing available funds in assets other than inventories. If the return that can be earned from investments in other than inventories is greater than the least cost credit alternative, then the financially prudent decision is to maintain the investment and finance inventories through the least cost credit alternative. That is, depending on cost, management should either take the discount and finance the purchase through an alternative source or, if less costly, finance it through the use of trade credit. If the opposite is the case, then the financially prudent decision is to take the discount and finance the purchase (inventories) through available funds or assets.

Example I

A. Assumptions
  1. $100 purchase at terms of 2-10, net 30.
  2. Alternative source A—sell two short-term investments yielding 12% payable annually, payment due in 10 days if investment is still held.
  3. Alternative source B—obtain a 30-day 9% bank loan for $150 (note the added $50 is for the required compensatory balance).

B. Costs
  1. Dollar = $2.00; interest rate = about 37%
  2. Dollar = $12.00; (lose year's earnings due to the terms of payment; interest rate = 12% yield (Alternative A)
  3. Dollar = $1.13; interest rate = 9% (Alternative B)

C. Decision
  The investments should be continued because the net loss exceeds any potential savings. However, the discount should be taken and the purchase financed through alternative source B because the bank loan represents the least cost alternative.

Example II

A. Assumptions
  Same as above, except earnings on investments are paid monthly.

B. Costs
  1. Dollar = $2.00; interest rate = about 37%
  2. Dollar = $1.00; interest rate = 12% (Alternative A)
  3. Dollar = $1.13; interest rate = 9% (Alternative B)

C. Decision
  The least cost alternative is to take the discount and finance the purchase through the sale of the short-term investments.

FIGURE 10.2 Working Capital Fluctuations

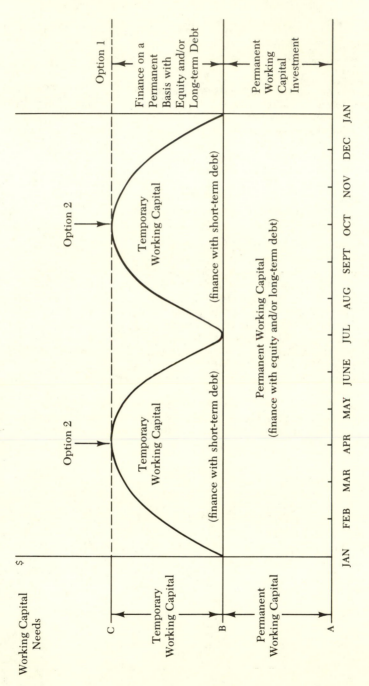

be stable over time and can only be altered through changes in the cash inflow or outflow cycles. An example of how a change in the cash inflow cycle can affect permanent working capital needs was described in Chapter 9.

Given that permanent working capital is a permanent asset (investment), it should be financed through a permanent source of funds. This approach to asset financing is consistent with the general financial management decision rule that holds that the timing of assets and their sources of financing should be matched. Thus, long-term or permanent assets should be financed through equity or long-term debt.

In the case of the hospital, the above general rule is not as applicable as it is in regard to commercial industry. This is the case because the hospital's ability to generate sufficient revenues to amortize any debt incurred for working capital purposes, due to the nature of cost-based reimbursement agreements, may be limited. However, as payment shifts to fixed price methodologies, the hospital's ability to generate operating margins to repay debt becomes related to the adequacy of the price. As payment programs become increasingly based on fixed prices, the general rule is increasingly applicable.

In addition to permanent working capital needs, the hospital, from time to time, will have to increase temporarily its working capital investment to meet the financial demands generated by temporary or cyclical increases in service volume. These supplementary working capital needs are depicted by the curve lying between points B and C in Figure 10.2.

It is important to realize that these temporary working capital needs are a byproduct of increases in production volume and can be considered to be temporary because they should be self-liquidating over the short run. The hospital, like almost all other industries, experiences certain periods during the year when the demand for services or products increases. To meet these increased demands, temporary additional personnel and supplies are often needed. However, as the discussion of the previous chapter should have made clear, if additional personnel and supplies are to be obtained, then—as a prerequisite—additional working capital is needed to finance these temporary increases in the factors of production. Admittedly, as Figure 10.3 makes clear, these financial needs can be met eventually with funds derived from internal operations. Due to the lag between cash outflows and cash inflows, though, the need for these funds occurs before they are available. Thus, management faces the problem of deciding how to finance these temporary needs until that time when internally generated funds are available.

The potential sources of funds for financing temporary working capital needs are the same as those discussed earlier in this chapter, that is, debt and equity. The decision management faces is that of determining which

FIGURE 10.3   Nature of Short-Term Working Capital Needs

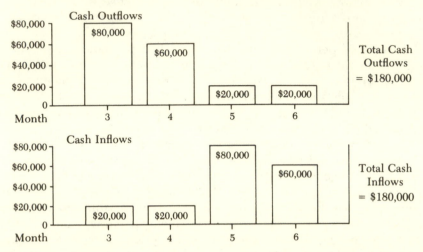

of these sources provides the least cost solution to the hospital's financing needs. Therefore, management must determine the costs of each of the financing alternatives.

COST OF FINANCING

Given this problem, consider the cost of equity. If equity is used as the source of financing, the accounting or out-of-pocket cost is any opportunity cost that occurs.

In a for-profit industrial firm, opportunity cost can be viewed as the full monetary return foregone by investing equity in working capital. Given a listing of alternative investments, the firm can quite easily calculate the returns foregone and, therefore, the cost of equity financing. Based upon this cost, the firm can then compare the cost of equity to the cost of other financing alternatives to determine the least cost source of financing.

In the case of a hospital, the same opportunity cost notion exists, but because of the nature of the hospital's investment alternatives, the value or magnitude of this cost is difficult to calculate. Nevertheless, the concept of opportunity cost can provide a useful approach to evaluating the relative cost of equity financing.

In the previous discussion of working capital financing, equity was recommended, for financially pragmatic reasons, as the most desirable source of funds for permanent working capital financing. The desirability of equity as the source of permanent working capital financing can also be justified in terms of an opportunity cost argument. The argument can be stated briefly as follows:

1. Permanent working capital funds are necessary if the hospital is to be able to operate.

2. Additionally, if the hospital is to be able to operate over the long run, permanent working capital funds cannot be obtained by means of debt financing, for at some point the debt must be repaid, and the hospital will be deprived of its permanent working capital funds.

3. Therefore, equity should be used as the source of financing, for it is the only permanent source of funds available and, thus, the only source that can ensure the continued availability of permanent working capital.

4. Consequently, the rate of return from investing equity in this manner is greater than that which can be obtained from an investment in any other alternative because the return is the hospital's ability to operate.

5. Therefore, the opportunity cost attached to not investing equity in permanent working capital is greater than the opportunity cost attached to not investing equity in any other alternative.

6. Thus, if management is to minimize costs, it must use equity to finance permanent working capital needs.

The same type of argument, however, cannot be made for the use of equity as the source of financing for temporary working capital needs. Temporary working capital needs are, over time, self-liquidating. Therefore, equity is not the only potential source of funds that can be used to finance these needs. Thus, the opportunity cost of not using equity as the source of funds is less in this case than it was in the previous one, for alternative sources are available and financially practicable. The decision as to whether or not equity should be used in this manner, therefore, should be based on an analysis of the cost of equity versus the cost of alternative sources.

If debt is used as the source of funds, then the cost can be said to be equal to the interest cost on that debt. If equity is used, then the cost is equal to the return foregone by not investing equity in another manner, such as lifesaving equipment or patient care programs. Admittedly, the rate of return on a piece of lifesaving equipment or a patient care program is difficult to determine. Intuitively, though, one would think that it is high and, certainly, at least higher than the interest rate on debt. If the rate of return from investing equity in other than temporary working capital is greater than the interest rate on debt, then the opportunity cost of financing temporary working capital needs through equity is greater than the cost of financing through debt. Therefore, equity is not the least cost financing alternative and should not be management's primary choice as the means of financing temporary working capital needs.

Long- versus Short-Term Debt

Given that equity should not be the primary financing choice for temporary working capital, hospital management must evaluate the remaining alternatives for least cost. The alternatives available to management are limited to either long-term or short-term debt. Short-term debt is a feasible alternative in this instance, for the working capital needs are only temporary. The problem facing management is simply that of determining which of the two alternatives has the least cost.

If long-term debt is used as the source of funds then, as is depicted by Option 1 in Figure 10.2, total working capital funds are increased for the entire period. However, due to the seasonal nature of the working capital needs, funds are not needed for the entire period. Thus, if long-term debt is used as the source of funds, the hospital is paying for the use of working capital funds during periods in which they are not needed. It is, therefore, unnecessarily incurring additional operating costs.

Admittedly, the excess funds can be invested during the periods in which they are not needed for working capital purposes. It is unlikely, though, that the returns from such investments will equal the interest costs of the debt. The financial implication of using long-term debt, therefore, is that it results in unnecessarily increasing the cost of financing working capital, for it does not match the need for funds with the availability of funds. Consequently, if management is to finance temporary working capital at least cost, it must use short-term debt.

Table 10.9 illustrates the cost advantages of short-term debt as the source of temporary working capital funds. As is clear from the table, the cost advantage of short-term debt is due to the ability of management to synchronize the timing of the debt with the timing of the hospital's need for temporary funds.[3] One might conclude, therefore, that the management decision rule for the financing of temporary working capital needs would be to finance these needs through short-term debt that has a maturity schedule matched exactly to the fluctuations in working capital. In theory, this decision rule is basically correct. Unfortunately, in an actual operating situation this rule is inappropriate, for it does not take into account the matter of uncertainty in regard to the timing of cash inflows.

Debt, whether long- or short-term, represents a fixed obligation whose timing and amount are both certain, that is, both the exact amount and the exact date of payment are known in advance. However, the cash inflows, which are the source of funds for servicing and retiring debt obligations, are uncertain. The approximate timing and amount of cash inflows are known, but due to various factors, the exact timing and amounts cannot be

---

[3]It should also be noted that, due to the term structure of interest rates, short-term debt is a less costly source of funds, for long-term rates are generally higher than short-term rates.

TABLE 10.9   Cost Advantage—Short-Term Debt

Assumptions
1. Hospital needs $100,000 for only a single three-month period per year.
2. Long-term debt can be obtained for a period of three years at 12%.
3. Short-term debt can be obtained for a period of three months at 12%.

Annual Operating Costs—Assuming excess long-term funds not invested
1. Long-term debt: due to the nature of the debt contract—three years—interest expense is incurred for the entire year. Cost, therefore   = $12,000
2. Short-term debt: interest expense is only incurred for the three months that the debt is used. Cost, therefore   = $3,000
3. Conclusion: operating costs can be reduced by $9,000 if short-term debt is used as the means of financing temporary working capital needs. Operating savings/year   = $9,000

Annual Operating Costs—Assuming excess long-term funds invested
1. Long-term debt: gross cost   = $12,000
   Investment income (assuming invest for
   9 months @ 8%)   =   ($6,000)
   Net cost   = $6,000
2. Short-term debt: gross cost   = $3,000
   Investment income   =   0
   Net cost   = $3,000
3. Conclusion: short-term debt is still the least cost alternative.
   Operating savings/year   = $3,000

accurately projected. Thus, the situation is one wherein a fixed obligation must be met through uncertain income flows.

This type of situation presents a substantial and costly hazard to the hospital, for if the timings of working capital fluctuations and debt maturity are exactly matched and cash inflows are slower than anticipated, the hospital will be unable to pay its obligation and will be forced to default on the debt. Default is an expensive action, for at best it casts doubt on the hospital's credit standing and, at worst, it can result in failure and dissolution. Thus, the hospital must attempt to minimize the probability of default.

This, however, does not mean that the hospital should forego the use of debt. Rather, it means that management should adjust or schedule the timing of the maturity of the debt to provide a margin of safety. This can be done by allowing the maturity date to overlap or extend a short period beyond the exact time for which the additional funds are needed. Figure 10.4 illustrates this scheduling strategy.[4]

---

[4]The appropriate length of the overlap period varies with the degree of cash inflow fluctuations and management's willingness to accept uncertainty. Therefore, no meaningful general rule can be applied. Each instance must be determined individually based upon a study of historical cash inflows and estimates of future events.

FIGURE 10.4   Short-Term Debt Maturity Schedule

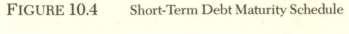

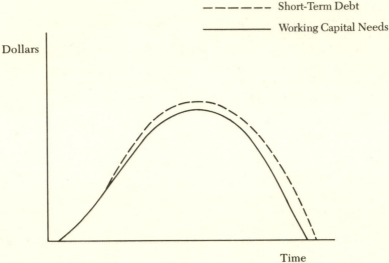

In addition to scheduling debt maturities, management must consider whether the debt must be secured or unsecured. Ordinarily, it is desirable to borrow on an unsecured basis, for in this way not only can the book-keeping and administrative costs attached to a secured loan be avoided, but also maximum financial flexibility can be maintained.[5] However, if the hospital's credit rating is weak or if the hospital has other debt obligations outstanding, it may be necessary either to pay a premium (higher rate of interest) or to provide some assets as collateral or security in order to obtain the loan.[6]

Several different types of asset are acceptable forms of collateral. Marketable securities are generally considered excellent collateral, as is real property such as buildings and equipment. Unfortunately, most hospitals do not hold large portfolios of marketable securities, and real property is usually reserved as security or potential security for long-term debt. Thus, the bulk of secured short-term financing involves the use of short-term assets—accounts receivable or inventories—as collateral.

Accounts receivable, in addition to serving as collateral for short-term

---

[5]The hospital may elect to secure the loan if it finds that a secured loan will result in a lower interest rate. However, in making this choice the hospital should consider the trade-off between the reduced interest rate and the loss of financial flexibility.

[6]Generally, as part of the loan approval process, a bank or any other lender will evaluate the hospital's capital structure, that is, existing mix of long-term financing. Based on this evaluation, the bank may, at the extreme, refuse the loan, grant it only at a higher than usual rate of interest, or require that it be secured.

debt, can play another role in regard to short-term financing. The pledging of accounts receivable as security for a loan is commonly known as discounting accounts receivable. In this process, an agreement is made between the borrower and the lender wherein the lender takes the receivables, but has recourse to the hospital if a patient defaults on an account; that is, the risk of default of an account remains with the hospital. Alternatively, in some instances accounts receivable, instead of being pledged, can be sold at a discount to the lender without recourse, that is, the hospital is not responsible for defaults. This process is known as factoring accounts receivable and, although in legal terms it is not a loan arrangement, it can be conceptualized for our purposes, since cash is obtained for a price, as a hybrid form of debt.

While no statistics are available as to the number of hospitals that factor their accounts, it is unlikely that it is a large proportion. This is probably due to both the relatively poor quality of a hospital's self-pay accounts receivable and the adverse public relations effects that can arise if the purchaser of the accounts pursues collection too vigorously. Nevertheless, the existence of this source of short-term financing should be known.

It should be noted also that one other source of short-term financing may be available. Hospitals may obtain payment advances from third party payers in order to meet temporary working capital needs. The nature and availability of these advances vary with the specific third party and the specific reimbursement contract. Thus, there is little value at this point in discussing this source in detail. It should suffice just to realize that advances may be available and that, if utilized, they represent a liability obligation or debt of the hospital.

Given the foregoing discussion, the critical point for management to understand is simply that, if costs are to be minimized, short-term financing (debt) must be used to meet temporary working capital needs. The form that this financing should take is a separate question that management can answer only after examining the cost of each alternative in order to establish which represents the least total cost to the hospital.

CONCLUSION

The discussion of the previous pages can be summarized in the following financial management decision rules:

1. Permanent working capital needs should be financed through equity.
2. Temporary working capital needs should be financed through short-term debt.
3. Trade credit (accounts payable) should be used as a source of working capital financing (either permanent or temporary) only when it is the least cost financing alternative.

Given these guidelines and the discussion in Chapter 9, the stage is now set for examining each of the primary components of working capital—inventories, accounts receivable, and cash. The management of each of these components is examined in the following chapters.

SUGGESTED READINGS

Archer, Stephen H. and D'Ambrosio, Charles A. *The Theory of Business Finance*, Chapters 26, 27, and 30.

Cleverley, William O. *Financial Management of Health Care Facilities*, Chapter 8.

Healy, Sister Mary Immaculate. "An Analysis of Accounts Receivable with Emphasis on Factoring."

Lindsay, J. Robert and Sametz, Arnold W. *Financial Management: An Analytical Approach*, Chapter 6.

Van Horne, James C. *Financial Management and Policy*, Chapter 15.

Weston, J. Fred and Brigham, Eugene F. *Managerial Finance*, pp. 445–51.

11

Inventory Management

The operating costs of a hospital can be segmented into the following expense categories:[1]

Expense Category		Approximate Percent of Total Cost	
Personnel Costs			
Nursing	=	30%	
Other	=	33%	
Total:			63%
Nonwage Costs			
Supplies	=	12%	
Depreciation	=	5%	
Heat, light,			
maintenance, etc.	=	20%	
Total:			37%
		Total:	100%

Based on the above, it is clear that supplies expense is a large nonwage cost element and represents a significant cost factor. It is a factor that can result not only in the loss of nonoperating revenues, but also in unnecessary operating costs, if not properly managed.[2] Therefore, it is incumbent upon

---

[1]Department of Health, Education, and Welfare, *Medical Care Prices, A Report to the President*, pp. 27–34.

[2]The Research Institute of America has found that the cost of having inventories ranges from 8.6% to 40.5% annually of the total value of the inventory.

management to administer this element of cost carefully, if the hospital is to achieve operational efficiency.

The control of supplies expense lies to some extent in the areas of internal control, accounts payable management, and purchasing policies. However, the major potential for controlling this cost lies in the area of inventory management, for as basic accounting theory makes clear, supplies are current assets—inventories—until they are consumed in the production process. Thus, the control of supplies costs is actually a working capital management problem, for inventories are a basic component of working capital.

INVENTORY VALUATION

Inventory costs appear in two places in a hospital's financial statements. They appear as a current asset titled inventory on the balance sheet, with a dollar value that represents the unused portion of the inventory on hand. They also appear as an expense item on the income statement as they are utilized in the generation of goods and services.

All methods of valuing inventory are based on the cost principle. Inventory purchase cost is utilized initially to assign value. During a given production period, however, identical goods may be purchased at different actual costs. Management then faces a problem of determining which inventory items and which related costs have moved from current assets to expenses.

In selecting a valuation methodology, the major objective is the correct matching of the production costs of the period with the revenues being generated. The most prevalent methods of inventory valuation are

— First in, first out method (FIFO). The first in, first out method assumes a flow of costs based on the use of the oldest goods first. This assumption conforms closest to actual usage patterns, especially for dated inventory items.

— Last in, first out method (LIFO). The last in, first out method reverses the cost flow. The assumption in using the LIFO method is that the latest costs are those most closely related to current revenues.

— Weighted average method. The weighted average method is based on the assumption that all inventory goods are commingled. The valuation of the inventory is an average, weighted according to the quantity purchased at each price.

— Specific identification method. Specific identification assumes that each inventory item can be tagged with its actual cost and accounted for as utilized.

The choice of inventory valuation methodology will have an effect on working capital through the value it assigns to the goods remaining as a current asset at the end of the period. The FIFO method has the effect of assigning the most recently incurred costs to the current asset inventory, whereas the LIFO method assigns the earliest costs to inventory. Therefore, during periods of rising prices, FIFO will more closely approximate the market value of the inventories remaining on hand; LIFO will more closely approximate the value of the inventories consumed. This understatement of the on-hand inventory under LIFO reduces the hospital's working capital, current ratio, and inventory turnover values. However, the production capabilities of the hospital remain the same under any of the above valuation methods because the productive value of the on-hand inventory is unaffected by the financial statement value assigned to it.

WHY HOLD INVENTORIES?

Given that inventory management is a critical factor in controlling supplies expenses, how should management administer inventories to produce a least cost situation? That is, how does management determine the quantity or level of inventories that the hospital should hold? Before answering these questions, one should examine why it is necessary to hold inventories.

In the case of a commercial enterprise, three basic factors are generally suggested as the causes or justification for holding inventories. These factors can be listed as follows.[3]

A. Time

The production process is not spontaneous; time is required to move goods through the process from raw materials to finished goods. Thus, at any single point in time the firm will hold some inventories in the form of "work or goods in process."

B. Discontinuities

The total production process can be characterized as consisting of various subprocesses, each of which must be coordinated with the others to produce a final product. It is impossible, however, to plan with sufficient precision that goods will always move steadily from one process to another. Therefore, to prevent discontinuities in the produc-

[3]Lindsay, J. Robert and Sametz, Arnold W., *Financial Management: An Analytical Approach*, pp. 51–54.

C. Uncertainties

tion process from stopping the entire process, extra stocks or inventories must be kept available at the various stages of production.

Due to the independent and segmented nature of the decision-making process in the economy, an individual firm cannot always project with certainty the quantity of finished goods that will be demanded or the volume of raw materials that will be needed. Therefore, to meet demands for goods and to ensure continuation of the production process, buffer stocks or inventories of both finished goods and raw materials must be kept available.

The above causes for holding inventories appear to be more applicable to a manufacturing firm than to a retailing enterprise or a hospital. Factors A and B specifically relate to circumstances and problems inherent in the manufacturing process. However, factor C—Uncertainties—has a much wider applicability and is particularly germane in the case of the hospital.

The demand for hospital services has been shown to be highly unpredictable. Also, due to the lifesaving and health maintenance nature of hospital services, the cost of failing to meet demand can be quite high. Thus, management is confronted with both an uncertain situation and a situation wherein stoppages in the production process, due to shortages of supplies, can be costly. Therefore, hospital management must hold a buffer stock or an inventory of needed supplies to assure the continuous provision of services.

COSTS

Given the above need to hold inventories, management must determine both the quantity that should be acquired in any single order and the timing of that order if an optimal inventory is to be maintained and the cost of supplies is to be controlled. If the size of the order is to be determined knowledgeably, the costs involved in holding inventories must first be identified.

The economists, financial management experts, and business researchers who have studied inventory management generally have considered the following five categories or types of cost as relevant to determining the least cost order size, that is, the economic order quantity.

PURCHASING COST

This is the cost or price paid to suppliers for goods. This is an expense that cannot be avoided, for if the hospital is to be able to render services, goods must be obtained and be available. One might assume that this cost is not particularly relevant to the order size decision, since suppliers have to be paid their price and management has little option in this area. Even so, this cost may influence the quantity that should be ordered, for suppliers may offer quantity discounts that may make large orders attractive. Thus, this cost should not be ignored in determining the size of the order.

For purposes of later reference, this cost will be referred to as PD, where P equals the price or cost per unit and D equals the number of units purchased annually.

ORDER COST

This is the administrative cost of obtaining the desired goods. This is the cost of such activities as writing specifications, soliciting and analyzing bids, preparing the order, receiving the goods, accounting for the goods, and paying the invoice. This cost may be large or small, depending upon the item purchased. If the item is standardized and the purchasing process routine, then the order cost will be relatively small. However, if it is the first time the item is being purchased or if the item is not standardized and specifications have to be written and bids taken, then the order cost will be relatively large.

It should be noted that, regardless of whether order cost is large or small, it varies not with order size but rather with the number of orders placed: as the number of orders per year increases, total annual costs also increase. Therefore, the existence of this cost encourages large orders, for the larger the order, the fewer the orders that have to be placed.

Order cost will be symbolized for later reference as O. The average cost of placing a single order, therefore, is O. However, the total annual outlay for order cost is O times the number of orders placed for the year. If D equals the number of units annually purchased and Q equals the order size, then D/Q equals the number of orders placed in a year. Total annual order cost thus equals (D/Q)O.

CARRYING COST

This is the cost attached to holding inventories. This cost can be understood most easily perhaps if it is viewed as consisting of two interdependent segments: an opportunity cost segment and a holding or storage cost segment.

When a hospital decides to hold inventories, it implicitly is making a decision to invest some of its funds in inventories as opposed to some other investment alternative. This decision means that the hospital, at the very least, incurs an opportunity cost equal to the return that could have been obtained if the funds used to finance inventories had been invested in some other way. Opportunity cost varies directly with both the rate of return on the investment alternatives and the size of the inventory investment. The greater the inventory investment, the greater is the opportunity cost incurred by the hospital.[4]

In addition to opportunity cost, the carrying of inventories involves a holding or storage cost. If management is to avoid being accused of malfeasance or negligence, it must adequately protect inventory holdings. This means that inventory stocks must be stored, insured, and properly secured. Each of these responsibilities represents a cost that the hospital cannot avoid and that varies positively and incrementally with the level of inventory holdings. Thus, the holding of inventories involves a cost to the hospital that increases as the level of inventory stocks increases.

The existence of carrying cost supports an inventory decision that is exactly opposite to the decision that order and purchase costs encourage. Due to the relationship between the size of inventory holdings and the level of carrying cost, inventory stocks should be kept as small as possible if cost is to be minimized. This, in turn, means that order sizes should be small and that orders should be placed often. Thus, there is a conflict between order and purchase costs and carrying cost, which must be resolved if a least cost solution is to be obtained.

Carrying cost, for purpose of later use, will be referred to as the quantity

$$(HQ + IP\frac{Q}{2})$$

This approach to symbolizing carrying cost has been selected to make explicit the composite nature of carrying cost. The storage cost element of carrying cost is represented by the term HQ, where H equals the cost of holding or storage per item and Q equals the order size which, as will be clear later, usually represents the maximum number of items that will be stored at any given time.

The opportunity cost element is represented by the expression

$$IP\frac{Q}{2}$$

That is, opportunity cost is equal to the highest alternative rate of return that could have been obtained times the average amount of funds that are

---

[4]It should also be noted that if funds are borrowed to finance inventories, that a cash cost, as opposed to an opportunity cost, is incurred. This cost also varies directly with the size of the inventory investment and is equal to the interest expenses due the lender.

invested in inventories. Thus, if the highest obtainable alternative rate of return was 8% and the hospital's average inventory holdings were $10,000, then:

$$\text{Opportunity Cost} = IP\ \frac{Q}{2}$$

$$I = 8\%$$

$$P\frac{Q}{2} = \$10,000$$

$$\text{Opportunity Cost} = (8\%)\ (\$10,000)$$
$$\text{Opportunity Cost} = \$800$$

As is indicated above, I represents the highest obtainable alternative rate of return. Generally, unless other information is available, I is assumed to equal the interest rate currently available in the capital market. Average inventory holdings are represented by

$$P\ \frac{Q}{2}$$

where P equals the price per unit and Q the order size. It should be noted that

$$\frac{Q}{2}$$

is the average inventory holdings, for, in a case where demand is certain, at the beginning of a period inventory holdings should equal Q and at the end of the period they should equal zero. Therefore, average holdings for the period equal the initial inventory Q plus the final inventory (zero) divided by 2, or simply Q/2. The rationale supporting this assumption is graphically illustrated in Figure 11.1.

LONG OR OVERSTOCKED COST

This is the cost attached to holding unused or unnecessary quantities of inventory stocks. This cost can be understood most easily if it is viewed as potentially consisting of two elements: a carrying cost component, and a perishability cost component.

If goods are purchased for use in a particular period but are not used in that period, then surplus inventories exist, for more goods than are actually needed are being held. In this type of situation, the hospital is forced to hold or carry these surplus stocks (overstocks) until that time when they can be used. This additional carrying of inventories, however, has a cost equal to the extra carrying costs that must be incurred. For example, if goods are obtained in period 1 but are not used until period 3, then the

FIGURE 11.1   Inventory Depletion

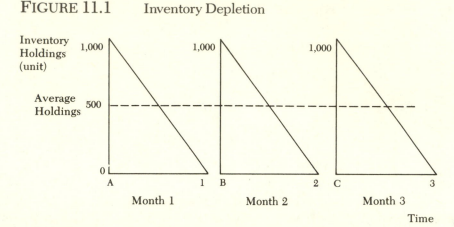

Assumptions: (1) Q = 1,000; (2) Demand per month equals 1,000 units; (3) Demand is constant over the month.

hospital has held the goods for two periods longer than actually necessary. This means that additional unnecessary carrying costs are incurred, for funds invested in inventories are committed (opportunity cost), and storage costs are incurred for a longer period than is ideally necessary.

The nature of this component of overstocked cost can be seen by referring to Diagrams A and A' in Figure 11.2. Diagram A represents the total carrying costs of holding goods. If, as is indicated in the diagram, 100 units are held, but only 50 units are used in the first period and the other 50 are not used until the third period, then unnecessary carrying costs equal to the vertically shaded areas are incurred. These costs can be considered unnecessary, for if perfect information were available regarding demand, only 50 units would have been obtained for use in period 1. Therefore, no surpluses would exist and no costs would be incurred for holding extra goods that are not immediately needed. Thus, to the extent that surpluses do exist, their cost can be viewed as not being necessary for the continuance of operations.

Diagram A' depicts this same cost notion from a somewhat different viewpoint. In this instance, the increasing nature of carrying cost is shown over several time periods. As is indicated, if goods are obtained in period 1 and used in period 1, carrying cost per unit, at a maximum, will equal OA. However, if goods are obtained in period 1 but not used until period 3, carrying cost per unit, at a maximum, will equal OB. Therefore, if overstocking or surplus inventories exist, the longer these inventories are held, the greater will be the carrying cost and, subsequently, the greater will be the overstocked cost.

The second component of overstocked cost—perishability—is perhaps

FIGURE 11.2   Overstocked Cost

1. Carrying Cost

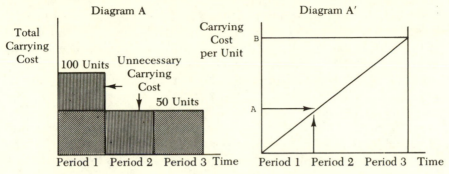

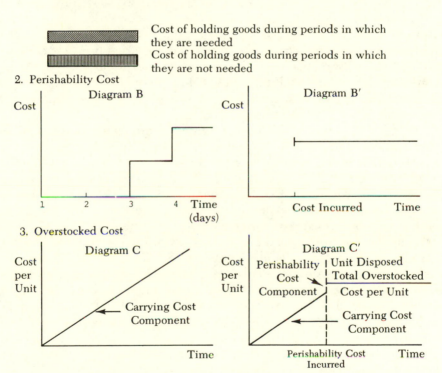

not germane to all hospital inventory stocks. Nevertheless, it should be discussed if the nature of overstocked cost is to be understood completely. Consider, for example, the case of a vegetable peddler and his perishable inventory of fresh vegetables. Prior to refrigeration, the peddler either had to sell his stock of vegetables in a day or two, or throw them in the garbage and incur the cost of the inventory that was disposed of as a loss. This loss, due to spoilage or perishability, can be considered as an overstocked cost.

A similar situation can be found in the case of some hospital pharmacy stocks that can be neither returned for credit nor dispensed after the expiration of certain time periods. In this instance, if the hospital is overstocked and unable to use the drugs before the expiration date, it incurs not only a cost for carrying the excess stock—carrying cost—but also a perishability cost equal to the cost of the drugs that have to be discarded. Diagrams B and B' in Figure 11.2 illustrate this cost.

It should be noted that perishability cost is pictured in Diagram B as a steplike curve due to the fact that the cost increases over time as price is lowered in an attempt to sell the perishable goods. For example, on the second day the vegetable peddler may, to increase sales and avoid a cash loss, reduce the price to just the cost of the vegetables. If surpluses still exist on the third day he may, to minimize his losses, reduce the price to less than cost. In this case, he will incur a perishability cost equal to the difference between the cost of the goods and the price he is charging. If surpluses still exist on the fourth day, he may have to discard the vegetables and thereby incur a perishability cost equal to the full cost of the goods that are discarded. Thus, perishability cost increases in steps over time, as the differential between price and cost changes.

Diagram B, however, is not an accurate representation of the perishability cost curve in the hospital situation. In the case of the hospital, the price of goods is not reduced in order to sell them before they become completely spoiled and unusable. Thus, as is shown in Diagram B', perishability cost for the hospital is a horizontal line. This is the case because perishability cost is equal to the cost of the goods that are no longer usable and this cost, once incurred, does not change over time.

Total long or overstocked cost for any given item is equal to the sum of the carrying and perishability costs for that item. This total cost, for purposes of later reference, will be symbolized as L and is shown in Diagrams C and C'. Diagram C represents the case wherein overstocking does not involve a perishability cost component, for example, unsterile dressings. In this case, overstocked cost is equal to just carrying cost. Diagram C' represents the case wherein overstocking involves both a perishability and a carrying cost component. In this instance, overstocked cost is equal to the sum of the two component costs.

SHORT OR STOCK-OUT COST

This is the cost attached to holding an insufficient quantity of inventory stocks. This is the cost that a firm incurs when it is not able to meet demands for goods from its inventory supplies.

In the case of a commercial enterprise, stock-out cost can be viewed as consisting potentially of two types of cost—an immediate cash cost and an intangible cost due to lost future sales. Assume that a customer demands an item which, at the time of his demand, is out of stock. If this is the case, the customer may be willing to wait a day or two for the item, but in all likelihood he will not be willing to wait as long as it would take to obtain the item through the normal delivery channels. Thus, the firm, if it is to avoid losing the sale, must go outside the normal delivery mechanism to obtain the desired goods. It may have to make special calls to its suppliers, assume the cost of an overtime production run, or arrange for special transportation. These activities represent a cash cost to the firm, which is reflected in terms of increased purchase and order costs and which cannot be avoided if the sale is to be saved. However, it must be realized that these costs arise due to a shortage of inventory stocks. Therefore, they can be considered to be the cost of stock-out or insufficient inventories.

Alternatively, a customer may not be willing or able to wait even a day or two for the goods. If this is the situation, stock-out has a cost equal not only to the current sale which is lost, but also to the discounted value (present value) of all future sales to that particular customer, which may be lost. Stock-out thus may entail a future cost to the firm in terms of lost sales due to customer dissatisfaction. This cost, though difficult to measure, is nonetheless a real cost that must be considered in inventory decisions.

In the case of the hospital, inventory stock-out is just one aspect of the more general and basic problem of allocating resources. For a hospital to be able to provide patient care, it must obtain and have available certain supplies. However, if the hospital is to operate efficiently, the quantities of these resources that are held available must be closely related to demand. The demand for hospital services, as has been indicated earlier, is highly unpredictable, and the costs of failing to meet demand are high. Thus, in the case of inventories, the cost of being unable to meet demand includes not only increased purchase and order costs, but also another far more significant intangible cost component.

The cost of inventory stock-out in the hospital situation should be measured both in terms of cash or monetary costs and also in terms of the intangible or nonmonetary costs of illness, pain, and death. Unfortunately for the decision maker, a market mechanism does not exist for measuring these nonmonetary costs. Their magnitude, therefore, must be subjectively estimated.

Usually, due to the nature of these factors, a high value is attached to stock-out cost, and the avoidance of any possibility of inventory shortages or stock-out is felt by many to be critical if not mandatory. However, from a pragmatic viewpoint it should be recognized that not only are there generally not enough resources available to guarantee that stock-out will never

occur, but also that it is excessively costly to maintain inventory levels that
will prevent any possibility of stock-out. Thus, a trade-off must be made or
a balance found between stock-out cost, service demands, and overstocked
cost if an optimal inventory management solution is to be obtained.[5]

Based on the foregoing, assuming stock-out is represented by S, the
total cost (TC) of obtaining and holding inventories can be expressed as
follows:

$$TC \;=\; \underset{\underset{\substack{\text{Purchase}\\\text{Cost}}}{\downarrow}}{PD} \;+\; \underset{\underset{\substack{\text{Order}\\\text{Cost}}}{\downarrow}}{\frac{D}{Q}O} \;+\; \underset{\underset{\substack{\text{Carrying}\\\text{Cost}}}{\downarrow}}{(HQ \;+\; IP\frac{Q}{2})} \;+\; \underset{\underset{\substack{\text{Overstocked}\\\text{Cost[6]}}}{\downarrow}}{L} \;+\; \underset{\underset{\substack{\text{Stock-out}\\\text{Cost[6]}}}{\searrow}}{S}$$

Given that these are the costs attached to inventories, the problem facing
management is simply that of determining how to obtain the minimum
value for TC. That is, determine the value of Q that will minimize TC.

INVENTORY DECISIONS—CERTAINTY

To understand how the above costs interact with one another and the
approach that management can use to minimize total inventory costs, it is
advantageous to begin with a relatively simple set of circumstances. Assume, for the sake of illustration, that a particular hospital operates in a
world of certainty. (The demand schedule facing the hospital is constant
and known.) Also, assume that the delivery of ordered goods to the hospital
is not instantaneous, but that the time lag between the placement of an
order and the receipt of goods is constant and known.

Given these assumptions, the inventory total cost equation can be re-
written as follows:

$$TC = PD + \frac{D}{Q}O + (HQ + IP\frac{Q}{2})$$

The equation can be written in this form because, in the world of certainty,
overstocked and stock-out costs do not exist. Thus, these two cost factors
for the moment can be ignored. They will, however, be considered below
as factors critical to the inventory management under conditions of
uncertainty.

---

[5]It should be noted that long and short costs involve a somewhat different type of
management decision than order and carrying costs. Long and short costs require that management balance the need for inventories against the level of stocks. Order and carrying costs
require that the size of orders be balanced against the frequency of orders.

[6]Due to the complex nature of these costs, they are expressed for the sake of simplicity
of illustration as just L and S. The reader should note, however, that these costs are a function
of such factors as order quantity and demand.

As indicated earlier, the first inventory decision that management must make is that of determining the quantity that should be acquired in any single order; that is, determination of the economic order quantity. In the above equation, order quantity is represented by Q. The problem facing management, therefore, is to determine the level of Q that corresponds to the lowest point on the inventory total cost curve, that is, TC $_{minimum}$.

At first glance, this may appear to be a difficult task. However, TC $_{minimum}$ can be found by differentiating the above equation as follows to establish the optimal order size, that is, Q_E :[7]

$$Q_E = \sqrt{\frac{2DO}{IP + 2H}}$$

Q_E is thus the economic order quantity or that order quantity that will result in total inventory costs being minimized. By solving the above equation, management can determine the optimal order quantity for its own particular operational situation. Tables 11.1 and 11.2 illustrate the use of this equation.[8]

Once the economic order quantity (Q_E) is established, it is a relatively simple task for management to determine the solution to the second inventory decision, that is, calculate the timing of when an order should be placed or the reorder point (R). Under conditions of certainty, the reorder point is simply equal to the number of units that will be demanded during the delivery time lag (D_L). That is, when the quantity of goods in stock is equal to the amount of goods that will be consumed in the time period between the placement and the receipt of an order, then the next order for additional goods should be placed.

The reorder point equation can be expressed simply as follows.

Reorder Point = Demand during Delivery Lag

or

$$R = D_L$$

Thus, if the delivery time lag is ten days and demand is 28 units per ten-day period, then the reorder point would be 28 units. Hence, returning to the foregoing example, when 28 units are left in stock an order for 58 units should be placed.

This same notion can be explained in a somewhat different fashion through the use of Figure 11.3. As is indicated in the figure, D (the slope of the curve) represents the rate of inventory use, line segment TE represents the time lag for deliveries, and E represents that point in time when

---

[7]Differentiation is a standard approach in calculus to solving a problem such as determining TC$_{minimum}$.

[8]Persons wishing to read a discussion of a more complex economic order quantity problem should refer to Appendix 11.

TABLE 11.1   Economic Order Quantity

Cost Factors

P = price/unit = $100*   I = interest rate = 5%
D = number of units purchased   H = storage cost/unit = $.50
  and used/year = 1,000   TC = total cost
O = cost of placing a single   Q = order size
  order = $10 Q_E = economic order quantity

Equations

$$TC = PD + \frac{D}{Q} O + (HQ + IP \frac{Q}{2})$$ where the minimum cost solution is

$$Q_E = \sqrt{\frac{2\,DO}{IP + 2H}}$$

$$Q_E = \sqrt{\frac{2(1,000)\,(10)}{.05\,(100) + 2.(.5)}}$$

$$Q_E = \sqrt{\frac{20,000}{6}} \text{ or } Q_E = \sqrt{3,333.33}$$

Q_E = 58 units (approximately)

$$TC_{minimum} = (100)(1,000) + \frac{1,000}{58} 10 + [(.5)(58)+(.05)(100)\frac{58}{2}]$$

$TC_{minimum}$ = 100,000 + 172 + (29 + 145)

$TC_{minimum}$ = $100,346

Conclusion
Total inventory costs will be minimized if the order quantity is set at 58 units.
Thus, 58 units is the economic order quantity.

---

*Changes in purchase price (P), due to quantity discounts, can be taken into consideration by simply using the lower value for P in the equation. However, the other cost factors in the equation must also be adjusted to reflect the impact of purchasing a larger quantity. Therefore, by solving a series of equations, each at a different purchase price, it is possible to determine the optimum quantity and price combination. It should be realized, however, since total demand is independent of inventory policy, that purchase price—including the amount of any quantity discount—is generally established at the outset and can be taken as a given.

inventory stocks are completely depleted. The inventory reorder date, therefore, is T, and the inventory quantity that signals the need to reorder is R.

The data that management needs in order to develop a least cost inventory management policy are now available. If a hospital were to operate in a world of certainty, all of the information, that is, how much to order and when to order, needed to minimize inventory costs and consequently supply costs would be known. Unfortunately, hospitals do not operate in a

TABLE 11.2   Proof of Table 11.1

Cost Factors
P = price/unit = $100
D = number of units purchased and used/year = 1,000
O = cost of placing a single order = $10
I = interest rate = 5%
H = storage cost/unit = $.50
TC = total cost
Q = order size

Equation

$$TC = PD + \frac{D}{Q} O + (HQ + IP\frac{Q}{2})$$

Solution*

Order Quantity	Purchase Cost	+	Order Cost	+	Carrying Cost	=	Total Cost
40 units	$100,000	+	$250	+	$120	=	$100,370
50 units	100,000	+	200	+	150	=	100,350
56 units	100,000	+	179	+	168	=	100,347
58 units	100,000	+	172	+	172	=	100,346
60 units	100,000	+	167	+	180	=	100,347
80 units	100,000	+	126	+	240	=	100,365

Conclusion
An order quantity of 58 units results in the least cost solution to the inventory total cost equation.

Note: The reader should note that the above technique can also be used as a trial and error approach to approximating the economic order quantity.
*Figures are rounded off.

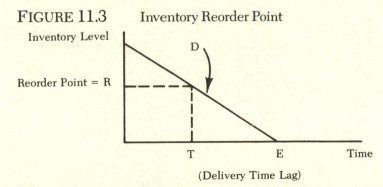

FIGURE 11.3   Inventory Reorder Point

Inventory Level

Reorder Point = R

D

T   E   Time

(Delivery Time Lag)

world of certainty. Therefore, if it is to be realistic, the foregoing inventory decision model must be expanded to take into consideration the uncertainty of actual hospital service demands.

INVENTORY DECISIONS—UNCERTAINTY

To expand the inventory decision model to allow for uncertainty, the two relevant inventory costs that were ignored in the previous model, that is, stock-out cost and overstocked cost, must be considered. Admittedly, these costs are difficult to measure. However, if management is to be able to make rational and intelligent inventory decisions, an attempt must be made, even if it is only subjective, to measure these costs. Thus, for purposes of this discussion, assume that stock-out (understocked) cost is equal to $75 per unit and overstocked cost is equal to $2.00 per unit.

In the world of certainty, when inventory stocks reached quantity R, management knew both that it was time to reorder and that the new order would arrive just as the last unit in stock was being consumed. In the world of uncertainty, however, the actual demand for goods after a new order has been placed may vary from the expected demand, leaving the hospital either over- or understocked.[9] Thus, the matter of concern is the variation in demand after the reorder point, for it is in this period that the hospital is exposed to the dangers of uncertainty. This situation is illustrated in Figure 11.4.

As should be clear from the figure, the issue is one of finding a compromise or balance between overstocking and its subsequent cost, and understocking and its cost. To determine this balance knowledgeably, that is, to determine the optimum reorder point, management must obtain two types of information: the probable variation in demand that can be expected

FIGURE 11.4   Demand Fluctuations and Inventory Stocks

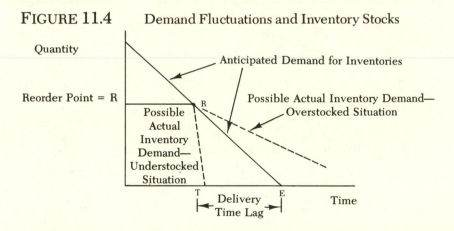

---

[9]It must be emphasized that hospitals, as well as all other businesses, operate in the world of uncertainty and that in the real world constant and predictable demand is seldom, if ever, found. Thus, if realistic and workable inventory decisions are to be made, the approach described in this section should be used as opposed to the more pedagogical and introductory approach of the previous section.

during the reorder period, and the costs attached to being either overstocked or understocked. The costs attached to being overstocked and understocked were previously assumed. Therefore, the problem is to develop some notion of the probable variation in demand that can be expected during the reorder period.

Assume that—based upon a study of historical records, information about future patterns of care, and subjective judgment—the following probabilities of various levels of demand can be developed.

DEMAND ESTIMATES

Probability	.20	.25	.20	.15	.10	.10
Demand	27	28	29	30	31	32

Based upon this demand information and the previously assumed costs, management can now calculate the expected value or cost under each reorder point strategy and determine which strategy results in the least cost solution. Table 11.3 illustrates the mechanics of determining the least cost reorder point.

Given the least cost reorder point (32 units), management now has available the information needed to develop its inventory policy. From the previous discussion of the economic order quantity, the size of each order is known (58 units).[10] Also, from the above discussion and Table 11.3, the reorder point, and hence, the timing of orders is known. Thus, all the information needed for managing inventories in a least cost manner under conditions of uncertainty is known.

PRAGMATISM

Admittedly, the foregoing model is a sophisticated management technique which necessitates not only a great deal of management skill and acumen in determining various inventory costs, but which also—if used indiscriminately for all stock items—can defeat its cost-minimizing purpose. The problems involved in measuring costs were alluded to previously in regard to short and overstocked costs. These same problems also apply to other inventory cost components such as order and carrying costs. Order cost is usually a minor cost that is both difficult and costly to measure precisely. Thus, for the sake of expediency and practicality, this cost should be estimated. The same policy should be followed in regard to carrying and overstocked costs, for these items are also costly to measure accurately.

---

[10]For our purposes, the economic order quantity can be considered to be the same under conditions of either certainty or uncertainty.

TABLE 11.3 Reorder Point—Uncertainty

Step 1. Assumptions
Understocked cost = $75/unit
Overstocked cost = $2/unit
Demand distribution:

Probability	.20	.25	.20	.15	.10	.10
Demand	27	28	29	30	31	32

Step 2. Overstocked and Understocked Cost Matrix—Unadjusted (see Step 4. Explanation)

Reorder Point Strategy (units)	Potential Demand 27	28	29	30	31	32
27	$ 0	$75	$150	$225	$300	$375
28	2	0	75	150	225	300
29	4	2	0	75	150	225
30	6	4	2	0	75	150
31	8	6	4	2	0	75
32	10	8	6	4	2	0

Step 3. Overstocked and Understocked Cost Matrix—Adjusted for Probability (see Step 4. Explanation)

Reorder Point Strategy	Potential Demand 27 (.20)	28 (.25)	29 (.20)	30 (.15)	31 (.10)	32 (.10)	Total Expected Cost
27	$ .00	$18.75	$30.00	$33.75	$30.00	$37.50	$150.00
28	.40	.00	15.00	22.50	22.50	30.00	90.40
29	.80	.50	.00	11.25	15.00	22.50	50.05
30	1.20	1.00	.40	.00	7.50	15.00	25.10
31	1.60	1.50	.80	.30	.00	7.50	11.70
32	2.00	2.00	1.20	.60	.20	.00	6.00

TABLE 11.3   Continued

Step 4. Explanation
Step 2. Unadjusted costs of various reorder strategies; for example:

Strategy	Demand	Cost
27 units	28 units	$75—1 unit short @ a cost of $75/unit
29 units	27 units	$ 4—2 units long @ a cost of $2/unit
31 units	31 units	0—supply equals demand

Step 3. Adjusted costs of various reorder strategies, that is, adjusted by multiplying value obtained in Step 2 by the demand probability assumptions set out in Step 1. This step is necessary because of the
unpredictable nature of inventory withdrawals.

Conclusion
An inventory strategy utilizing 32 units as the reorder point, that is, the
quantity that signals reorder, will result in minimizing total inventory costs.

Explanation
1. At point E, inventory stocks will be exhausted.
2. TE equals the delivery time lag where point T corresponds to an inventory
    level equal to R.
3. Thus, additional goods should be reordered when inventory stocks equal
    the number of goods that will be used during the delivery lag period.

Short cost, due to the nature of the hospital's service, is perhaps both
the most critical and the most difficult cost component to measure. It is
difficult, if not impossible, in the case of a lifesaving item or service, to
determine objectively the cost of being short. Thus, management must carefully evaluate both the patient care implications of stock-out for any given
item, and the problems, possibilities, and expenses involved in obtaining
an item on short notice. Based on this evaluation, the cost of being understocked should then be estimated as reasonably as is possible.

In addition to the cost measurement problems involved in using the
inventory decision model, management must determine which stock items
should be closely controlled. Indiscriminate application of the model to all
inventory stocks will only result in increasing total cost. This is due to the
fact that the expense of controlling low value items will exceed the expense
attached to holding excess stocks of those items. Thus, the model should be
applied only to those stock items that have a high potential for cost reduction. One technique that can be a useful aid in determining the appropriate
application of the model is the ABC stratification of inventory items.

ABC stratification of inventories is a method of separating stock items into various categories to determine which items require close control.[11] Of the 1,000 to 3,000 items that a hospital typically carries in inventory, 10% to 15% of the total number represent 60% to 70% of the total inventory value. These high value items are the A classification and should be managed through the use of the above model.

Correspondingly, another 10% to 15% of the total number represent 20% to 30% of the total inventory value. These medium value, B classification items should be managed through the use of the economic order quantity component of the model. Reorder points, however, should be subjectively determined. The remaining 70% to 80% of the items, C classification, should be managed through standardization and subjectively determined order quantities and reorder points.

Figure 11.5 illustrates the volume/value distribution of inventory items. The classification of any particular item, or group of items, should be based on an analysis of all inventory items in terms of item value, or cost per unit, multiplied by annual usage. The specific points of demarcation between A and B items and B and C items should be subjectively determined, based on management experience and the time and personnel available for inventory control.

INTERRELATIONSHIPS

The techniques for inventory management should now be understood. Application of the foregoing financial management tools will help management to minimize not only the total cost of inventories and consequently total supplies expense, but also the total quantity of working capital. This latter result is due to the fact that the inventory decision model will enable management to determine the optimum inventory quantity or investment. Thus, use of the above techniques will aid management in minimizing the total cost of working capital (see Chapter 9). The least cost method of financing inventories also should be clear from the discussion of the previous chapter.

PURCHASING AND MATERIALS MANAGEMENT

Much of the actual cost control and inventory management is left to the hospital purchasing agent. The administrator's interest should be directed to assuring that the proper purchasing policies are in place to protect the hospital's assets and that the purchasing agent's performance is of the highest possible caliber. The hospital's portfolio for inventory management

---

[11]Salling, Raymond C., "Can Your Inventory Control Be Scientific?" *Modern Hospital,* October 1964, pp. 34, 36.

FIGURE 11.5   Inventory Volume/Value Distribution

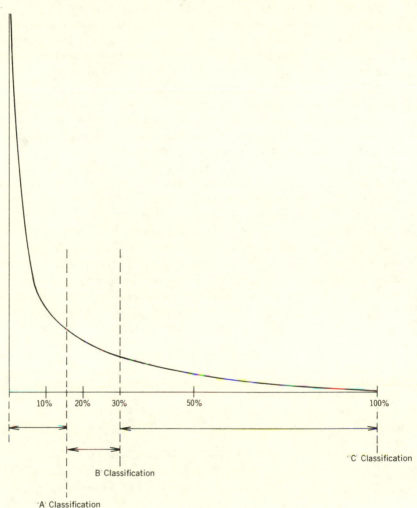

should include competitive bidding by contractors, periodic contract review, and periodic review of the inventory items utilized. These reviews are intended to assure not only that the hospital is getting the best item for an individual purchase but also that the items received are the best quality for the uses they are put to.

An inventory management technique that has become quite prevalent in its use by hospitals is group purchasing. According to a recent survey by *Hospital Purchasing Management,* almost every hospital participates in at least one group purchasing consortium, two-thirds participate in two or more consortia, and one-eighth participate in three or more.

A group purchasing consortium is a separate organizational entity that is formed through the cooperation of several hospitals in the acquisition, storage, and control of their inventories. The consortium may deal in a wide range of supply items or may specialize in one particular type of supply, for example, medical supplies or housekeeping supplies. This in part explains the multiple consortium membership of some hospitals. However, some of the multiple memberships are in competing group purchasing arrangements. The hospitals involved in this situation merely buy from the consortium that currently is offering the best price.

Group purchasing can occur in many types of arrangement. The most common arrangement is a partnership between hospitals. A second type of arrangement is a partnership between hospitals and the supplier. The supplier may be the actual manufacturer or a middleman who has inserted himself between the manufacturer and the hospitals. In such an arrangement, the group purchasing entity may be no more than a supplier or warehouser who guarantees availability and quick delivery. Many suppliers today are also making electronic order transfer available as a means of reducing ordering and warehousing costs and enhancing inventory control. More information on group purchasing and electronic order entry is available in the Suggested Readings and general literature.

SUGGESTED READINGS

Bursk, Edward C. and Chapman, John F. (eds.). *New Decision-Making Tools for Managers*, pp. 273–93.

Halse, David L. "Electronic Order Entry in Hospital Purchasing."

Hillier, Frederick S. and Lieberman, Gerald J. *Introduction to Operations Research*, Chapter 12.

Hopp, Michael. "Purchasing and Accounting Information System."

Kowalski, James C. "Strategic Planning for Hospital Materials Management."

Lindsay, Franklin A. *New Techniques for Management Decision-Making*, pp. 114–18.

Lindsay, J. Robert and Sametz, Arnold W. *Financial Management: An Analytical Approach*, pp. 51–67.

Raitz, Robert E. "The Effect of Using an Economic Order Quantity Formula and Exponential Smoothing to Reduce Hospital Purchasing Costs."

Seawell, L. Vann. *Hospital Financial Accounting: Theory and Practice*, Chapter 12.

APPENDIX 11
MULTIPLE-ITEM ORDERS—
JOINT REPLENISHMENT

The following material is adapted from *Production Planning and Inventory Control* by John F. Magee and David M. Boodman. It should be noted that while this material presents a more complex economic order quantity problem, the matter and technique of establishing reorder points are the same as discussed in the chapter.

MULTIPLE-ITEMS ORDERS

When an economic order is calculated, the controlling order cost may apply to the gross order size which can be split among a number of items. For example, central supply may obtain a large number of items from a single source. It may be desirable, in this instance, to have any shipment from the source to the hospital equal, in total, an economic size.

In cases of this type, the economic order quantity concept can be used to determine the size of the total order. Procedures can then be set up to determine (1) when to make an order and (2) how to balance the order among individual items. These procedures must meet the following requirements:

1. An order must be received before any individual item runs out.
2. The sum of the amounts of the individual items ordered must equal the total desired economic order size.
3. The quantity ordered should be balanced among individual items to delay need for the next order as long as possible.

An approach that can be used follows these lines:

1. A reorder point is set on each individual item. (This is set in the usual way to minimize total expected cost.)
2. A new order is made whenever the inventory on hand for an individual item reaches a reorder point.
3. The new order is distributed among items as follows:

Let I_i = inventory on hand of one item, the ith item

P_i = reorder point, the ith item

s_i = expected usage rate, the ith item

Q_i = amount of the order given over to the ith item

Q = total order size

I = total inventory, all items

P = total of the individual reorder points

S = total of the individual usage rates

Note that the quantities Q, I, P, and S must all be in common units. Then the amount of any individual product shipped would be

$$Q_i = s_i \frac{Q + I - P}{S} - I_i + p_i$$

This will result in an inventory on hand that will be balanced among all items in the following sense: the expected time before the inventory of an item reaches a reorder point will be the same for all items. This will put off the need for a new order as long as possible.

To illustrate how this procedure works, suppose an intravenous solution is available in three sizes: A, B, and C. Also, assume that the economic order quantity, as determined from the formula in the chapter, for total solution orders has been determined to be 400 quarts, total inventory on hand equals 270 quarts, total of individual item reorder points equals 240 quarts, and total usage is estimated at 150 quarts per week. Further assume that the inventory on hand for item B has reached the reorder point, thus signaling the need for an order.

Based on the above, the ratio

$$\frac{Q + I - P}{S}$$

can be calculated as follows:

Q = total amount of order	= 400 quarts
I = total inventory	= 270 quarts
P = total of individual reorder points	= 240 quarts
S = total usage per week	= 150 quarts

$$\frac{Q + I - P}{S} = \frac{400 + 270 - 240}{150} = \frac{430}{150} = 2.87$$

Given the foregoing ratio and the following individual usage rates, inventory levels, and reorder points, the individual orders can be calculated from the formula

$$Q_i = 2.87_{si} - I_i = P_i$$

Item = (2.87) (usage rate) − Inventory + Reorder Point = Order

	Item	Quarts
A(½ qt) = (2.87)	(100) − 32 + 20 = 275.0	137.5
B(qt) = (2.87)	(50) − 34 + 35 = 134.50	134.5
C(2 qt) = (2.87)	(25) − 30 + 25 = 66.75	133.5
		405.5[12]

The order that would be placed would be as follows:

Item	Order/Units
A	138
B	135
C	134

---

[12]Difference between economic order quantity of 400 and 405.5 due to rounding error.

The above procedure requires a calculation that can be added to the basic economic order quantity determination and that can be done in a straightforward way from data on the inventory record. Where balances of individual items are maintained on separate cards or records, a notation can be made on each record of the items to be ordered with it. In a mechanical system, using punched-card or internally programmed equipment, product codes designed to identify common-source groups are helpful in selecting the records for items to be ordered in conjunction.

CHAPTER

12

Accounts Receivable Management

Accounts receivable not only is the largest single component of working capital but also, with the exception of certain fixed asset holdings, is a hospital's largest single asset investment.[1] The magnitude of a hospital's accounts receivable holdings is primarily due to two factors: (1) the nature and cost of hospital services and (2) the third party payer system. The significance of these factors will become clear as the discussion progresses. However, at this point, it is sufficient just to realize that these factors necessitate both that a hospital hold accounts receivable and that its holdings be a substantial segment of its total assets. Given this set of circumstances, it is incumbent upon management, if the quantity of working capital is to be optimized and actual operating costs are to be minimized, to control the size of this asset carefully.

THE NATURE OF ACCOUNTS RECEIVABLE

Accounts receivable can be defined as the monies due from patients, or their agents, for services rendered to them by the hospital. As such, they can be considered to be the reciprocal of accounts payable, for the hospital's accounts receivable are a patient's or a third party payer's accounts payable. Furthermore, if accounts payable are viewed as business loans received (see Chapter 10), then accounts receivable must be viewed as business loans granted.

---

[1]In the case of the commercial enterprise, the ratio of receivables to total assets centers on about 16% to 20%. However, wide variations are experienced among firms, particularly when nonmanufacturing industries are included.

As was discussed earlier, accounts payable can represent a costly source of financing to the borrower.[2] Conversely, if accounts payable are costly to the borrower, then accounts receivable should represent an attractive investment alternative to the lender. If this were the case, it would seem reasonable to assume that the lending firms not only would be eager to extend credit, but also would gladly extend more if borrowers would want more accounts payable. However, this is not the case. The reason for this apparent inconsistency can be determined easily if one examines the business lending operations of a commercial firm.

COST OF ACCOUNTS RECEIVABLE

In Chapter 10, the interest rate on an account payable, with terms of 2-10, net 30, was determined to be, as of day 30, approximately 37%. This interest rate is obviously a substantial rate of return which lenders would be delighted to obtain. Unfortunately, 37% is not the actual rate of return that a lender receives, for the costs involved in granting credit are not considered. Thirty-seven percent is a gross rate of return that must be adjusted if the net or true rate of return on accounts payable is to be determined.

Judging from the actions of most nonfinancial commercial enterprises, the net rate of return on accounts payable is insufficient to make the granting of credit a profitable investment alternative. Admittedly, financial enterprises, such as banks and commercial credit companies, find the granting of credit to be an attractive line of trade. However, for the nonfinancial firm there are costs attached to granting accounts receivable which a bank can avoid through economies of scale, specialization, and expertise, but which make the granting of credit financially unattractive to the nonfinancial firm. The costs attached to accounts receivable can be identified and separated into three general categories: (1) carrying cost; (2) routine collection and credit costs; and (3) delinquency cost.

In the previous chapter, carrying cost was defined as the cost of holding inventories and was viewed as consisting of two independent cost segments—storage cost and opportunity cost. In the case of accounts receivable, the storage cost segment can be ignored for the most part, for elaborate warehousing and security mechanisms are not needed to hold or store accounts receivable. Carrying cost can thus be equated to the opportunity cost that arises due to the fact that the lending firm, in granting credit, is committing a part of its assets to an accounts receivable investment as opposed to some other investment alternative. Therefore, by definition, the lending firm incurs an opportunity cost equal to the return that could have

---

[2]See Chapter 10.

been obtained if the funds invested in accounts receivable were invested instead in some other manner.[3]

It should be realized that carrying cost exists during the entire credit period, for the firm's funds are committed for the entire period. However, to the extent that some borrowers do not take the discount and prefer instead to pay for the use of credit, this cost is offset. In fact, as Table 12.1 illustrates, if carrying cost were the only cost attached to extending credit, the use of accounts receivable could possibly be profitable for the lending firm. As was mentioned earlier, however, there are other costs.

In addition to carrying cost, the second major category of costs that are attached to the use of accounts receivable are routine collection and credit costs. These costs are operating expenses that arise due to the fact that if a firm is going to extend credit it must, in order to make knowledgeable credit decisions and to protect its revenue and operating position,

1. Operate a credit department—to identify those purchasers who are poor credit risks and, hence, should not be granted credit; and

2. Operate a collections department—to keep track of invoice, discount, and due dates; send payment reminders; and, when necessary, take follow-up action on unpaid accounts.

The operation of these departments can obviously be quite expensive. Therefore, since these departments are only needed if the firm extends credit, one can reasonably ask, why should a firm extend credit? Why is it either necessary or advantageous to a firm to incur the additional costs inherent in offering credit? These questions can be answered in two ways.

First, it can be argued that credit exists due to business necessity. Consider, for a moment, the tremendous operational problems that would be created if credit were not available and all business transactions had to be conducted on a cash-and-carry basis. Without the existence and reasonable availability of credit, it would be impossible to create or to operate a diverse, multibillion-dollar economy such as exists today. Admittedly, small items can be handled on a cash-and-carry basis; however, if constant production is to be maintained, if the economy is to grow, and if the wheels of commerce are to turn smoothly and efficiently, credit must exist. Thus, due to business and economic practicality, firms must extend credit if the economy is to operate and grow to its full potential.

The necessity and advantage of credit can also be explained in terms of sound and astute business practice. The extension of credit obviously

---

[3]It should also be noted that if funds are borrowed to finance accounts receivable that a cash cost, as opposed to an opportunity cost, is incurred. This cost also varies directly with the size of the accounts receivable investment and is equal to the interest expense due the lender.

TABLE 12.1   Accounts Receivable and Carrying Costs

Assumptions
1. Firm makes two separate sales of $1,000 each.
2. Terms of purchase are 2-10, net 30.
3. If the discount is taken—cost to the purchasers is $980 each.
4. The highest available rate of return from an alternative investment is 12% per year.
5. All receipts from sales are immediately invested.

Alternative A—Purchasers pay cash upon delivery.
(No accounts receivable—firm is paid cash, which it invests at 12%)
    Cash receipts = $1,960 (net receipts from two $1,000 sales)
    Income = $1,960 invested at 12% per year for 30 days
            = $19.60 (approx.)
        Total income $19.60

Alternative B—Purchasers pay at the end of the discount period.
(Hold accounts receivable for 9 days—on day 10 firm is paid $1,960)
    Cash receipts = $1,960 (received on day 10)
    Income = $1,960 invested at 12% per year for 20 days
            = $13.07 (approx.)
        Total income $13.07

Alternative C—One purchaser takes the discount, and one pays at the end of the net period.
Purchaser 1—takes discount. Therefore, firm receives $980 on day 10 which it
                invests at 12% for 20 days = $6.53
Purchaser 2—pays at the end of the net period. Therefore, firm receives a $20 return
                for the granting of credit = $20.00
        Total income $26.53

Alternative D—Purchasers pay at the end of the net period.
Firm receives a return of $20 on each purchase, that is,
        Total income $40.00

Conclusion
Given the above discount terms, the granting of credit can be profitable; that is, the
return obtained from extending accounts receivable will exceed the opportunity or
carrying cost if at least 25% of all purchasers elect not to take the discount.*

---

*Determined by solving the following set of equations which assume:
100 sales at terms of 2-10, net 30
$980 = the opportunity cost of 100 sales (see Alternative A)
$6.53 = return on sales wherein discount is taken (see Alternative C)
$20 = return on sales wherein discount is not taken (see Alternative C or D)
X = number of sales on which discount is taken
Y = number of sales on which discount is not taken
$$980 = 6.5X + 20Y$$
$$100 = X + Y$$

involves a cost to the lending firm. However, the availability of credit also widens the potential market for a firm's product, for both purchasers with ready cash and those without ready cash can buy goods. The availability of credit can thus act to increase sales which, in turn, can increase profits. Therefore, if the availability of credit results in sales and profits increasing by more than costs, it is incumbent upon management, if it is to achieve its primary objective of maximizing owner's wealth, to offer credit. Table 12.2 describes this type of situation. The critical point to be realized is that firms offer credit not only because it is an operational necessity, but also because it is a potentially sound strategy for increasing profits.

TABLE 12.2   Impact of Credit Availability on Profits

Assumptions
Situation A—Firm does not offer credit; all sales made on a cash basis.
  1. Sales = 100,000 units
  2. Profit per unit—$2 (cost per unit = $3; selling price = $5)
  3. Total profit = $200,000
Situation B—Firm changes policy and offers credit; terms net 30.
  1. Sales = 150,000 units (100,000 units sold on a cash basis and 50,000 sold on credit)
  2. Gross profit per unit = $2
  3. Total gross increase in profits due to the availability of credit = $100,000 (50,000 × $2)
  4. Increase in costs due to policy change:
      a. *Carrying Cost.* Assuming the 50,000 additional units are sold on credit, the firm incurs a total annual production cost, due to these sales, of $150,000 ($3 × 50,000 units). To support this additional cost, assuming receivables are paid monthly and will be self-sustaining after the first month, that is, the cash received in the second month for the first month's sales will support the second month's production, the firm must invest $12,500 or 1/12 of this total cost.* If the firm could earn 10% per year by investing these funds in some other manner, then the carrying cost (opportunity cost) attached to offering credit would be $1,250.
      b. *Routine Credit and Collection Costs.* The change in policy requires that the firm establish credit and collection departments. Assume the cost of these departments is $45,000.
  5. Total additional cost = $46,250
  6. Net increase in profits due to credit availability—$100,000 less $46,250 = $54,750
  7. Total profit = $253,750

Conclusion
The availability of credit results in sales and profits increasing by more than the costs attached to the offering of credit. Therefore, if management is to increase total profits, it should make credit available.

*This assumes that sales are constant over the entire year.

In viewing the impact of the availability of credit on profits, a third cost to the lending firm must also be considered, if an accurate and complete analysis is to be obtained. In addition to carrying and routine credit and collection costs, the extension of credit carries with it another category of cost which can be identified as delinquency cost. Delinquency cost arises due to the uncertainties inherent in the credit screening and granting process.

It is unreasonable to believe that all purchasers will always pay their bills on time or even that all bills will always be paid. If buyers could be completely trusted to pay their accounts, there would be no need for a credit department to screen applicants and identify poor credit risks. It is equally naive to believe that a credit department will be infallible in its screening process. Despite the most careful work and screening by the credit department, some purchasers will invariably fail to pay their bills. When this situation occurs, the selling firm must take certain steps to collect its past due accounts. It is at this point that delinquency cost begins to emerge, for the actions that the seller must take will add to the total cost of extending credit.

When an account becomes overdue, the first step that generally is taken is simply that of allowing the collection department to follow-up on the account by reminding the purchaser that he is past due. If, as is often the case, this is all that is necessary to collect the account, then delinquency cost will not be significant.

However, if the reminders of the collection department are insufficient to cause payment, other, more costly, steps must be taken. For example, the account may be turned over to a collection agency which may charge 10% to 12% (or more) of the amount outstanding for its efforts, or a lawyer may be retained at a fee of at least 10% of the outstanding balance, or—as a last resort—the account may have to be written off as a bad debt with a resultant additional cost equal to the cost of the goods. Regardless of which specific step or steps are taken, the fact should be clear that delinquency cost can be quite expensive. In fact, it is largely due to this cost factor that credit extension, in and of its own right, is not an attractive business opportunity for a nonfinancial firm.

Figure 12.1 illustrates the costs of credit to the lending firm and the potential impact of credit on profits. As is clear from the figure, the availability of credit can result in a large increase in gross profits while, at the same time, due to its costs, having only a limited effect on net profits and, subsequently, a relatively low rate of return. However, even with its low rate of return, a firm may choose to make credit available due to the necessities of business, to protect its market position, or for other reasons. Whatever the specific reason, it must be realized that credit, though perhaps necessary, is costly, and, therefore, should be judiciously managed and controlled.

FIGURE 12.1   Credit and Profit

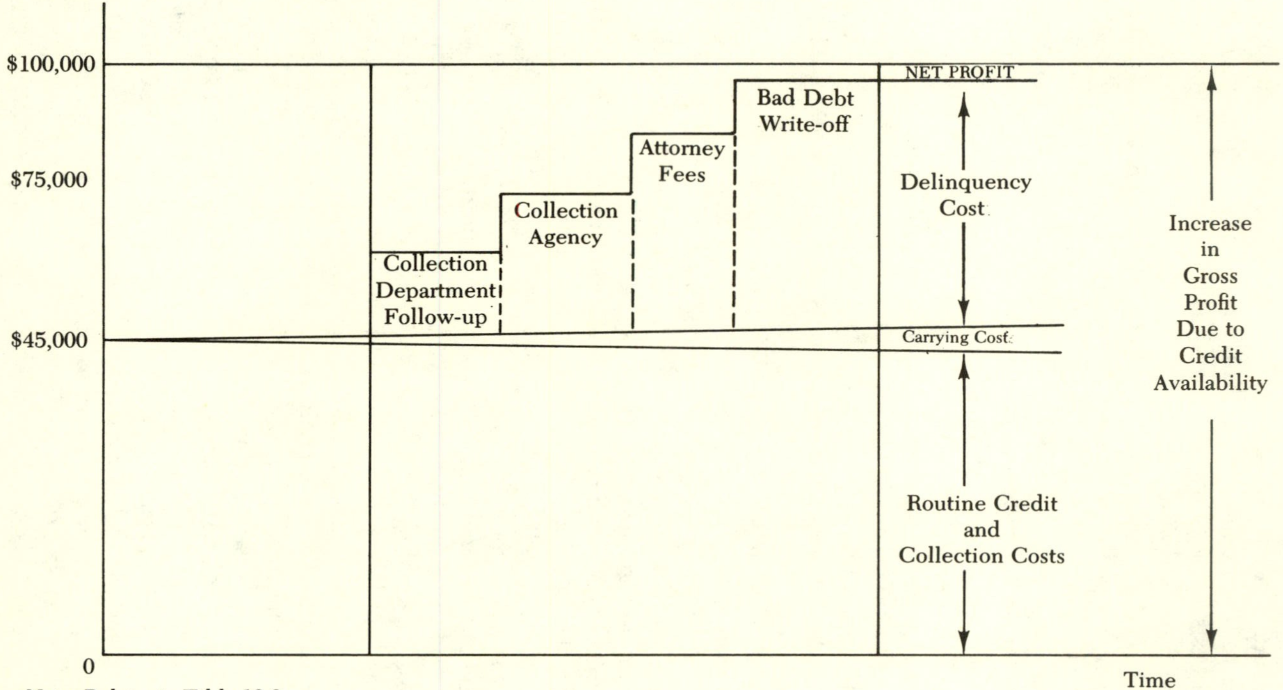

$100,000

$75,000

$45,000

NET PROFIT

Increase
in
Gross
Profit
Due to
Credit
Availability

Bad Debt
Write-off

Attorney
Fees

Collection
Agency

Collection
Department
Follow-up

Delinquency
Cost.

Carrying Cost.

Routine Credit
and
Collection Costs

Time

0

Note: Relates to Table 13.3

MANAGEMENT GUIDELINE

Based on the foregoing discussion, the following guideline can be inferred for the management of accounts receivable.

General rule:

The extension of credit is a costly undertaking for the lending firm and, hence, should only be utilized to the extent that it increases profits.

Interpretation:

The extension of credit, while not in its own right an attractive line of trade for the nonfinancial commercial enterprise, can help to increase sales and can, therefore, act to enhance profits. However, if credit is granted indiscriminately, the costs incurred due to its extension can exceed the increased profits obtained due to an expanded sales volume. Thus, credit or accounts receivable should be kept to a minimum, with the minimum being that point where the marginal increase in profits equals the marginal increase in costs.

In summary, credit extension, though a costly operation to the lending firm, has a profit-increasing potential and therefore should be utilized to the fullest extent of that potential.

HOSPITAL ACCOUNTS RECEIVABLE

Based upon the above material, the reader should now have an understanding of the potential and costs of accounts receivable in the commercial setting. With this understanding in mind, it is now possible to turn and examine the role of accounts receivable in the hospital setting.

Hospitals are by necessity in the credit business. A hospital, even if well managed, can typically expect to hold about 25% of its total assets and 75% of its current assets in accounts receivable. This is obviously a substantial investment. However, this investment is, at least in part, unavoidable.

A hospital is a community resource whose primary objective is that of providing the community with the services that it needs. In the strictest sense, this objective means providing services to any and all patients without regard to their financial situation. In practical terms, from either a public relations or, as some courts are attempting to establish, a legal standpoint, a hospital cannot refuse care to a patient in need.[4] Given this fact, and the additional facts that hospital care is costly and that the need for hospital care is generally both emotionally and financially unexpected, it is not

---

[4] One could also argue this point in terms of the Internal Revenue Service regulations that require that a hospital, in order to retain its tax exemption, cannot be operated exclusively for those who are able to pay.

difficult to understand why a hospital cannot operate on a cash-and-carry basis and, hence, must extend credit to self-responsible (self-pay) patients.

The nature of hospital–third party payer relationships also forces hospitals into the credit business. It is impossible, if only due to the quantity of transactions and distance considerations, for hospitals to deal with third party payers on a cash-and-carry basis. Thus, credit granting is an intrinsic and unavoidable operational fact of life for hospitals.

Since hospitals are in the credit business, they incur the same credit extension costs as do commercial firms. However, unlike commercial firms, hospitals cannot use the profit-generating potential of credit to justify the costs of credit, nor have they chosen to offer their services on terms in order to offset the costs of credit.

The commercial firm can use the availability of credit to increase sales and, consequently, profits. A hospital, however, due to the nature of the demand for its services, cannot significantly increase its patient days either by making credit available or by liberalizing its credit terms.[5]

Additionally, hospitals have traditionally felt that it would be unwise to charge interest, either in the form of offering services on terms or in the form of a lending or handling charge, on accounts receivable. Hospital managers have long held the position that charging interest will result in adverse public relations and also, due to the nondiscretionary nature of the bulk of hospital demand and the community resource position of hospitals, that it is morally wrong. Recently, though, some managers have taken the position that charging interest is both justifiable and necessary if tbe hospital is to be competitive for the debtor's dollar. However, it remains questionable whether the revenues from these charges will outweigh the costs of extending credit or whether the public is ready to accept this practice by hospitals.

Appendix 12.A discusses the above matter in greater detail. Readers desiring additional information should refer to the appendix and the Suggested Readings at the end of the chapter. At this point, it should be realized that hospitals, for the most part, do not specifically charge for the credit that they make available to patients.

The implications of this situation are quite clear. Since hospitals cannot use the availability of credit as a mechanism for increasing sales and profits, the advantage or value of credit does not exist for the hospital as it does for the commercial firm. In the case of the hospital, the extension of credit only results in additional operating costs being incurred. Therefore, if part

---

[5]Some hospitals have begun to offer pricing discounts in an attempt to attract patients and increase sales. Primarily, the discounts are being operationalized through the waiver of the patient's deductible or coinsurance obligation. This goes beyond the granting of credit because the expectation of payment is actually waived. Additionally, the acceptance of this practice by the public and third party payers is still undergoing debate.

of management's goal or objective is to provide services at least cost, the operational guideline for managing accounts receivable can be stated simply as follows:

Accounts receivable, and the granting of credit, should be kept to a minimum if costs are to be minimized.

Admittedly, as has been discussed, the holding of some accounts receivable is an unavoidable part of hospital operations. Management, however, can and must exercise some control over this amount if it is to minimize costs. Thus, the question that can be asked at this point, and the realistic problem that faces management is, what can be done to minimize the costs of accounts receivable? That is, given the constraint of operational necessity, what management actions can be taken to minimize the costs of accounts receivable?

MANAGING ACCOUNTS RECEIVABLE

The management of accounts receivable is a complex problem that begins not when a patient is discharged but rather with the preadmission of a patient and continues through until the account is paid or a decision is made to write off the account as uncollectable. Between these points, management is confronted with numerous internal and external operational problems and decisions, each of which requires definite management action if costs are to be minimized.

Basically, the problem of controlling the costs of accounts receivable centers on the matter of controlling the time or the length of the accounts receivable payment cycle. As was discussed in Chapter 9, the longer this payment cycle, the larger must be the hospital's working capital investment in accounts receivable. Consequently, the more assets that are involved, the greater will be the carrying cost. Also, the larger the amount of accounts receivable, the greater will be the routine credit and collection costs, for more people will be needed to keep track of the accounts and, probably, the greater will be the delinquency cost, for older accounts are less likely to be paid.[6] Thus, if costs are to be minimized, it is imperative that the payment cycle be kept as short as is pragmatically feasible. The question confronting management is, how can this be done?

Viewing the problem realistically, hospital management, due to the presence of third party payers, is limited in regard to the amount of control it can exercise over the accounts receivable payment cycle. It is unreasonable to believe that a single hospital can force a Blue Cross plan or the

---

[6]The American Credit Indemnity Company suggests that an account that is 90 days past due will be diminished in value by 10%, an account 120 days past due 15%.

government (Medicare or Medicaid) either to reduce the amount of paper work involved in billing for a covered patient or to increase the speed with which it pays its debts, that is, pays accounts receivable. A hospital, however, can improve its own in-house (internal) processing procedures and thereby accelerate the rate at which it is able to submit bills to both third party payers and self-responsible payers and receive payments. Obviously, to the extent that a hospital can reduce its in-house processing time, it can reduce the amount of its accounts receivable holdings and carrying cost.

To accelerate in-house processing time, management must design an accounting system that ensures not only that all requests for services are registered, but also that all services rendered are *promptly* and *accurately* charged to the appropriate patient's account for subsequent transmission to the payer. The importance of these two factors should be clear. If extra time has to be spent in trying to identify services that have been rendered, internal processing time must increase. Also, processing time must increase if the correct charges are not promptly entered into a patient's account and billed. The system should be designed to ensure that adequate internal control checks and balances exist. The in-house processing of service requests is often referred to as order entry. Order entry represents the initiation, assembly, and forwarding of all patient "charge tickets" to the hospital business office for incorporation into the patient's billing record. The system captures the necessary information on the services requested and on those provided. Order entry may be performed manually or through a computerized entry system. In a manual system, the capture is performed on paper charge tickets prepared in the service department. Although manual systems have been utilized effectively for years, the trend is now toward computerized systems because of the number of distinct services provided by hospitals and the amounts of data required by payers in the adjudication of the patient's bill. Hospitals attempting to continue to utilize manual systems may experience high volumes of lost and late charges, high processing costs, and a high volume of bills returned by payers because of insufficient or inaccurate data. Computerized order entry involves the use of computer terminals at the hospital nursing stations and in the ancillary service departments. The service request, pricing, and charge record are all handled by the computer. The major problem with a computerized system relates largely to the initial employee education and acceptance at the entry stations. However, once this is overcome, many hospitals feel that the systems are cost justified in that previously unrecognized revenues are identified and a reduction in processing costs occurs.

Paperless billing is another technique that can be applied once all the billing information is in the business office. It utilizes cassette tapes or other electronic media to transfer necessary information to the third party payer. Medicare, Blue Cross, and some commercial payers currently use paperless billing in varying degrees. For a hospital, the use of paperless claims requires a computer capability, a fixed and known data format for payment, and the ability to sort patient data by payer. Paperless billing provides the hospital with operating efficiencies in processing and storage of data, gives edit controls for bills, and can potentially accelerate cash flows. A checklist of internal control requirements for accounts receivable is presented in Table 12.3.

The length of the payment cycle can also be reduced by improving the efficiency of the credit and collection function and by developing a system-

TABLE 12.3   Accounts Receivable—Internal Control Checklist

1. Are all charges made in accordance with the rate schedule?
2. Is a ledger account established for each patient admitted, and is it checked against the admission register?
3. Are satisfactory procedures followed in service departments to ensure the prompt reporting of *all* services involving charges?
4. Are charges for services checked for accuracy of:
   a. Period covered?
   b. Type of services?
   c. Rates used?
   d. Extensions?
5. Are control totals developed from the charge media and balanced against the accounts receivable posting?
6. If statistical data are maintained, are they correlated with recorded revenues?
7. Is a reconciliation of the total of the individual accounts in the accounts receivable ledgers with the general ledger control:
   a. Prepared periodically?
   b. Reviewed by a responsible person?
8. Are statements of all accounts receivable mailed regularly?
9. Are aging schedules:
   a. Prepared periodically?
   b. Reviewed and tested periodically by a responsible person?
10. Are the following functions handled independently:
   a. Posting?
   b. Credit?
   c. Development of control totals?
   d. Cash receipts?
   e. Allowance approval?
11. Do persons independent of accounts receivable personnel and credit department personnel confirm accounts by mail and by:
   a. Checking patients' statements with accounts?
   b. Keeping statements under control to assure mailing?
   c. Receiving reported differences directly?
   d. Investigating reported differences?

Note: Partial listing, adapted from American Hospital Association, "Internal Control and Internal Auditing for Hospitals" (American Hospital Association, 1969).

atic credit granting and follow-up procedure. Improving the efficiency of the credit and collection function will also reduce routine operating costs. Additionally, delinquency cost will be reduced by: implementation of a system for granting credit based on information necessary to evaluate a patient's credit status and a system with follow-up procedures for accounts receivable; proper organization and timing of collection efforts; use of collection agencies and legal assistance when necessary; and adoption of criteria for writing off an account as uncollectible.

The credit and collection function should begin, whenever possible, with the preadmission or preregistration processing of a patient. Through preadmissions, the hospital can obtain, prior to admission, the information necessary to confirm a patient's insurance coverage or analyze his credit status systematically, and it can inform a patient of any required deposit. Preadmission of patients can also aid the hospital in the early identification of free service patients, for it enables the hospital to obtain the financial information needed to determine a patient's credit status. (See Figure 12.2.)

Many hospitals have incorporated financial counseling services for patients who are expected to experience payment difficulties. These services can be a benefit to both the hospital and the patient. Effective financial counseling benefits the hospital by improving the probability of payment. The hospital's payment and credit policies are presented "up-front" so that increased understanding and receptiveness occur. Counseling is used to direct patients to funds established for charity care recipients or to local lending institutions where commercial credit arrangements are available or to help the hospital and patient establish a budget payment plan.

The fact that an account receivable goes unpaid does not, by definition, mean that the account should be classified as a bad debt. If, from the outset, the possibility of ever collecting on a particular account is zero, that account should not be classified as a regular or normal account receivable. Rather, the account should be classified as a free service account. The misclassification of free service accounts results only in wasted collection effort and expense, inflated accounts receivable balances, and a distorted picture of the hospital's collection efforts and results. Thus, if a true picture of the hospital's accounts receivable situation is to be obtained and if unnecessary collection efforts are to be minimized, free service accounts should be identified as early as possible.

Finally, the hospital can shorten its payment cycle by taking advantage of any periodic advance or interim payment program offered by a third party payer. Traditionally, periodic advance payment programs were available from cost-basis payers because of the absence of a working capital factor in the cost-based payment formula. The basis of the payment is a mutually agreed upon amount of cash which is transferred to the hospital at fixed periodic intervals. The amount of the payment usually is based on

FIGURE 12.2 Patient Preadmission Form

Patient name_____

Address_____ County_____ Township_____

Place of birth_____ Date of birth_____ Age_____

Marital status_____ Religion_____ Telephone_____ S.S. #_____

Have you ever stayed overnight at_____ Hospital?_____

Patient's employer_____ Occupation_____

Employer's address_____ Telephone no._____

Spouse's name_____ Occupation_____

Spouse's employer_____ Address_____

Patient's father's name (if minor)_____ Mother's maiden name_____

Person responsible for bill_____

Address_____

Employer name and address_____

Physician name_____ Expected date of hospitalization_____

Reason for hospitalization_____

Hospital bill will be paid by the following (check one):

_____ Blue Cross—Name of subscriber_____ Name of Blue Cross plan_____

Contract number_____ Code number_____

_____ Other group insurance—Name of company_____

Address_____

Policy number_____

_____ Medicare—Medicare number_____

_____ Patient

_____ Other—_____

_____

Signature_____

Unless other arrangements are made with the hospital, the hospital bill is payable in full upon discharge.

Please complete this form and return at once to:

_____

_____

historical billing data for the utilization of services by the payer's subscribers at the individual hospital. When using a periodic advance payment approach, the cash payment to the hospital is made prior to the final adjudication of the claim. In some instances, the cash payments in aggregate may also exceed the aggregate billings for the period, resulting in a temporary liability to the payer. At year-end a reconciliation between the periodic payments and the actual payments due is made to settle the payer's account. These programs are quite effective for smaller hospitals with limited administrative capabilities and for hospitals with widely fluctuating patient volumes. However, in order to be effective from the payer's viewpoint, the historical billing estimates must be modified to account for changes in traditional subscriber utilization patterns. Because of the shift to prospective fixed price methodologies and the obvious working capital cost these programs incur for the payer, the use of periodic advance payment is being reevaluated. In all probability the option of periodic advance payments will be sharply curtailed in the near future.

Numerous texts and articles have been written on the specific mechanics of hospital credit and collection techniques and systems. Given the volume and quality of the existing literature, there is little value and insufficient space to repeat or summarize that material in this text. Additionally, the mechanics of operating the credit and collections function should not be a primary concern of the hospital's administrator.

The reader should realize that the design of the accounts receivable system is basically a systems analysis problem that should be solved by the hospital's industrial engineer, internal auditor, and controller. The role of general hospital management in this area is limited to reviewing the system design and its results, to ensure that the system is functioning properly. Readers interested in further information on the design of accounts receivable systems should refer to the Suggested Readings at the end of this chapter.

CREDIT CARDS

Commercial firms have found that the acceptance of bank and commercial credit cards can be a useful mechanism for accelerating the accounts receivable payment cycle. Credit cards, such as Visa and MasterCard, are held by millions of persons and are accepted by most businesses, including some physicians and hospitals.

The advantage to a hospital of accepting these credit cards for payment of accounts centers on both the acceleration of the payment cycle and the reduction of collection efforts and subsequent costs. The key characteristics of a credit card acceptance agreement are that

1. The hospital agrees to accept the patient's credit card for payment of amounts owed;

2. The hospital pays a fee—service charge—to the issuing bank for each charge submitted;

3. The hospital must maintain an account at the bank issuing the credit card;

4. The issuing bank agrees to pay all accounts to the hospital quickly by depositing funds in the hospital's account at the issuing bank; and

5. The bank determines the patient's creditworthiness and has no recourse for uncollectible accounts.

In essence, a credit card acceptance agreement allows a hospital, for a fee, both to accelerate its payment cycle by shifting the problem of collection lags to the issuing bank, and to transfer a portion of its credit investigation and collection efforts (and costs) to the issuing bank.

Given the nature of the agreement, the financial decision rule as to whether or not to accept credit cards is quite simple. If the benefits (savings) in terms of reduced working capital needs and reduced credit investigation and collection costs exceed the sum of the costs of the fee and the tangible and intangible costs of either holding a subsidiary account at the issuing bank or transferring an entire account to the issuing bank, then the hospital should consider more than just financial implications.

The use of credit cards by hospitals raises both public policy and philosophical issues. Stated simply, a hospital must weigh the internal financial implications against

1. The potential increased cost of care to the patient, due to the interest charge that the bank or credit company adds to accounts that it finances over time, that is, that patients pay in installments; and

2. Its obligation, as a vital community resource, not to shift the burden of collection or of loss to another party (the card-issuing bank or company) or, through the bank or company, to patients financially unable to pay for needed care. In addition to these factors, the matters of image and patient reaction must be taken into account.

Obviously, each hospital must balance these issues in terms of its own environment and financial requirements. However, as a middle ground, it may be judicious management, if the acceptance of credit cards is financially justified, to limit acceptance either to certain services, for example, emergency department or outpatient, or to charges that are less than a predetermined level—less than $100.

CREDIT AND COLLECTION COSTS
AND TOTAL COST

Intuitively, it would seem that one approach to reducing the total cost of accounts receivable would lie in reducing credit and collection costs to a minimum. In some instances, however, the hospital may be able to decrease total cost by increasing credit and collection costs. It has been found that as collection efforts increase, with an increase in credit and collection costs, that the average collection time and bad debt losses decrease, that is, carrying and delinquency costs decrease. Figure 12.3 illustrates this situation.

As can be seen from the figure, the initial increments in credit and collection expenditures (Y to Y_1) have no effect on carrying and delinquency costs. However, as more is spent (Y_1 to Y_2), carrying and delinquency costs begin to fall and continue to fall until a saturation point (Y_3) is reached. As the figure indicates, additional expenditures (Y_3 to Y_4) beyond the saturation point have no cost reduction impact.

How much a hospital should actually spend on credit and collection efforts is an empirical problem that can be solved only by examining the costs and savings attached to different levels of expenditure. Ideally, funds should be invested until that point is reached at which the marginal savings equal the marginal cost. That is, credit and collection expenditures should increase until that point at which the savings from an additional expendi-

FIGURE 12.3   Credit and Collection Expenditures and Carrying
                 and Deliquency Costs

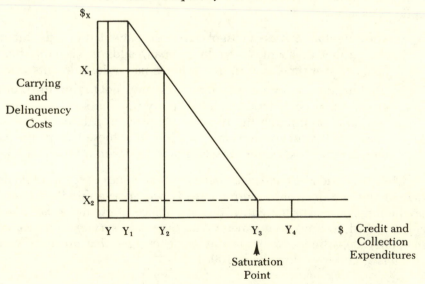

ture just equal the cost of that expenditure. Table 12.4 illustrates this general rule.

ACCOUNTS RECEIVABLE AND FINANCING

A discussion of accounts receivable management would be incomplete without an examination of the role and usefulness of accounts receivable in providing short-term financing for a hospital's temporary working capital needs. This material was discussed in part in Chapter 10. However, this topic is also important to accounts receivable management and, therefore, bears reiteration. The use of accounts receivable in short-term financing centers around either the pledging of accounts as security or collateral for a loan or the selling of the receivables. The pledging of accounts receivable is known as discounting accounts receivable. In this process the lender takes the receivables, but has recourse to the hospital (the borrower). That is, if an account is not paid, the lender can hold the hospital responsible for the account, and the hospital—not the lender—must absorb the loss.

In the case of hospitals, the discounting of accounts receivable can take one or both of two forms. The hospital may discount the accounts directly with a bank or finance company. In this instance, the hospital deals directly with the lender, and the patient generally is unaware of the fact that his account has been discounted. If the patient defaults on the account, the lender obtains payment from the hospital and the hospital, in turn, attempts to collect from the patient.

As an alternative to the above, the hospital may develop an arrangement with a bank wherein the bank will make loans to patients for medical expenses. In the strictest sense, this arrangement does not actually involve the discounting of accounts receivable. However, it is similar to discounting in that the bank, as a prerequisite to such an arrangement, will generally require that it have recourse to the hospital if the patient defaults on the loan. Thus, under either alternative, the risk of default remains with the hospital.

A direct bank-patient loan arrangement is probably of most benefit to the hospital in regard to self-pay patients. Also, to the extent that it can provide a means of financing the self-responsible portion of a patient's bill, such an arrangement can be of value relative to patients who are covered by third party payers. However, its use in regard to accounts due from third party payers does not appear to be practical. Alternatively, the discounting approach is practical for both third party and self-pay accounts and, depending on the costs, may be the most desirable short-term financing alternative if substantial amounts are needed.

Accounts receivable can also play another short-term financing role. Receivables can be sold or factored to a lender. In this process, the hospital

TABLE 12.4   Credit and Collection Expenditures and Accounts Receivable Costs

General Assumptions

Average accounts receivable holdings	=	$500,000
Cost of operating credit and collections department (annual)	=	$100,000
Carrying cost per year (assuming opportunity cost at 6%)	=	$ 30,000
Delinquency cost (average annual cost)	=	$150,000
Total accounts receivable cost		$280,000

Situation A

Employ an additional person in the collections department:
cost = $12,000
Projected effects:

Cost of credit and collections department	=	$112,000
Carrying cost per year	=	30,000
Delinquency cost	=	150,000
Total		$292,000

Decision

Do not hire additional person. Expenditure increases costs by more than the savings. This situation is similar to a move from Y to Y_1 in Figure 12.3.

Situation B

Develop and implement systematic credit and collection procedure that requires a staffing increase of three positions: cost = $50,000
Projected effects:

Cost of credit and collections department	=	$150,000
Carrying cost (reduce average accounts receivable holdings to $300,000)	=	18,000
Delinquency cost	=	100,000
Total		$268,000

Decision

Implement the above actions. This situation is similar to a move from Y_1 to Y_2 or perhaps from Y_2 to Y_3 in Figure 12.3.

Situation C

Assume present situation is as described in Situation B above. Given this situation, the credit manager requests the hiring of an assistant credit manager at a cost of $15,000.
Projected effects:

Cost of credit and collections department	=	$165,000
Carrying cost	=	18,000
Delinquency cost	=	100,000
Total		$283,000

Decision

Do not hire the assistant credit manager, for it does not produce a savings over Situation B. This situation is similar to a move from Y_3 to Y_4 in Figure 12.3.

sells, without recourse, its receivables to a bank or finance company. That is, the hospital not only transfers the receivables to the lender, but also transfers the risk of default to the lender. Generally, when receivables are factored, the patient is notified of the transaction and makes payment directly to the bank or finance company.

Accounts receivable factoring is a common practice in some hospitals. However, its value can be questioned. Factoring, due to the fact that the lender bears the risk of default, is more expensive than discounting. Also, if the lender harasses the patient during the collection process, factoring can have adverse public relations effects. Thus, accounts receivable factoring is not recommended as a primary means of financing temporary working capital needs.

CONCLUSION

The role of accounts receivable in hospital operations should now be clear. It should be borne in mind that the granting of credit and the holding of some accounts receivable are a necessary and unavoidable part of hospital operations. However, the extension of credit and the holding of receivables are costly and, to the extent that the amount of accounts receivable can be reduced, the costs of operation can also be reduced. Therefore, the operational guideline for the management of accounts receivable is simply that, given the necessities of operation, accounts receivable should be kept to a minimum.

SUGGESTED READINGS

Barnes, E. H. *Barnes on Credit and Collection.*

Freeman, Gary and Allcorn, Seth. "Examine the Balance Fraction Method: Improving Receivables Management."

Fritz, Michael H. "Collection Techniques."

Healy, Sister Mary Immaculate. "An Analysis of Accounts Receivable with Emphasis on Factoring."

Lippold, Ronald C. *Hospital Credit Training Manual.*

Markstein, David L. "The Pros and Cons of Credit Cards for the Hospital Field."

Massachusetts Hospital Association. "Follow Up Analysis: Methods and Procedure for Minimizing Financial Loss Risk and Accounts Receivable."

Seawell, L. Vann. *Hospital Financial Accounting: Theory and Practice*, Chapter 11.

Weston, J. Fred and Brigham, Eugene F. *Managerial Finance*, Chapter 13.

APPENDIX 12.A
INTEREST CHARGES AND ACCOUNTS RECEIVABLE

I.   Carrying Cost

An opportunity cost equal to the revenue foregone by investing funds in accounts receivable as opposed to some other investment alternative. It should be noted that carrying cost is an economic cost of operations. However, it is not an out-of-pocket cost since it is revenue foregone.

A. Current Status

1. Third party payers
Presently do not include carrying cost as an allowable cost.

2. Self-responsible patients
For the most part, hospitals presently do not charge interest on late payments. However, these charges could be added to the bills of self-pay patients who are late in payment and to the self-responsible portion of accounts due from patients who are covered by third party payers.

B. Conclusion

1. This cost, though not an accounting cost, is an economic and real operational cost. Therefore, revenues to compensate for the income foregone (opportunity cost), due to the holding of accounts receivable for the usual or customary carrying period, should be obtained as part of normal operations.

2. Revenues to compensate for income lost (opportunity cost) due to payments that are delayed beyond the usual or customary carrying period should not be obtained from normal operations. These costs should be viewed as being due to unusual or abnormal events that are the responsibility of particular debtors. Thus, they should be treated as abnormal and neither be aggregated into normal operating costs nor be offset through normal operating revenues. Instead, separate late or interest charges should be used to compensate for these costs. Such charges not only are economically justified, but also are mandatory if an economically sound financial position is to be maintained.

II.   Credit and Collection Costs

The routine operating costs incurred in the operations of the credit and collections department. As such, these costs are part of the normal day-to-day operations of the hospital.

A. Current Status

1. Third party payers

An allowable cost that is included in the third party reimbursement formula.

2. Self-responsible patients

A real cost of operations that should be included in the hospital's charge structure.

B. Conclusion

Revenues to compensate for these costs can and should be obtained as part of normal operations. Therefore, late or interest charges are not needed to provide revenue for these costs.

III. Delinquency Cost

The cost that arises due to patients' defaulting on their debt obligations. The magnitude of this cost, for each account that becomes delinquent, can range from just a small amount, for extra collection efforts on the part of the hospital's collection department, to—at the extreme—the writing off of the entire account as uncollectible. Historically, third party payers have not defaulted on their agreed-to obligations. Therefore, this cost is attributable entirely to obligations that the patient has to pay himself.

A. Current Status

1. Third party payers

A disallowed cost that is not included in the reimbursement formula. (As discussed in Chapter 7, Medicare allows bad debt costs [for its patients] as a reimbursable item, if a reasonable collection effort has been made.) It is, in effect, a price discount that is given to third party payers in recognition of the reduced business risk that they represent.

2. Self-responsible patients

A real operating cost that should be recognized in the hospital's charge structure.

B. Conclusion

Revenues to compensate for this cost can and should be obtained as part of normal operations. Therefore, late or interest charges are not needed to provide revenues for this cost.

APPENDIX 12.B
THE UNIFORM HOSPITAL BILL (UB-82)
HISTORY

For over 25 years, attempts have been made at designing a national uniform billing form. The goal has been to develop a standard data set and format that can be used by health care providers to transmit charge and claim information to all third party payers. Several versions of a uniform bill have been developed and implemented with varying degrees of success in a number of states. The National Uniform Billing Committee (NUBC), which is chaired by the American Hospital Association (AHA), was organized formally in 1975. The NUBC includes representatives from the Health Care Financing Administration (HCFA), the Blue Cross and Blue Shield Association (BCBSA), the Health Insurance Association of America (HIAA), the Office of Civilian Health and Medical Programs of the Uniformed Services (CHAMPUS), the Federation of American Hospitals (FAH), the Healthcare Financial Management Association (HFMA), and state hospital associations.

Before the formation of the NUBC, the AHA had worked closely with the HFMA and the federal government to develop a uniform hospital bill. Between 1968 and 1972, 13 different form designs were developed and discarded as unsatisfactory. The 14th version was field tested in Georgia in 1973. The form was modified and introduced for a second trial in Wyoming. In 1978, the HCFA agreed to participate in a pilot test in five states of the then latest version of a uniform hospital bill, the UB-16-78. An independent consultant evaluated the pilot project and the uniform bill UBF-1 used in New York. As a result of this evaluation and the subsequent deliberations of the NUBC, the UB-82 emerged as the uniform hospital bill endorsed by provider and third party representatives on the NUBC. The UB-82 format and data specifications were finalized at the May 1982 NUBC meeting. The focus has now shifted to the state level for implementation of the UB-82.

DATA SPECIFICATIONS

The UB-82 is intended to be used for summary billing of inpatient and outpatient hospital services and, at the option of the hospital, for hospital-based skilled nursing facilities and home health agencies. In determining the data to be included on the UB-82, the NUBC attempted to balance the payers' need to know certain information against the burden of providing that information. Data elements identified as necessary in most cases to process a hospital bill for payment are assigned designated spaces on the form (for example, patient name, insurance certificate number, or diagnosis). Elements needed occasionally by a limited number of payers are incorporated into general fields and are assigned numeric codes (for example, the value code: "most common semiprivate room rate," the occurrence code: "date of accident," and the condition code: "patient is full-time student"). Both unassigned codes and undefined spaces are included in the UB-82 data set to meet unique hospital or payer needs at the state or local level. This built-in flexibility is intended to promote the greatest use of the data

FIGURE 12.B-1 HCFA Form 1450—National Uniform Bill

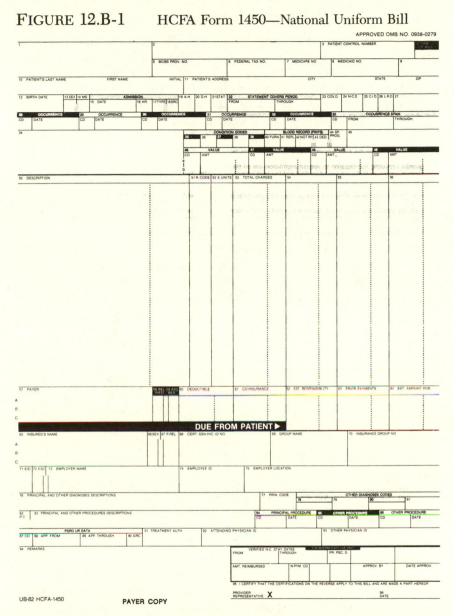

set and to eliminate the need for attachments to the billing form. The data specifications manual contains national requirements for preparing Medicare, CHAMPUS, and commercial insurance claims. Decisions regarding local Blue Cross and state Medicaid requirements are made at the state level.

PAYER IMPLEMENTATION PLANS

The HCFA required that the UB-82 (HCFA-1450) replace the current Medicare billing forms HCFA-1453 and HCFA-1483 for inpatient and outpatient hospital billing by October 1, 1984. Hospitals must submit claims via either the paper copy UB-82 or electronic data set. Certain data elements not required for claims processing by Medicare but necessary for the fiscal intermediaries to meet their contractural obligations to provide patient abstracts to peer review organizations must also be submitted on the UB-82.

October 1, 1985 was the target date set by Medicare for providers other than hospitals, although fiscal intermediaries have been instructed to implement the UB-82 for skilled nursing facilities, home health agencies, and end-stage renal disease facilities as soon as feasible even if after the deadline. The UB-82 is required for all hospice claims.

The April 19, 1983 *Federal Register* contained a proposed rule requiring state Medicaid programs to use the UB-82 by October 1, 1985, or risk a reduction in the 75% federal financial participation rate for costs of operating a Medicaid Management Information System (MMIS). States with approved MMIS would receive 90% federal matching funds for their UB-82 conversion costs if they were implemented by January 1, 1986.

The BCBSA is working with its local Blue Cross plans to coordinate UB-82 implementation for the private business side with that of the fiscal intermediary. The commercial insurance industry strongly supports the UB-82 and welcomes a standardized billing form. CHAMPUS is also working with its intermediaries to promote UB-82 implementation. In addition, the federal Black Lung Program has adopted the UB-82 for its billing form.

STATE RESPONSIBILITIES

Each state has established a State Uniform Billing Committee (SUBC) for implementation of the UB-82 within the state. The SUBC membership is modeled after that of the NUBC with both payers and providers represented. The SUBCs are largely chaired by the state hospital association or a representative from an individual hospital. The SUBC is responsible for reviewing the national UB-82 data specifications manual; adding billing requirements for the local Blue Cross plan or plans, state Medicaid program, and other significant payers, for example, workers' compensation; agreeing on the use, if any, of the unassigned data fields to capture state-specific information; and, where needed, defining state-specific codes using code values set aside for that purpose. The SUBC or other designated organization is also responsible for the distribution of the state UB-82 manual to payers and providers within the state.

13

Cash and Short-Term Investments

Most financial management authorities and practicing administrators would agree that cash is the lifeblood of the hospital. The strong and steady circulation of cash is as critical to the good health of a hospital as is the proper functioning of the circulatory system to the health of a human organism. Given this importance, it is incumbent upon management to manage cash effectively. This chapter is devoted to examining cash management and the investment of excess cash holdings.

WHY HOLD CASH?

The reason why a hospital, or for that matter any other firm, holds cash can be explained in several ways. Perhaps the most sophisticated explanation is the Keynesian approach which identifies three motives for holding cash: transactions, precautionary, and speculative.

The transactions motive can be defined as the need to hold cash in order to meet payments (demands for cash) that arise out of the ordinary course of conducting business, for example, supplies purchased, labor costs, insurance costs. The precautionary motive explains the need to hold cash in terms of the necessity of having a cash buffer or cushion available to meet unexpected cash demands or requirements. Finally, the speculative motive can be defined as the need to hold cash in order to be in a position to take advantage of changes in security prices. According to the Keynesian hypothesis, all cash holdings can be explained and justified as being a function or result of these three factors.

If the Keynesian approach represents one extreme, the other is represented by the practical businessman who would explain the need for holding cash in terms of business necessity. Quite simply, if a firm is to be able to pay its bills as they come due, it must hold some cash balances. Regardless of which approach is used, the underlying reason is the same. Hospitals must hold cash due to the lack of synchronization between cash inflows and outflows.

If cash inflows and outflows could be synchronized, there would be no need for a hospital to hold any cash. In a synchronized situation, cash would just pass through the hospital. Cash, in effect, would go directly from the hospital's sources of revenue to its creditors. However, due to the uncertain character of cash inflows and the unexpected nature of some cash outflows, it is impossible to synchronize the two flows either consistently or precisely. Thus, if management is to avoid having to default on obligations, it must hold a stock of cash available as a reserve.

Perhaps the simplest way to understand the effects of cash flow synchronization is to view cash holdings as a reservoir or pool into which flow revenues and from which drain payments to creditors. Figure 13.1 (Case 1) utilizes this approach to illustrate the implications of synchronization. The critical point to be realized is that, due to a lack of synchronization, hospitals must hold some cash balances.

COST OF HOLDING CASH

Given that a hospital must hold some cash balances, the obvious question is, what are the costs of holding cash? Generally, two categories of cost are associated with a hospital's cash holdings—a short cost and a long or carrying cost. As Case 2A in Figure 13.1 illustrates, short cost arises when a hospital's cash holdings are insufficient to meet all of its cash outflow demands.

The magnitude of short cost can vary markedly with the extent of the cash shortage and the frequency of occurrence. If the shortage is an occa-

FIGURE 13.1   Cash Flow Synchronization: Implications

Case 1—Cash Flow Synchronized
   Inflows—$100,000 Received on Day 20
   Outflows—$100,000 Due on Day 20

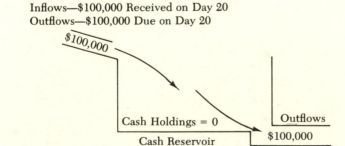

FIGURE 13.1   Continued

Case 2—Cash Flows Unsynchronized
    Inflows—$115,000 Received on Day 30
    Outflows—$100,000 Due on Day 15

A. Day 15

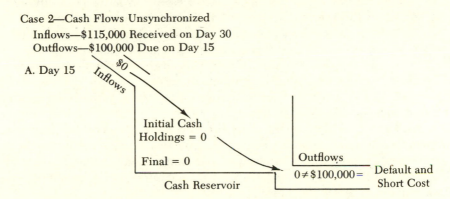

B. Day 15

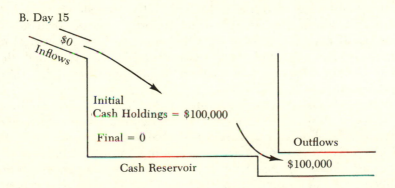

C. Day 30

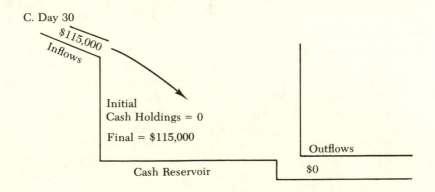

sional or infrequent event, it can be easily met, in most cases, at a small cost through borrowing on an open line of credit or, if available, through the selling of short-term investments. If the shortages are either large or frequent, they will result in loss of discounts on purchases, short-term borrowing at high interest rates, a poor or deteriorating credit rating, or insolvency. Any of these consequences obviously is costly and should be avoided. Therefore, management should attempt to maintain a cash balance sufficient not only to meet routine transactions, but also to provide protection against unexpected cash requirements.

As was the case in regard to inventories, the existence of a short cost argues for a hospital to hold a large cash inventory or balance. However, in addition to a short cost, hospitals must also contend with a long or carrying cost. This latter cost encourages a cash balance decision exactly opposite to the decision that a short cost supports.

Carrying or long cost can be defined as the opportunity cost attached to holding cash balances. When a hospital decides to hold any given amount of cash, it is in effect electing to invest some of its funds in cash holdings as opposed to some other investment alternative. This decision means that, at the very least, the hospital will incur an opportunity cost equal to the return that could have been obtained if the funds had been invested in some other way. The magnitude of this cost varies directly with both the rate of return on the investment alternatives that are available and the size of the cash investment.

For purposes of analysis, the opportunity cost attached to cash holdings can be segregated into two components. As has been discussed, a hospital must hold some level of cash balances to be able to operate (see Case 2B, Figure 13.1). This basic operational cash holding can be defined as the hospital's minimal cash balance. Since this minimal cash balance represents an investment it, by definition, has an opportunity cost that varies proportionately with the size of the minimal balance, that is, the greater the balance, the greater the cost.

In addition to its minimal cash balance a hospital may, from time to time, due to the lack of synchronization between cash inflows and outflows, find itself holding cash balances in excess of the minimal level. An example of this situation is represented by Case 2C in Figure 13.1. These excess cash holdings, like the minimal cash balance, represent an investment on the part of the hospital. Hence, they have an opportunity cost attached to them that varies directly with the magnitude of the holding.

Given that these are the costs attached to cash holdings, the issue facing management can be stated simply as that of determining how to minimize the total cost of holding cash. Actually, the problem can be most easily understood if it is viewed not as a single question, but rather as three interrelated problems. First, to minimize the opportunity cost attached to the minimum cash balance, management must develop the operating conditions necessary for minimizing the absolute amount of this investment. Second, based on the actual operating conditions, the magnitude of long and short costs, and the probability of incurring these costs, management must determine the optimal minimum cash balance, that is, the amount of cash holdings that will minimize the total expected value of long and short costs. Finally, based on the minimum cash balance, management must determine both how to finance additional cash requirements and how to invest any excess cash holdings. Since this is a multipart problem, let us first consider the matter of how to minimize the level or amount of the hospital's basic operational cash needs, that is, how to create the operating conditions necessary to minimize the absolute amount of the hospital's minimum cash balance.

MINIMIZE CASH HOLDINGS

As Case 1 in Figure 13.1 illustrates, it is not necessary for a hospital to hold any cash balances if cash inflows and outflows are synchronized. Therefore, if management is to minimize the size or amount of the hospital's basic operational cash requirements, it must attempt to synchronize cash flows. This point, while perhaps obvious, is much easier to deduce logically than to achieve operationally. The difficulty lies in the fact that hospitals have relatively little control over either cash inflows or cash outflows.

The bulk of a hospital's cash outflows involves payments for personnel—salaries, taxes, fringe benefits. The timing of these payments is fixed by the government, union contracts, insurance companies, or tradition, and little can be done to alter the due dates for these payments. The remainder of a hospital's cash outflows generally involves payments for purchases of supplies and materials—food, drugs, electricity. The timing of these payments is, for the most part, fixed by contract or convention. It is in regard to these outflows, however, that management may be able to exercise some discretion and thereby affect the timing of cash outflows. Therefore, to the extent possible, management should attempt to slow down the pace of cash outflows, while at the same time trying to minimize costs of the operation.[1]

Decelerating the pace of outflows is advantageous in that it allows more time for

1. Cash inflows to be received—thus increasing the probability of being able to match or synchronize inflows with outflows; and

---

[1]As was discussed in Chapter 10, financing cash needs by foregoing the discount on accounts payable can be quite costly. Therefore, if total cost is to be minimized, financing should be obtained from the least costly source, which may not necessarily be accounts payable.

2. Cash holdings to be invested—thus reducing the opportunity cost attached to holding cash balances.

Management's strategy, therefore, should be that of carefully examining payment dates and alternative costs in order to decelerate cash outflows as much as is practical.

The management of cash outflow may be enhanced by relating the conversion of funds from the hospital's interest-bearing accounts to cash to the day the check or demand voucher is presented at the bank rather than relating the conversion to the day the check is mailed. This procedure is known as a "book overdraft" since it involves the commitment of funds via the check which are not as yet present in the bank account being drawn upon. The invested funds continue to earn interest during the "float" period. These additional earnings can be material depending on the hospital's level of invested funds and on current investment rates. At a minimum, the additional earnings will make a contribution to offsetting some of the hospital's banking charges.

The key to the successful management of the book overdraft is an accurate projection of the float period. The projection requires both an estimate of how long the float will exist and an estimate of the percentage of dollars presented at the bank each day of the float. The method of predicting the pattern of demand is based on historical information. The information is available from the hospital's cash reports and bank statements. Additional data and assistance may also be obtained from the bank. If managed poorly, this practice can result in strained relations with the bank and suppliers due to insufficient demand funds on hand. The risk of insufficient funds may be alleviated by establishing a line of credit with the bank in the operating account. With a line of credit, payment is made upon the presentation of the hospital's check. If insufficient funds are present to cover the check's value, a liability is created and charged to the hospital along with current level interest on the funds overdrawn.

The control that a hospital may be able to exercise over cash inflows, though perhaps greater than that which can be exercised over outflows, is also limited. Due to its relative economic size and power, a single hospital cannot bring sufficient pressure to bear on third party payers to force them to accelerate or even to change the timing of their payment schedules. Also, a hospital's influence over the payment schedules of self-pay patients, because of the restricted financial resources of these patients, is limited. However, though a hospital's ability to control cash inflows by influencing payers is restricted, it can—through its in-house processing and internal control procedures—still have a substantial impact on the timing of cash inflows. Figures 13.2 and 13.3 illustrate the impact that these two elements can have on cash balances.

FIGURE 13.2   In-House Processing Time and Cash Balances

CASE 1

Assumptions:
1. Bill preparation and submission processing time = 14 days
2. Payer processing time = 21 days
3. Cash conversion processing time = 7 days
4. Cash outflows = $100.00 due on Day 30
5. Cash inflows—patients discharged, representing $100,000 in revenue, on Day 1

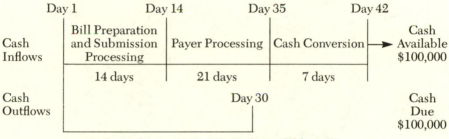

Cash Outflow = $100,000: Cash Available = $0

Implications
Due to the length of the in-house processing time, cash flows are not synchronized and the hospital is unable to meet its obligations. Therefore, a short cost is incurred.

CASE 2

Assumptions: same as above, except—
1. Bill preparation and submission processing time reduced to 6 days
2. Cash conversion processing time reduced to 2 days

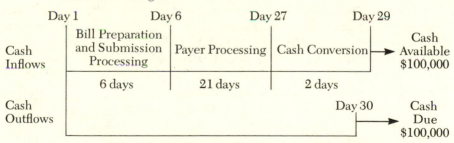

Cash Outflow = $100,000: Cash Available = $100,000

Implications
Due to the shortening of the in-house processing time cycle, the hospital is able to meet its obligations.

FIGURE 13.3   Internal Control and Cash Balances

Case 1

    Inflows—$100,000 Received on Day 20

    Outflows—$100,000 Due on Day 20

    Thefts—$2,000

    Other Losses—$3,000 = Due to Negligence and Carelessness

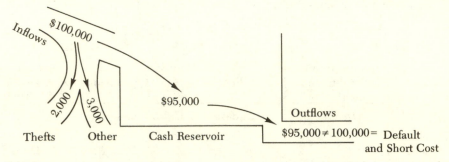

It is axiomatic that the longer the in-house processing time, the longer a hospital must wait until cash inflows will be available to meet cash outflow demands. Conversely, the shorter the in-house processing time, the sooner cash inflows will be received and the greater the probability that cash will be available to meet outflow demands. Management must attempt to accelerate the pace of cash inflows by reducing the length of in-house processing time if it is to minimize its basic operational cash needs.

The shortening of the in-house processing time period can be viewed as a two-part problem. It involves not only the preparation and submission of patient bills but also the processing of revenues, once received, into cash.

Hospital management should consider the use of a "lock box" and electronic funds transfers to accelerate the processing and posting of cash receipts. When using a lock box, the hospital's cash payments are sent directly to the bank. At the bank, the checks and accompanying media are separated; the checks are deposited to the hospital's account; and the receipt media along with a copy of the checks are forwarded to the hospital. This places the cash received in the hospital's account and makes it available for use while the in-house processing of the accounts receivable proceeds. Electronic funds transfer has the same advantage. It is available for large deposits from a single source such as a third party payer. In utilizing electronic transfer, the payer wires the funds from its bank via computer terminals to the hospital's bank. This eliminates both the mailing and the in-house processing time that delay the deposit of large cash receipts. Separately, by mail, the hospital receives any payment media directly from the payer.

Primary responsibility for the development and the day-to-day operations of the in-house revenue processing and internal control systems not only is beyond the scope of general management's knowledge, but also is an inappropriate use of its time and unique talents. Management's responsibility in this area should be *just* that of ensuring that the hospital's revenue systems result in minimizing both processing time and revenue losses.

The management strategy for cash inflows can thus be summarized as one of attempting both to accelerate the pace of cash inflows, through efficient in-house processing systems, and to protect revenue receipts through effective internal control measures. Accelerating the pace of inflows is advantageous in that it

1. Increases the probability of being able to synchronize cash inflows and outflows, for inflows will be received at a faster rate; and
2. Provides the potential for reducing opportunity cost, for cash may be invested for longer periods.

The advantage of effective internal control lies in the fact that by preventing leakages or losses from the revenue system it increases the probability that cash will be available as needed. Hence, it enables management to maintain a smaller cash balance. Management, therefore, if it is to create the operating conditions necessary to minimize the absolute amount of the hospital's minimum cash balance, must decelerate cash outflows and accelerate and protect inflows.

DETERMINING THE MINIMUM CASH BALANCE

Assuming that management has created the necessary operating conditions, its next problem is actually to determine the minimum cash balance. This problem is quite complex due to the uncertainty inherent in cash flows, the difficulties involved in accurately measuring long and short costs, and the numerous other factors that must be considered. However, it is a problem that must be solved if management is to administer its cash investment effectively.

The size of a hospital's minimum cash balance can be a function of either a self-imposed or an internal constraint or an externally imposed constraint such as a working capital agreement with a commercial bank. In this latter case, a formal or informal agreement may require the hospital to hold compensating cash balances, that is, required levels of deposits in the bank, as partial payment for services. Alternatively, a hospital may hold a cash balance in its bank in order to improve its banking relationships or to maintain an option for future borrowing. Regardless of the specific reason, the critical point is that a hospital's minimum cash balance may be established by an external constraint, such as a banking requirement. However, establishing a minimum cash balance on the basis of *just* external factors ignores the real issue in the cash management decision.

A decision about a hospital's minimum cash balance should depend primarily on the implicit or intangible return that is obtained from holding cash and the cost of holding cash. The return obtained from holding cash can be understood most easily if it is viewed simply as a short cost that is avoided. Up to certain levels of cash holdings this return is quite high. Hence, up to certain levels, the benefits obtained from holding cash—the avoidance of a short cost—will exceed the opportunity or long cost attached to holding cash, that is, the implicit return from holding cash is higher than any return that can be obtained by investing cash in an alternative manner.

As cash balances increase, the intangible return declines, for the probability of cash shortages and a short cost is lessened. Consequently, at some point the opportunity cost of holding cash will exceed the benefits obtained from such holdings. The problem facing management is simply that of determining this marginal point.[2] Management must calculate the level of cash holdings that provides the optimal trade-off between long and short costs. This level of cash is, by definition, the minimum cash balance.

Since cash flows are uncertain, the approach that should be used for calculating the minimum cash balance is the same as that which was used for determining the inventory reorder point under conditions of uncertainty.[3] As was the case in regard to inventories, long and short costs are again difficult to measure. Nevertheless, if rational and intelligent cash decisions are to be made, management must attempt to measure these costs even if it does so entirely on a subjective basis.

For purposes of illustration, it can be assumed that long or opportunity cost equals 5% of any excess cash balance, and short cost equals $200 per shortage occurrence plus, on average, 6% of the shortage. It should be noted that short cost is expressed in terms of both a fixed and a variable cost component. This has been done to reflect the fact that each time a hospital is forced to obtain a loan or defer payments, it must invest a certain amount of time and effort in soliciting and arranging the financing mechanism. This investment is approximately the same regardless of either the amount or the maturity schedule of the financing and, hence, can be viewed as a fixed cost. In addition to this fixed cost, the hospital incurs a cost for the use of the funds that it obtains. This latter cost, since it varies with the amount and maturity of the financing, can be viewed as a variable cost.[4]

---

[2]The marginal point is where the additional or marginal return from holding another dollar of cash just equals the marginal cost of holding that dollar.

[3]Readers desiring a further discussion of the application of inventory techniques to cash management should refer to Appendix 13.A.

[4]To simplify the presentation, only an average variable short cost figure has been assumed. Some might argue that this is inappropriate due to the fact that it does not specifically

Along with estimates of long and short costs, management must also develop some notion of the probable variation in monthly net cash flows, that is, cash inflows less cash outflows, that can be expected during the year. Net cash flows are the critical factor, for the matter of concern is not the individual inflows or outflows, but rather the effect of these flows on the hospital's cash position. To determine this effect, it is necessary to consider both flows, and this can be accomplished most readily and efficiently through an examination of the net flows.

Based upon a study of historical records, projections of future volume and patterns of patient care, estimates of third party payment practices, and subjective judgments, assume that the following probabilities of various amounts of net cash flows can be developed.

NET CASH FLOW ESTIMATES

Probability	.20	.30	.10	.20	.20
Net Cash Flow	+ $5,000	+ $3,000	+ $1,000	− $3,000	− $5,000

Given this information and the previously assumed costs, it is now possible, by calculating the expected value or cost of various cash balance strategies, to identify the least cost cash balance. Table 13.1 illustrates the mechanics of determining the least cost minimum cash balance.

As is indicated in Table 13.1, $3,000 is the least cost minimum cash balance strategy. However, before management adopts this strategy it should consider several other factors. For example, if this strategy is accepted, there is a 20% probability that cash needs will exceed the available cash balance and that some type of financing will have to be arranged. Management should thus consider its willingness to bear the risk of being out of cash. Also, it should consider the governing board's attitude toward cash shortages and its willingness to borrow. Additionally, the previously discussed external factors or banking relationships and requirements should be included in the decision process.

The critical point to understand is that the cash balance decision should be made on the basis of various considerations. The most important of these is probably the least cost minimum cash balance factor, for it indicates not only the least cost strategy, but also the costs of other strategies. However, the final decision should not be made on *just* the basis of any *one* factor.

---

indicate the individual impact of both financing maturity and amount on variable cost. However, inclusion of both variable cost elements on an individual, as opposed to a consolidated average basis, greatly complicates not only the measurement aspects of the problem, but also the practicality of calculation. Thus, it is questionable if the benefit received from such a refinement would exceed its costs.

TABLE 13.1   Minimum Cash Balance

Step 1. Assumptions
Short cost = $200 plus 6% of the shortage
Long cost = 5% of any excess minimum cash balance
Net cash flow distribution:

Probability	.20	.30	.10	.20	.20
Net cash flow	+5,000	+3,000	+1,000	−3,000	−5,000

Step 2. Cost Matrix—Unadjusted (see Step 4. Explanation)

Minimum Cash Balance Strategy \ Net Cash Flow	+ $5,000	+ $3,000	+ $1,000	− $3,000	−$5,000
$1,000	$ 50	$ 50	$ 50	$320	$440
2,000	100	100	100	260	380
3,000	150	150	150	0	320
4,000	200	200	200	50	260
5,000	250	250	250	100	0
6,000	300	300	300	150	50

Step 3. Cost Matrix—Adjusted for Probability (see Step 4. Explanation)

Minimum Cash Balance Strategy \ Net Cash Flow	+ $5,000 (.20)	+ $3,000 (.30)	+ $1,000 (.10)	− $3,000 (.20)	−$5,000 (.20)	Total Expected Cost
$1,000	$10	$15	$ 5	$64	$88	$182
2,000	20	30	10	52	76	188
3,000	30	45	15	0	64	154
4,000	40	60	20	10	52	182
5,000	50	75	25	20	0	· 170
6,000	60	90	30	30	10	220

Continued

Instead, it should be based upon an evaluation of the total situation—including, but not just limited to, the costs of the various cash balance strategies.

THE CASH BUDGET

Once the minimum cash balance decision has been made, the stage is set for solving the third aspect of the cash management problem. Specifically, management must determine how to finance additional cash requirements and how to invest any excess cash holdings. That is, if management

TABLE 13.1   Continued

Step 4. Explanation

Step 2. Unadjusted costs of various minimum cash balance strategies, for example:

Strategy	Net Cash Flow	Cost
$1,000	+5,000	— Positive net cash flow; therefore, long $1,000 at a cost of 5% per $1,000 or $50.
$3,000	−3,000	— Negative net cash flow equal to the cash balance; therefore, cash needs equal available cash and cost is 0.
$3,000	−5,000	— Negative net cash flow which exceeds the cash balance; therefore, short $2,000 at a cost of $200 plus 6% of shortage, i.e., $200 plus 6% of $2,000 or $320.
$5,000	+1,000	— Positive net cash flow; therefore, long $5,000 at a cost of 5% per $1,000 or $250.

Step 3. Adjusted costs of various minimum cash balance strategies are obtained by multiplying the values calculated in Step 2 by the probability assumptions set out in Step 1. This step is necessary because of the unpredictable nature of cash flows.

Conclusion

A strategy involving a minimum cash balance of $3,000 will enable management to minimize total cash holding costs.

---

is to minimize the total cost of needing and holding cash, it must determine not only the least cost method of financing cash needs, but also the most advantageous investment opportunities for any temporary excess cash balances. If these decisions are to be made knowledgeably, however, more information is needed than just data on the desired level of the minimum cash balance.

The necessity of additional information can be seen clearly in the hypothetical case described in Table 13.2. As should be apparent from the table, management must have information on both the desired minimum cash balance level and future cash flows. Information on the minimum cash balance can be obtained through use of the techniques discussed in the previous section and is necessary in order to determine if a cash surplus or an additional cash requirement exists. Data on future cash flows can be obtained through the development of a cash budget. This latter information is needed in order to determine the appropriate investment strategy—or financing strategy, if necessary.

A cash budget can be defined as a forecast or a schedule of future cash receipts and disbursements. Quite simply, it is a projection of future cash flows. It is designed to assist in controlling the hospital's cash position by enabling management to

TABLE 13.2   Cash Management Information Needs: Hypothetical Case

1. *Month 1*
   Operating Results
   The hospital generates a positive net cash flow that leaves it with an excess cash balance, that is, a cash surplus over the minimum cash balance of $15,000.
   Action
   Based upon an evaluation of available investment alternatives, management decides to invest the excess funds in a six-month bank note paying 12%. The terms of the note stipulate that interest will be paid only if the note is held to maturity.

2. *Month 2*
   Operating Results
   The hospital incurs a negative cash flow that results in its needing $10,000 to meet its immediate cash obligations and restore its cash position.
   Action
   After reviewing all available financing alternatives, management decides to redeem the bank note—incurring the early redemption interest loss penalty—and then proceeds to meet its obligations.

3. *Evaluation*
   At first glance, the Month 1 action appears to be reasonable. In the light of later cash flows, though, the inappropriateness of such action becomes obvious. If management had had more information available regarding future cash flows, it could have planned its investment strategy differently so as to maximize revenues while still being able to meet cash needs. For example:
   1. Hypothetical case   Total revenues = $ 0
   2. Possible alternative—assuming management had projections of future cash flows, it could have invested its excess funds as follows:
      —$5,000 in the six-month note
      —$10,000 in a Treasury bill yielding 8% and due in 30 days
      Total revenues = $368
   As the results of the alternative make clear, given information about future cash flows, management is able to make better cash decisions.

4. *Conclusion*
   To make cash investment or financing decisions wisely, management must not only have data on the desired level of the minimal cash balance, but also on future cash flows.

1. Predict the timing and amount of future cash flows, net cash flows, cash balances, and cash needs and surpluses; and

2. Examine systematically the cost implications of various cash management decisions.

The cash budget is thus an invaluable management tool, for it provides a substantial portion of the information necessary to protect the hospital's cash position and to ensure that it invests its assets appropriately.

A sample budget procedure, describing in detail the mechanics of preparing a cash budget, and an example of a cash budget's decision-making usefulness, are presented in Appendix 13.B. This material should provide the reader with a thorough understanding of the nature and potential management value of a cash budget. The only additional point that is worthy of emphasis is the fact that a cash budget is not a primary budget. A cash budget is constructed from information obtained from the revenue, expense, and capital budgets as opposed to being derived directly from basic operating decisions and forecasts.[5] Thus, the cash budget is actually a summary budget obtained by converting the foregoing budgets from an accrual to a cash basis. Figure 13.4 illustrates the relationship of the cash budget to the hospital's other budgets.

INVESTING TEMPORARY CASH SURPLUSES

Based upon the desired minimum cash balance level and the information obtained from the cash budget, management now has available the data necessary to determine knowledgeably how either to finance additional cash needs or to invest excess cash balances. The matter of financing additional cash or working capital requirements was discussed in Chapter 10. Thus, the nature of the available financing alternatives and the cost of those alternatives should be clear to the reader. The matter of investing excess cash balances, however, has not yet been examined. Therefore, before completing this discussion of cash management, the problem of investing excess cash balances should be considered.

FIGURE 13.4   Cash Budget

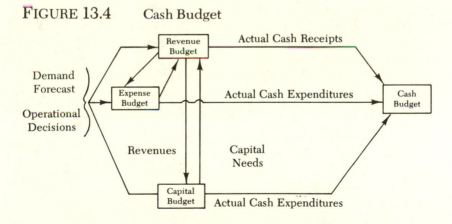

_____

[5]The accurate development of the hospital's expense, revenue, and capital budgets is obviously critical to the construction of a sound cash budget. A discussion of the techniques and mechanics of preparing these budgets is included in Chapters 15 through 20 of this book.

Due to any of a number of factors—seasonal occupancy fluctuations, delays in billings from suppliers, unexpected contributions, and so forth—a hospital may find itself with cash that is temporarily not needed for operations. These excess cash holdings represent an investment on the part of the hospital which, by definition, has an opportunity cost attached to it. Thus, if management is to minimize the cost of holding cash, it must invest its excess cash balances in revenue-generating securities as opposed to holding them as idle cash. The issue, therefore, is one of selecting the appropriate investment alternative—based on the amount of cash available, the length of time the excess will exist, and the financial situation of the hospital.

Numerous potential investment opportunities are available to a hospital. Marketable securities (short-term investments), however, generally present the most advantageous possibilities. This is due to the fact that these investment instruments, though producing a relatively low yield, provide an almost riskless investment that is both highly liquid (marketable) and available in various maturities. These latter two points are particularly important.

Liquidity can be defined as the ability to sell an investment instrument rapidly without incurring a loss in principal. Due to the uncertain nature of cash flows, management may be forced to sell securities to meet unexpected cash needs. If the securities can be sold rapidly without a loss in principal, they obviously provide a better investment opportunity than alternatives that lack this characteristic.

The availability of numerous maturities is also advantageous. A wide range of maturity dates provides management with the flexibility needed to synchronize investment maturities with future cash needs. Such synchronization is vital if cash holdings are to be as productive as possible and if investment revenues are to be maximized. Thus, the guideline for the investment of excess cash balances can be set out as follows:

> Excess cash balances should be invested in marketable securities, with the actual investment selection based on the maturity schedules, yields, and risks that are most appropriate to a particular hospital's financial situation.

Table 13.3 lists the most common marketable security investment alternatives.

One additional point is worthy of note. The administration of a marketable securities portfolio is a complex and highly specialized task. A discussion of the specific techniques and mechanics of portfolio management is beyond the scope of this text. However, the task of administration is an integral part of the cash management process and as such should be the primary responsibility of the hospital's controller or financial manager. The

TABLE 13.3   Marketable Security Investment Alternatives

Securities	Comments
Treasury bills: 91-day maturity, issued weekly.	These are popular investments since they combine security (as obligations of the U.S. government) with liquidity (because of the frequency and regularity of their issuance).*
Money market funds: No fixed maturity, available daily.	Relatively new financial instrument, having a variable yield* and a high degree of liquidity, i.e., redeemable on demand. Degree of risk is theoretically higher than Treasury bills.
U.S. Treasury notes, certificates of indebtedness, and tax anticipation certificates: More than 91-day but less than five-year maturities.	Also popular, these are useful for companies that wish to invest to meet specific cash requirements (dividends, taxes, and capital expenditures).
Federal agency securities: Offerings of five federally sponsored credit agencies (federal land banks, banks for cooperatives, federal home loan banks, federal intermediate credit banks, Federal National Mortgage Association), that issue their own securities and borrow directly from the public. Most corporate portfolios are restricted to nine-month to 1½ year maturities.	These securities are not guaranteed by the federal government, and their yield is generally just above that of Treasury securities. However, they are considered very safe investments.
Public Housing Authority notes: Issued to finance various government land development projects. Most corporate portfolios are restricted to one-year maturities.	These securities have the double advantage of being guaranteed by the federal government and of being tax exempt. The latter feature makes the effective yield to a corporation roughly double that quoted. The strong demand for these notes makes them very liquid in the secondary market.
State and local bonds: One-year and longer maturities. (A number of states will provide almost any maturity required by a corporate buyer.)	Those rated AA and AAA are considered very safe investments. Their tax-exempt status makes them the highest-yielding security in the money market. They are sometimes used to meet specific cash requirements.

Continued

TABLE 13.3   Continued

Securities	Comments
Bankers' acceptances: One-month to six-month maturities (usually three months).	A bankers' acceptance is a time draft, drawn on a large bank by a trader, that becomes a negotiable instrument and can be discounted for resale to investors. It is considered a very safe investment.
Commercial certificates of deposit (CDs): Activity is generally restricted to prime certificates with a maturity of 90 days. However, maturities of up to three years are available.	The CD is a receipt given by a bank for a time deposit of money. The bank promises to return the amount deposited plus interest to the bearer of the certificate on the date specified. The certificate is transferable and may be traded before its maturity date. Because the denominations offered are large and Federal Deposit Insurance Corporation protection is limited† the size and reputation of the issuing bank are imporant.‡
Finance company paper: Short-term maturity, usually 90 days. (A number of finance companies will provide almost any maturity required by the corporate buyer.)	These obligations of companies financing consumer appliances and automobiles are reasonably safe, but much depends upon the reputation of the issuing company. They are traded on the secondary market, and maturity dates are usually very flexible. Yield is generally high.
Commercial paper: Usually four-month to six-month maturities but sometimes as short as five days. (Purchasers usually intend to hold such obligations until maturity.)	Commercial paper today consists mainly of short-term, unsecured promissory notes issued by a relatively small group of highly rated companies. The yield is usually the highest of those that can be obtained from any short-term security, except tax-exempts.

Source: E.J. Mock. "The Investment of Corporate Cash," *Management Services*, Vol. 4, No. 5 (September-October 1967), p. 55.

*This rate changes quite frequently depending on the market's demand for money. In the mid-1970s and early 1980s the rate ranged from about 5½% to almost 20%.

†Insurance protection provided by the Federal Deposit Insurance Corporation was increased gradually from the original coverage of $10,000 for each depositor to the current limit of $100,000 for each.

‡It may also be possible to obtain consumer certificates of deposit. These carry a lower yield, but may be available in denominations of as low as $500 with a maturity of six months.

role of general management in this area is limited to ensuring that the financial manager is carrying out his responsibility properly. This can be acccomplished quite easily by comparing maturity schedules with the cash budget (to examine synchronization), by comparing the composite portfolio yield to yields available in the market (see Chapter 14), and by subjectively evaluating the portfolio in terms of the hospital's financial situation and willingness to bear risk.

COMPENSATING BALANCES AND BANK SERVICE CHARGES

Banks and most other commercial banking entities have recently adopted more explicit fee schedules for assessing their service charges. Minimum balances, check cashing and processing fees, and interest-bearing demand accounts have replaced the more traditional noninterest checking account.

Hospital management should not take service charges for granted. One means of minimizing service charges is to establish an arrangement with the bank under which the excess funds in the account are invested by the bank in short-term investments or an interest payment is made on the daily account balance at a predetermined rate. The earnings from the excess funds are then accumulated over some time period, normally a month or a quarter, and are offset against the bank's service charge arising during the same period. The interest earnings act as a compensating factor to reduce or eliminate the bank's service charge. If the service charge exceeds the compensating balance from the interest earned, a debit to the hospital's principal funds is created; if the compensating balance exceeds the service charge, the hospital receives a credit to its account or a carry-forward to the next period. (See Figure 13.5.)

CONCLUSION

The basic principles and mechanics of not only cash management but also working capital management should now be clear. The reader should now have a general understanding of both the factors that should be considered in arriving at working capital decisions and the techniques that financial managers can and should utilize as aids in making these decisions. Given this understanding, a manager needs only one other bit or type of information to evaluate a hospital's performance in these areas. He must have available certain informational reports. The following chapter is devoted to a discussion of the reports needed to evaluate the efficiency and effectiveness of a hospital's working capital performance.

FIGURE 13.5   Stanley Beach Community Hospital—Analysis for
March 1985

Average Funds on Deposit

Account balance	$ 2,103,435
Value dated transaction float	(11)
Deposit float (uncollected funds)	(467,175)
Net compensating balance	$ 1,636,249

Collected Balance Required

For credit	$ 0	
For measured services performed (based on banks fee schedule)	1,912,641	
Total collected balance required		$ 1,912,641
Account balance after credits and measured services		$ −276,392

Apr 85 9.00%	Apr 85 9.00%	Earnings allowance on investable portion of collected balances (net of reserve requirements)
$152	$152	Multiplier (average monthly collected balance required per $1.00 fee)

Summary of Analysis (YTD)

Month	Ledger Balance	Collected Balance	Collected Balance Required	Excess (or Deficit) Balance	Interest Rate	Rate Valued Monthly Excess (or Deficit)	Cumulative Rate Valued Excess (or Deficit)
01/85	1,746,710	1,414,216	1,666,730	−252,514	10.00	−2,104	−2,104
02/85	2,132,240	1,651,672	1,449,908	201,764	9.25	1,369	735
03/85	2,103,435	1,636,249	1,912,641	−276,392	9.00	−2,073	−2,808

SUGGESTED READINGS

CASH MANAGEMENT

Frank, C. W. *Maximizing Hospital Cash Resources.*
Orgler, Yair E. *Cash Management: Methods and Models.*
Van Horne, James C. *Financial Management and Policy,* Chapter 16.
Weston, J. Fred and Brigham, Eugene F. *Managerial Finance,* Chapter 13.

SHORT-TERM INVESTMENTS

Cannedy, Lloyd L. "How Hospitals Use Money Market Instruments."
Markstein, David L. "How to Make Short-Term Cash Work at Full-Time Rates."

APPENDIX 13.A
CASH MANAGEMENT MODELS

"Inventory control techniques dominated the early cash management models. The application of inventory theory to the management of cash was first explored by [W. J.] Baumol." The Baumol model is based on the assumption that payments are known and have to be made at a constant rate and that there are no cash receipts during the payment period. Additionally, the model is static in that it does not consider the interrelationships between subsequent time periods and is limited to the interval between two successive cash receipts. Consequently, this model is an oversimplification of reality and has limited applicability.

A second type of inventory model emphasizes the probabilistic nature of cash flows. An example of this type of model is the Miller and Orr model, which assumes that net cash flows fluctuate in a completely stochastic manner as opposed to the deterministic cash outflows of the Baumol model.

The essential elements of both these models are summarized below.

THE BAUMOL MODEL

The basic Baumol model is the standard inventory sawtooth model (see [Figure 13.A-1]). The inventory item is cash which flows out at a constant rate and is restocked instantaneously by borrowing or by withdrawing from an investment [that is, selling the investment]. Total cash outflows are assumed to be known and are made at a constant rate over a given period. The size and timing of cash inflows are completely controllable and are associated with a fixed cost per order and a variable cost per dollar (interest on a loan or the yield lost by selling securities). Since cash outflows are given, the only cash management decision is how much cash to obtain and at what frequency, assuming that the objective is to minimize total costs.

Based on these assumptions, which also underline the standard inventory model, Baumol solves his model and obtains the famous square-root formula for the optimal order size:

$$C = \sqrt{\frac{2bT}{i}}$$

FIGURE 13.A-1   Pattern of Cash Receipts and Expenditures—
Baumol Model

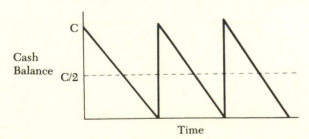

Source: Yair E. Orgler, *Cash Management: Methods and Models*, Belmont, CA: Wadsworth Publishing Company, Inc., 1970, p. 38. Reprinted with permission of the author.

where b is the fixed cost per order (transaction), T is the total amount of payments (cash flows), and i is the variable cost per dollar per period (interest rate). Since in this model the average amount in stock is half the order quantity, the average cash balance is:

$$\frac{C}{2} = \sqrt{\frac{bT}{2i}} \; ^6$$

THE MILLER AND ORR MODEL

[The model] is designed to determine the time and size of transfers between an investment account and the cash account according to a decision process illustrated in [Figure 13.A-2]. Changes in cash balances are allowed to wander until they reach some level h at time t_1; they are then reduced to level z, the "return point," by investing h−z dollars in the investment portfolio. Next the cash balance wanders aimlessly until it reaches the minimum balance point, r, at t_2, at which time enough earning assets are sold to return the cash balance to its return point, z. The model is based on a cost function similar to Baumol's, and it includes elements for the cost of making transfers to and from cash and for the opportunity cost of holding cash. The upper limit, h, which cash balances should not be allowed to surpass, and the return point, z, to which the balance is returned after every transfer either to or from the cash account, are computed so as to minimize the cost function. The lower limit is assumed to be given, and it could be the minimum balance required by the banks in which the cash is deposited.

The cost function for the Miller-Orr model can be stated as E (c) = bE (N)/T + iE (M), where E (N) = the expected number of transfers between cash and the investment portfolio during the planning period; b = the cost per transfer; T is the number of days in the planned period; E (M) = expected

FIGURE 13.A-2   Miller and Orr Cash Management Model

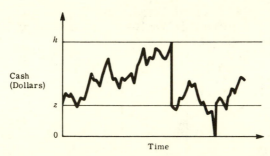

Source: *Quarterly Journal of Economics* Vol. 80, No. 3, August, p. 420. Copyright 1966. Reprinted with the permission of John Wiley & Sons, Inc.

---

[6]The Baumol Model section is from Orgler, Yair. *Cash Management: Methods and Models.* Belmont, CA: Wadsworth Publishing Company, Inc., 1970.

average daily balance; and i = the daily rate of interest earned on the investments. The objective is to minimize E (c) by choice of the variables h and z, the upper control limit and return point, respectively.

The solution as derived by Miller and Orr becomes

$$z^* = \left(\frac{3\, b\sigma^2}{4i} \right)^{1/3}$$

$$h^* = 3z^*$$

for the special case where p (the probability that cash balances will increase) equals .5, and q (the probability that cash balances will decrease) equals .5. The variance of the daily changes in the cash balance is represented by σ^2. As would be expected, a higher transfer cost b, or variance σ^2, would imply a greater spread between the upper and lower control limits. In the special case where $p = q = \frac{1}{2}$, the upper control limit will always be three times greater than the return point.

Miller and Orr tested their model by applying it to nine months of data on the daily cash balances and purchases and sales of short-term securities of a large industrial company. When the decisions of the model were compared to those actually made by the treasurer of the company, the model was found to produce an average daily cash balance which was about 40% *lower* ($160,000 for the model and $275,000 for the treasurer). Looking at it from another side, the model would have been able to match the $275,000 average daily balance with only 80 transactions as compared to the treasurer's 112 actual transactions.

As with most inventory control models, this model's performance depends not only on how well the conditional predictions (in this case the expected number of transfers and the expected average cash balance) conform to actuality, but also on how well the parameters are estimated. In this model, b, the transfer cost, is sometimes difficult to estimate. In the study made by Miller and Orr, the order costs included such components as "(a) making two or more long-distance phone calls plus fifteen minutes to a half hour of the assistant treasurer's time, (b) typing up and carefully checking an authorization letter with four copies, (c) carrying the original of the letter to be signed by the treasurer, and (d) carrying the copies to the controller's office where special accounts are opened, the entries are posted and further checks of the arithmetic are made."[7] These clerical procedures were thought to be in the magnitude of $20 to $50 per order. In the application of their model, however, Miller and Orr did not rely on their estimate for order and costs; instead, they tested the model using a series of assumed order costs until the model used the same number of transactions as did the treasurer. They could then determine the order cost implied by the treasurer's own action. The results were

---

[7]Miller, Merton H. and Orr, Daniel. "An Application of Control Limit Models to the Management of Corporate Cash Balances." *Proceedings of the Conference on Financial Research and Its Implications for Management, Stanford University.* Alexander A. Robichek, ed. New York: Wiley, 1967.

used to evaluate the treasurer's performance in managing the cash balances, and, as such, provided valuable information to the treasurer.

The treasurer found, for example, that his action in purchasing securities was often inconsistent. Too often he made small-lot purchases well below the minimum of h−z computed by the model, while at other times he allowed cash balances to drift to as much as double the upper control limit before making a purchase. If it did no more than give the treasurer some perspective about his buying and selling activities, the model was used successfully.[8]

In addition to these inventory models, the techniques of dynamic programming and linear programming have been applied to the cash management problem. A discussion of these more sophisticated models, however, is beyond both the scope of this work and the typical needs of the operating hospital manager. Readers desiring information on how these latter techniques can be utilized should refer to:

Baumol, William J. "The Transactions Demand for Cash: An Inventory Theoretic Approach."

Beranek, William. *Analysis for Financial Decision*, pp. 345–81.

Calman, R.F. *Linear Programming and Cash Management: Cash ALPHA.*

Miller, Merton H. and Orr, Daniel. "An Application of Control Limit Models to the Management of Corporate Cash Balances."

Miller, Merton H. and Orr, Daniel. "Model for the Demand for Money by Firms," pp. 413–35.

APPENDIX 13.B
CASH AND SHORT-TERM INVESTMENT

Due to its operational importance, cash management is a complex problem that has attracted a great deal of management science interest in recent years. Various authorities have examined the problems involved in managing cash and have developed intricate analytical models designed to provide quantitative solutions for cash management problems. These models generally involve a large number of variables and constraints and require sophisticated computer knowledge and capacity if they are to be used. Also, these models, because of the abstraction requirements of constructing mathematical models, have limitations that restrict their operational application. It is the feeling of the authors at this point in time that the models are not appropriate hospital operational tools. Instead, the use of a cash budgeting technique that allows for the development of multiple budgets and the simulation of various cash management decisions appears, at least for the present, to be a more feasible and practical approach to hospital cash management. A step-by-step description of such a technique is presented below.

---

[8]The Miller and Orr Model section is from Weston, J. Fred and Brigham, Eugene F. *Managerial Finance, Fifth Edition.* Hinsdale, IL: The Dryden Press, 1975.

PART I. CASH BUDGET PREPARATION

A. Step 1

The budget officer should obtain the information needed to convert the accrual-based primary budgets, from which the cash budget is derived (see Figure 13.4), to a cash basis.

1. Information needed to convert primary budgets from an accrual to a cash basis

   a. Revenue Budget

      1) Percent of total service revenue, both inpatient and outpatient, by source of payments, that is, what percent of total revenues are received from Blue Cross, Medicare, self-pay patients

      2) Average timing of accounts receivable cycle by source of payment, including self-pay patients, that is, time period or lag between patient discharge and receipt of payment by source of payment

      3) Percent of billed charges paid by the various third party payers; for example, Medicare may pay 90% of billed charges, Blue Cross, 95%

      4) Timing of receipt of all other revenues, for example, when income from investments will be received, when grants from the United Fund will be received

   b. Expense Budget

      1) Salary and wage payment periods

      2) Timing of quarterly and other nonmonthly expense payments, that is, F.I.C.A. payments, insurance premiums, federal withholding tax

      3) Percent of purchases for which trade credit is offered

      4) Average nature of trade credit terms

      5) Average payment terms for all other purchases

      6) Timing of purchases, that is, purchases made evenly throughout the month or on a specific day of the week

   c. Capital Budget (Plant and Equipment Budget)

      1) Timing of plant and equipment expenditures, that is, the month(s) in which a capital expenditure appropriation is actually to be paid

2. Technique for obtaining necessary information

a. Revenue Budget

The data needed to convert the revenue budget should be obtainable from two sources—a sampling study of revenues and the information available in the controller's office.

1) Sampling study of revenues

To determine the percent of total revenue by source, percent of total revenue paid in cash, and the timing of the accounts receivable cycles, a special study of both inpatient and outpatient revenues should be conducted, under the supervision of the budget officer, by the business office. The methodology for this study can be as follows:

a) Establish a log for recording all charges made for patient services (see Figure 13.B-1);

b) Each time a patient bill is prepared, an entry should be made in the log indicating the name and identification number of the patient, date of discharge or, for ER and OPD services, the date of service, source of payment, and amount of bill;

FIGURE 13.B-1   Sample Revenue Log Form

Billing Data			
Patient Name	*I.D. No.*	*Date of Discharge*	*Amount of Bill (Total)*
Sample Entry Ban, Unger	325362125	6-3-84	$2,480

Payment Data						
Source of Payment				*Cash Receipt Data*		
Primary Source	*Amt.*	*Secondary Source*	*Amt.*	*Payment Amt.*	*Record Date*	*Source*
Blue Cross	$1,904	Self-Pay	$576	$250 (cash)	6-3-84	Self-Pay
				$326	7-1-84	Self-Pay
				$1,904	8-5-84	Blue Cross

Note: This form can be used for recording both inpatient and outpatient revenues. If it is used for outpatient revenues, the column headed "Date of Discharge" should be changed to "Date of Service."

c) Each time a bill is paid, an entry should be made in the log indicating the amount, date, and source of payment; and

d) Using the above information, the budget officer should determine the foregoing items.

A study of this nature should be performed annually for both inpatient and outpatient revenues and should encompass a period of at least three months.

2) Information available from the controller's office

The controller should have available information on the percent of billed charges paid by the various third party payers. Additionally, the controller should have knowledge as to the timing of the receipt of investment income, United Fund grants, nursing school tuition. The controller, based on historical experience, should estimate the timing and amount of any third party payment adjustment.

3) Other information

a) Emergency room and outpatient revenues. These are patient service revenues and should be handled by means of the above special study.

b) Deductions from revenues. See comment 2 above (A-2: a-2).

c) Miscellaneous revenues, other operating revenues, and other revenues. If information in regard to the timing of the receipt of revenues budgeted for these items is not available from the controller, then, if acceptable subjective estimates cannot be made, sampling studies, similar to those described above, should be conducted.

b. Expense Budget

The data needed to convert the expense budget should be obtainable from two sources—a sampling study of expenses and the information in the controller's office.

1) Sampling study of expenses

To determine the percentage of purchases for which trade credit is offered, the average nature of trade credit terms, and the average terms for all other purchases, that is, for purchases wherein trade credit is not offered, a special study should be conducted (under the supervision of the budget officer) by the purchasing department and any other departments that purchase goods directly. The methodology for this study can be as follows:

a) Establish a log for recording the receipt of all goods;

b) Whenever goods are received, an entry should be made in the log indicating: type of item, total cost of the goods, and the terms of purchase; and

c) Using the above information, the budget officer should determine the foregoing items.

A study of this nature need be performed only annually and should encompass a two-month period.

2) Information available from the controller's office

The controller should have available information on the timing of all regular nonmonthly payments and the salary and wage payment policies of the hospital.

Some hospitals also adjust their cash budget for the time that will elapse between the date the disbursement is recorded by the hospital and the date it actually is paid out of the hospital's account at the bank. This refinement enables management to invest available funds in interest-yielding securities until the last possible day before they are needed to cover operating disbursements. It also, however, increases the probability of an overdraft due to a miscalculation or a change in historical demand patterns. The method for estimating the delay is similar to the method of estimating cash receipts in accounts receivable.

c. Capital Budget (Plant and Equipment Budget)

The data needed to convert the capital budget to a cash basis should be obtained by the budget officer from the information available in the capital budget.

B. Step 2

The budget officer, in consultation with the controller and the director of the hospital, should determine the horizon or the planning period of the budget. Generally, cash budgets are prepared based on a planning period of one year which, in turn, is segmented into 12 monthly subperiods. This general approach is compatible with the hospital's other budgets; that is, they are also constructed using monthly subperiods and appear to be acceptable at this point in time. However, the budget officer should periodically review the length of the cash budgeting period and limit it to only that future time span beyond which additional information will not affect decisions made in the first subperiod.

C. Step 3

The budget officer, using the data determined in Step 1 and the revenues budget, should convert the revenue budget to the cash receipts segment of the cash budget. This is simply a mechanical task of applying the timing data obtained in Step 1 to the accrual-based projections of the revenue budget (see Table 13.B-1).

D. Step 4

The budget officer, using the data determined in Step 1 and the expense budget, should convert the expense and capital budgets to the cash disbursements segment of the cash budget. This is sim-

TABLE 13.B-1   Conversion of the Revenue Budget to a Cash Basis

The conversion of inpatient revenue projections to a cash basis is presented below as a means of illustrating the mechanics of converting the revenue budget to a cash basis.

1. Assume the following inpatient revenue projection:

May	$100,000
June	$ 90,000
July	$ 80,000

August	$ 90,000
September	$100,000

2. Based on the data presented earlier in regard to the percent of total inpatient revenue by source, the figure in "1" above can be recast to a cash basis as follows.

Revenue by Sources (Inpatient)

Month	40% Blue Cross	20% Medicare	10% Medicaid	10% Comm. Ins.	15% Self-Pay	5% Other	Total
May	$40,000	$20,000	$10,000	$10,000	$15,000	$5,000	$100,000
June	36,000	18,000	9,000	9,000	13,500	4,500	90,000
July	32,000	16,000	8,000	8,000	12,000	4,000	80,000
Aug.	36,000	18,000	9,000	9,000	13,500	4,500	90,000
Sept.	40,000	20,000	10,000	10,000	15,000	5,000	100,000

3. Cash receipts in September

Blue Cross	=	95%* of July billings† of	$32,000 =		$30,400
Medicare	=	90%* of July billings† of	16,000 =		14,400
Medicaid	=	90%* of June billings† of	9,000 =		8,100
Comm. Ins.	=	100% of ½ Aug. billings†		$4,500	
		100% of ½ Sept. billings†		5,000	
				=	9,500
Other	=	100% of July billings† of	14,000 =		14,000
Self-pay	=	15% of Sept. billings of	15,000 =	2,250 (cash)	
		20% of Aug. billings† of	13,500 =	2,700	
		40% of July billings† of	12,000 =	4,800	
		15% of June billings† of	13,500 =	2,025	
		5% of May billings† of	15,000 =	750	
				=	12,525
		Total cash receipts inpatient revenue			$88,925

*Adjustment made for the percent of billed charges paid.
†Adjustment made for timing of the accounts receivable cycle.

ply a mechanical task of applying the data obtained in Step 1 to the projections of the expense and capital budgets (see Table 13.B-2).

E. Step 5

The budget officer should consolidate the data obtained in Steps 3 and 4 into the completed cash budget. A sample budget is illustrated in Table 13.B-2.

At this point, the cash budgeting process is completed. A comprehensive cash budget should now be available for management's use as a decision-making tool. An in-depth discussion of the managerial usefulness of the cash budget is beyond the scope of this text. However, Part II of this appendix briefly examines the decision-making potential of the cash budget.

TABLE 13.B-2   Conversion of the Expense Budget to a Cash Basis

The conversion of supplies expense projection to a cash basis is presented below as a means of illustrating the mechanics of converting the expense budget to a cash basis.

1. Assume the following supplies expense projections.
   August   = $10,000
   September   = $15,000

2. Based on the data presented earlier in regard to supplies purchases, the figures above can be recast to a cash basis as follows.

| | Purchases 2-10, net 30 | Net 30 | |
Month	Terms	No Terms	Total
August	$4,000	$6,000	$10,000
September	$6,000	$9,000	$15,000

3. If all purchase discounts are taken and supplies are purchased evenly over the month, then cash payments in September will be as follows.
   August Supplies
   One-third of supplies purchases for which terms are offered—supplies received on or after the 20th of the month   = $ 1,333 (approx.)
   All of the supplies purchases for which no terms are offered   = $ 6,000
   September Supplies
   Two-thirds of supplies purchases for which terms are offered—supplies received prior to the 20th of the month   = $ 4,000

   Total cash disbursements supplies: $11,333 (approx.)

PART II. DECISION-MAKING POTENTIAL OF THE CASH BUDGET

To examine the potential of a cash budget in aiding management to make cash-related decisions, assume the following budget, as shown in Table 13.B-3.

Based on the above assumptions, a $230,000 surplus exists in month 1, a $160,000 deficit exists in month 2, and a $15,000 surplus exists in month 3. Implicit in the above is a sequential approach to cash management, that is, a two-step approach wherein the first step involves estimating the cash surplus or deficit and the second step involves an investment or borrowing decision. The sequential approach, however, is limited in that it fails not only to consider the interrelationship of the two steps, but also to use the

TABLE 13.B-3   Example of a Cash Budget (in thousands of dollars)

	Month 1	Month 2	Month 3
Cash Balance			
(beginning)	$ 450	$ 500	$ 500
Receipts			
Inpatient	$ 750	$ 550	$ 825
Outpatient	360	300	300
Other operating	50	150	50
Nonoperating	25	20	0
Total receipts	1,185	1,020	1,175
Total cash available	$1,635	$1,520	$1,675
Disbursements			
Salaries and wages	$ 600	$ 650	$ 650
Supplies	230	330	250
Plant and equipment	75	200	100
Other (notes payable)	0	0	160
Total	$ 905	$1,180	$1,160
Cash Balance	$ 730	$ 340	$ 515
(ending)			
Less: minimal cash balance*	500	500	500
Cash Surplus (shortage)	$ 230	$ (160)	$ 15
Borrowing		$ 160	
Investment	$ 230		$ 15

*Assume that the minimum cash balance is determined through the techniques described in Chapter 13.

information available in the cash budget to make least cost decisions. This point can be illustrated as follows:

Assume: return on investments = 9%
                                 cost of borrowing = 15%

Therefore: 1. $230,000 surplus in month 1 can be invested at 9% for months 2 and 3. The resulting income will be $3,900.

                                 2.$160,000 will be borrowed at the beginning of month 2, for months 2 and 3, at a cost of $4,000.

                                 3. The cost of managing cash in the above manner will be $100 ($4,000 − $3,900 = $100).

However: Assume that management uses the foregoing budget as the means of simulating various cash management decisions in order to determine the least cost decision, that is, uses the foregoing budget as the basis for developing alternative budgets that will reflect different cash management strategies.

For example:

Alternative 1

Based on the above budget, management decides to change the timing of the capital expenditure tentatively planned for month 2 to month 1. If this were done, then the cash surplus in month 1 would be reduced from $230,000 to $30,000, the cash deficit in month 2 would be reduced from a deficit of $160,000 to a surplus of $40,000 and the surplus in month 3 increased, due to not having to pay the note payable, to $175,000. Thus, $30,000 would be available for investment in months 2 and 3 and $40,000 would be available for month 3. At 9% these surpluses would result in an income of $750 for the hospital as opposed to an expense of $100 as was shown in the previous case.

Alternative 2

Based on the above budget, management decides to invest only $70,000 of the month 1 surplus and hold the remaining $160,000 in cash. If this were done, then $70,000 would be available for investment during months 2 and 3, the month 2 deficit would be 0, and the month 3 surplus would be $175,000. At 9% this cash management strategy would result in an income of $1,050, as opposed to the $750 income of Alternative 1 and the $100 cost of the original case.

Other examples could be used to explain the same point. However, the critical matter is not the exploration of various examples, but a realization that the cash budget is useful for more than just projecting cash surpluses and deficits. As has been illustrated, the cash budget not only can project surpluses and deficits, but also can be used as the basis for simulating various cash management decisions in order to determine the least cost management alternative.

CHAPTER

14

Management Reports: Working Capital

Hospital managers, like their counterparts in commercial industry, have found that two steps must be taken if operational efficiency is to be maintained as the scope of operations increases beyond the management capacity of a single individual. First, in order to share the load and provide sufficient coverage, management must delegate the responsibility for the operation of certain areas or functions to subordinates. Second, in order to judge how well or poorly these subordinates are carrying out their responsibilities, management must receive reports from them. These two management principles are applicable to any area of hospital operation—including financial operations.

Financial reports generally are categorized as being either planning and informational reports or performance reports. Planning and informational reports can be described as statements designed to aid and enable management to recognize overall trends and determine long-range policies and actions. Performance reports are documents designed to assist management in controlling current operations and expenditures; they can be conceptualized as consisting of two subcategories—stock reports and flow reports.

Stock reports are statements that describe the performance of management in relation to the stock or inventory of values, that is, the group of assets and liabilities that the hospital has at any particular point in time. Examples of this type of report are the hospital's balance sheet (position statement), aged accounts receivable report, and cash position report. Flow reports are statements that describe management's performance relative to the flow or movement of values, that is, the stream of revenues and expenses that the hospital incurs over time. The best examples of this type of report are a hospital's income (operating) statement, departmental performance reports, and Hospital Administrative Services (HAS) reports.

A discussion of flow reports is more germane to the matters of cost accounting and operational budgeting than to the topic at hand. They are discussed in Chapter 21. The focus of this chapter will thus be limited to the stock reports needed for the management of working capital.

FUNDAMENTAL PRINCIPLES

Before actually discussing the various financial stock reports that management should receive, it would be worthwhile to review several fundamental reporting principles. These principles are basic not only to financial reporting, but also to management reporting in general. As such, they must be observed by the financial manager if he is to provide effective management reports. These basic reporting guidelines are presented below.

TIMELINESS

If reports are to be of value to management in controlling current operations, they must be current and up-to-date. A late report is almost as useless as no report at all. Hence, if reports are to be effective management tools, they not only must be prepared as frequently as necessary, but also must be promptly available. Only through timely reports can management obtain the information that it needs to control and guide operations.

ACCURACY

The need for accurate reports should be obvious. If management is to have confidence in reports, and if reports are to act as an aid in controlling operations, they must be understandable, reliable, and valid. Late reports may be almost useless, but inaccurate reports are detrimental.

CLARITY

Accuracy will create confidence in the reports that are provided. However, if reports are to be used to their fullest extent, management must feel comfortable with them. Reports should be clearly and simply designed, be expressed in language and terms familiar to the reader and, to the extent possible, be standardized. Through these considerations, reports not only can be tailored to management's desires and peculiarities, but also can be designed so that their usefulness will be maximized.

COMPARABILITY

Actual performance data alone usually are of relatively little worth, for they do not provide management with a frame of reference or a bench mark from which to base analysis and evaluation. If management is to place actual performance in the proper perspective, it must be able to compare it either to past performance or to reasonable standards. Only in this way is it possible to judge current performance adequately, identify trends, and determine the appropriate nature of any future actions.

Figure 14.1 presents examples of two types of comparative statement. Part A depicts a "simple" comparative report wherein current performance is presented alongside of either the previous year's performance or some standards. Statements of this type facilitate the identification of changes over time and enable management readily to discover trends that otherwise might go unnoticed. Thus, they improve the general usefulness of reports as a control device and should be used whenever possible.[1]

FIGURE 14.1   Comparative Reports

Part A. Simple Comparative Report

A and L Millstone General Hospital
Comparative Working Capital Report
As of February 28, 1984
(dollars in thousands)

	Assets				Liabilities		
	1982	1983	1984		1982	1983	1984
Cash	$ 150	$ 170	$ 200	Accounts			
Marketable				payable	$300	$320	$350
securities	30	10	50	Salaries and			
Accounts				wages payable	100	120	50
receivable	1,200	1,300	1,600	Accrued			
Inventories	170	130	150	interest	50	30	30
Total	$1,550	$1,610	$2,000	Total	$450	$470	$430

Part B. Common Size Report

A and L Millstone General Hospital
Common Size Working Capital Report
As of February 28, 1984

	Assets				Liabilities		
	1982	1983	1984		1982	1983	1984
Cash	9.7%	10.6%	10.0%	Accounts			
Marketable				payable	66.7%	68.0%	81.4%
securities	1.9	.6	2.5	Salaries and			
Accounts				wages pay.	22.2	25.6	11.6
receivable	77.5	80.7	80.0	Accrued			
Inventories	10.9	8.1	7.5	interest	11.1	6.4	7.0
Total	100 %	100 %	100 %	Total	100 %	100 %	100 %

[1]Comparative data are unquestionably of value. However, caution must be exercised in drawing conclusions from these data, for price level and volume changes can distort their validity.

Part B illustrates another type of comparative report that can be helpful. To identify and evaluate relative changes in performance, managers, together with accountants, have developed "common size" reports. A common size comparative report differs from a simple comparative statement in that items are presented in terms of a percentage of the total instead of in absolute dollars. The advantage of this modification lies in the fact that it pinpoints relative changes and thereby allows management to evaluate the distribution of items and their implication.

Common size reports are not used as extensively as simple comparative statements. However, they do have some value for internal management purposes and should be used whenever they will add to management's decision-making capabilities.

COMMENTARY

Reports are communication devices used to transmit information and ideas to management. To accomplish this task effectively, reports should include explanatory comments designed both to direct the user's attention to important items and to interpret the significance and meaning of those items.

The commentary segment of a report should be aimed at expediting management by exception. It should distinguish between functions that are progressing satisfactorily and those that need management attention and concentrate on only the latter. This approach will result in both better reports and an improved utilization of management time and talent, for attention can be immediately directed and concentrated on only exceptional areas and problems.

MEANINGFULNESS

The foregoing has pointed out the basic elements necessary for effective and usable reports. However, if the value of reports is to be maximized, one other overriding standard must also be met. They must provide meaningful and needed information.

Managers need performance data if they are to carry out their responsibilities successfully. However, the case of the manager who receives so many reports that they must be delivered on a hand truck too often approaches reality. A data overload is just as counterproductive as insufficient data, for in both instances the manager will be inadequately informed. Hence, if reports are to be useful, they must concentrate on the critical or key variable that must be controlled—if the item under question is to be controlled—and not just provide a mass of words and figures that are either ill-focused or beyond a reader's absorption level.

This last standard is particularly important and merits careful consideration. Simply, reports must focus on problems as opposed to symptoms of problems. To accomplish this, they must provide data not on the elements of working capital per se, but rather on the process that underlies, and thereby controls, each element. This distinction should become clear through the following discussion.

BALANCE SHEET

Given an understanding of the above principles, the stage is set for considering the various financial stock reports that management should receive. Of these reports, the most basic and comprehensive is the balance sheet or position statement.

A balance sheet can be viewed as being analogous to a photograph. A photograph depicts action, an event, or a subject at a particular point in time. Correspondingly, a balance sheet depicts the results of a number of financial events and actions at a particular point in time. It shows as of a specific date (point in time) the accepted monetary value of both the hospital's assets and its obligations or liabilities. The difference between these two categories of item—assets and liabilities—is the hospital's capital or net worth. Due to the fact that the statement portrays a balance between assets and the total liabilities and net worth, it is commonly referred to as a balance sheet.

Figure 14.2 illustrates a sample hospital balance sheet. As can be seen, the statement is presented in the traditional corporate finance format. The rationale for this approach should be clear from the discussion in Chapter 2. In addition to this basic change in presentation form, it should be noted that prepaid expenses are shown in an asset category entitled "Deferred Charges." This was done to reflect the particular "near" expense nature of these assets and to distinguish them from current assets that can be readily converted into cash.

Balance sheets should be prepared for management's use no less frequently than annually and no more frequently than monthly. Monthly reports represent one extreme, for any period less than one month is generally too short a time span either for trends to appear or for management to act. Conversely, annual reports represent the other extreme, for if management is to avoid the allegation of fiscal negligence, it must review the financial position of the hospital at least annually. It is the authors' opinion that monthly or, at the extreme, quarterly is the preferable reporting frequency.

As indicated earlier, the balance sheet should be presented in a comparative form so that management can more readily evaluate its significance. Additionally, a technique known as ratio analysis can be used by management to evaluate a balance sheet.

Ratio analysis is the financial tool that is most commonly used in com-

FIGURE 14.2 Lindsay Memorial Hospital—Statement of Financial Position As of December 31, 1984

	1984	1983
Assets		
Current assets		
Cash	$ 125,000	$ 27,000
Marketable securities	20,000	115,000
Accounts receivable—patients	175,000	200,000
Accounts receivable—others	25,000	20,000
Inventory	40,000	45,000
Total current assets	$ 385,000	$ 407,000
Fixed assets		
Land	$ 50,000	$ 50,000
Equipment (net of depreciation)	825,000	875,000
Buildings (net of depreciation)	1,750,000	1,700,000
Total fixed assets	$2,625,000	$2,625,000
Other assets		
Endowment Fund A—unrestricted	$ 75,000	$ 90,000
Endowment Fund B—restricted	1,000,000	1,000,000
Total other assets	$1,075,000	$1,090,000
Deferred charges		
Prepaid insurance	$ 5,000	$ 7,500
Total deferred assets	$ 5,000	$ 7,500
Total assets	$4,090,000	$4,129,500
Liabilities & Net Worth		
Current liabilities		
Accounts payable	$ 138,000	$ 150,000
Accrued wages	22,000	30,000
Total current liabilities	$ 160,000	$ 180,000
Long-term debt		
Mortgage—Building A	$1,000,000	$ 950,000
Loan	300,000	300,000
Total long-term debt	$1,300,000	$1,250,000
Net worth	$2,630,000	$2,699,500
Total liabilities & net worth	$4,090,000	$4,129,500

mercial industry as a mechanism to aid management in interpreting a firm's balance sheet. Quite simply, ratios are a means of expressing, in quantitative terms, the relationships between various items in the balance sheet. These actual relationships can be compared to standard or normal ratios which can be used as guidelines to estimate financial performance and identify areas of inadequacy. The existing literature contains many alternative categories of financial ratios and numerous individual ratios. These and other techniques of financial analysis are discussed in detail in Chapter 21.

In addition to a balance sheet, management should utilize several other stock reports. These basic reports are examined in the following sections. It is important to realize that, depending on a hospital's particular operating situation and management's desires and style, reports other than those discussed may be utilized in some instances. The task of describing all possible working capital reports and their variations, however, is obviously beyond the scope of this text. Therefore, only those reports that are commonly used for working capital management will be discussed.

CASH REPORTS

Traditionally, daily cash reports have been used by administrators as their primary cash management report. These reports usually consist of just a summary listing of both cash receipts—by source—and cash disbursements by item. As such, their usefulness is quite limited, for they encompass too short a time span for management either to make an evaluation or to act. However, for hospitals with chronic cash shortages or with sharply fluctuating cash balances these reports can be a valuable aid. Figure 14.3 illustrates a modified cash report that can be used to project cash flow and monitor weekly activity.

Generally, comparative reports, which both contrast actual cash flows with the cash budget and estimate the next ending cash balance, are more useful to upper management than are simple daily cash reports. This type of report is of more value, for it not only provides an analytical frame of reference for control decisions, but also, if prepared weekly or monthly, allows management to identify and evaluate trends. With this information, management can more knowledgeably select cash investment or financing strategies.

The usefulness of this type of comparative cash statement should be clear. In the authors' opinion, this report should be used by most hospitals as their basic management report. Figure 14.4 presents an example of this statement.

In addition to the above, management should receive, at least monthly, a listing of the hospital's short-term investments. This report, as Figure 14.5 illustrates, should indicate the nature of the investment, date purchased,

FIGURE 14.3   Havens General Hospital—Modified Weekly Cash Report

for week ending: _____

	Monday	Tuesday	Wednesday	Thursday	Friday	Total	In-Process
Beginning daily balance	___	___	___	___	___	___	
Cash receipts							
Source							[received/not processed]
Blue Cross	___	___	___	___	___	___	___
Medicare	___	___	___	___	___	___	___
Medicaid	___	___	___	___	___	___	___
Commercial	___	___	___	___	___	___	___
Self-pay	___	___	___	___	___	___	___
Other	___	___	___	___	___	___	___
Total receipts							
Total cash available							
Cash disbursements							
Item							[written/not cashed]
Payroll	___	___	___	___	___	___	___
Accounts payable	___	___	___	___	___	___	___
Capital purchases	___	___	___	___	___	___	___
Other	___	___	___	___	___	___	___
Total disbursements							
Ending cash balance	___	___	___	___	___	___	___

FIGURE 14.4   Lanoff County Hospital—Monthly Cash Report for the Month Ending

week of:

	Actual	_Budget_	_Actual_	_Budget_	_Actual_	_Budget_	_Actual_	_Budget_	Total _Actual_	_Budget_
Beginning cash balance										
Cash receipts										
Inpatient										
Outpatient										
Other operating										
Nonoperating										
Total receipts										
Cash disbursements										
Payroll										
Accounts payable										
Capital purchases										
Other										
Total disbursements										
Ending cash balance										

FIGURE 14.5   M. Cohn General Hospital—Investment Report As of July 31, 1984

Security	Date Purchased	Cost	Market Value	Maturity Date	Yield	Income to Date
Hosp. Credit Corp.—Note	5-1-84	$10,000	$10,000	10-1-84	6%	$150
U.S. Treasury Bills	6-15-84	19,750	19,860	9-15-84	7%	—
Certificate of Dep.—Consumer	7-1-84	5,000	5,000	12-1-84	8.25%	—
Hosp. Credit Corp.—Note	7-15-84	5,000	5,000	3-1-85	7%	—
		$39,750	$39,860		6.88%	$150

Other Information

Investment balance last month	$45,000
Income this month	50
Total investment income (all investments) this year =	$ 1,750

purchase cost, present market value, maturity date, yield, income received year-to-date, total investment balance for both the current and previous months, and composite portfolio yield. With this information, management can evaluate the quality and profitability of the hospital's short-term portfolio. Also, based on this report and the monthly cash reports, management can assess the appropriateness of both the short-term investment balance and the minimum cash balance.

ACCOUNTS RECEIVABLE REPORTS

As was indicated in Chapter 12, accounts receivable are the biggest single component of working capital. Hence, if for no other reason than size, they should merit management's concern and attention. Accounts receivable, however, are critical for another reason. If receivables are not collected and are allowed to increase, it is not only possible but also likely that a hospital will not have sufficient cash available to pay its obligations as they come due.[2] Thus, if management is to maintain the financial integ-

---

[2]The research department of the American Collectors Association reported the following dollar values in delinquent accounts:

Age	Value
Current	$1.00
Two months old	.80
Six months old	.67
One year old	.49
Two years old	.27

The Association also reported that an overall recovery of 40% occurred during the first 90 days that the accounts were being worked on a collection basis.

rity of the hospital, it must be sure that the accounts receivable collection function is performed as effectively and efficiently as is possible. There are five methods of monitoring accounts receivables: the gross accounts receivable method, the aged accounts receivable schedule, the percent of collections method, the average days outstanding method, and the balance fraction method.

The gross accounts receivable method requires management to monitor the gross accounts receivable recorded in the hospital's periodic financial statements. An increase in the accounts receivable is viewed as a loss of liquidity; although working capital is unaffected, cash collections have not kept pace with billings for new accounts arising in the last period. A decline reflects an acceleration in cash collections and is advantageous. Because of its focus on the gross level of accounts receivable, interpretation of the gross accounts receivable method is susceptible to distortions caused by seasonal fluctuations in billing volume and cash collection. Both situations are common to the hospital field. To be meaningful, therefore, the gross accounts receivable method must be applied over many reporting periods to avoid these short-term fluctuations (see Figure 14.6).

The aged accounts receivable schedule monitors the age composition of the accounts receivable over time. This is accomplished by grouping the individual patient accounts into similar age categories and determining the percentage relationship of each category to the total accounts receivable outstanding (see Figure 14.7). Interpretation of the aging schedule facilitates management's understanding of the effectiveness of its payment and collection policies. An increase in the proportion of newer accounts indicates improved cash flow; an increase in the older accounts indicates a deterioration in payments. A focused analysis of the older accounts may also identify problems that management can control through changes to its credit and payment policies. However, like the gross accounts receivable method, the aged accounts receivable schedule must be interpreted carefully to avoid misinterpretation.

The percent of collections method provides management with a measure of the rate of actual cash inflow. It is calculated by dividing cash collections for the period by the revenue generated during the same period.

$$\text{Collections percentage} = \frac{\text{Cash collected during period}}{\text{Revenues recorded for period}}$$

The percent of collections method adds additional insights to management's analysis because it separates cash reductions from other types of account receivable credit, that is, write-offs or discounts.

The average days outstanding method is the most widely used by hospitals. It provides a bench mark of the amount of average daily charges left

FIGURE 14.6 Lindsay Memorial Hospital—Gross Accounts Receivable Report As of December 13, 1984

	January	February	March	April	May	June	July	August	September	October	November	December
Current month billings	$100,000	$120,000	$100,000	$100,000	$100,000	$100,000	$ 80,000	$100,000	$100,000	$100,000	$100,000	$100,000
Beginning accounts receivable balance	100,000	114,000	104,000	102,000	100,000	100,000	100,000	86,000	96,000	98,000	100,000	100,000
	200,000	234,000	204,000	202,000	200,000	200,000	180,000	186,000	196,000	198,000	200,000	200,000
Cash received	106,000	120,000	102,000	102,000	100,000	100,000	94,000	90,000	98,000	98,000	100,000	100,000
Ending accounts receivable balance	114,000	104,000	102,000	100,000	100,000	100,000	86,000	96,000	98,000	100,000	100,000	100,000
Aged account receivables												
0–30 days	84,000	70,000	70,000	70,000	70,000	70,000	56,000	70,000	70,000	70,000	70,000	70,000
31–60 days	20,000	24,000	20,000	20,000	20,000	20,000	20,000	16,000	20,000	20,000	20,000	20,000
61–90 days	10,000	10,000	12,000	10,000	10,000	10,000	10,000	10,000	8,000	10,000	10,000	10,000
	$114,000	$104,000	$102,000	$100,000	$100,000	$100,000	$ 86,000	$ 96,000	$ 98,000	$100,000	$100,000	$100,000

FIGURE 14.7   Israel General Hospital—Aged Accounts
Receivable Report, January 31, 1984

A. General (all dollars in hundreds)

Time Outstanding	Amount Current Month	Amount Last Month
0–30 days	$12,500	$10,000
31–60 days	9,750	9,000
61–90 days	7,000	8,500
91–120 days	5,000	4,000
121–180 days	3,000	—
Over 180 days	—	—
Total outstanding	$37,250	$31,500

B. By Payer (all dollars in hundreds)

Percentage of Revenue by Payer	40% Blue Cross		20% Medicare		10% Medicaid		30% Other	
Time Outstanding	Current	Last	Current	Last	Current	Last	Current	Last
0–30 days	$ 5,000	$ 4,000	$2,500	$2,000	$1,250	$1,000	$ 3,750	$3,000
31–60 days	$ 3,900	$ 3,600	$1,950	$1,800	$ 975	$ 900	$ 2,925	$2,700
61–90 days	$ 2,800	$ 3,400	$1,400	$1,700	$ 700	$ 850	$ 2,100	$2,550
91–120 days	$ 2,000	$ 1,600	$1,000	$ 800	$ 500	$ 400	$ 1,500	$1,200
121–180 days	$ 1,200	—	$ 600	—	$ 300	$ —	$ 900	—
Over 180 days	$ —	—	—	—	—	—	—	—
	$14,900	$12,600	$7,450	$6,300	$3,725	$3,150	$11,175	$9,450

uncollected. The resulting indicator of days outstanding is useful because
it provides a measure of the financial investment that management has in
the receivables on a current basis. The average days outstanding is derived
by dividing the accounts receivable balance outstanding at the end of the
period by an estimate of the average revenues per day during that same
period.

$$\text{Average days outstanding} = \frac{\text{Receivable balance}}{\text{Average daily revenue for period}}$$

The interpretation of the average days is applied in the same manner as the
gross accounts receivable method. An increase reflects a slowing in cash
collections and an increased investment in the receivables; a decrease indicates an acceleration in payments and is desirable. Use of the average
days outstanding method is further enhanced when it is calculated individually for each class of third party payer. The average days outstanding
should be viewed cautiously, however. The write-off policy of the hospital

and the relative weighting of the aged accounts at the end of an individual period have the ability to skew a comparison of the index between different reporting periods.

The balance fraction method combines the indexing qualities of the average days outstanding method and the aging qualities of the aged accounts receivable schedule. An example of the computation of the balance fraction method is presented below.

Month	Receivable Balance Outstanding	Total Revenue Billed
October (61–90 days)	$10,000	$100,000
November (31–60 days)	60,000	120,000
December (0–30 days)	75,000	150,000

To obtain the balance fraction, the total accounts receivable balance for the current month is aged by category. The receivable balance outstanding for each category is divided by the total revenues for the month in which the billings were made.

$$\text{October} \quad \frac{\$\ 10,000}{100,000} \quad = \quad .1$$

$$\text{November} \quad \frac{\$\ 60,000}{120,000} \quad = \quad .5$$

$$\text{December} \quad \frac{\$\ 75,000}{150,000} \quad = \quad \underline{.5}$$

$$\text{Total balance fraction index} \quad = \quad \underline{\underline{1.1}}$$

The principal advantage of the balance fraction index is that, unlike the other methods, it relates the accounts receivable outstanding at the end of a specific period to the revenues of the period from which they arose.

Because of the significant and growing influence of contractual allowances and pricing discounts, management should also receive information on the difference between the gross revenues reflected in the hospital's accounts receivable and the cash received as net revenue. This information is obtained from a report of net revenues and billing such as illustrated in Figure 14.8. From the information presented, management can obtain measures of the billings actually required to support a predetermined level of cash flow and the cost shift or markup experienced by the hospital's retail customers. This presentation, like so many others of interest to management, is further enhanced by adding payer, product, or comparative data identifiers into the format.

FIGURE 14.8   Unger Memorial Hospital—Monthly Net Revenues
                     Billed for Budget Year 1984

Month	Gross Revenues Patient Services	Deductions from Revenue	Net Revenues Patient Services	Cash Trans- actions	Total Revenue Anticipated
January	$ 1,988,310	$ 189,344	$ 1,798,966	$ 20,000	$ 1,818,966
February	1,963,670	180,818	1,782,852	25,000	1,807,852
March	1,852,360	197,182	1,655,178	21,000	1,676,178
April	1,746,210	188,244	1,557,966	20,000	1,577,966
May	1,774,590	192,925	1,581,665	19,000	1,600,665
June	1,936,110	188,144	1,747,966	27,000	1,774,966
July	1,855,440	199,280	1,656,160	18,000	1,674,160
August	1,637,540	199,880	1,437,660	19,000	1,456,660
September	2,773,370	201,690	2,571,680	20,000	2,591,680
October	1,774,590	192,925	1,581,665	21,000	1,602,665
November	1,765,440	199,280	1,566,160	21,000	1,587,160
December	2,078,370	201,690	1,876,680	25,000	1,901,680
Total	$23,146,000	$2,331,402	$20,814,598	$256,000	$21,070,598

Based upon these reports, management has available the data necessary both to evaluate the overall effectiveness of the hospital's credit and collection efforts and to pinpoint any troublesome areas. Using this information, management should be able to assure that accounts receivable remain at acceptable levels.

ACCOUNTING RECOGNITION OF BAD DEBTS

An estimate of the amount of bad debts should be made periodically to adjust the hospital's accounting records to reflect management's judgment of collection probability. One method of making this adjustment is by a direct write-off. Accounts that are believed to be uncollectible are simply eliminated from both the accounts receivable records and the financial statement balances as individual account determinations are made.

This is an acceptable approach for maintaining accounts receivable records. However, conservatism requires that the financial statements reflect a more current estimate of total collectibility than is practical under specific identification procedures.

An alternative procedure is to estimate the total amount of uncollectible accounts and to show this estimate as a deduction from accounts receivable on the balance sheet. This balance sheet contra account is labeled "Allowance for Doubtful Accounts" or "Allowance for Uncollectible Accounts." It normally appears as a parenthetical note on the accounts receivable line of the balance sheet. Various methods may be used to estimate the amount of the bad debt:

1. Estimate bad debt as a percentage of total revenues for the period.
2. Estimate bad debt as a percentage of the revenues from credit sales for the period.
3. Adjust the prior period's allowance for doubtful accounts so that it equals a prescribed percentage of the accounts receivable recorded at the end of the reporting period.

The percentage in each case depends in part on what the records show is the entity's experience in past collections and in part on management's judgment of whether that experience will continue. The allowance should be sufficient at all times to absorb the total of all accounts that are suspected to be uncollectible.

It is advisable to develop different percentages for the different age groups of the accounts receivable and for different types of account receivable. The collectibility of the account and the experience of the hospital may be different in each case. Separate estimates add to the accuracy of the overall estimate. An example of estimating doubtful accounts by age category based on the outstanding accounts receivable balance at the end of a period is shown in Figure 14.9.

INVENTORY REPORTS

The nature and mechanics of inventory management were examined in detail in Chapter 11. Given that material, the first step that must be taken is to assure that the hospital's actual inventory practices are as consistent as practicable with the ideal guidelines that were set out. In addition to this initial control step, management should receive reports, such as the inventory turnover report, which will aid it in continual evaluation and control of the hospital's inventory practices and position.

FIGURE 14.9   Aging Schedule for Estimating Bad Debts

Status	Amount Outstanding	Estimated % Uncollectible	Allowance for Doubtful Accounts
Current billings	$200,000	1	$2,000
Accounts receivable			
0–30 days	26,000	1	2,600
31–60 days	10,000	5	500
61–90 days	7,000	10	700
91–120 days	3,000	20	600
Over 120 days	6,000	30	1,800
Total	$252,000		$8,200

Inventory turnover can be defined as the number of times during a given period, usually a month, that the existing inventory stocks would be depleted and replaced. This statistic can be calculated for each cost center by simply dividing the dollar amount of supplies and other inventory items that are expected to be used in a month by the dollar amount of inventories on hand.

$$\text{Inventory turnover rate} = \frac{\text{Value of inventory used}}{\text{Average inventory on hand}}$$

Generally, a low turnover rate indicates excessive inventory holdings and poor working capital management. A moderately high or high turnover rate usually indicates a desirable situation. An extremely high turnover rate often indicates insufficient inventory stocks. What a particular turnover rate specifically means can be determined either through an analysis of historical data and current operating conditions or through inventory control studies. Based upon these judgments, management can assess both a department's and the total hospital's inventory position. Figure 14.10 illustrates a monthly inventory turnover report.

Management may also find that other reports can be useful in evaluating a hospital's inventory position. For example, reports on actual and maximum inventories, on averages and shortages in physical holdings, or on comparisons between actual and budget, may be of value. Therefore, the financial manager, in conjunction with administration, should determine the type of information needed, review the reporting options available, and provide those reports that will be of most value to management.

ACCOUNTS PAYABLE RECORDS

In contrast with the above items, control of both accounts and wages payable is not obtained through the direct management of the items per se, but rather through the controls exerted on the underlying processes that produce these liability accounts. Specifically, accounts payable are a function or a direct product of the purchasing process. Therefore, if the level of accounts payable is to be maintained at acceptable and manageable limits, the purchasing process must be controlled through the establishment of and the adherence to sound inventory and purchasing policies and procedures.

The same situation is true in regard to wages payable. These payables are a function of the personnel process and can be controlled only through the proper management of that process. Thus, to maintain wages payable at financially reasonable limits, management must establish policies and procedures that assure that sound internal control exists over both hours worked and wage payments.

FIGURE 14.10   Lindsay General Hospital—Monthly Inventory Turnover Report, May 31, 1984

(1) Cost Center	(2) Expected Monthly Usage	Inventory Holdings (3A) Current Month	(3B) Last Month	(4) Turnover Rate (Col. 2 ÷ Col. 3A) Current Month	Last Month*	Annual Average†
1. Central Supply	25,400	5,000	20,000	5.1	2.7	2.6
2. Dietary	102,700	32,000	45,000	3.2	3.2	3.0
3. Pharmacy	37,800	3,100	5,000	12.2	10.8	9.5
17. Nursing Unit-A	6,500	2,000	4,000	3.2	2.1	1.8

*From last month's report.
†Arithmetic average of turnover rates for the last 12 months.

Hence, to control and evaluate the financial performance or position of the hospital relative to the above liabilities, management, for the most part, must examine the performance of the underlying processes. The balance sheet report and ratio analysis can provide some insight into the appropriateness of the relative size of these items. Also, a monthly report indicating the amount of purchase discounts lost (see Figure 14.11) can be useful in evaluating the accounts payable payment function. It must be realized, however, that control over these items can be obtained only through the control of the processes of which they are a function.

CONCLUSION

Given the foregoing material, the discussion of working capital management is now complete. Based on the discussion in Chapters 9 through 13, the reader should have a sound understanding of the financial tools and techniques that can be of value in minimizing the size and, consequently, the cost of working capital. The discussion in these chapters has, the authors hope, made clear the reports needed to evaluate a hospital's working capital position. Therefore, if all has gone according to plan, the reader should now have the knowledge necessary not only to evaluate a hospital's working capital performance and position, but also to correct any deficiencies.

Admittedly, there is more to hospital financial management than has been discussed in the foregoing chapters. The topics of operational bud-

FIGURE 14.11   Anders General Hospital—Purchase Discounts Lost Report, Month Ending January 31, 1984

	Current Month		Last Month	
1. Total purchases	$25,000		$30,000	
2. Purchases offered with discounts	$10,000	40%	$20,000	66.7%
3. Dollar value of discounts available	$ 150		$ 400	
4. Dollar value of discounts taken	$ 100		$ 400	
5. Dollar value of discounts not taken	$ 50		0	
6. Explanation of discounts not taken:				

Cash shortage in the last quarter of the month—due to insurance premium payment—resulted in the need to defer payment on several large accounts.

geting, investment decisions, and responsibility accounting are all critical areas that are, unfortunately, beyond the introductory nature of this volume. The intent of this text has been to provide an initial orientation to the financial environment of the hospital and to build a foundation for examining these more complex topics.

SUGGESTED READINGS

Choate, G. Marc. "Financial Ratio Analysis."
Esmond, Truman H., Jr. *Budgeting Procedures for Hospitals,* Chapter 9.
Heckert, J. Brooks and Wilson, James D. *Controllership.*
Seawell, L. Vann. *External and Internal Reporting by Hospitals,* Chapter 12.
Seawell, L. Vann. *Hospital Accounting and Financial Management,* Chapter 11.
Van Arsdell, Paul M. *Corporate Finance: Policy, Planning, Administration,* Chapter 6.
Young, D.E. "Effective Presentation of Reports: Information for Understanding."

Resource Allocation Decisions: Corporate Planning, Budgeting, and Control

Planning: the half science of
breathing operational form and life into dreams;
of applying the art of the possible
to merge concept and operations
into a single, cohesive, reality.

N. S. Hinkle

15

Strategic Planning

Corporate planning has long been viewed as a basic component of effective management. However, the practice of corporate planning has often been focused on its mechanics and techniques rather than on a systematic implementation of its precepts. The pendulum now may be swinging in the other direction. Corporate planning is becoming, at many hospitals, a principal management tool. Hospital corporate planners are becoming part of the senior management team.[1]

Although hospital managers have only relatively recently come to recognize the need for corporate planning, their dilatoriness may be a blessing. In examining the practice of corporate planning in commercial industry, for example, one is struck with a feeling that planning may have evolved along intellectually interesting but operationally less than optimal lines. Planning may in effect have become not only an end unto itself, but also a barrier to expeditious corporate decision making.

In reaction to this perhaps natural evolutionary tendency, some firms have begun to assess the effectiveness of their planning programs. The goal of this review has been both to streamline the planning process and to harness the process to assure that it serves the larger corporate interests, not simply the interest of the planners.

Special thanks to Edwin Tuller for assistance with this chapter.

[1]It is worthwhile to note that hospitals have long done facilities and services planning. Corporate planning includes facilities and services planning, but also goes beyond it. Corporate planning focuses on the role of the hospital—in all its aspects—as a "market-driven" community resource.

As the hospital field embraces the concepts of corporate planning, it can be the beneficiary of the experience of commercial industry. The major lesson of that experience is the reaffirmation that planning is an instrument of management to assist the hospital in operationally fulfilling its responsibilities to its community.

Corporate planning consists of two major elements. The first is strategic planning—the process by which an organization determines the overall direction in which it will be moving in the future. The end result of strategic planning is a corporate strategy (see Figure 15.1). The second element is operational planning and budgeting—the process by which an organization allocates resources to implement effectively the corporate strategy. The end result of this is an operating plan and budget (see Chapters 16, 17, and 18). Together, these two elements enable the hospital to ask systematically and answer comprehensively its two most basic operational questions:

1. What should its overall future direction be?

2. How should its resources be used within that overall direction?

The essence of corporate planning, however, is not the articulation of the above questions. Nor is it the defining and implementing of a particular planning process to answer these questions. Rather, it lies in the analysis and evaluation of the past, present, and future as viewed from the perspective of a hospital's mission and role in its community and of its community's needs. More precisely, the essence of corporate planning is the "thinking" necessary to answer the foregoing questions in relevant and even creative ways. The planning and budgeting systems underlying such a thought process should stimulate thinking. They should not be complicated or complex, lest they discourage thinking in the face of the burden of filling out forms and crunching numbers. Planning and budgeting systems, however, demand rigorous thinking.

The purpose of Part IV is to lay a foundation for these planning and budgeting processes. By design, the emphasis has been given to clarifying the thought process, identifying key decision points in that thought process, and establishing an integrated set of conceptual bench marks. These bench marks can in turn be used for "tailoring" general planning and budgeting process principles to fit and work well in various hospital settings. This chapter focuses on the first phase of corporate planning—strategic planning. The following chapters address the remaining phases, that is, operational planning, budgeting, and reporting.

STRATEGIC PLANNING

As described above, strategic planning is the process of establishing the organization's future direction. The managerial values of such a process

FIGURE 15.1   Strategic Planning Process

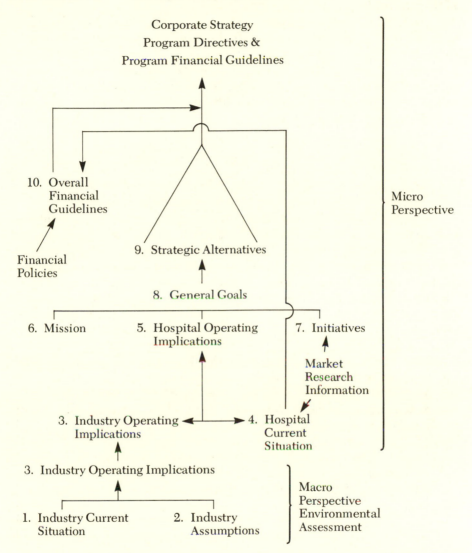

Corporate Strategy
Program Directives &
Program Financial Guidelines

10. Overall Financial Guidelines

Financial Policies

9. Strategic Alternatives

8. General Goals

6. Mission   5. Hospital Operating Implications   7. Initiatives

Market Research Information

3. Industry Operating Implications   4. Hospital Current Situation

3. Industry Operating Implications

1. Industry Current Situation   2. Industry Assumptions

Micro Perspective

Macro Perspective Environmental Assessment

are several. Principally, however, strategic planning provides both the opportunity and the procedural and thought discipline for management to examine systematically the future—its challenges, demands, threats, and opportunities—in order to sort out the path, that is, set the program priorities and financial limits, that will enable the hospital to utilize effectively its human, financial, and plant resources to meet the health services needs of its community.[2]

Strategic planning consists of two major components: an externally oriented macro facet and an internally focused micro element. Of the two, the second is obviously of more direct concern to the individual hospital. However, for the individual hospital's strategic planning to be relevant, it must be built upon the first component—the assessment of the larger, external environment in which it currently exists and within which it must operate in the future.

ENVIRONMENTAL ASSESSMENT

As illustrated by Figure 15.1, the macro portion of strategic planning is encapsulated within the notion of an environmental assessment.

The process of assessing the environment involves explicit identification, analysis, and evaluation of those factors external to the hospital that will affect—or may affect—its operations or performance. This process, as well as the product of this effort, serves two key purposes. First, it provides vital information about the trends and challenges that will be influencing the hospital and that must be taken into account, if the resulting work is to be relevant. Second, it provides a common information base and a communication vehicle that are essential in the development and implementation of the hospital's strategy, operating plan, and budget.

The importance of this latter role should not be underestimated. Because of its usefulness in establishing a common information base, the environmental assessment is perhaps the keystone element in the entire corporate planning process. However, if its potential is to be realized fully, its development must be characterized by broad staff involvement and full debate. Moreover, if it is to be a helpful communication device, it must be kept current. Therefore, the environmental assessment must be reviewed, at least annually, and appropriately modified and updated.

As shown in Figure 15.1, the environmental assessment process can be viewed as being the sum of three steps. Two of these steps, industry current situation (Step 1) and industry assumptions (Step 2), are essentially independent variables. The third, industry implications (Step 3), is a dependent amalgam, flowing from the analysis and evaluation of the data provided by Steps 1 and 2. Together the three yield the hospital's environmental assessment statement.[3]

---

[2]See Chapter 16 for a discussion of the value of planning and budgeting as management tools. The comments regarding the usefulness of operational planning apply to strategic planning as well.

[3]Operationally the three components can be presented separately or blended into a single statement.

STEP 1. INDUSTRY CURRENT SITUATION

The industry current situation is a straightforward summary of the present status of the hospital field. It should reflect both the general socioeconomic environment as well as those factors that are of particular relevance to the hospital field itself. Its purpose is to provide an objective statement of reality. Therefore, as painful as it might be, it must be written with candor, avoiding the traps of unproven conventional wisdom, professional rhetoric, and wishful thinking about what one would like reality to be. Broad discussion within the hospital respecting the industry current situation usually provides an excellent opportunity and test for candor and sound thinking.

STEP 2. INDUSTRY ASSUMPTIONS

Industry assumptions stand in counterpoint to the current situation. Assumptions can be described generally as statements that project future events and the resulting future environment. In the context of strategic planning, they can be defined operationally as statements describing future major developments that will affect hospital operations but whose occurrence is beyond the direct control of the individual hospital, for example,

1. Enactment of national health insurance or state rate review; or

2. Shift in the demographic character of the hospital's market area.[4]

As indicated, assumptions are by definition projections or estimates of the future. As such, they may well prove to be erroneous in the final analysis. At their inception, however, they represent management's "best judgment" as to what will happen. Hence, their development should be based on a careful analysis and evaluation of objective and subjective data concerning both local and national legislative and operating environments. Also, they should project events into the future up to the point of the hospital's planning horizon, that is, up to that point in the future wherein the availability of additional information will neither improve nor change any current operational decisions.[5] For this same reason, assumptions need to

---

[4]The fact that these developments are beyond the direct control of hospital management does not mean that they are events that cannot be influenced. For example, hospitals—both singularly or as a group—may oppose federal revenue caps. The opposition of the field may prevail in terms of the ultimate legislative result. The field, however, does not unilaterally control the final decision; it can only act to influence it. Similarly, while a shift in the hospital's traditional market area may be beyond its direct control, the expansion and reshaping of the market area, through new products and services, are within the hospital's control.

[5]The length of a hospital's planning horizon will differ both with the nature of the hospital's environment and the type of assumptions being considered. The general principle, however, is to limit the length of assumptions to that point in the future wherein additional input will not change current decisions. For example, if, in terms of day-to-day operational

Continued

be only as precise as necessary to shape the decisions that flow from them. Precision beyond the necessary level is not only irrelevant but potentially damaging to sound thinking.

STEP 3. INDUSTRY OPERATING IMPLICATIONS

The principal benefit of the assumption setting process is not the seemingly academic exercise—the hypothesizing, debating, and testing—involved in determining the assumptions themselves. Instead, the value of assumptions lies in their conversion into pragmatic statements reflecting operating implications.

Operating implications can be defined, in working terms, as simply the operational impact or meaning of the assumptions and current situation. They are the opportunities and threats presented by the combination of the current situation and environment translated into the actions that must be taken to capitalize on the environment described by the assumptions. Without translation into operating implications, the assumptions seem, and in fact are, irrelevant to the planning in the hospital. In stating the operating implications of the assumptions and current situation, the hospital is able to establish both the point of departure and the direction for all the decisions that follow in the planning and budgeting processes.

The notion of a planning horizon complements this translation process. It sets the outer time limit for projections. A planning horizon reinforces the current situation–assumptions–implications process by providing a constant reminder of the limits on the operational usefulness of remote possibilities. Therefore, as opposed to setting assumptions as far into the future as the imagination can wander, one needs only to make projections and determine their implications up to the point of the planning horizon.

The existence of a planning horizon is also important in terms of long-range planning. The length of long-range planning cannot exceed the planning horizon, for no assumptions upon which to base the plan exist beyond the planning horizon. Hence, one can only plan ahead, that is, develop a long-range plan, as far into the future as realistic and usable assumptions extend.[6]

If, for example, a hospital's planning horizon is three years, a long-range plan extending three years into the future could be developed. Based

---

[5]*Continued*

decisions, events four years into the future have no effect on current operating decisions, there is no need to project operational assumptions four years ahead. Typically, a hospital's planning horizon is three to five years. However, in the case of capital decisions the horizon might be longer. In each instance, assumptions must be tested in terms of their impact on current decisions. If there is no impact, then, at least at that point in time, the assumption is not needed.

[6]The planning horizon must, at times, be stretched to the far limits of the assumptions. As noted in footnote 5, an especially long lead time is required, for example, in the planning of physical requirements.

on the assumptions and their operating implications, the results desired to be achieved three years into the future could be defined. These results would represent the objectives or goals of the long-range plan. The activity which must be undertaken in the first year of the plan, if the objectives are to be achieved by the third year, represents the current operating plan and budget. Thus, the operating plan and budget for any single year are a consistent part of a larger (longer) plan. This longer-range plan extends as far into the future as the hospital's assumptions extend—to the planning horizon—and, if necessary, is modified as assumptions are modified and revised goals are established.

MECHANICS

The foregoing reflects the steps involved in preparing an environmental assessment. The mechanics of preparation, while perhaps more involved than the simple description of components, need not be difficult.

The most pragmatic approach to developing an initial environmental assessment is to build on the work of such organizations as the American Hospital Association. AHA provides annually a national level environmental assessment. This document can be used as a starting point which then can be modified as necessary to be appropriate. (See Appendix 17 for an excerpted example of an environmental assessment.)

The modification process should focus on building a consensus among the hospital's staff on their appraisal of the environment confronting their institution. To this end, both objective and subjective data should be welcomed, with consensus emerging through the process of testing, by debate, the facts and impressions being presented.

The development of subsequent (that is, succeeding years') environmental assessments should follow the same general pattern. The only difference is that the starting point should involve the hospital's previous environmental assessment.

PLANNING AND MARKETING

Before narrowing the focus of the strategic planning process to the hospital specific level, it is worthwhile to consider first the role of marketing and market information and their relationship to corporate planning. Like accounts receivable and the credit business, hospitals are involved in some marketing activities whether or not they explicitly recognize it or even wish to be. An involvement in marketing cannot—and if the hospital is to serve its community effectively should not—be avoided.

In the current environment, with increased competition and newly emerging alternative forms of health services and health care delivery, marketing can be a particularly helpful hospital management tool. The only real questions therefore are how thoughtful the hospital's involvement in marketing will be and how marketing technology will be applied to help the hospital identify and better serve the changing needs of its market (community) and patients (clients).

An in-depth discussion of the mechanics of marketing tools and techniques is beyond the scope of this book. An understanding of the marketing concept, however, is important both to productive corporate planning and more broadly to effective hospital management. Corporate planning can be viewed—and the term is so used in this text—as an umbrella notion, encompassing traditional facilities planning, operations planning, budgeting, and market research, as well as strategic planning.

Market research falls within this umbrella notion because it is a direct source of basic data for the strategic planning process. For purposes of strategic planning, marketing provides insights as to: the needs and wants of the community; preferences as to how the identified desires might best be satisfied, for example, how products and services should be packaged, where they should be located, how they should be distributed and priced; and the community's attitude toward the hospital and its current services. This kind of information is obviously critical to the hospital's planning process. As a management discipline, marketing has a usefulness beyond this strategic planning role. Marketing tools and techniques can help to stimulate demand for the hospital's services, contributing in a "business sense" to the achievement of the institution's overall mission.

It is in this latter regard—of demand stimulation through such activities as advertising, promotion, and sales efforts—that marketing is most often thought of. Marketing, however, must be understood to be more than simply selling. Demand stimulation and its various component elements are part of a total marketing effort. The components of demand stimulation must be done well if the hospital is to be successful. The activities, though, are derivatives of other decisions and needs, for example, strategic planning decisions and cash flow and operating margin requirements, not ends in themselves.

The aim of hospital marketing must be to understand the hospital's clients—community, patients, and medical staff—so well that products and services seem to sell themselves. Ideally, marketing through market research, product development and testing, and product distribution should result in a consumer who is ready to buy a needed service. All that should be required is to make the consumer aware of the availability of the product or service. The "end game" to the transaction, that is, the "purchase" should be a matter of logistics, not salesmanship.

The foregoing is not meant to deny that effective promotional activity can increase service demand. Advertising can, for example, increase patient volume for some discretionary services by creating an awareness of service availability. However, neither advertising nor other promotional activities can create long-term needs that do not legitimately exist. Demand stimulation techniques, no matter how effective, cannot overcome a lack of consumer need for a service.

Too often the tendency has been to try to "save" ill-conceived or unplanned projects through promotional activities. Marketing has in effect been called in to rescue poorly planned initiatives. Frequently, these initiatives have high visibility and high personal as well as corporate costs if they fail. In such circumstances marketing is little more than dignified peddling and has unavoidably often appeared to fail. A natural consequence has been a questioning by management of the utility of marketing and the rate of return on marketing expenditures.

In part, marketing "rescue" efforts have failed because of the situation and circumstances. Projects that are out of sync with the community's needs will almost always result in market failures regardless of what efforts are made to promote them. Marketing efforts also have fallen short because of health care marketing's own limits.

Application of marketing as a management discipline within health care began to emerge in the middle 1970s. Since then, considerable progress has been made in extending marketing techniques to the health care setting. Quite reasonably the starting point for health care marketing's development was the knowledge base that had been established in the commercial sector for consumer goods. This base of theory and experience, while a useful starting point, did not provide a precise fit for the health care marketplace. For example, the lack of understanding of the health care consumer and the health care exchange transaction has been an important contributing factor in the failure of many preventive health care and health responsibility programs to achieve their goals. As a result, if significant progress is to be made in the health industry, health care marketing must evolve from this initial knowledge transference phase to the development of its own body of theory and practice. Obviously, this is a long-term task. However, it must continue to be pursued if health care marketing is to achieve its full potential.

At the individual institutional level, if the marketing function is to be successful, a marketing orientation must permeate the entire hospital. Operationally, this involves more than just the establishment of a marketing department. Marketing must become a way of day-to-day management and operational thinking. The hospital must become a market-driven organization, more concerned with patient or client attitudes and satisfaction than with professional convenience and imperatives. Within the hospital, serving and satisfying patient and community needs must become the prevailing attitude and the management instinct. Attention to community satisfaction must rival attention to clinical quality as the hospital's motivating force. In a marketplace characterized by alternatives and competition, no other approach will enable the organization to flourish, let alone survive.

With respect to corporate planning, the marketing process must begin within the planning process. This does not mean that marketing is, or should be, subsumed within the planning function. Like other disciplines within the hospital, marketing has a role and mission of its own. In fact, effective technical marketing performance is as important to the hospital's achieving cost effective results as is effective technical performance in any other program area or department. It does mean that marketing must be part of strategic planning, contributing to determining the needs of the community and shaping the hospital's response to meeting those needs. It is in this context that marketing is viewed in this chapter.

Appendix 15 describes in some depth one element of the marketing and planning process—demand analysis and projection. As indicated above, marketing research and marketing involve more than just demand forecasting. Demand analysis, however, is a beginning point from which other planning decisions and marketing actions must flow. Therefore, special attention is given to it in this appendix.

NARROWING THE FOCUS

As discussed earlier, the environmental assessment provides the overall foundation for the individual hospital's strategic plan. At this point in the planning process, however, the usefulness of the environmental assessment to hospital specific planning is limited. This is the case for, by design, the environmental assessment's focus is macro in nature. To be useful for an individual hospital's strategic planning, its perspective must be narrowed from the industrywide environment to the hospital's specific environment. This narrowing of focus is done in Steps 4 and 5.

STEP 4. HOSPITAL CURRENT SITUATION

Step 4, hospital current situation, is the institution specific analogue to Step 1, industry current situation. In this step, the specific strengths and weakness of the hospital are identified and assessed.

Such an appraisal of performance and status can be done informally through management review of goals and progress toward achieving goals, analysis of major accomplishments and shortfalls, and appraisals of individual or departmental performance. An informal approach, while doable and of benefit, represents less than the ideal model. Ideally, the assessment of the current situation should be a part of the hospital's ongoing market research and management control processes. It should be accomplished through the formal and systematic process of program evaluation, wherein the assessment is derived from the disciplined examination of the adequacy of programs,[7] organization, staffing, policies, procedures, level of resources, and results.[8] Appraisal of patient and community attitudes toward the hospital and its services should be included in this formal process.

Like Step 1, the purpose of Step 4 is to provide an objective picture of reality. Therefore, it should be developed with a careful avoidance of wishful thinking and unproductive charity relative to either management or performance shortfalls.

STEP 5. HOSPITAL OPERATING IMPLICATIONS

Step 5, hospital operating implications, is essentially a continuation of the translation process begun in Step 3. The comments that were made above, therefore, also apply here.

While generically similar, the two steps differ with respect to the degree of institutional specificity that they provide. Step 3 defines operating implications at the industrywide level. Step 5 pares these industrywide implications to provide a set of operating implications that are specific to a particular hospital.

In carrying out this step, management should bear in mind two points. First, as discussed above (see "Mechanics"), the results of Step 3 are a hybrid. That is, they are industrywide implications in the sense that they apply in general and in aggregate to the field. However, they are less than national in scope. The consensus-building approach that was suggested requires that the implications be modified to reflect the local environment that faces the hospital. Thus, the results of Step 3, while not being hospital specific, are reflective of the local environment.

Second, hospital specific operating implications are derived by comparing, or more accurately contrasting, the demands of the environment (Step 3) with the institution's specific attributes, resources, and talents (Step 4). In comparing an attribute with aspects of the environment, strategies and weaknesses *for the future* are determined. It does not necessarily follow that a current strength will be a strength in the future. Where the hospital's specific attributes meet or compare favorably with environmental implications or demands (strengths), the hospital specific operating implications focus on how to capitalize on that strength. In contrast, when there is a mismatch, that is, an attribute of the hospital's current situation does not fit with a demand in the environment (a weakness), the hospital's specific operating implication focuses on developing the needed attribute. Taken

---

[7]As discussed in the following chapter, programs are groups of activities that are all directed toward the same goal or end.

[8]The American Hospital Association's Program for Institutional Effectiveness Review (PIER) is a useful tool for aiding management in conducting a formal assessment of the hospital's status and performance.

as a whole, these findings are the hospital's operating implications.[9] These implications are the sum of each individual matching of attributes and needs. However, the hospital's operating implications should give explicit consideration to the implication(s) of some or all of these individual implications when taken together.

Figure 15.2 illustrates the above process. In reviewing this figure, the reader should recognize that the specific operating implications for a particular hospital are those operational actions that are necessary to enhance an existing area of performance weakness, as identified in the current situation, to the level where it meets the anticipated needs of the environment.

EXPANDING THE BASE

Hospital specific operating implications are obviously major considerations in shaping the hospital's strategy. They are not, however, the exclusive considerations. To reflect the unique character as well as the particular goals of the hospital, two additional types of information must be included as basic forces in the design of the institution's strategy. These additional considerations are depicted in Figure 15.1 as mission (Step 6) and initiatives (Step 7).

FIGURE 15.2   Step 5: Hospital Operating Implications

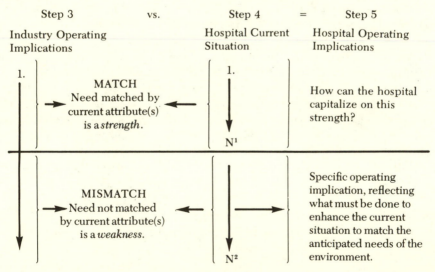

Step 3	vs.	Step 4	=	Step 5
Industry Operating Implications		Hospital Current Situation		Hospital Operating Implications

MATCH
Need matched by current attribute(s) is a *strength*.

How can the hospital capitalize on this strength?

MISMATCH
Need not matched by current attribute(s) is a *weakness*.

Specific operating implication, reflecting what must be done to enhance the current situation to match the anticipated needs of the environment.

---

[9]It is logically conceivable, though not realistic, that there could be no mismatches. If such were the case, the weakness as identified in Step 4 would serve as the product of Step 5.

STEP 6. MISSION

In the simplest sense, mission can be viewed as the broad, timeless definition of the scope and purpose of the hospital. It is typically given concrete form through the hospital's mission statement or statement of purpose. Such a statement is a formal document that expresses, in language for both internal and external audiences, the identity, function, and community or public service goals of the hospital. Table 15.1 presents examples of mission statements.

The process of defining and refining the hospital's mission is complex and interactive, with implications and importance beyond just the needs of corporate planning. However, in viewing the mission statement within the context of the planning process, several points should be emphasized.

1. In terms of presenting the hospital to the public as well as to the medical staff and employees, the mission statement is the hospital's fountainhead. It in effect defines the hospital's market niche. Therefore, not only should it be a product of careful board deliberation, but it should also be expressly ratified by the board.

TABLE 15.1   Examples: Mission Statement

1. Hospital Association
   The purpose of the Hospital Association is to help hospitals serve their communities.

2. Major Medical Center
   The purposes and objectives of the Dillon–Graszer Hospital Medical Center shall be as follows:
   a. To own, operate, support, and maintain the Dillon–Graszer Hospital Medical Center
   b. To furnish the patients of every race, creed, or nationality medical, clinical, and surgical attention and care; nursing, medical, social, and dietary services; and all other affiliated and related hospital and medical services
   c. To conduct educational and training activities in the field of medicine and medical care, including nursing, medical, and paramedical training, and education and training of medical students and graduate doctors
   d. To participate, so far as circumstaces may warrant and permit, in any activity designed and carried on to promote the general health of the community and the improvement thereof

3. Urban Teaching Hospital
   The Mackie Hospital is an urban teaching hospital whose primary purposes are to enhance the health status of its urban community, to provide health services to any member of the Jewish community of Metropolitan Middletown in need of such services, and to provide the nation with skilled health manpower to meet the health needs of urban communities.

2. In keeping with the above, neither the language of nor the concepts inherent in the mission statement should be allowed to be changed cavalierly. This does not mean that the mission statement is either above review or beyond modification. Just the opposite is the case. A hospital's mission statement should be examined regularly as an explicit step in the corporate planning process. Changes to the mission statement, however, should only be made after a careful evaluation of the health care environment and the needs of the hospital's market as well as a thorough consideration of the hospital's service philosophy. Within the review process, the prejudice should be toward maintaining continuity and consistency.

3. The review of the mission statement need not be a sequential component of the planning process. Rather, it can proceed simultaneously with the other early steps. In fact, a simultaneous approach may make the entire process more productive, for it provides an early opportunity to involve the board in the planning process.

In addition to the above, a final point should be highlighted. The mission statement serves as a means for adding unique direction and shape to the hospital's strategic plan, while at the same time serving as a device for delimiting the plan. It does this by setting out a guideline for determining what generic activities the hospital should as well as should not pursue. Using the example of Table 15.1, the Dillon–Graszer Hospital Medical Center mission statement allows the hospital to become directly involved in community redevelopment activities. At the same time, by inference, it directs it away from pursuits such as pure biomedical research and commercial business ventures.

STEP 7. INITIATIVES

When compared to the mission statement, initiatives represent what can be viewed as a countervailing philosophical pressure. They provide the means for pragmatically shaping and reshaping the operational character of the mission statement to reflect the changing needs of the community (market) and the resulting new operating goals of the hospital. Viewed less philosophically and more mechanically, initiatives are an explicit mechanism for forcing the planning process to remain vital, flexible, and responsive to the needs of patients and the community.

In their most basic form, initiatives are ad hoc, direct perceptions of what the organization should do. These perceptions, however, are neither established nor defined in a vacuum. As illustrated by Figure 15.1, they flow from and are in large part dependent upon two previous steps as well as market research information.

Hospital operating implications (Step 5), along with market research information, provide direct insight as to what activities the hospital should be undertaking to meet its internal operational as well as its community's needs.[10] It in effect provides a broad menu of potential initiatives that the hospital might justifiably pursue. Hospital current situation (Step 4) acts as a filter with respect to the range of possible initiatives. It establishes programmatic boundaries as to what can be done, in the sense of resources and of management change.

Recognizing the limits of the organization is a significant management understanding. While it is important that the hospital be able to move forward in a manner that is responsive to its emerging needs, such movement must be undertaken within a context of operational reality. Management must, therefore, strike a balance that judiciously uses initiatives to move the hospital forward without either overwhelming it or pulling it in what might appear to be conflicting directions.

INTEGRATION AND REFINEMENT

All of the foregoing can be viewed as establishing a base for the corporate strategy. Step 8, general goals, builds on this base.

STEP 8. GENERAL GOALS

Step 8 is an integrating step wherein the information and results of the previous steps are reviewed and distilled into a comprehensive set of general goals. These general goals in turn form the framework around which the actual strategy is built.

General goals can be defined as broad and enduring statements of significant end conditions or results that the hospital wishes to achieve. They are, in effect, the outcomes that the hospital establishes as its long-run targets for accomplishment.

The distillation process for the setting of general goals is procedurally simple but intellectually complex. The process is not a matter of mechanics. It is instead an exercise in rigorous thinking. Its focus is on sorting out, from within the fabric of the demands of the environment, those directions or accomplishments whose attainment will achieve, or help to achieve, the hospital's mission.

No procedural tricks or short cuts are involved in setting goals; hard work is essential. Functionally, management must first establish tentative goals and then sharpen them. The sharpening is done through a reiterative objective as well as subjective testing and modification of the initial goals to assure that within the context of its mission statement and environment,

---

[10]Marketing, through its product development and demand-stimulation components, also contributes to the ultimate success of initiatives.

that is, operating implications and initiatives, they move the hospital forward in a manageable manner. Table 15.2 presents examples of general goals.

In setting and testing its proposed goals, management should bear in mind three caveats. First, the number of goals should be limited. General goals are not departmental objectives. Rather, they are basic pillars or themes around which program directives, and later operating objectives, cluster. Second, while not having as acute a continuity and consistency bias as the mission statement, general goals should be relatively stable and enduring. Third, they should be sufficiently comprehensive that, taken as a whole, the goals provide meaningful end results for all aspects of the hospital's mission. Thus, while goals should be reviewed and established as part of the overall planning process on a year-to-year basis, they should be changed only after careful thought and with great care.

STEP 9. STRATEGIC ALTERNATIVES

Step 9, strategic alternatives, flows from both the previous step and Step 4, hospital current situation. Its focus is on identifying the strategy or strategies that might be employed by the hospital in pursuing its general goals.

This step, like the previous one, is also more a matter of management thinking than of procedural mechanics. Management must carefully define the range of alternatives available for meeting the hospital's goals and then

TABLE 15.2   Examples: General Goals

1. Hospital Association
    General goals 198X–199Y
    a. To preserve the ability and the opportunity of hospitals to fulfill their responsibilities for the delivery of health care
    b. To enhance the effectiveness of hospitals in improving the health status of their communities
    c. To assert leadership in stimulating the role of the hospital as the center for community health
    d. To establish the Association as a central figure in the development and implementation of health policy

2. Urban Teaching Hospital
    Over the next ten years, the general objectives of Mackie Hospital will be
    a. To establish itself as the preeminent urban community teaching hospital in the country
    b. To improve its effectiveness in enhancing the health status of its community
    c. To assert leadership in stimulating the development of its community

weed out those that, from the prospective of the hospital's real capacity and capability, are impractical. The informational basis for these decisions is obviously the data from Step 4 as well as all of the other foregoing steps. The actual decision process, however, cannot be effectively reduced to a formula. Rather, it relies on management's thoughtfully cataloging and shifting alternatives to deduce a realistic general set of operational approaches to achieving the hospital's goals.

For example, if one goal of a hospital is "to assert leadership in stimulating the development of its community" (see Table 15.2), then the alternative strategies that might be employed for accomplishing this could include

1. Purchasing property, renovating it, and then selling or leasing it

2. Making low-interest loans to small, community-based businesses

3. Aiding existing community groups to obtain urban development grants from either the government or private foundations

4. Constructing senior citizens housing

5. Approaching private foundations directly for community development grants

Based on the current situation (data from Step 4), several or all of these potential strategies might be eliminated. Assuming that the hospital had little or no endowment, alternatives 1, 2, and 4 would likely have to be disregarded, because none matches with a current attribute of the hospital. Strategies 3 and 5, on the other hand, might capitalize on the hospital's present talents in community relations and fund raising; both strategies might be accepted.

The refinement of strategic options process is depicted in Figure 15.1 by the narrowing of alternatives to form the corporate strategy.

STEP 10. FINANCIAL GUIDELINES

The general or overall financial guidelines (Step 10) are a prospective bench mark setting out both expenditure limitations and revenue targets for the planning and budgeting period. As illustrated in Figure 15.1, Step 10 is a product of the current situation (Step 4) and the hospital's financial policy decisions.

The current situation provides information as to the hospital's operating, nonoperating, philanthropic, reimbursement, and revenue environment. Those data provide the basis for projecting initial revenues. The financial policies are reflected in the hospital's long-range financial plan and specify operating margin rates and reserve levels and growth rates.[11] These policy decisions generally are established by the finance committee

---

[11]See Chapter 16 for a further discussion of long-range financial planning.

(of the governing board) and should be ratified by the full governing board. Together these two sources establish the basis for the initial budgetary guidelines, that is, expenditures limitation as well as operating margin and reserve targets (see Table 15.3).

Before leaving this step, it is important to recognize and understand the tentative nature of the initial financial guidelines. These financial decisions cannot be made in an operating vacuum. In fact, there is a reiterative relationship between the financial plan and the operating plan, with the two coming together when the revenue, expense, and capital budgets are integrated and brought into balance. As part of this balancing, the financial plan, and therefore the overall financial guidelines, may be revised. Even so, an initial plan and accompanying guideline are necessary in order to provide basic guidance.

CORPORATE STRATEGY

With the completion of Step 10, the stage is set for linking all the pieces together and formulating the hospital's specific strategy. This final step involves

1. Translating the strategic alternatives (Step 9) and the overall financial guidelines (Step 10) into program directives and corresponding initial program area guidelines

TABLE 15.3   Cleves Hospital Financial Guidelines

General Financial Policy 198X–199Y

Expenditures
For 198X expenses should increase by no more than 4.8%. By 199Y expenses should increase at a rate equal to the rate of growth in the gross state product.

Operating Margin
Operating margin should increase to an aggregate level of 6% by 199Y.

Operating Margin	198X	199Y
Patient care services	1%	4%
Nonpatient care services	3%	10%

Reserves
Current contingency revenue levels are adequate. Reserves, therefore, should be held constant.

Program Area Financial Guidelines
Program Area: Community Relations and Education
    For the coming year, resources should expand.
Program Area: Corporate Development
    For the coming year, resources should remain at the current budget level.

2. Reviewing, and if necessary modifying, the total corporate strategy to assure that it is financially and operationally balanced.[12]

Program directives are explicit statements of desired results and constraints by program area, that is, objectives by program area. They flow naturally from Step 9 in that they define, within the context and parameters of the selected strategic alternatives, the operational direction and expected accomplishments of each program area.

Using the previous example from Step 9, partial program directives for two of the hospital's program areas might be

—*Program Area: Community Relations and Education*
Utilize existing community relationships to identify and pursue urban redevelopment projects focused on improving housing.
—Aid at least two existing 501(c)(3) community groups in developing and submitting proposals to private foundations within the next year.

—*Program Area: Corporate Development*
Identify and develop relationships with private foundations interested in supporting voluntary initiatives aimed at community development.
—Submit at least three proposals to various foundations within the next 24 months.

These examples are presented as only partial program directives because other strategic alternatives might also affect these program areas. If such were the case, these directives would be expanded to encompass additional desired results.

Program area financial guidelines are the last component of the corporate strategy. These guidelines flow from the general constraint of the overall financial guidelines. They differ, however, in that at this point in the process they are not specific quantitative bench marks. Rather, they are statements of relative emphasis, indicating not a program dollar limit but whether a program area should expect to grow, remain constant, or contract. Due to the reiterative relationship of the operating and financial plans (see Chapter 16), this degree of financial guidance is all that is necessary at this point.[13] Table 15.3 illustrates general and program area financial guidelines.

The corporate strategy is now functionally complete. However, before implementation as the basis for operational planning and budgeting, it

---

[12]See Chapter 16 and Glossary for definition and discussion of programs.

[13]If quantified guidelines are available, they would be useful. However, given the reiterative nature of the process and, as discussed later, the pragmatic limits to either growth or contraction, it is counterproductive, in terms both of the added work needed to develop the detail and of the behavioral reaction to later changes, to push at this point for specific quantification.

should be reviewed to assure that it is financially and operationally balanced. This procedural check is recommended as a means of avoiding later the wasted effort and frustration that will result if the strategy is not internally coordinated and consistent.

The financial review is simply a testing of the program area financial guidelines against the overall financial guidelines. Its purpose is to assure that, when aggregated, the program area guidelines are consistent with the overall guidelines. For example, this review should identify situations where directed program area growth, net of directed program area contractions, exceeds the total growth anticipated by the overall financial guidelines. The importance of identifying and correcting this kind of inconsistency, before operational planning and budgeting begin, is obvious.

The purpose of the operational review is similar. Its scope, however, is broader, encompassing all aspects of the corporate strategy development process.

Figure 15.3 uses a wheel to illustrate the concept of operational review. The wheel in the figure depicts the components of, as well as the interrelationship of the components to, the totality of the corporate strategy. The point of using a wheel is to emphasize the need for internal consistency between general objectives and the environment, coordination between general objectives and program area directives, consistency among program area directives, and balance between program areas, resources, and organization.[14]

Operational review is the means for assuring the coordination, consistency, and balance of the corporate strategy. It provides an opportunity for a final check to guarantee that: all aspects of the strategy have been addressed; at all levels, internal consistency has been built into the strategy; and resources, organization, and program areas are coordinated and balanced.

The mechanics of conducting both of these reviews is not involved. Essentially, all that is required is that management, using a template like that of Figure 15.3, take a holistic view of the corporate strategy and examine each piece of the strategy against both itself and the whole. Depending upon how the hospital's corporate planning process is structured, this can be done either by a desk audit or, probably more productively, through the use of a planning and budgeting committee. Table 15.4 presents a summary of organizational accountabilities for this as well as the other steps in the strategic planning process.

---

[14]"Resources" refers to the financial, human, and physical plant "raw material" available for use in implementing the program area directives. "Organization" refers to the hospital's internal arrangements of functions (for example, departments), its governance structure and relationships with operating subsidiaries (if any exist), and relationships with external organizations and agencies (for example, a university, voluntary health agencies, government). Both resources and organization include the underlying policies and strategies (for example, a financial policy).

FIGURE 15.3   Operational Review

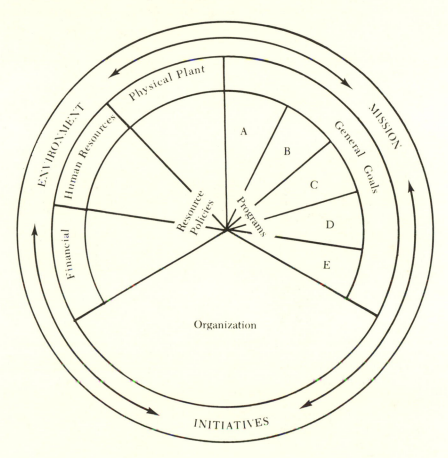

CONTINGENCY PLANNING AND MODELING

Before leaving strategic planning, the matters of contingency planning and modeling should be touched upon. The two topics are not directly related in a substantive sense. They are linked, however, by the common risk of quantitative analysis obscuring or confusing in meaningless detail careful decision making. They are also joined in that if not controlled they both will contribute to planning becoming an end to itself, with management relying on "scenarios" and the "numbers"—instead of clear-headed judgment—to make decisions.

With respect to contingency planning the foregoing has set out an ap-

TABLE 15.4   Strategic Planning Accountabilities

Board	Exec. Mgmt.*	Senior Mgmt.*	Staff Planning & Budgeting Committee	Corporate Planning	Budget Director	Fiscal Service
	---	---		1. Current Situation	Industry	
	---	---	---	2. Industry Assumptions	---	
			---	3. Industry Operating Implications		
	---	---	---	4. Hospital Current Situation	---	
	---	---	---	5. Hospital Operating Implications		

6. Mission

7. Initiatives
8. General Goals

9. Strategic Alternatives

Financial Policies

10. Financial Guidelines

11. Program Directives
    Program Financial Guidelines

Strategy Review

Approach

—————— Primary Accountability

---------- Supporting (staff or participative) Accountability

*See Chapters 16 and 17 and Glossary for definitions as well as discussion of function.

proach to planning that appears to establish a single strategy. This is partly true. However, it is misleading to view a single strategy as a fixed strategy.

Effective planning requires that the environment be continually monitored and that an assessment be continually made as to whether any significant changes either are emerging or have taken place. To the extent that the environment has changed, the hospital's strategy must also change. Thus, while the hospital, at any point in time, has only a single strategy, that strategy is not inalterably set in time duration or substance. Instead, it is a strategy built on a dynamic base, reflecting the current best estimates of the demands and pressures of the environment; it changes as those demands and pressures change. The environmental assessment process, notably the hospital operating implications element, should have provided a sense of areas in which the hospital is vulnerable. Unexpected changes in these areas should stimulate a prompt review of the hospital's strategy.

The alternative to this approach to accommodating change is to develop explicit contingency plans. The risk of this option is twofold. First, it is an unending process, limited only by one's imagination as to the number of possible alternatives that can be conceived. Second, it draws energy and attention away from the critical matter of monitoring the environment. The hospital does not need volumes of contingency plans. Rather, it needs a sensitive measure of the environment and a planning process that enables it to reformulate its strategy quickly to capitalize upon both emerging environmental trends as well as explicit changes in the environment.

This does not mean that a hospital should not have any contingency plans. Plans for potential events such as community disasters or labor disruptions are a necessary part of hospital management. Anticipating and planning for such explicit contingencies is markedly different from trying to anticipate an endless array of unknown contingencies.

Modeling—particularly with the advent of low cost, high power computers—represents a different aspect of the same danger. Models and modeling offer a seductive but nevertheless false promise of precision and certainty. If the promise is uncritically accepted, the model's judgment will be allowed to replace management's analysis, knowledge of the market, intuition, and experience. Such a trade-off may seem to work for a time in a steady state environment. However, in a changed and changing environment such as that now confronting hospitals, abdication of management judgment to the simplistic mechanics of a model will only result in missed opportunities, lost services, and, perhaps, even financial failure.

Nothing is inherently wrong with models and the use of models in the planning process for such elements as demand forecasting, financial projections, and "what if" questioning. In fact, models can be beneficial if they force management to make explicit its assumptions and to clarify operating cause-and-effect relationships. If used in this manner they can be helpful, bringing rigor and discipline to the planning process. At the same time, they can eliminate some of the number-crunching tedium. However, if models are used to avoid clarifying assumptions and to obscure the basic operating relationships that determine performance and results, then they represent a danger.

The lesson is simple. Models are not necessarily to be avoided. Rather, they should be used as a tool, employed either after assumptions and underlying processes and relationships have been made explicit or as an aid in helping management to make these factors explicit. Models must not, however, be allowed to replace an understanding of the anatomy of the planning and operating processes or management judgment.

EVOLUTION

A closing point should be noted. The previous sections have outlined a comprehensive approach to developing a hospital's strategic plan. Full implementation of these decision processes and concepts is an involved and complex task, which should typically not be attempted in a single stage. Rather, the hospital's strategic planning process should evolve, with each succeeding cycle becoming more refined.

The key to the long-run acceptance and successful operation of any corporate planning process is controlled management impatience combined with a clear understanding of where one wishes to be in the end. The foregoing has defined the end. Management must provide its own sense of pace, recognizing the evolutionary nature of change.

SUGGESTED READINGS

American Hospital Association. *Environmental Assessment of the Hospital Industry.*

Hofer, Charles W. and Sahendel, Dan. *Strategy Formulation: Analytical Concepts.*

Kotler, Philip and Murray, Michael. "Third Sector Management: The Role of Marketing."

Lorange, Peter and Vancil, Richard F. *Strategic Planning Systems.*

MacStravic, Robin E. *Marketing Health Care.*

Mintzberg, Henry. "Planning on the Left Side and Managing on the Right."

Peters, Joseph P. A *Strategic Planning Process for Hospitals.*

Peters, Thomas J. and Waterman, Robert H., Jr. *In Search of Excellence.*

Steiner, George A. *Strategic Planning.*

Tuller, Edwin and Kozak, David. "Logical Thought Process Key to Corporate Plan."

APPENDIX 15
MARKET RESEARCH: COMMUNITY DEMAND
ANALYSIS FOR HOSPITAL
AMBULATORY CARE SERVICES[15]
BY SIMONE TSENG[16]

Strategic planning has become an essential management tool to assess the hospital's current and future environments and identify strategies that coordinate its mission and goals with its strengths, weaknesses, opportunities, and threats. Community demand analysis is an integral component of the hospital strategic planning process and an important market research tool that determines the types of service needed and estimates the magnitude of market shortages in the service area. Data limitations will continue to frustrate efforts to analyze community level demand for specific ambulatory care services. However, the estimates of market shortage and surplus that result from community demand analysis can provide useful guidance to hospital decision makers and can assist them in identifying new opportunities to serve the community.

The term market research covers a variety of tools and techniques for systematically and objectively developing useful information relevant to identifying and solving marketing and planning problems. Demand analysis or demand forecasting is just one of these techniques. Other types of market research not covered in this discussion, but which offer useful information for hospitals considering developing new services or changing existing services include pricing studies, consumer attitude surveys, and service acceptance focus groups.

ANALYSIS OF COMMUNITY CHARACTERISTICS

Before a hospital can define a service area for a particular ambulatory care program, the characteristics of the surrounding geographic region must be examined. The term community refers to the population unit that is most convenient for preliminary analysis and within which the users of the hospital's ambulatory care services are located. Whether it is defined by zip code, city, county, or other boundaries, the community must be large enough to include the relevant populations and to furnish adequate data to complete a community profile, and yet be small enough to reveal distinct character-

---

[15]Adapted, with permission, from Chapter 4 of *Hospital Ambulatory Care: Making it Work,* ©1983 by American Hospital Publishing, Inc.

[16]Simone Tseng is currently the Director of Marketing at the University of Chicago Medical Center. At the time she developed this material she was on the staff of the Division of Hospital Planning, American Hospital Association.

istics. On the basis of physician-utilization patterns and other factors, a service area within this broader community is then defined.

Political and Economic Profile. The hospital should be aware of the perspectives and future expectations of the community leadership, such as officials of local government and health planning and regulatory agencies, civic groups, and individual community leaders. The economic component of the community profile should address the state of the local economy and major sources of employment. Land use considerations, including the current and projected degrees of residential and commercial development, are important because of their impact on population and health care manpower growth. For ambulatory care services, the transportation systems (major highways and public transportation) strongly influence the choice of providers and should be documented. Housing characteristics also yield useful information about the local economy and health status of the population.

Demographic Profile. A thorough investigation of demographic characteristics is essential to gain an understanding of the community's health needs and the unique factors that determine the population's demand for services. The characteristics of greatest importance include

—Population size and rate of growth

—Age distribution, or proportion of the population within each age group

—Sex ratio, or proportion of males to females

—Racial, ethnic, and religious composition, in terms of percentage of each and geographic distribution in the defined community

—Psychosocial/cultural characteristics, including attitudes toward seeking medical care, physicians, illness, self-care

—Education levels and health awareness

—Mobility, in terms of immigration and emigration rates, as an indicator of population shifts and community stability

—Fertility

—Health status, in terms of mortality, morbidity, and disability

Health Services Inventory. The community profile must include descriptions of the health care resources of the community, that is, the facilities and manpower available to meet the health care needs of the population. The ambulatory care services provided by each hospital or by independent physicians' offices and clinics in the community should be charted. After the specific service area is defined, a more detailed analysis of demand versus supply should be conducted for individual services, and data regarding office-based individual and group practitioners should be compiled.

DEFINITION OF THE SERVICE AREA

The techniques used in defining an ambulatory care service area are less sophisticated than those used for inpatient care because of the lack of areawide utilization data for physician services. As briefly described in the following section, the market share approach to defining inpatient service areas is not applicable to ambulatory care services. Because definition of an ambulatory care service area must rely on incomplete and frequently subjective information, a combination of analytical approaches is advocated. Where historical data are available, the service area can be defined on the basis of the hospital's historic dependence on (or proportion of patient visits from) specific communities, supplemented by travel time and distance limits and knowledge of the locations of alternative sources of care. If patient origin information is not available, as in the case of a proposed new service, a greater reliance on the travel time and distance limit approach is necessary.

Successful market research necessitates an empirical rather than a normative approach to service area definition. All relevant factors and assumptions that might influence a resident's choice of a particular facility should be explicitly stated. The primary service area for a particular ambulatory care service should be defined to include those residents who view the hospital in question as a major source of care. The majority of the hospital's patients for the service in question will be drawn from the primary service area, and a large segment of the remaining patients will come from surrounding regions referred to as the secondary service area. Given a high probability of error in predicting the actual behavior of residents, it is wise to consider several different definitions of the service area, or to examine primary and secondary service areas simultaneously. Separate demand analyses for the two adjacent regions provide the opportunity to examine and forecast the utilization behavior of two distinct populations.

The Market Share Approach. The service area population can be estimated without rigid geographic boundaries in a market share analysis of inpatient services when reliable patient origin data are available. For example, the relevance index approach determines the market share of each facility for specified zip codes, census tracts, or minor civil divisions. Service area boundaries are then drawn for each facility to include the regions of high and/or moderate relevance. The contribution of each region to the service area population is calculated by applying the relevance index or market share percentage to the total population of the region. However, this method is not applicable to ambulatory care services because the denominator of the market share measure, or the total number of physician visits from an area, usually cannot be estimated.

Patient Origin Approach. Patient origin data by zip code should be available at the individual institution for ambulatory care services. The service area boundaries are drawn to include the areas from which the majority of the outpatient visits originate. The hospital may determine that the service should draw at least 75% of its total visits from its primary service area. Alternatively, or in addition, the service area boundaries may be drawn to include each zip code or locality that contributes at least 5% of the hospital's total visits to the particular service. The commitment index, which is defined as the percentage of the facility's total outpatient visits that originate from a specific area, is useful in these determinations:

$$\frac{\text{Commitment}}{\text{index}} = \frac{\text{Number of visits from area to hospital service}}{\text{Total hospital visits}}$$

This index examines the facility's degree of dependence on a given community, that is, the proportion of the facility's ambulatory care resources that is committed to the community. Its perspective differs from that of the relevance index, or market share, which indicates the degree to which a community depends on a particular facility, that is, the relevance of the facility to that population. Calculation of the commitment index for ambulatory care services is based on the individual hospital's patient origin data, as illustrated in Figure 15.A-1. In this figure, the primary service area would include zip code areas 00002 and 00003, which contributed 75% of the family practice clinic's visits over a one-year period. The inclusion of other areas is based on the consideration of other relevant factors (such as travel time and distance and the proximity of alternative sources of care) in the assessment of the degree of reliance of each area on the hospital service. The degree of dependence of individual communities on the hospital is an important subjective consideration in the determination of an ambulatory care service area.

The locations of all ambulatory care providers of the service in question, including physicians' offices, should be marked on a detailed map of the region. Ultimately, the definition of service area boundaries involves the examination of patient origin data and consideration of the location of

FIGURE 15.A-1   Example of Calculations of Commitment Indexes

Zip Code	Number of Visits to Family Practice Clinic in One Year	Commitment Indexes (Percent of Provider's Visits from Zip Code Area)
00001	240	240/2000 = 0.12
00002	860	860/2000 = 0.43
00003	640	640/2000 = 0.32
00004	160	160/2000 = 0.08
00005	100	100/2000 = 0.05
Total	2,000	1.00

the facility in relation to other ambulatory care providers, travel flow and accessibility by public transportation and highways, and the shopping habits and community loyalties of local residents. In addition, geographic barriers, such as rivers or mountains, and socioeconomic and cultural barriers, such as the income level, race, ethnic background, language, and religious preferences of various segments of the population, should be considered in the determination of service area boundaries.

Travel Time and Distance Limits. A very simple approach to service area determination is to set travel time and/or travel distance limits for specific services provided by a particular facility, and to draw boundaries accordingly. Travel time is a more justifiable measure of convenience than travel distance to a particular facility, but the use of both measures can be effective. Theoretically, the travel time or distance limit would be higher for more specialized services than for primary care.

To place a high emphasis on travel time or distance factors implies a normative determination, that is, the setting of standards for the desired availability of services. However, if the limits are determined by consideration of actual or probable utilization and other relevant factors, they are simply an index of physical accessibility or convenience. The distance traveled to the hospital by patients currently using the ambulatory care unit can be determined from patient origin data. A chart similar to that shown in Figure 15.A-2 can be used to examine patient load by service. As seen in the figure, a service such as ambulatory surgery may draw patients from a larger radius than a more available service such as internal medicine. Service area size is likely to vary for the different ambulatory care services provided by the hospital, depending on the availability of alternative sources of care and other relevant factors that determine the demand for specific services.

A critical factor in determining the boundaries of the service area is

FIGURE 15.A-2   Example of Data Showing Distance between
                   Hospitals and Patients' Homes

Outpatient Service	*Percentage of Patients*		
	0–5 Miles	*5–10 Miles*	*Over 10 Miles*
Internal medicine	65	30	5
Ambulatory surgery	50	30	20
Pediatrics	65	25	10
Family practice	60	30	10
Obstetrics/gynecology	70	25	5

Adapted from N. H. McMillan, *Planning for Survival: A Handbook for Hospital Trustees.* (Chicago: American Hospital Association, 1978), p. 43.

the extent of population concentration and urbanization. Clearly, service area definition is most difficult in urban areas where the effect of distance is less important in the patient's choice of a source of care. Socioeconomic, ethnic, and religious factors as well as perceptions of quality, access, and overall convenience (for example, waiting times in clinics and for appointments) determine utilization patterns when multiple resources are available. Thus, the concept of nonoverlapping service areas in urban areas is far from reality. At best, service area boundaries can be drawn with an effort to cluster resources that are geographically proximate. Decisions on the quantity of services to provide must then be based on assumptions regarding the relative use of those multiple resources by the defined population. The risk of error can be minimized only by the review of actual utilization data for those resources.

In summary, the approaches to service area definition for ambulatory care are largely subjective, combining available data on utilization and community characteristics with judgments on the behavior of residents. Because of the limited availability of ambulatory care utilization data, the assumptions that are made in drawing service area boundaries must be conservative.

DEMAND ANALYSIS MODEL

The determination of area boundaries for a particular ambulatory care service enables the hospital to estimate the population-based demand and physician supply of that service area, from which the market shortage or surplus of physicians is determined. The methodology discussed below can then be used to estimate the future utilization of the hospital's existing ambulatory care services and to assess the current and future community demand for potential new services. If a market shortage of physicians is believed to exist and the service in question is consistent with the hospital's mission and strategy for services delivery, initiation or expansion of the service becomes a strategic option for the hospital. Before the hospital can commit itself to a new service, the financial feasibility and the effects on hospital utilization, case mix, medical staff, and other personnel must be assessed.

The obstacle to community-based analysis that is most frequently mentioned is the lack of areawide ambulatory care utilization data. With few exceptions, the absence of areawide physician utilization data has prevented planners from determining local physician use rates. However, state and national utilization data can be used effectively to produce local demand estimates and forecasts that provide guidance in strategic decision making. The methodology summarized here attempts to factor in the unique characteristics of the local area.

The following key units and measures are defined to facilitate the reader's understanding of the methodology:

—*Active physician full-time equivalents (FTEs)*. The *physician* category includes all duly licensed and currently practicing doctors of medicine and doctors of osteopathy who spend some time in caring for ambulatory patients at an office location. Hospital-based physicians (residents or full-time hospital staff) are excluded. The term *active* refers to physicians who are professionally active as providers of patient care. Inactivity for physicians may be a shift to research, teaching, or administrative duties or to retirement or temporary leave. Estimates of the number of active physician FTEs should ideally be based on the numbers of active full-time and part-time physicians. Frequently, these data are not available. However, an assumption may be made that the large majority of physicians are in full-time practice and provide the normal amount of ambulatory care services at an office location.

—*Annual physician productivity rate*. The productivity rate refers to the average number of visits per year provided per physician in each of the specialties.

—*Physician use rate*. The use rate relates the use of physician services to the population, in terms of physician visits per person per year. It excludes physician visits to hospital inpatients.

—*Visit*. This term is used to refer to a direct, personal exchange between an ambulatory patient and the physician (or members of the physician's staff) for the purpose of seeking care and rendering health services.

Overview of Methodology. Before a hospital can estimate the future demand for specific ambulatory care services in a service area, the current-year physician demand must be determined. The current-year demand analysis methodology is presented, followed by guidelines for forecasting future market shortages and surpluses of physician services. The key factors in this method are the service area population, physician supply, physician use rates (visits per person per year), and annual physician productivity rates. To determine the current-year demand, the challenge is to arrive at the best possible estimates of these four factors.

To forecast the future service area demand, the assumption is made that both physician use rates and physician productivity rates will remain constant, based on current-year estimates. Emphasis is placed on obtaining population projections that are based on conservative assumptions. In addition, the difficult task of forecasting the future physician supply may necessitate the use of several supply projections based on alternative assumptions. In general, the time horizon for physician demand and supply forecasts may extend to ten years. However, it must be emphasized that the accuracy of such estimates beyond five years is highly questionable as a result of the changing environment and the impact of unforeseeable socioeconomic forces. The current-year demand analysis model for a specific service area is summarized in Figure 15.A-3 and consists of the following components:

—*Current-year physician demand*

Step 1. Service area population estimation—current year, by age and sex (cohort groups)

Step 2: Determination of physician use rates (visits per person per year)—by age and sex

Step 3: Estimation of population-based demand for visits—by age, sex, and physician specialty, derived from Steps 1 and 2

Step 4: Determination of annual physician productivity rates—by physician specialty

Step 5: Estimation of population-based demand for physicians—by physician specialty, derived from Steps 3 and 4

—*Current-year physician supply*—active FTEs, by specialty and by age

—*Current-year market shortage or surplus*—the difference between population-based demand for physicians (Step 5 of demand estimate) and the physician-supply estimate, by specialty

—*Hospital service objectives and ambulatory care requirements*—for those services in which a market shortage is determined, feasible objectives for new or expanded hospital services specified in terms of the estimated shortage. Physician requirements for the services are derived from those objectives for the current year

FIGURE 15.A-3 Summary of Current-Year Demand Analysis

Demand Step 1 Population estimates for service area, by age and sex	×	*Demand Step 2* Physician use rates, by age and sex	=	*Demand Step 3* Total physician visits required to meet service area demand, by specialty
Demand Step 3 Total physician visits required to meet service area demand, by specialty	÷	*Demand Step 4* Annual physician productivity rate, by specialty	=	*Demand Step 5* Total physicians required to meet service area demand, by specialty
Demand Step 5 Total physicians required to meet service area demand, by specialty	−	*Supply Estimate* Total physician FTEs, by specialty	=	Current market shortage (or surplus), by specialty

Current-Year Physician Supply. To estimate the current supply of physicians in the defined area, data must be gathered from several sources. State licensing agencies generally provide the most complete and up-to-date information on physicians practicing in the state. The types of data collected and tabulated vary from state to state. The data from licensing agencies can be supplemented with data from local medical societies and by checking telephone listings and hospital mailing lists.

Supply should be estimated in terms of active full-time-equivalent physicians. State level or county level average percentages of active physicians and active physicians by type of practice can be applied to the total physician equivalents in the service area when local breakdowns are not available. The current-year supply estimates will serve as the basis for projecting future physician supply.

Current Market Shortage or Surplus. For the current year the physician supply estimates are compared to the demand projections by specialty. The difference between the demand for and supply of physicians is taken as a measure of the ability of the service area to support a new or expanded source of ambulatory care services (see Figure 15.A-4).

| Total physicians required to meet service area demand, by specialty (demand estimate) | − | Total active physician FTEs, by specialty (supply estimate) | = | Current market shortage (or surplus), by specialty |

It is critical to note that the estimated excess demand is not necessarily unmet, but may be unexpressed within that service area. Where a resource shortage exists, causing such inconveniences as long office or clinic waiting times or difficulties in obtaining appointments, residents may seek care outside of the service area. In areas with high migration rates, a large percentage of estimated excess demand may be unexpressed due to the tendency of new residents to retain former sources of care. Patients are often willing to spend a longer time traveling to maintain a strong primary care physician-patient relationship.

FIGURE 15.A-4   Example of Current-Year Market Shortage or Surplus of Physicians, by Specialty

Specialty	Demand	Supply	Shortage (or Surplus)
General practice	32.9	25.0	7.9
Internal medicine	10.5	4.0	6.5
General surgery	8.1	4.0	4.1
Obstetrics/gynecology	10.7	8.0	2.7
Pediatrics	6.3	5.0	1.3

Forecasting Community Demand   The method used to forecast the market shortage or surplus of physician services parallels the current-year demand analysis model (Figure 15.A-5). In fact, each step of the demand analysis can be performed for each of the current and future years before proceeding to the next step. For example, Step 1 might be performed for 1982, 1984, and 1986, and then Step 2 would be performed for those years, and so on. The only difference in the demand analysis methodology for future years is the use of a range of physician supply estimates for each projection year.

Physician-demand projections.

FIGURE 15.A-5   Summary of Demand Forecasting Methodology

Demand Step 1 Population projections for service area, by age and sex (future)	×	*Demand Step 2* Physician use rates, by age and sex (current)	=	*Demand Step 3* Total physician visits required to meet service area demand, by specialty (future)
Demand Step 3 Total physician visits required to meet service area demand, by specialty (future)	÷	*Demand Step 4* Annual physician productivity rate, by specialty (current)	=	*Demand Step 5* Total physicians required to meet service area demand, by specialty (future)
Demand Step 5 Total physicians required to meet service area demand, by specialty (future)	− − −	*Range of Projections* *Supply* Total physician FTEs, by specialty (assumption 1) Total physician FTEs, by specialty (assumption 2) Total physician FTEs, by specialty (assumption 3)	= = =	*Range of Market* *Shortage Forecasts* Future market shortage or surplus, by specialty (assumption 1) Future market shortage or surplus, by specialty (assumption 2) Future market shortage or surplus, by specialty (assumption 3)

Physician-supply projections.   Unlike the demand for physician services, there is no clear relationship between the supply of physicians and the size of the service area population. That is, an increase in the population does not necessarily imply a proportional increase in the number of physicians. The assumption that the service area will sustain a constant physician-to-population ratio should be made only if the physician supply trends in the past and an examination of service area characteristics support that assumption.

The use of several physician supply projections allows one to examine a range of possible outcomes contingent upon various conditions that may occur in the service area. Each projection yields different combinations of active physicians by specialty for each projection year. Once specified, the planner may choose to endorse one of the supply projections as having the highest probability of occurrence or assign probabilities of occurrence to each projection.

All projections are derived from current estimates of the physician supply and an analysis, by specialty, of the age distribution of these physicians. If the age distribution is accurate, the loss of physicians through retirement or death can be forecast. Such an analysis may demonstrate a need for active recruitment efforts. For example, the age distribution in Figure 15.A-6 indicates that a large number of active physicians can be expected to retire in the next five to ten years and that there are few young physicians establishing practices in the area. Such warning signs must be addressed if the hospital is to maintain its referral base and its ability to meet the needs of the community. A potential shortage of ambulatory care physicians in the community clearly demands the formulation of strategic actions by the hospital.

In addition to examining the age distribution of physicians, it is necessary to consider the following factors:

—Supply of medical graduates from educational programs in the area

—Residential characteristics of the service area, for example, standard of living and cultural attractions

FIGURE 15.A-6   Age Distribution of Active Physicians in Hypothetical Service Area

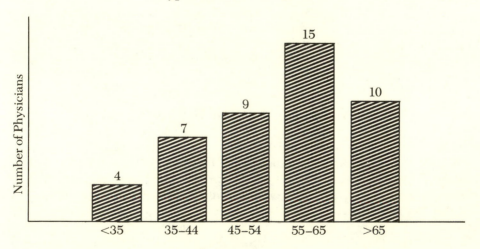

—Available opportunities for physicians to join group practices

—Projected growth of the service area population

—Projected residential and/or commercial development of the service
area

These and other interrelated factors determine the ability of the service
area to recruit and maintain physicians. After a study of such factors, assumptions may be made regarding the expected inflow and outflow of physicians. The physician supply projections would be based on different
assumptions for key factors. For example, three different supply projections
might correspond to a constant physician supply, a constant physician-to-
population ratio, and an increasing physician-to-population ratio based on
assumptions regarding the success of hospital recruitment efforts, future
commercial development, and potential development of new health facilities and services, respectively (Figure 15.A-7). If reliable historical data
can be obtained, identifiable trends in service area physician supply are
often the best predictors of the short-term future. However, service area
characteristics should be considered in developing all supply projections
regardless of historical data availability, as significant new forces may become apparent.

Service Objectives and Physician Requirements. To take the demand
analysis a step further, it is essential to translate the number of additional
physicians or physician visits required to meet the service area demand
(the estimated market shortage) into realistic objectives for the hospital-
based service in question.

The determination of utilization objectives for a given service is highly
dependent on the characteristics of the individual community and its residents. It is critical to consider such factors as the tendency of residents to
retain former sources of care, the availability of transportation, and the time
lag to be expected in the development of community awareness of the
service. In addition, it is critical to examine the capacity of existing re-

FIGURE 15.A-7   Example of Physician Supply Projections for
Pediatricians in Primary Service Area, Based
on Alternative Assumptions

	Supply of Pediatricians		
Assumptions	*Current*	*Year 3*	*Year 5*
Supply unchanged	15.0	15.0	15.0
Physician-to-population ratio unchanged	15.0	17.5	21.0
Increase of two pediatricians/year	15.0	21.0	25.0

sources in the service area. To a large extent, the achievement of projected utilization levels will depend on the plans for growth of neighboring providers. Consideration of the plans and potential capacity of local providers to expand and or initiate ambulatory care programs provides a well-informed basis on which utilization objectives can be determined.

Given the uncertainty in predictions of consumer behavior, it is advisable to examine several alternative sets of feasible utilization objectives for the hospital's outpatient service over a three-year to five-year period. It is inappropriate to assume that a high percentage of the estimated excess demand in the service area will be captured immediately by a proposed new service. The wisdom of conservative estimates cannot be overemphasized.

Each utilization objective for a given service should be stated with its associated assumptions. In a hypothetical case, Hospital A might set an objective for a new internal medicine clinic to meet 20% of the market shortage of internal medical services in its first year, 30% by its third year, and 40% by its fifth year. Figure 15.A-8 illustrates the method used to estimate the clinic's physician requirements.

Finally, the analyst should recommend the most realistic set of utilization objectives for the hospital, based on intuition and understanding of the community. Such a recommendation may assist hospital decision makers in examining the range of potential outcomes. If the hospital adopts a set of objectives for the provision of ambulatory care services based on the demand analysis, a program for evaluating progress toward meeting those objectives should be established. Periodic reports should be reviewed to compare actual utilization with expected or forecasted utilization. Demand projections can be adjusted as necessary.

Assumptions, Caveats, and Adjustments of Method.

Physician demand. In using state and national average use rates, this methodology assumes that an individual service area that has been properly categorized (rural or urban, high or low income, and so on) will be *average* in its demand for physician services. To minimize the risk of error, a thorough understanding of community residents is crucial. The psychosocial char-

FIGURE 15.A-8   Example of a Physician-Requirement Estimate for Hospital Outpatient Service in Internal Medicine

Projection Year	Service Area's Market Shortage	Hospital Objective (%)	No. of Internists Required
Current	5.0	20	1.0
Year 3	7.0	30	2.1
Year 5	10.0	40	4.0

acteristics, that is, attitudes toward seeking medical care and toward self-care, and the lifestyles of residents have a profound effect on the utilization of ambulatory care services.

The key question of the demand projection is, How will utilization rates change over time? In a rapidly changing environment, it is unlikely that utilization levels will be stable. Growth is expected in ambulatory care utilization as cost containment pressures encourage the provision of lower-cost alternatives to inpatient care. However, it is difficult to quantify the potential impact of external forces on future use rates. Examination of national survey data from the past ten years indicates that use rates have fluctuated within a narrow margin without a clear pattern. The analyst can make only a "best guess" about the future based on historical information and an understanding of the factors affecting demand. National level and state level trends in the organization and financing of ambulatory care services should be followed closely. If it is assumed that the service area use rates will remain stable, the risks of error must be examined.

In addition, a key assumption of this methodology is that the demand for visits is distributed evenly over time. Certain services, such as pediatrics and obstetrics, will typically exhibit a seasonal fluctuation in volume. However, because demand estimates generally are calculated for a full year, this assumption should not contribute significantly to error.

Physician supply. In a service area where the number of physicians is small, an error of one physician in the supply estimate may have a significant impact on estimates of unmet demand. Physician supply information must frequently be pieced together from multiple and noncomparable data sources. Adjustments in the data that are made to resolve inconsistent time frames, different measures or units of supply, and different geographic breakdowns, for example, zip codes versus census tracts, must be clearly specified.

The impact of substitute services for each specialty should be examined and, where significant, should be accounted for in the physician supply estimates. Midlevel health practitioners play an increasingly important role as providers of ambulatory care services, particularly in rural and underserved areas. When local data are not available, data from recent studies assessing the productivity and percentage of physician visits delegated to midlevel health practitioners can be incorporated into estimates of the physician services supply. Also, specialty substitution will occur in some cases. For example, in a demand analysis for pediatric services, general and family practitioners should be included with pediatricians in estimating the available supply of pediatric visits. In such cases, where the focus of analysis is services used by a particular population group rather than services provided by a particular specialty, the methodology should be adjusted to use the physician visit as the unit of analysis.

Physician productivity.   The organization of the area's health care delivery system must be studied to ensure that selected or surveyed physician productivity rates reflect the local conditions. The physician productivity rates will differ for a system based on physicians in individual practices as compared to one based on clinics, HMOs, and group practices. Differences in these rates can also be attributed to the use of physician extenders, involvement in medical education programs, the type of physician compensation, for example, fee-for-service versus salary versus capitation, and various other factors.

Out-of-area utilization.   Finally, the utilization by service area residents of physician services located outside of the primary area should be estimated to assist in the interpretation of market shortage estimates. The market shortage of ambulatory care services may be overestimated if this effect is not accounted for, particularly in underserved areas. However, a local population survey may be necessary to estimate the actual level of out-of-area utilization, which may differ for each physician specialty, and to determine the magnitude of access problems in the area. Where time and resource constraints prevail, the conventional assumption is made—that the supply as well as demand for physician services are confined by the geographic boundaries of the service area.

16

Operational Planning

This and the following chapters in Part IV address what can be characterized as a translation process. In sum, they focus on the process of converting the corporate strategy into health and patient care programs.

Statements of purpose and strategy, as discussed in the foregoing chapter, can set the basic direction for the hospital. However, if the strategy statement is to be managerially useful, it must be given what philosophers and scientists call operational definition. That is, it must be expressed as specific, measurable activities and desired results. Thus, translated, strategy becomes objectives that when implemented become health services.

For purposes of understanding and discussion, the translation process can be viewed as consisting of two primary steps:

1. Converting the corporate strategy into an operating plan; and
2. Expressing the operating plan as a budget.[1]

---

[1]Like other words in the English language, the word "budget" has, to some extent, been slandered. A negative connotation—emphasizing repressive control and also, in some instances, laborious and often useless preparation—has attached itself to the word.

The word budget is derived from the Old English word *bougette*. A *bougette* was a small bag or pouch that was used to carry items of value needed for daily business. When a trip was planned, the *bougette* was packed with the essentials for the journey. Thus, a budget is actually nothing more than a collection or list of items needed for carrying out some planned activity.

The traditional literature has been faithful to this definition. A budget is generally defined as a comprehensive plan or guide for some future period of time—usually, by convention, a year.

Plans can be expressed in a variety of ways, for example, manhours, dollars, outputs. A budget, however, is primarily a financial plan and is, therefore, expressed in dollars. Thus, the term budget might be defined more explicitly as a comprehensive financial plan, based upon anticipated outputs and predetermined hospital goals and policies for future operations, that is expressed in dollars of expense and corresponding dollars of revenue.

The first step involves defining the specific workloads, projects, and other operating activities that must be undertaken to transform the corporate strategy into reality. The second step focuses on expressing the operating plan in financial terms, for example, dollars of expense, capital purchases, revenues.

It should be recognized that in practice, these two steps are intertwined as financial data are used to make decisions about alternative projects and activities. For purposes of discussion, however, it is useful to untangle the two. Therefore, this chapter addresses operational planning. Its focus is on planning at the micro level, that is, at the division, department, responsibility center, and cost center level. It is in effect the micro level analogy to strategic planning. It is strategic planning at the operational level.

The following chapters address budget preparation, focusing on the process of expressing the operating plan in quantified financial language. To the extent possible, duplication of the existing substantial body of technical and mechanical literature has been avoided. Forms, calculation methodologies, and other technical concerns will, from time to time, creep into the discussion. The main thrust of these chapters, however, will be identifying and describing the principles and relationships that underlie successful budget preparation.

PLANNING AND BUDGETING

Historically, operational planning has either been ignored, done implicitly, or subsumed within the generic notion of budgeting. While it may be argued that planning is a part of the larger budgetary process, it must also be recognized that planning is distinct from simply preparing a budget. One can plan without translating that plan into financial terms. Similarly, one can budget without planning. The fallacy of the latter alternative, however, should be obvious.

Blind luck may allow success for a time, but without planning, managers have no basis for testing whether decisions will move the hospital toward achieving its long-term goals and fundamental purposes. Management without planning degenerates into expediency and opportunism. In contrast, management with planning enables one, as both a visionary and a pragmatist, to create a hospital that adds value to its community, serving that community as a basic health and social resource.

Operational planning is set out in this text as the first step in the budgetary process to reflect the authors' belief that planning, rather than being separate and distinct from budget preparation, is the keystone to meaningful budget preparation.[2] Planning is the catalyst that changes bud-

---

[2]The budgetary process or budgeting is defined as having two basic components: (1) operational planning; and (2) budget preparation, that is, construction of a comprehensive financial plan, based upon anticipated outputs and predetermined hospital goals and policies, that is expressed in dollars of expense and corresponding dollars of revenue.

get preparation from an arithmetic exercise to a substantive management activity. It is the vehicle for sorting out the variety of basic alternatives and new project and activity ideas to hone in on those that will best serve and meet the hospital's goals. This sorting process avoids both the pitfalls of rising but unmet expectations and the frustrations of having line management prepare budgets for activities that, because they are either inconsistent with or peripheral to the hospital's goals and strategy, will not be funded.

It is only within the context of the hospital's operational plan that the budget is functionally useful. As such, it must always be borne in mind that the plan "drives" budget preparation. It is the budget that must be tailored to the plan—not the plan to the budget.

MANAGEMENT TOOL

The foregoing "begs" a basic question. Operational planning may well be the keystone to making budgeting a substantive process. However, why should management plan and budget? This fundamental question can be answered from either an external or an internal perspective.[3] Regardless of the view, the answer is the same.

Planning and budget preparation are necessities for successful hospital operations. They provide management with its most powerful operational tools and techniques: for first identifying the future activities that will provide the greatest community benefit and for then guiding the hospital in implementing and operating those selected activities in a manner that is least disruptive to the fabric of the total organization.

Management is continually confronted with a variety of alternative activities and courses of action. Each of these alternatives has some cost and some corresponding related level of community benefit attached to it. If a hospital is to achieve its goals, management must select from among the alternative demands on the institution for its limited resources. This selection must be done in a way that produces a combination of activities that yields, in total, the greatest amount of community benefit (see Chapter 1).

In a micro economic context, management must move the hospital to

---

[3]According to the Medicare Program, Section 234, an overall plan and budget of a hospital, extended care facility, or home health agency shall be considered sufficient if it

1. Provides for an annual operating budget that includes all anticipated income and expense . . .;
2. Provides for a capital expenditures plan for at least a three-year period . . .;
3. Provides for review and updating at least annually; and
4. Is prepared, under the direction of the governing body of the institution or agency, by a committee consisting of representatives of the governing body, the administrative staff, and the medical staff (if any) of the institution or agency. Also, states with a rate setting or rate review program require that hospitals prepare a budget.

the margin. Optimally, this would mean that expenditures for any particular activity should be continued until the point where the marginal cost, that is, additional cost, equals the marginal benefit to the community. In the less than optimal, but more realistic instance, where resources are limited, the same principle of moving to the margin applies. However, in this case, management must invest its limited financial resources in a manner that places priority on those alternatives that produce the greatest community benefit. It must fund projects in such a manner that, even though the marginal point might not be obtained for any particular project, the sum of realized benefits is maximized.

The budgetary process, that is, operational planning and the translation of that plan into a budget, provides not only the tools to enable management to move to the margin, but also an important part of the total control mechanism needed to monitor the hospital's progress toward achieving its objectives. How the budgetary process does this can be understood if one examines the relationship of the total process to each of the functions of management. The traditional literature identifies these functions as consisting of: planning, organizing, coordinating and controlling operations, and motivating employees. To these traditional functions should be added, at least for today's chief executive officer, political involvement and public service.

PLANNING

As discussed, the budgetary process consists of two major components. The first is the operational plan. The second, the budget, is the operational plan expressed in dollars.

Of these two components, operational planning can be viewed as the decision-making or management function. In contrast, budget preparation is a financial function, involving the restatement of the plan in dollars. As emphasized earlier, the primacy of the management function over the financial function must always be borne in mind. If the direction of the flow or order of importance is allowed to be reversed, then budget preparation becomes little more than a paper exercise. It becomes a task that fulfills the demands of the finance staff, but has little operational value to management.

The budgetary process can aid management in planning in two ways. First, it provides the opportunity to plan. Systematic planning is a task that is often viewed as not requiring management's immediate attention. Thus, despite its importance, planning is often pushed aside in favor of seemingly more pressing operational issues. The budgetary process, however, requires that management both direct its attention to the future and plan for it. It, in effect, raises the priority of planning by making it a required component of an operational problem—preparing a budget. By raising the priority of planning, the budgetary process forces management to devote attention to planning. It provides at least one opportunity in the course of the year to plan.

The budgetary process also aids management in planning by providing a structure in which to plan. It forces management to view the future, and its plans for the future, in terms of operating expense, revenues, capital expenditures, and cash flows.[4]

ORGANIZING

The budgetary process is an aid to management both in organizing operations and in organizing resources. Effective budget preparation and management control require a clearly defined, responsibility centered organization structure with corresponding cost centers. The organizing of operations along distinct cost/responsibility center lines is necessary to ensure that the initial costs of each distinct function are identified correctly and to enable the accurate computation of the total cost of final cost centers (see Chapter 5). It is only through this cost/responsibility center approach to the organization of operations that actual and planned performance can be meaningfully compared, evaluated, and, most important, controlled.

The budgetary process assists management in achieving this kind of organization structure by providing an incentive—in terms of the potential for improved operational control—for a carefully defined organization, with clear assignments of responsibility and lines of control. Additionally, the budget preparation process aids management in organizing operations by providing documentation and a periodic opportunity for management to correct organizational overlaps or gaps.

The budgetary process is also the primary tool available to management for purposes of organizing resources. As discussed earlier, management must strive to move the hospital to the margin, that is, management must attempt to organize or allocate its resources such that the greatest total community benefit is obtained. To accomplish this goal, alternative expenditure opportunities must be evaluated and funding priorities established so that those projects with the greatest benefits are funded first and, if need be, to the exclusion of other projects with lesser benefits.

In the abstract, the necessity of this kind of conceptual approach to resource organization is easily understood. Moving from the abstract level

---

[4]A hospital's annual budget is the sum of four separate, but mutually dependent budgets: the expense budget, the revenue budget, the capital budget, and the cash budget. These four budgets, in addition to their critical role in assuring financial coordination, provide a framework for guiding the planning process, for they force management to consider each of its intended actions in terms of expense requirements, revenue-generating potential, capital needs, and cash flows.

to operational reality, however, creates somewhat of a problem. This is due to both the number of alternatives that must be compared and evaluated and the relative uniqueness of the benefits of each alternative. However, as will be discussed later, procedural tools are available that management potentially can use to move from concept and theory to practical, operational implementation.

COORDINATING

Obviously, by providing a mechanism for comparing revenues and expenses, the budget is a key tool in assuring financial coordination. The budgetary process, however, is also a useful tool for assuring the coordination of operations.

The budgetary process provides the vehicle for establishing common goals and communicating those goals between and within operating programs. The process of common goal setting and communication provides the basis for operational coordination. Moreover, the budget preparation component of the process, by requiring that each responsibility center's plans be examined, allows management to evaluate (in terms of the common goals) planned operations and, if necessary, to make adjustments.[5] Management can then assure that activity overlaps are eliminated, gaps are filled, and total operations are meshed into a coordinated result.

The budgetary process can also aid management in coordinating the allocation of resources among major expenditure areas. Through a technique known as program budgeting, management has available a tool, or more accurately a structured thinking and decision-making process, for coordinating the apportionment of resources among programs. That is, it allows coordination of the allocation of resources among groups of activities that are all directed toward the same goal or end result.

Program budgeting gained wide recognition when it was introduced into the Department of Defense in 1962 by then Secretary of Defense Robert McNamara. It was extended by presidential directive to all other federal agencies in 1965.

As developed originally, program budgeting was intended to serve as a management tool for the purpose of systematically and rationally identi-

---

[5]There is no one right way to organize or structure any given institution. What works best is a function of the organization's history, the line management's skill and experience, and the style of the chief executive officer. Nevertheless, for purposes of simplified discussion, observe the following organization hierarchy:

Program Area:
1 or more Divisions—Program Area
1 or more Departments—Division
1 or more Responsibility Centers—Department
1 or more Cost Centers—Responsibility Center

fying the costs, consequences, and trade-offs among alternative programs all directed to a similar objective.[6] For example, program budgeting could be used to examine and evaluate the relative benefits and consequent trade-offs of inpatient care versus ambulatory care in terms of the hospital's objective of providing the community with needed patient care. It is by design a tool that is macro in nature. Its primary value lies in aiding management to achieve, over the long run, a rational balance (coordination) in allocation of its limited resources.

Unfortunately, program budgeting has not realized all of its hoped for value. The reasons for this shortfall are open to speculation. However, the difficulties and problems appear to have centered on implementation barriers and mechanical/procedural weakness.

Deterministic program evaluation has proved difficult, if not impossible to accomplish. Also, implementation has been hampered not only by resistance to change but also by the need to "fit" the system into a political decision process that is often economically irrational. Nevertheless, program budgeting has produced some positive accomplishments in terms of improved information and decision making. Moreover, if used in a pragmatic manner, with a careful recognition of its limitations as a tool for detailed resource allocation decisions, it can be a useful management technique for evaluating and coordinating general resource expenditure choices.

CONTROLLING

A budget is, perhaps, the most critical element in a management control system. As such, it acts as both an indirect and a direct aid in the controlling of operations. In a simplistic sense, the budget is the key component of the monitor portion of a control system.[7] A control system can be defined as a set of activities or devices that maintains, in terms of previously established goals, an ongoing assessment of the achievements of a process, and that attempts to correct the process when actual achievement is different from planned (expected) performance. Its purpose is twofold:

1. To provide control of a process so that results are consistent with expectations; and

2. To generate a warning signal when control is not being achieved.

Mechanically, a control system can be viewed as consisting of three basic parts:

---

[6]The conceptual innovation in program budgeting is a simple idea, reflecting little more than basic common sense. In its essence, program budgeting is nothing more than disciplined thinking, in broad strokes, about what it is that an institution produces or does.

[7]The following material on control systems has been based on *Quantitative Techniques for Hospital Planning and Control* by John R. Griffith. Readers interested in more information on management control systems should refer to this work, particularly Chapters 1 and 10.

1. Sensor—the reporting mechanism that identifies the actual state of the process or operation under control; the output of the sensor is a reference signal.

2. Monitor—the process of comparing the reference signal (actual performance) against the expectations for the operation (the budget); the output of this process is an error signal—the measure of the difference between actual performance and expectations.

3. Controller—the mechanism for taking corrective action aimed at the reduction in the magnitude of the error signal, if the error signal exceeds a predetermined tolerance limit.

The interrelationship of the components is illustrated in Figure 16.1.

As the figure illustrates, the budget is the "expectations" portion of the control system. The budget provides the basis for management control, for it establishes the standard (the expectation) to which actual performance must be compared in order to identify out-of-control operational processes. Obviously, more than just a budget is needed if management control is to be successful. As discussed in Chapter 20, feedback or reports identifying, to the person responsible, the status of actual performance are needed at frequent intervals. It must be recognized, however, that operational control cannot be effective unless there is a standard—the budget—against which actual performance can be measured and evaluated.

In addition to the need for feedback, if maximum operational control potential is to be obtained, the budget should be constructed on the basis of organizational responsibility centers. That is, it should be constructed as a responsibility budget, identifying performance expectations in terms of the individual accountable for the management of each activity and group of activities within the hospital.

FIGURE 16.1   Management Control Systems

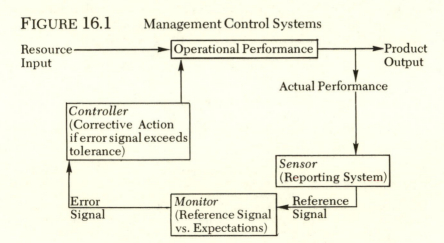

It is important to note that a responsibility budget is not an approach or a technique for making resource allocation decisions. Rather, it is a way of organizing the data that are the outcome of resource allocation decisions. Resource allocation decisions are made using tools and techniques, such as program and zero base budgeting, incremental increase (decrease) guidelines, management interaction and negotiation, and/or arbitrary decisions.

The principle that underlies the construction of a responsibility budget is the same as that which guides the development of a chart of accounts (see Chapter 2) and that establishes the structure for cost analysis (see Chapter 5). The goal in all three instances is to categorize financial data in a manner that recognizes the hospital's organization structure and that consequently reflects the allocation of responsibility for operational performance.

The benefits of this approach to budget organization are threefold. First, it identifies performance expectations in terms of the person responsible for managing the operation. Hence, it allows any needed corrective action to be precisely directed. Second, it links the budgeting and reporting process by accumulating expected and actual performance data on the same basis. Finally, as is discussed below, it provides a steppingstone for motivating employees.

The budgetary process is also an indirect aid to management in the control of operations. The indirect role that the budget plays can best be described as that of creating or adding to a sense of performance and cost consciousness. The managerial discipline and thought involved in operational planning and budget preparation, together with the presence of the budget document, tend to make the entire organization think in terms of costs and to be sensitive to the relationship of current performance to budget expectations. Moreover, by linking operational planning, budget preparation, and performance reporting to the person accountable for the operation of a given responsibility center, the sense of performance consciousness is heightened. Not only is the entire organization captured in a sense of consciousness, but the focus of accountability and performance is directed to those individuals with the ability to guide and control actual outcomes.

MOTIVATING

Both operational planning and budget preparation present the opportunity to apply positive and negative motivational stimuli. Certainly, as should be apparent from the foregoing discussion, the role of the budget in controlling operations also involves motivational implications. For the most part, the stimuli produced by the control functions of the budget are negative: incorporating either real or imagined incentives not to exceed the budget. The strength of these negative stimuli should not be underestimated. It is because of their existence that management must administer the budget with a sense of caution and humility.

The budgetary process also provides the opportunity for applying positive motivational stimuli. In fact, budgeting represents, perhaps, the simplest and easiest vehicle for implementing a program of management by objectives (MBO).

Management by objectives is an approach to managing that makes goals or objectives the heart of the practice of management. It is not a new concept, having been used in a variety of forms and with varying degrees of success for over a quarter of a century.

Regardless of the details of a particular hospital's MBO program, all MBO or MBO-like programs involve the following generic steps:

1. Supervisors provide subordinates with a framework reflecting the hospital program area's larger purposes, goals, and objectives (see following discussion of program and division directives).

2. Within the framework, subordinates propose objectives for themselves.

3. The proposed objectives are reviewed, modified if necessary, and finally agreed upon as a set of operating objectives.

4. The agreed upon objectives are converted into a responsibility center budget.[8] (It should be noted that there is some circularity between Steps 3 and 4, as financial data may be used in the process of reviewing and modifying objectives.)

5. Financial and operating feedback is provided.

6. Based on the feedback, subordinates review their performance and periodically report back to their supervisors.

7. If actual performance differs significantly from the original proposed objective(s), then corrective action is proposed by the subordinate. It is then reviewed, modified if necessary, and agreed upon by both the subordinate and supervisor.

8. Steps 5 and 6, and Step 7 as necessary, are repeated throughout the year.

Intuitively, it would seem that the MBO process of involving the person who is going to be accountable for performance in making decisions and setting the goals by which performance will be evaluated would improve

---

[8]The linkage between control and motivation should be recognized. The "linking pin" is the responsibility budget that results in objectives being established and financial data being organized on the basis of responsibility centers, that is, clear, single points of management accountability. The responsibility center budget is fundamentally nothing more than a statement of performance goals for a particular responsibility center and individual, expressed in dollars.

motivation and enhance performance. This intuitive sense is supported both by empirical observation and by a number of systematic research investigations. In general, the benefits of MBO can be summarized as follows:

1. It directs work activities toward organizational goals.
2. It reduces conflict and ambiguity.
3. It helps provide clear standards for control and performance appraisal.
4. It provides improved motivation.

In practice, however, it is not surprising that the benefits of MBO are often not fully realized. The MBO process is often flawed by such problems as

1. *Burdensome Procedures.* To be done properly, MBO takes time. Time is always a scarce management commodity. If these inherent time demands are compounded either by an overly rigid, bureaucratic approach or by the MBO process becoming just a paper work exercise, then line management will rebel, prostituting the system not only to wipe out any potential benefits, but also to produce negative results. This behavior, while perhaps not justifiable, is understandable. It reflects the price that an organization might have to pay if it forces or overlays an artificially complex process on itself. With common sense and sensitivity to the limits of line management's time, this price can be avoided or at least minimized.

2. *Overemphasis on the Quantification of Objectives.* Not all results or objectives lend themselves to meaningful quantification. This point, while appearing obvious, is often lost in a doctrinaire approach to MBO. As a result, means and ends become confused, MBO syntax requirements replace operating needs, and line management feels forced by the procedure to compromise the system. The results of this situation are the same as described above.

   The principle to be remembered is that not all objectives have to be quantified. Objectives should be specific statements, permit clear verification, focus on the user or receiving system and specify the point in time by which they will be achieved. If they can also be quantified, so much the better. Quantification, however, is not a prerequisite for an objective to be either accepted or effective.

3. *Suboptimization.* MBO's focus on the setting of objectives at the responsibility center level carries with it the risk of an overemphasis on individual objectives. The hazard attached to this risk is that the organization's larger goals will be lost as managers strive to meet their agreed upon responsibility center commitments. To protect against this risk, supervisors must:

a) Assure that individual responsibility center objectives are set within the framework of the hospital's, as well as the specific program area's, larger goals and objectives; and

b) Review each subordinate's objectives against those of organizationally adjacent subordinates to assure not only that they are not in conflict, but also that they are at least compatible, if not mutually supportive.

4. *Illusionary Participation.* The point here should be obvious. If positive motivation is to be achieved, all levels of management must be given meaningful roles in the objective setting as well as the overall budgetary decision-making process. It is only through this real involvement that managers will be committed and motivated to perform in accord with the operating plan and budget. If such involvement is not fostered, the value of budgeting in motivating employees, and also to a large extent the usefulness of the budget in controlling operations, will be substantially lost.

POLITICAL INVOLVEMENT

The last decade has been marked by a seemingly endless flow of legislation, regulation, and judicial rulings that affect not only the "nuts and bolts" of doing business, for example, location and height of fire extinguishers, but also fundamental business policy decisions such as divestitures and acquisitions. Because of the large amount of governmental funds flowing to hospitals and government's concern about the public health and welfare, the hospital field has been particularly affected by federal and state legislation and regulation. As a result, if not as a survival reaction to the pressure of existing as well as the threat of future legislation and regulation, every hospital manager in the nation is either involved in, or being pressed to become involved in, the political process.

There is nothing inherently inappropriate in such involvement. In fact, it is to be encouraged. It is only through the jousting, within the political process, of the countervailing powers of interest groups that sound public policy is created and workable regulations are promulgated.

The budgetary process aids hospital managers in engaging in the political process in two ways. First, operational planning and budget preparation provide the manager with the opportunity and the means to define the issues and understand their operating implications. The result of this is a knowledgeable advocate: a person who can explain, with more than just rhetorical fluff, the public policy, health economics, and community welfare implications of proposed legislation and regulations.

Second, the budgetary process provides management with the time, and raises the priority of management taking the time, to become involved in the political process. The point here is the same as that made earlier with respect to planning. The budgetary process forces management to direct its attention to political issues, for these matters affect the operating environment of the hospital. Further, by giving management the opportunity to plan and anticipate events, as opposed to just reacting to crises, the budgetary process provides management with the time to channel its increased political attention into constructive involvement.

PUBLIC SERVICE

At first glance it might seem unusual to consider public service as one of management's functions. However, if one looks at the calendars of most senior and executive managers, it becomes clear that a substantial amount of time is spent in giving speeches to public groups, service on public boards, and support to various community projects.

The contribution of the budgetary process to enabling managers to carry out this function is straightforward. Simply put, by enabling management to plan and anticipate events, the budgetary process allows management to reallocate its time away from the resolution of crises to other matters. Like political involvement, public service is one of the ways that managers can reinvest their available time.

Whether such an investment is beneficial might arguably be an open question. The weight of at least subjective evidence, however, seems to support the continuation of public service as a management function. This is particularly true in the case of the hospital. In many localities, hospital managers are among the most skilled and experienced resources in the community. The involvement of these people in community affairs brings not only talent to the project, but also an added dimension to the entire fabric of the community.

AXIOMS

In reflecting on the foregoing, it would seem reasonable to conclude that the budgetary process would be the centerpiece of a hospital's management system. Unfortunately, this is often not the case. In one form or another, most hospitals typically have some type of budgetary process. Often, however, the budgetary process, due to insensitive design or clumsy implementation, acts only to overburden or intimidate the management staff. The net result in such circumstances is that budgeting often becomes little more than a paper exercise. More important, line management's focus shifts from using budgeting as a means for achieving the hospital's goals to subverting the process so as to blunt its influence on operating decisions.

For the value of the budgetary process to be realized, its management power, as well as its psychological, operational, and interpersonal relationship subtleties, must be recognized. In broad terms, this means that the design and implementation of the budgetary process must be guided by common sense and an operational understanding that all processes have a set of biases (implicit as well as explicit) to which managers will respond.

Common sense is a phenomenon that is so simple and obvious in its conclusion, and so elegant in its presentation, that until it directly confronts one it is often difficult to see. To facilitate this confrontation, the following principles or budgetary axioms are postulated.

AXIOM I. EVOLUTIONARY PROCESS

Budgetary processes can be designed with varying degrees of complexity and sophistication. The complexity of the process should not, however, exceed either the sophistication of the organization or the skill and experience of line management. If the process is more involved than the experience of management can understand and accept, it will fail in a managerial sense.

To avoid this pitfall, the process should be tempered so as to stretch, but not overreach, the experience of the organization. Similarly, as organizational experience is gained, the budgetary process should evolve, becoming increasingly precise and rigorous in its anticipation and quantification of community needs, planned operational response, financial planning, and performance monitoring and feedback.

It also should be recognized that the budgetary process—at whatever the level of sophistication—is basically a human system. Therefore, it should neither be surprising nor frustrating, particularly since the process should try to stretch the organization to increasingly better performance, if implementation does not proceed exactly as laid out in the hospital's budget manual. As long as the organization is moving consistently in the correct direction, progesss is being made.

AXIOM II. TIME TO PLAN

At this point it might seem obvious that the budgetary process can neither proceed nor succeed without planning. However, if broad scale planning is to take place, a specific time in the process must be allocated to planning. This means that a step in the early stages of the process must be identified as the point where operational planning is done. Additionally, this step must have sufficient time allocated to it to enable managers to think through the operational implications and requirements of the hospital's goals and strategy.

The importance of adequate time to plan should not be underestimated. Often there is a tendency or pressure to sacrifice time at the front end of the process in order to leave more time for budget calculations, fiscal services' preparation of detailed accounting data, or unexpected delays and slippage. The dangers of this strategy are twofold.

First, if there is too little time to develop an adequate managerial plan, then the budget, regardless of its level of precision and detail, will be inadequate. From a management perspective, it makes little sense to have a precise budget if its underlying foundation is valueless. Functionally, if a timing sacrifice has to be made, it is better to squeeze the accounting calculations or the end of the process than it is to eliminate the time needed for sound planning.

Second, if inadequate time is provided for planning, an implicit signal is given to operational management that the process is a sham. The result is that the motivational and control benefits of budgeting are seriously eroded, if not lost. The conclusion here is the same as above: provide a specific as well as adequate time to plan.

AXIOM III. HUMAN NATURE

As indicated above, all processes have an implicit as well as explicit set of behavioral biases. If the budgetary process is to be effective, it must not only recognize this fact but also capitalize on it. It makes little common sense and less operational sense to ask line managers to do things that are contrary to their best interests. To make such requests is to fly in the face of both human nature and economically rational behavior.

The design of the budgetary process, and particularly the budget preparation component, should use human nature as an ally by building positive biases into the process wherever possible. Operationally, this means that every step in the proposed process should be examined from the perspective of how line management will respond psychologically as well as functionally to the requested action. Similarly, the process should be designed to emphasize giving line managers positive feedback; allowing them to feel that their work and, if necessary, sacrifices are recognized and contribute to the achievement of the hospital's goals.

A corollary to this point should be noted: The process should be kept as simple as possible. The reasons for this are several:

1. The simpler the process, given the variances and vagaries of human behavior, the less is the exposure to and the subsequent risk of counterproductive managerial reaction.
2. The opportunities to subvert the process are reduced in direct proportion to its simplicity.
3. The appearance as well as the reality of make-work is avoided by simplifying the process.
4. A positive bias is signaled by a simple, readily understandable, and workable process.

Keeping the process simple does not mean that it cannot be rigorous. Even sophisticated processes can be made simple. The key is to review each step and ask if it is necessary. Only those steps that provide information that can be used to make or change decisions should be viewed as necessary and be kept in the process.

AXIOM IV. MATCHING DETAIL
TO DECISION NEEDS

A common failure of budgetary process designs is that they require managers to produce overly detailed documentation at the initial stages of the process.

The level of detail should be matched to the rigor of the decisions that are going to be made. If only general management or policy decisions are required at the outset, then the level of detail should be kept general. Operationally, this means that managers should be asked to do no more work than is necessary to support the level of decision that is to be made. To ignore this point not only unproductively complicates the process, but also needlessly frustrates line management by creating false expectations and unnecessary work.

A corollary to the principle of matching detail to decision needs is the notion that information should build upon itself. As the planning and budget preparation process proceeds, decisions will have to be more precise. Detail will thus need to be more precise. The expanded amount of information should be developed on an additive basis, growing like a series of concentric circles that become larger with each succeeding budgetary step. The goal must be to avoid procedural redundancy and duplication of effort by designing a process that utilizes the data and results of preceding steps as the foundation for the next step—and the next decision.

AXIOM V. KEYSTONE DECISIONS—
THE RULE OF BEGINNINGS

All things have a beginning. However, beginnings are often the most difficult of all the steps that must be taken. Creating a hospital's budget is no exception to the rule of beginnings.

As is discussed in more detail later, the keystone decisions in the budgetary process are top management's providing guidance relative to program direction and fiscal limits. Whether implicitly or explicitly at the beginning, middle, or end of the process, decisions on both these issues ultimately have to be made. Because these questions reflect difficult decisions, management often tries to shy away from them, seemingly hoping that through some magic the questions will resolve themselves. In practice, magic generally fails. Management, however, often procrastinates until the final stages of the budget preparation process, where these decisions, if revenues and expenses are to be balanced, become unavoidable.

It is generally a sound management principle to delay making decisions until they are needed. In this instance, the point to be recognized is that these decisions are needed at the beginning: to give line management the information it needs to plan; to avoid raising false hopes; to limit or eliminate unnecessary work; and to simplify the total process.

AXIOM VI. CERTAINTY AND UNCERTAINTY

Establishing operational direction and setting fiscal limits add a level of certainty to the budgetary process. Budgeting, however, is a process that is unavoidably characterized by a high degree of uncertainty. Throughout the process managers are asked to make projections, rank order activities, provide alternatives, and accept risk. These requests are not unreasonable. They represent the means for identifying and evaluating the organization's options. They are, however, in conflict with a manager's desire to limit surprise and uncertainty.

To an extent, this conflict between a manager's desires for certainty and the budgetary process's inherent uncertainty cannot and should not be eliminated. In the short run, however, this conflict, unless it is carefully monitored, can become dysfunctional. Over the long run, as management gains more experience and a greater understanding of the subleties of the budgetary process, the potential negative aspects of this conflict will diminish.

Procedurally, the counterpoint to the inherent uncertainty of the process is its reiterative nature. As managers proceed through the budgetary process, they will find that the same matters are being questioned at each step. This continual review allows for a check and balance on decisions and should act to reduce managerial anxiety.

As noted earlier, more detailed information should be added to both the line manager's and the decision maker's data base with each succeeding step. With more information, not only is clarity obtained and uncertainty reduced, but the data needed for sound decisions are provided.

AXIOM VII. SENSITIVITY

The budget is obviously a potent tool for management's use in guiding and controlling operations. However, if its value is to be fully realized, management must use it with care and with a sense of empathy both for the reality of operations and for the potential adverse effects of heavy-handed management intervention. To be effective, the budget must be viewed by management as an indicator of the relationship between expected and actual performance, not as a disciplinary mechanism or as an arbitrary whipping post. If management fails to use the budget with caution and sensitivity, not only will its management benefits be negated, but also, and more important, the budget will act to produce counterproductive results. An improperly administered budgetary process will result in an organization focusing on "beating" the budget as opposed to meeting its responsibilities to its community.

PREREQUISITES

The foregoing has provided a context in which to place the budgetary process. Effective budgeting, however, requires three additional factors: (1) a series of internal operating prerequisites must exist; (2) management must make several budgetary design decisions; and (3) a systematic operational planning and budget preparation procedure must be developed and implemented. Factors one and two are discussed below. Factor three is addressed in both the final section of this chapter and in the following chapters.

The operating prerequisites for budgeting are similar to those that a hospital faces for other management functions such as cost analysis (see Chapter 5). Budgeting, in common with cost analysis, requires

1. A well-designed organization structure that eliminates overlapping responsibility and clearly defines all accountabilities
2. A chart of accounts that corresponds to the organization structure and allows for the accumulation of actual cost data by cost and responsibility center
3. An accurate accounting system capable of accumulating and appropriately assigning all financial data
4. A comprehensive management information system capable of collecting nonfinancial data relative to total volume of services demanded and cost center workloads

In addition, because it is both a time series process and a process that involves the entire management structure of the hospital, budgeting requires

1. Historical and current actual performance data for use in projecting future volumes and costs
2. A formal feedback reporting mechanism
3. A high level of management staff capability and sophistication

Historical and actual performance data are necessary for purposes of establishing the basis for projecting future workloads and cost behavior. Generally, unless some phenomena are involved that act to alter the historical relationships that characterize the operations of any given environment, the best estimates of the future are past performance and past performance trends. By its definition as a plan, the budget is future oriented. Thus, its usefulness is heavily dependent on accurate estimates of the future. If these estimates are to be attained with any degree of confidence, historical data are a necessity.

A formal feedback reporting mechanism is also a prerequisite condition. The role of reporting, in the generic context of management control systems, was discussed above. In the specific case of budget operations the role of reporting is critical, for it is the linking pin between expectations (the budget) and reality (actual performance).

Formal, detailed reports, incorporating responsibility reporting and reflecting variances from originally budgeted activity, should be prepared on a monthly basis, unless circumstances require increased frequency. These reports should be provided to all responsibility center managers. The level of detail provided should be tailored to the level of management, with increasing levels of supervision being given summary reports, unless they request more detail. Management reporting, reporting procedures, and report analysis are discussed in detail in Chapter 20.

The final prerequisite of staff capability is, perhaps, the most important element in the successful preparation and use of a budget. As emphasized earlier (see "Axioms"), effective use of budget requires that management appreciate the subtleties of motivating employees and maintain an empathy for the reality of day-to-day operations. Only a sophisticated management team has the sensitivity necessary to capitalize on the opportunities presented by both the budgetary process and the resulting budget document.

It is critical to recognize that while organization structures, data, and procedures are all necessary, they are all of secondary importance when compared to capable management. Budgeting is fundamentally a people-moving as opposed to a paper-moving process. If budgeting is to be successful, all levels of management must understand its value and limitations, how the budget is to be developed and used, and their own specific roles and responsibilities. These latter items will be discussed in the following chapter. At this point, it is sufficient merely to appreciate the pivotal role that management plays.

BUDGETARY DESIGN DECISIONS

In addition to assuring that the internal mechanics and management capabilities exist, management must make a series of budgetary design or policy decisions. These decisions are preconditions to actual budget preparation, for they define the specific character of the budget that is to be constructed. In broad terms, management, in addition to determining the basic structural design of the budget, must decide whether the budget is to be

1. Incremental or zero base
2. Comprehensive or limited in scope
3. Focused on only a fixed volume or workload estimate or be capable of accommodating varying levels of workload
4. A discrete or continuous process

STRUCTURAL DESIGN

As is the case in architecture, the structural design decision is a fundamental choice in terms of determining the final shape and ultimate usefulness of the budget. Essentially, the design decision comprises two parts. Whether the designer is an architect or a manager, he must determine

1. How to organize the material or resources at his disposal. (In the case of designing a home, is it to be a colonial or a split-level? In the case of the budget, is it to be organized on the basis of discrete activities or programs?)
2. How to put together, within the established organization, the various components. (In the case of a home, is it prefabricated or built on site? In the case of a budget, does one adopt a piecemeal or a holistic approach to determining the allowable expenditure level of various responsibility centers?)

With respect to budget organization, management is confronted with the need to make both macro and micro level decisions. At the micro level, it must be decided how costs are to be grouped. Costs can be grouped on the basis of line items (natural cost accounts, such as salaries, medical supplies, drugs, laboratory supplies, travel, consulting fees) and/or on the basis of organizational work units. Also, within organizational work units, costs can be grouped on the basis of cost centers or on the basis of both cost and responsibility centers.

The need for some form of cost grouping should be clear. The magnitude of a hospital's budget operation is such that if all appropriate requests were treated in a disparate manner it would be difficult, if not impossible, for management either to obtain a realistic picture of the total operation or to control ongoing operations. Hence, the question to be resolved is not the need for grouping but the method of grouping.

If costs are grouped on the basis of line items only, management can identify and control hospital expenditures. It cannot, however, identify or control the costs or the results (performance) of a specific function, that is, the performance relative to the agreed upon objectives of any particular work unit. Therefore, in addition to grouping on the basis of natural account, management must design the budget so that costs are categorized by work unit.

The basic work unit is a cost center. When cost and responsibility centers are synonymous, grouping on the basis of cost centers and natural accounts provides management with the information necessary both to visualize clearly and understand hospitalwide expenditure patterns and to control work unit and total hospital cost and performance. However, when cost and responsibility centers are not synonymous, then in addition to cost center grouping, the grouping or aggregating of cost centers into a responsibility center is necessary. That is, the natural costs of the various involved cost centers must be grouped to show both total natural costs and the total costs of the responsibility center.

The importance of grouping costs on the basis of responsibility centers cannot be overemphasized. As the earlier discussion under "Management Tool" emphasized, organizing the budget so that it reflects the management allocation of responsibility for operational performance is essential if the control potential of the budget is to be realized. The only way the budget can be organized to accomplish this is to group costs on the basis of responsibility centers.

At the macro level, management is confronted with a similar problem. The question in this instance centers on how responsibility centers should be grouped or organized. Should they be grouped on an activity or department basis or should they be grouped by program area? The solution of choice is to organize along both approaches, with departments ultimately being aggregated into program area groupings.[9]

If the budget's organization is limited to only an activity or departmental orientation, it is difficult for management to evaluate the scope and direction of the total hospital's planned activities with respect to either coordination of effort or conformance to stated policy objectives. Organizing the budget on a program basis, however, enables management to accomplish both these evaluative functions readily. Hence, in terms of organization, the structural design of the budget can be described as a program budget organized at the micro level by line item and responsibility center, with responsibility centers then grouped into programs at the macro level.

Management's choices are relatively limited in terms of how to put the budget together. Essentially, the budget can be constructed either on a piecemeal basis, where projects are reviewed and funded on their ad hoc merit, with only passing regard to corporate direction and the merits of other projects, or on a holistic (that is, total entity) basis.

Obviously, the holistic approach is the alternative of choice. It allows

---

[9]See footnote 5 for organizational flow.

project and activity alternatives to be examined within a framework of program priorities and relative cost/benefit analysis. As a result, it enables resource allocation decisions to be made in a manner that increases the probability of the total benefit to the community being maximized (as opposed to the random probability of the piecemeal approach). One of the two generic techniques or tools for implementing the holistic approach, program budgeting, has been discussed above. The other, zero base budgeting, is discussed below.

INCREMENTAL OR ZERO BASE

As discussed earlier, program budgeting is a tool whose primary value lies in aiding management to achieve, over the long run, a rational balance in the allocation of its resources. If used in a pragmatic manner—without overemphasis on requiring that all functions in the hospital, including those whose value is primarily subjective, be deterministically quantified and with a careful understanding of its limitations as a tool for detailed resource allocation decisions—program budgeting can be a useful technique for evaluating and coordinating general resource expenditure choices.

Program budgeting, however, is of little help in determining the allocation of resources within, as opposed to between, any given program area. Because of this limitation, management must use another technique for determining allowable expenditure levels for the responsibility centers within each program area. Typically, an incremental approach is used to resolve this problem.

The weakness of an incremental approach should be apparent. The requirement that only the incremental expenditure request be evaluated and justified ignores the opportunity to evaluate all proposed expenditures and make the trade-offs that will result in the greatest total benefit being achieved. To capitalize on this opportunity, a zero base approach to budget construction must be used.

Zero base budgeting is an approach to budgeting that has been used successfully in both industry (Texas Instruments, Inc.) and government (state of Georgia).[10] Essentially, zero base budgeting is a process wherein all future expenditures are evaluated and rank ordered.

As indicated above, in the traditional budget process managers responsible for established (ongoing) activities generally have to justify only the incremental portion of their proposed budget. That is, they only have to defend the increase that is being sought over the previous year's appropriation. Customarily, what is already being spent is accepted as necessary and is implicitly approved as a continuing expenditure. Zero base budget-

---

[10]Readers interested in further information relative to the philosophy and mechanics of zero base budgeting should consult *Zero Base Budgeting* by Peter A. Pyhrr, New York: John Wiley & Sons.

ing differs from the traditional approach in that it requires every department to defend its entire budget request each year, just as if all its activities were entirely new.

By taking this perspective, zero base budgeting allows management to examine expenditure alternatives in their total portion, as opposed to just their incremental portion. Management can thus select those alternatives that provide the greatest total benefit.

Procedurally, there are two basic steps in zero base budgeting:

1. *Developing Decision Packages.* This step involves the operating manager describing and evaluating each of the activities—both ongoing and proposed—for which he is responsible.

2. *Ranking Decision Packages.* This step involves senior management's analyzing and ranking, through cost/benefit analysis and/or subjective judgment, the decision packages developed in the first step.

Once decision packages are developed and ranked, management can allocate resources, funding the projects having the greatest net benefit, regardless of whether they are existing or new activities. The final budget is produced by taking the activities that have been accepted for funding, sorting them into their appropriate organizational units, and then summarizing the costs identified to produce the budget for each responsibility center, department, division, and program area, as well as for the entire hospital.

Essentially, a decision package is nothing more than a form that contains the programmatic and gross financial information necessary to describe a specific activity and its alternatives so that management can[11]

1. Analyze the activity and its alternatives and decide whether to approve or disapprove it; and

2. If the decision is to approve, rank order the activity or the approved alternative against other expenditure requests.

Within a decision package the identification of alternative means of accomplishing the proposed activity or project is critical. It is only through the presentation of such alternatives that management can consider the full range of available choices, that is, both intra and inter decision package alternatives, and make decisions that will produce the greatest total benefit.[12]

Two types of alternative should be presented in each decision package. The first should examine alternative ways of accomplishing the same ob-

---

[11]See Chapter 17 for an example of a decision package.

[12]Given a limitation on funds, if management is not presented with internal alternatives for an activity, it might elect not to fund a particular activity as opposed to funding it—if it were performed at a different level of effort or in a different manner. By either ignoring, or not being aware of, these internal alternatives, management makes less than the optimal choice. To avoid this pitfall, alternatives for accomplishing the desired objective, if they represent realistic options, must be presented as part of an activity's decision package.

jective. The decision package should highlight the recommended way of performing the activity, with the alternatives being identified and briefly explained.

A second category of alternatives focuses on different levels of effort. In this instance, a minimum level of effort should be identified as should the current and requested levels, presuming they are different. A separate decision package can be developed for each level of effort, or a single package can be used with each level of effort being identified, briefly discussed, and rank ordered against the others.

Decision packages should initially be developed at the lowest practicable level within the organization. At a minimum, the manager accountable for each responsibility center should develop the decision package for the activities within that center. Ideally, however, the person responsible for each discrete activity, function, or operation within the responsibility center should develop the decision package for his programs. Details concerning the mechanics of preparing decision packages are set out in the following chapter.

The second step in zero base budgeting is the rank ordering, based on the alternative of choice, of decision packages. The ranking process provides management with a vehicle for allocating its limited resources. Essentially, a rank ordering is a listing of all decision packages, that is, alternative projects, in order of decreasing cost/benefit to the total organization.

Initial ranking selections should be made by the manager responsible for developing the decision packages. Managers at each succeeding level in the organization should consolidate the decision packages and rankings received from their subordinates and produce their own ranking for all the packages presented to them. Finally, senior and/or executive management should consolidate all decision packages and rankings into a final total institutional ranking. This last ranking can then be compared to revenue projections to determine "how far down" the ranking list the hospital can go. The result, that is, the aggregate expenses of the funded decision packages (the alternative project choices that are to be funded), represents the hospital's total expense budget.

In theory, ranking decisions should be made on the basis of cost/benefit analysis. However, in the reality of the actual hospital operations, the role and value of the subjective judgment process should not be underestimated.

For purposes of initial rankings, quantitative techniques can provide useful information. At the senior and executive management level, however, the emphasis should primarily be on broad distinctions of relative order: assuring that package 5 is more important than package 35, and on determining the action to be taken in regard to discretionary as opposed to required activities. In both, subjective judgment, honed by experience, and a detailed knowledge of the environment are perhaps the best tools available. Figure 16.2 graphically illustrates the ranking process.

Before proceeding further, several cautionary points are worthy of note. First, the foregoing discussion has approached zero base budgeting from the perspective of its being both a concept and a mechanical process. As will be reiterated, a procedure—whether presented as a model approach or as the unique approach utilized by a particular organization—should never be arbitrarily superimposed upon an organization.

If successful results are to be obtained, mechanical procedures must be tailored to the unique character, history, and style of the user organization. In some instances this tailoring may mean that some procedural components should be eliminated. Such deviation from a prototype procedural approach may be anathema to particular managers. It should be remembered, however, that the emphasis must be on substance and results—not on form and process. In the case of zero base budgeting, the important element is the basic concept of examining both the ongoing need for current activities and the alternatives available for conducting needed activities, not the process to be employed or the forms to be used.

FIGURE 16.2   Decision Package Ranking Process

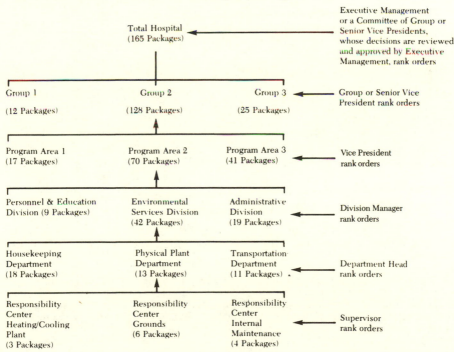

Second, it should be recognized that zero base budgeting, though reasonable in theory, will be a threatening concept for some managers. Therefore, its implementation should reflect an appreciation of the preceding discussion (see "Motivation" and "Axioms") and a careful application of the principles of management of change.

This point is particularly germane in the application of zero base budgeting in the hospital setting. Clearly, there are a number of hospital activities wherein management's options to expand, contract, or eliminate a function are limited.[13] The existence of these activities does not invalidate the concept of zero base budgeting. However, it does require, as was the case above, that the procedural mechanics of the concept be modified to reflect operational reality. If used pragmatically, zero base budgeting will provide management with a workable mechanism for evaluating alternative expenditure opportunities and selecting those that, in sum, produce the greatest total benefit.

Finally, it should be noted that zero base budgeting complements program budgeting. Program budgeting is fundamentally a macro level application of the principles of zero base budgeting. It is the evaluation of the relative benefits of program areas as opposed to projects or specific activities. Zero base budgeting supports program budgeting by acting as a review mechanism on the priorities that have been determined. That is, by determining the specific expenditures that are to be undertaken within each responsibility center, zero base budgeting acts as a check on program budgeting decisions. The interrelationship of zero base and program budgeting is illustrated in Table 16.1

COMPREHENSIVE OR LIMITED SCOPE

A comprehensive budget can be defined as a budget system wherein all planned capital and operating costs and all anticipated revenues are projected and then incorporated into a single, integrated budget document. In contrast, a limited scope budget is a budget system that includes only a particular element (or elements) of the total budgetary process. A limited scope budget, for example, may be a salary budget only or it may be an expense and revenue budget, ignoring projected capital expenditures.

From the perspective of management efficacy, a comprehensive budget is the budgeting system of choice. It is only through a comprehensive budget, wherein all phases of the hospital's production and physical and finan-

---

[13]Zero base budgeting was not designed primarily for health services management applications. Therefore, a too rigorous application of the principles requiring the presentation of alternatives for either services such as the emergency room and the general surgery operating rooms, where the possibility of implementing the alternatives is unlikely, or functions where the interchange of resources is impossible, will result in only unproductive and needless work and a loss of confidence and support of the staff for the budget program.

TABLE 16.1   Zero Base Budgeting and Program Budgeting:
             Decision Process Interrelationship

Step 1

Activity (Responsibility Center)[1]	Program[1]	Program budgeting evaluation is used to determine the relative contribution and priority of activities toward achieving a specified objective. Once relative priorities are established the next step is to determine activity priorities, both within and
Activity (Responsibility Center)[n]	Program[n]	between programs. Zero base budgeting can be used for this.

Step 2

Program[1] Activity[1]	Zero base budgeting is used to rank activities based on costs and benefits. It focuses not on what will be done, but rather on how it will be done. Program[1], Activity[1] would be funded first in priority to Program[1], Activity[2]. Program[2], Activity[1] would
Activity[n]	generally be funded in priority to Program[3], Activity[1]. However, if analysis shows that Program[3], Activity[1] has the greater
Program[n] Activity[1]	benefit, it would be funded in preference. In this way, a check exists to allocate to broad priorities and then to assure that within and between priorities activities of the greatest benefit
Activity[n]	are funded.

cial operations are examined, planned, and budgeted that the full operational value and management usefulness of the budgeting process can be realized.

Though the method of choice is clear (a comprehensive budget), recognition must be given to the problems inherent in the management of change when implementing a comprehensive budgetary system (see Axiom I). In some hospitals, movement from a position of either no or a minimal budgetary process to a comprehensive budget may well create too much organizational trauma to be accomplished effectively in one step. In such instances, a limited scope budget can play an important role as an evolutionary measure providing management with the opportunity to control and spread the dislocation effect, intrinsic in any change, over a longer period of time. Whether such an evolutionary approach is necessary will depend on the history and current status of the organization and the skills and capacity of its personnel. In relatively weak organizations, or organizations that have just completed or are in the process of implementing other major change activities, an evolutionary approach may well represent the most desirable and pragmatic way of achieving an effective comprehensive budgeting system. In each instance, however, management must evaluate its own situation and design an implementation plan accordingly.

FIXED OR FLEXIBLE

As its name implies, a fixed budget is one that is developed on the basis of a single estimate of expected workload or volume.

After considering past levels of workload, demographic factors, and changes in the hospital's range of services, management can estimate either a range of expected workloads or a single level of volume. If only a single volume estimate is made or if only a single volume estimate is used in preparing the budget, the resulting budget is said to be fixed. To the extent that the single workload estimate is correct, a fixed budget is both an accurate budget and a highly reliable management tool. Even if projected and actual volumes differ, to the extent that a hospital's costs are fixed; that is, either they do not vary directly with changes in workload or the volume change is too small to cause a change to the hospital's production function, a fixed budget can be a reliable management tool. Unfortunately, it is unusual in either a hospital or any other type of enterprise to find an operating situation that is so static that estimates of demand can routinely be made with perfect precision. Moreover, hospital costs are not entirely fixed. While no completely definitive data are available, it is generally agreed that over the near and long term as much as 50% to 60% of operating costs may be subject to variation. (The degree of short-run variability may be quite limited; over a period of a month or several months only 10% to 20% of total costs may either vary proportionately with volume or be susceptible to management efforts to vary with volume.) Given this kind of operating environment, a fixed budget, while of value, has certain implicit limitations. To correct for these limitations, a tool known as a flexible budget is available.

A flexible budget can be defined as a statement of expected performance that can be adjusted to reflect the effects of operating at different levels of volume. Essentially, a flexible budget is a series of fixed budgets covering a specified range of volume alternatives. The size of the relevant range of alternatives will differ with each particular situation. However, as a rule of thumb, the accuracy of workload estimates for most hospitals should be within 5% to 10%. Therefore, the range of a flexible budget should be no more than 10% to 20%.[14]

Also within the relevant range, budget alternatives should be developed only to reflect those changes in volume that will materially affect the budget (see Axiom IV). That is, if a 1% change in workload will neither significantly change unit cost nor materially influence the way management

---

[14]In establishing the range for a flexible budget, recognition should be given to the probability as well as the possibility of volume changes. If a hospital has operated for the last three years at between 95% and 97% occupancy, then the relevant range might be 90% to 100%—not 75% to 115%. The point to be noted is that in selecting flexible budget ranges the principle of common sense should be applied.

would plan or make decisions, then it is not necessary to prepare an alternative budget for each 1% change in volume. Typically, the traditional literature uses a 5% change in workload as the incremental volume change sufficient to justify the development of an alternative budget. However, the principle of a 5% volume change should not be taken as an absolute rule. The level of incremental change that should signal the need for an alternative budget varies with each situation (production function) and must be determined for each hospital on the basis of an individual analysis and understanding of its cost behavior.

In theory, to determine the critical level of incremental change, management must first define the cost structure of each department. That is, it must identify those costs that: over the budget period, regardless of volume, remain constant (fixed costs); remain constant relative to day-to-day volume changes, but that can vary due to management decisions such as the opening or closing of a wing or nursing station (semifixed costs); vary on less than a proportional basis with volume changes (semivariable costs); and vary directly and fully with volume changes (variable costs). Given this analysis, the next step is to determine to what extent costs will change with various changes in volume. This evaluation could begin by determining the minimum level of volume that could be expected with a high degree of confidence and then proceed to a similar estimate of maximum volume. Based on this information, management can both identify the incremental volume levels requiring alternative budgets and determine the relative degree of cost variability from one level to the next.

Though accurate, the theoretical approach is cumbersome. Therefore, as an alternative, historical data can be reviewed and analyzed to determine at which levels of volume unit cost markedly changed, and to establish the relative percentages of fixed and variable costs. Given these data, management then can identify the volume levels requiring alternative budgets.

Clearly, a flexible budget is the approach of choice. It provides a more valid and reliable internal management tool and is more defensible in terms of rate review, prospective payment, and external price control negotiations. A flexible budget, however, requires a degree of sophistication, knowledge, and skill that a hospital just beginning a comprehensive budgeting program may not possess. In such instances, an evolutionary approach, relying on a fixed budget and volume variance analysis, may be a more prudent choice.[15] As was the case earlier, in each instance, management must evaluate its own situation and design a unique implementation plan.

---

[15]Variance analysis is a technique for evaluating differences between actual and planned performance. Briefly, volume variance analysis is a device for identifying how much of a total variance is due to the difference between planned and actual volume. The calculation, using assumed data, can be illustrated as follows: *Continued*

CONTINUOUS OR DISCRETE

In addition to the foregoing, management must determine if it wants a continuous (rolling) or a discrete (periodic) budget. A discrete or periodic budget is one that is prepared at one point in time and applies to a fixed future period. Usually a periodic budget is a budget that is prepared annually and that encompasses in its projection a 12-month time period.

In contrast, a continuous budget is one that is updated routinely so that at any point in time the hospital is operating under approximately a 12-month plan. Typically, a continuous budget is updated on a quarterly basis, i.e., as a quarter ends the remaining three quarters of the budget year are reviewed and, if necessary, revised and another quarter is added. However, a monthly updating cycle can also be used if the operating environment warrants budget review and revision at greater frequency.

A continuous budget is the method of choice. Although in an absolute sense a continuous budget may require a bit more work, it

1. Allows for a more even spreading of the planning and budget preparation workload;
2. Provides for the ongoing maintenance of a full 12-month detailed financial plan; and, most important,
3. Replaces the crisis environment that typically surrounds planning and budget preparation with an ongoing process that integrates the budgetary process into routine general operations.

It should be recognized, however, that continuous budgeting involves both a high degree of familiarity with the process and mechanics of budget preparation and a sophisticated management team. As was the case with other policy decisions, an evolutionary approach that begins with a periodic budget and then proceeds to a continuous budget may be the more pragmatic and effective decision. Again, management must make its decision based on the specific operating situation.

As a related issue, management must also determine the period to be covered by the budget. The above discussion presumed a 12-month budget

---

[15]*Continued*

Budget = $10,000
Projected Volume = 5,000 units
Cost/Unit = $2/unit
Actual Cost = $12,000
Actual Volume = 5,500 units

(Actual Volume) − (Budget Volume) × Budget Unit Cost = Volume Variance

$$5,500 - 5,000 \times \$2 = \$1,000$$

Based on the above example, of the total variance of $2,000 ($12,000 − $10,000), $1,000 is due to an increase in volume. Therefore, presumably if unit costs do not decrease with volume, only $1,000 is due to increased supply prices or production inefficiencies.

period, for a 12-month period is the generally accepted convention. A 12-month period may not, however, be appropriate to all instances.

Probably the best answer, however inconclusive, to the question of how long the budget period should be is: long enough, but not too long. That is, presuming there are no statutory requirements, the budget period should cover a time span sufficient in length to allow for effective planning. Operationally, this means that it should be long enough to

1. Discount for unusual short-term variations in demand and/or the nature of the operating environment; and

2. Take into account events in the future whose outcome will affect current decisions. (That is, it should extend to the planning horizon or that point in the future wherein additional information will not affect current decisions.)

This last point is a key concept, for it acts to place a single period's budget preparation effort into a larger and longer term context and to emphasize the need for not only a current operating plan and budget, but also for a multiyear or long-range plan.

Simply, if management is to be able to make sound current operating decisions, it must weigh and evaluate those decisions against future needs. Also, if management is to achieve the hospital's longer-term strategic goals, it has to begin to make preparations and take the initial steps toward those goals in the current period. Both these circumstances or requirements make clear the need for a multiyear plan that can be used both as a bench mark and as an indicator of future direction.[16]

Given the availability and use of a multiyear plan, the question of the period to be covered by the budget becomes somewhat of a moot point. A 12-month period, however, synchronized with the hospital's fiscal year and set within the context of an overall multiyear plan, generally should be an acceptable and a workable period.

The mechanics of developing a multiyear plan are discussed in the following sections.

THE CONVERSION PROCESS

The foregoing has set the stage for the conversion of the corporate strategy into a multiyear operating plan. The corporate strategy is the product of the strategic planning process. Functionally, it is the hospital's statement of purpose and the program directives that flow from and are held together by the statement of purpose (see Figure 16.3 and Table 16.2).

---

[16]As discussed later the development of a multiyear plan, aside from its financial implications, is an essential task of prudent management. Such a plan should be coordinated and consistent with the areawide plan developed by the hospital's local health systems agency.

Program directives establish objectives, that is, specific desired results and constraints, by program area. Assuming that these objectives are congruent with the hospital's purpose and are mutually reinforcing or, at least, not contradictory, they in sum

1. Define the hospital's operational direction
2. Provide an initial framework for operational planning and budgeting decision making

FIGURE 16.3 Hospital Corporate Organization Model

It should be recognized that though there is no simple best way to structure a hospital organization, common patterns of organization seem to emerge. This figure illustrates a basic corporate style approach to organization structure. It should be recognized that in any particular hospital the allocation of responsibilities as well as the title may differ from that depicted here.

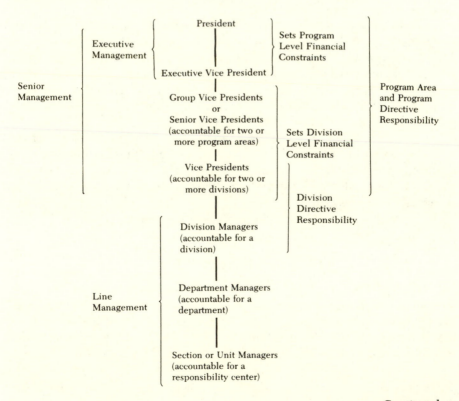

Continued

FIGURE 16.3   Continued

Examples of the functional areas, that is, programs, divisions and departments, that match the foregoing general organization structure are listed below. These examples are only a partial listing, intended to provide a fuller sense of the organization—not complete detail.

The caveats that are set out above also apply to the following:

Program Areas	Divisions	Departments
Inpatient Acute Services	Nursing Services: Units	ICU
	Nursing Education	CCU
	Nursing Administration	Medicine
	Operating Rooms	Surgery
Environmental Services	Housekeeping	Carpentry Shop
	Physical Plant	Paint Shop
		Power Plant
Fiscal Services	Accounting	Third Party Payment
	Data Processing	Budgeting and Payroll
	Admitting	Credit and Collections
Clinical Services	Laboratories	Outpatient Radiology
	Radiology	Diagnostic Radiology
	Physical Medicine	

Included as part of the corporate strategy should also be an overall financial guideline as well as a financial guideline for each program directive. The overall financial guideline should set a limit on the total expense budget for the future year, for example, growth of 4.8%. The specific quantification of the limit should flow from an estimate of revenues and the decisions incorporated in the hospital's long-range financial plan relative to operating margin rates and reserve levels.[17]

Just as a hospital should have a multiyear operating plan, it should also have a multiyear financial plan. Due to the unique financial environment of hospitals, developing such a plan is a relatively straightforward task. Essentially, all that is required is a set of explicit decisions as to: operating margin rates for each revenue center; the level of restricted and unrestricted reserves that are desired; and the rate at which reserves are to be either

---

[17]It should be recognized that, due to the dominance of third party payers and contract payment arrangements, the matter of projecting revenues is less speculative for the hospital than it is for the typical commercial corporation. For further discussion of this point, see Part II.

TABLE 16.2   Example: Brumlik County Hospital Corporate Strategy

Mission Statement
To deliver health services to the residents of Brumlik County with the primary purposes of: improving health status of individuals and continuing to increase the value of the community's health services expenditures.

Financial Guideline
For the coming year, expenses should increase by a maximum of 4.8%. Additionally, a positive operating margin of 4% should be generated.

Program Area I: Inpatient Acute Services
   Maintain the hospital's traditional standards of patient care services while at the same time reducing bed capacity in order to produce an 87% occupancy rate.
   1. Control nursing vacancies to a level equal to no more than 10% of approved professional staff complement.
   2. Review procedures and performance re JCAH standards, and implement necessary corrective action prior to accreditation review.

   For the coming year, resources should remain at the current budget level.

Program Area II: Ambulatory Care Services
   Maintain existing emergency services program. Add outreach programs that will make the hospital's services more conveniently accessible to the community.
   1. Outreach program emphasis should be on
      a.   Worksite services
      b.   Services to the aged
      c.   Pediatric services

   For the coming year, resources should expand.

Program Area III: Environmental Services
   Maintain current quality standards while continuing to increase productivity by 1.5%.

   For the coming year, resources should be maintained at a current services level, adjusted for productivity improvement.

Note: This table represents an excerpt from the hospital's corporate strategy—not the entire strategy.

increased or decreased. Given these decisions the data necessary to establish financial guidelines, as well as, if desired, develop pro forma projected financial statements, are available.

   It should be recognized, however, that these financial decisions cannot be made in an operational vacuum. In fact, there is a reiterative relationship between the financial plan and the operating plan, with the two coming together when the revenue, expense, and capital budgets are integrated and brought into balance. As part of this balancing, the financial plan may be revised. Even so, an initial plan is necessary in order to provide basic guidance. The process of integrating and balancing the budgets and making "adjustments to plan" is discussed in the following chapter.

At this point in the process, the financial guideline for each program area (see Figure 16.3 and Table 16.2) is more a statement of emphasis than a quantitative bench mark. That is, the program level financial guidelines should indicate relative emphasis among program areas—not specific dollar amounts—signaling which program areas should grow, which should remain relatively constant, and which should contract.

On a year-to-year basis, the corporate strategy, unless major changes take place in the hospital's purpose or environment, should remain relatively constant. Each year it should be reviewed and refined for a better fit with the hospital's evolving environment. The year-to-year changes, however, should reflect only a fine tuning of the basic strategy.

The objectives set out in the corporate strategy, while adequate for setting the hospital's general direction, are not sufficient for operational management purposes. To meet the needs of line management, more detailed and specific objectives are required. It is a difficult process, however, to move from basic organizational objectives, that is, program directives, to operating objectives in a single step. To facilitate this transition a linking pin is needed. The division directive (see Figure 16.3 for the organizational location of divisions) serves this linking function.

A division directive is simply a specific, measurable, or verifiable statement of desired results or accomplishments for a program area subunit, that is, a division. It is in effect a statement of "contributing objective" in that if each division in a program area achieves its directive, then the program area, in total, will accomplish its objectives.[18]

Moving from program directives to division directives is basically a deductive question-and-answer process. A program directive presents a statement of where the hospital wants to be for a particular aspect of its operations, that is, a program area. A division's current situation and level of performance represent where it is. The division directive sets out what the division must do within its scope of activities this year and, if necessary, in subsequent years, to contribute fully to the achievement of its program directive. It is a gap-filling statement, defining what must be done, year by year, to proceed from where the division and hospital are, to where they want to be. (See Table 16.3 for examples of division directives.)

As illustrated in Figure 16.4, division directives are shaped by the hospital's environmental assessment and management's decisions with respect to financial constraints. Also, as illustrated, it is from the division

---

[18]A division, though organizationally located in a single program area, might contribute to several program directives. If this is the case, the division directive must identify what must be accomplished with respect to each program directive to which it contributes. For purposes of this discussion, it is simpler to view a division as contributing only to a single program directive.

TABLE 16.3   Example: Brumlik County Hospital Division Directives

Program Area I: Inpatient Acute Services

Program Directive
Maintain the hospital's traditional standards of patient care services while at the
same time reducing staffed bed capacity in order to produce an 87% occupancy
rate.

1. Maintain on a continuing basis nursing vacancies at a level equal to no more
    than 10% of approved professional staff complement.
2. Review procedures and performance re JCAH standards, and implement
    necessary corrective action prior to next year's accreditation review.

For the coming year, resources should remain at the current services level.

Division Directives
Nursing Services
Maintain current nursing hours and staff mix to patient day ratios. Design and
implement, prior to year-end and in conjunction with Social Services Division,
a discharge planning program. By year-end, close nursing units 3 West and 3
North.

Resources should remain at the current services level/patient day. (This, however, should reflect a reduction in total budget as compared to current year.)

Nursing Administration

Implement nurse recruitment program designed to generate in year 1 a net
increase in the nursing staff of 35 professional nurses. In year 2 and beyond,
the program should generate 25 new nurses.

Implement salary and career ladder program that reduces turnover to 15% in
year 1 and maintains it at 10% in year 2 and beyond.

Resources should grow by 5% in year 1 and remain at the current services level
in year 2.

Note: Excerpt from division directives.

directives that department and, subsequently, responsibility center objectives flow. Establishing these later objectives is addressed below. Before
proceeding to that discussion, it is important to note several points.

First, the foregoing discussion of how to develop division directives
has been brief. This has been by design in order to emphasize that establishing division directives is neither a quantitative nor a magical process.
Senior management must take the initiative and provide the leadership in
guiding and shaping the development of division directives. Actual specification of the directives, however, should be done: (1) in partnership with
line management; and (2) through a process that is characterized by common sense, rigorous thinking, and imagination.

FIGURE 16.4   Division Directives

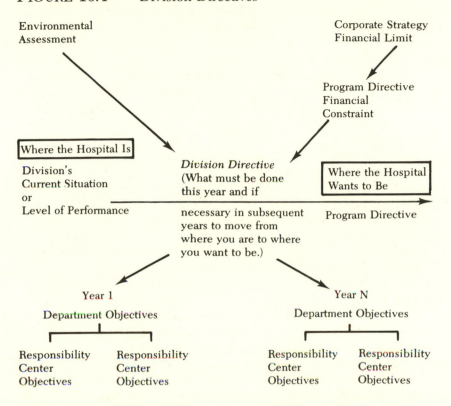

Second, like program directives, division directives must also have a financial component.[19]

A program directive provides financial guidance with respect to the total budgetary limits for the aggregate expenditures of all the divisions within a program area. However, depending on the program directive and the financial requirements placed on the other divisions in a program area,

---

[19]For those organizational units that are capable of controlling revenues, a revenue goal should also be established. Typically in the hospital setting individual cost centers and departments have relatively little, if any, control over revenues. Revenue centers are basically creations of the accounting cost-finding system and are not functional organizational units. Even when a revenue center is also a final cost center, that is, a specific organizational unit to which costs can be allocated and for which management responsibility can be identified, there is little that such a cost center can do directly to influence its revenue performance. Therefore, it is rare to set revenue goals on less than a total hospital basis. Goals should, however, be established for the total institution.

a particular division can grow, remain constant, or contract.[20] Given this potential for variation, if division level management is to be able to plan, it needs guidance as to the level of resources that will be available. Because of the trade-offs that must be made among divisions, the setting of division level financial constraints must be directed by program level management.

In keeping with the concept of the matching of detail to decision needs (see Axiom IV), financial constraints or guidelines in division directives must be more precise than those in program directives. At first glance, it may appear that setting a more precise financial limit is, or should be, a complicated task. In reality, it need not be difficult. The key is the same notion of a relevant range that was discussed earlier.

Unless an explicit management decision has been made to the contrary, the ability of a division, department, or responsibility center significantly to expand or contract is operationally and pragmatically limited (see Figure 16.3). That is, the relevant range of potential expansion and contraction is limited in one direction (upward) by the ability to acquire and absorb resources productively and in the other direction (downward) by the need to maintain production stability and employment security.

Given inflation, and assuming a constant volume, if a division is to remain constant, it must grow budgetarily by an amount equal to the level of inflation. If it is to grow in "real terms," it must increase its budget by an amount sufficient to compensate for inflation, plus a "real" increase beyond that amount. Similarly, if a division is to contract, its budget might just remain at a constant dollar level, resulting in shrinkage equal to the level of inflation.

Based on the above, and an understanding that organizational units, regardless of size, are complex, dynamic organisms that in a short period of time can expand or contract productively by only a limited amount, a set of decision guidelines or rules of thumb can be set out. Simply put, the relevant range is generally from zero growth to inflation plus 10%.

Assuming that no explicit decision has been made to eliminate all or part of an activity, zero growth represents a real reduction in operations equal to the level of inflation. Such a level of shrinkage generally can be accommodated on a single-year basis without destroying a sense of organizational stability and security. In contrast, given an organizational unit's limits in assimilating new personnel and constructively spending new resources, growth may well be limited to real expansion of no more than 10%.

---

[20]For example, if a program directive specifies that the program area, in total, is to remain at a constant level of service, then the sum of the program area's division directives must total a dollar level equal to the previous year's program area budget plus an amount sufficient to compensate for inflation, less productivity increases. This can be done by all of the program area's divisions remaining at a constant level of service, some divisions growing while others contract by an equal amount, or a combination of the two.

Some organizational units can obviously accommodate larger levels of either growth or shrinkage. Therefore, the above rules of thumb are not set out as indelible propositions. Rather, they are just a starting point. Like all other general management rules, they must be tested against the character and abilities of the particular organization and management team and tailored accordingly.

It should be recognized that there is a countervailing philosophy to the above approach. Some argue that the foregoing technique for establishing financial constraints does not place adequate pressure on line management to perform efficiently. To the extent that executive management feels that there is "organizational slack," pressure can be exerted by allowing for only a partial pass through for inflation. Such a strategy forces line management both to increase efficiency and, as is consistent with zero base budgeting, to consider which tasks should be continued or discontinued.

Finally, division directives should often encompass multiyear periods.[21] The reasons for this are several. From a pragmatic point of view, the fit between what must be done to achieve a program area's objectives and the available financial resources may be mismatched. This will often be the case, for resources are limited. In such instances, the two can be meshed by lengthening the time period available to accomplish the necessary tasks. The systematic lengthening of the time period requires a multiyear directive and plan.

A multiyear directive is also needed to provide continuity. The separation of the planning and budgeting cycles into 12-month periods, though conventional, is arbitrary. The flow of work does not always conveniently divide itself into 12-month spans. Some activities are ongoing while others, regardless of the availability of resources, require multiyear periods to accomplish. A multiyear directive recognizes both these operating realities as well as the need for succession from period to period.

Third, like a continuous budget, a multiyear directive and corresponding plan help to smooth the workload inherent in planning. Also, they help to make planning a more routine part of management, as opposed to a special, ad hoc activity.

Creating a multiyear directive, like establishing financial constraints, need not be difficult. Essentially, it involves two steps. Both of these steps can be incorporated into the initial development of the division directive.

The first is the "stretching" of the directive to encompass all the activities that must be accomplished to achieve the program area's objective. The second is the addition of time frames by subdividing the directive into

---

[21]In some instances, where the production process is routine and performance is expected to continue at a constant level, a multiyear directive is not necessary. Where, however, change is being planned or performance standards are being raised, multiyear directives should be developed.

sequential activities by year, that is, identifying what has to be done in year 1, as well as what has to be done in year 1 in order to provide the base for year 2 activities.

Admittedly, the requirements that division directives have a financial component and a multiyear planning horizon add a degree of rigor to the planning process. The key, however, to developing even these more complex and comprehensive directives is the same as that which was emphasized earlier. Establishing division directives is neither a quantitative nor a magical process. Rather, it is the application of common sense, rigorous thinking, and imagination.

DEPARTMENT OBJECTIVES

Department level objectives flow from the division directives. The process of establishing these operating level objectives is similar to the foregoing. That is, it is a deductive process aimed at identifying what must be done, by year, to fill the gap between where the division currently is and the goals that the division directive establishes. The relationship between the two is one where the division directive defines what has to be done and department objectives define the contribution that the component units of the division (departments) will make toward achieving the specified ends.

In setting department objectives, the division's financial constraint must also be recognized. The approach here is the same as that described above. The guiding principle is that the sum of the department financial constraints (projected budgets) cannot exceed the financial level established by the division directive. Department level financial constraints should be established by division level management.[22]

Where organizationally appropriate, the same process is repeated at the responsibility center level. Responsibility center financial constraints should be established by department level management. The sum of the total projected expenses of the responsibility center financial constraints should not exceed the department level constraint.

The hospital's budget flows directly from department and responsibility center objectives and financial constraints. The budget specifies in quantified financial terms how each department or responsibility center will accomplish its objectives. The preparing of the budget increases the specificity of detail by another step. By this point, however, the level of certainty is also increased. Objectives have been reviewed and approved, and financial constraints (projected aggregate budgets) have been summed—and, if

---

[22]The process of setting objectives should be participative. However, because of the trade-offs involved in establishing financial constraints, division level management must assume a leadership role.

necessary, adjusted—to assure that they are consistent with the corporate strategy's financial target. Thus, wasted effort and unfulfilled expectations are kept to a minimum.

The following chapter addresses the mechanics of budget preparation, as well as the application of the concepts of zero base budgeting to "test" if particular activities should be either continued or continued at the same level of expenditure. The preparation of the budget is actually the final operating step in the planning process, for it refines the process by: (1) adding quantitative precision; and (2) forcing an examination of the alternatives available for how to accomplish, within the financial constraints, the agreed upon objectives.

Before proceeding to this discussion, three points should be noted with respect to setting department or responsibility center objectives. First, the objective-setting process should be participative. Though the empirical evidence is mixed as to whether subordinate involvement in setting objectives makes any difference in motivation and performance, the character of the entire planning process, that is, that it is an important management activity, demands that subordinates be involved. Moreover, genuine commitment is seldom achieved when objectives are externally imposed.

Second, the more difficult the objective, the higher is performance, so long as the objective is mutually set and agreed to. If objectives are too easy, they are less likely to engage one's urge to achieve. Similarly, if they are too difficult, they will be passively ignored. Only if the difficult objective is accepted and becomes the individual's level of aspiration does it tend to lift performance.

In this context, a shortfall, in terms of fully accomplishing a difficult objective, should not be viewed as prima facie evidence of performance failure. Part of the purpose of establishing objectives is to stretch the organization. By stretching, the organization may accomplish more than it would have if it had adopted easier objectives, which it could have fully met. The use of objectives in this manner is part of the managerial dynamics of taking full advantage of the opportunities for improving performance that are inherent in the planning process.

Third, objectives should be as specific as possible. This does not mean, as discussed earlier with respect to management by objectives, that all objectives must be quantified. Rather, it requires that objectives be set out in such a manner as to be verifiable. That is, they should be defined in a way that provides a bench mark for assessing performance.

THE PLAN

Through the foregoing process the hospital has constructed its operating plan, except for one step. It has built a multiyear plan that identifies:

the hospital's goals; what each organizational unit within the hospital must do to achieve those goals; and the resources, both in total and by organizational unit, available to accomplish the goals. The remaining step is a consistency check of the total plan.

As mentioned above, the plan must be reviewed to assure that it is both internally consistent as well as consistent with the corporate strategy, and then it must be approved. The process is essentially the reverse of the foregoing. Each level of management aggregates its established objectives and projected budgets for the units reporting to it. Objectives are reviewed to assure that they

1. Contribute to the hospital's goals

2. Are mutually supportive, or, at least, not in conflict with each other

If both of these criteria cannot be met, objectives must be renegotiated. Projected budgets are reviewed to assure that they are consistent with each level of financial constraint. If an inconsistency is found, the budget target must be revised to bring it into accord.

Following consistency review, and any necessary revision, the plan is complete and ready for approval.[23] The approval process will vary with each organization. Regardless of the process and route, the plan must be approved by the hospital's board. The board-approved operating plan provides the foundation for the hospital's budget.

The significance of the board's role in operational planning should not be underestimated. The board certainly cannot, nor should it, attempt to take the place of an aggressive and imaginative management team. The board, however, through its experience and perspective, can bring to the operational planning process a unique character and insight that will enhance the ultimate result. Additionally, the board's involvement in the process provides the touchstone for its commitment to and support of the plan and its implementation. The value of this latter asset, though intangible, is great.

The specific steps and accountabilities in the operational planning process are summarized in Table 16.4.

SUGGESTED READINGS

Anthony, Robert N. *Management Accounting.*
Deegan, Arthur. *Management by Objectives for Hospitals.*
Esmond, Truman H., Jr. *Budgeting Procedures for Hospitals.*
Griffith, John R. *Quantitative Techniques for Hospital Planning and Control.*

---

[23]Forms have intentionally been omitted from this chapter. This has been done to emphasize that planning is a thinking process. Tables 16.2 and 16.3 provide examples of format. Appendix 16 presents a sample form that illustrates the projected budget.

TABLE 16.4   Operational Planning Accountabilities

	Board	Executive Management	Senior Management	Line Management	Corporate Planning
Phase I	--------	Corporate strategy / Overall financial constraints	--------		--------
	Approval of corporate strategy	--------			--------
		Program level financial constraints	--------		--------
			Program directives / Division level financial constraints	--------	--------
				Division directives (division managers) / Departmental financial constraints (division managers) / Departmental objectives (department managers)	--------
Phase II	Approval of operating plan	--------			Consistency review

-------- Primary accountability
- - - - - - Supporting (staff or participative) accountability

Latham, G.P. and Yukl, G.A. "A Review of Research on the Application of Goal Setting in Organizations," pp. 824–45.

McConkey, Dale D. *MBO for Nonprofit Organizations.*

McGregor, D. "An Uneasy Look at Performance Appraisal," pp. 89–94.

Mintzberg, Henry. "Planning on the Left Side and Managing on the Right."

Odiorne, G. *Management by Objectives.*

Selznick, Phillip. *Leadership in Administration.*

Silvers, J.B. and Prahalad, C.K. *Financial Management of Health Institutions.*

Vraciu, Robert A. "Programming, Budgeting, and Control in Health Care Organizations: The State of the Art."

APPENDIX 16
SAMPLE OPERATIONAL PLANNING FORM

Program Directive—Program Area I

    1. Directive

    2. Financial Constraint

Division Directive—Division I-A

    1. Directive

    2. Financial Constraint

Department Objectives

Department I-A-1

    1. Financial Constraint

    2. Objectives

       —

       —

       Current Budget _____

       Projected Budget*_____

Department I-A-2

    1. Financial Constraint

    2. Objectives

       —

       —

       Current Budget_____

       Projected Budget*_____

*Projected department budgets must be consistent with their financial constraints. The sum of department financial constraints cannot exceed, unless specific exception has been granted, the division financial constraint. Similarly, division financial constraints must be, in aggregate, consistent with the program area constraint.

17

Budget Preparation: Procedure, Organization, and Accountabilities

The corporate strategy and the operating plan provide the foundation that the hospital needs to build its budget. Before constructing the budget, an additional element is necessary. Simply, if the budget is to be developed successfully, management must establish and implement a budget preparation procedure.

Generally, a procedure can be defined as a system or a systematic way of accomplishing an identified objective. As is the case in most complex management processes, the budget preparation procedure involves two fundamental components. One part is essentially technical in nature, focusing on the mechanics, that is, the mathematics of calculating expected expenses. It addresses the techniques and technology of such activities as

1. Projecting workload (volume)
2. Converting volume estimates into resource requirements and revenue estimates
3. Converting resource requirements into direct cost estimates
4. Calculating indirect costs
5. Adjusting revenues and total costs to obtain the necessary equality

The other component of a procedure can be viewed as being basically behavioral in character. It addresses both the organizational and interpersonal relationship aspects of the preparation process as well as the management of the entire process.

The technical aspects of budget preparation have been described in substantial detail by other authors. To avoid unnecessary duplication, the focus of this chapter will be on the behavioral component of the procedure, emphasizing the organization and management of the process.

From time to time, the discussion unavoidably will touch on technical and mechanical issues. This material will be introduced to add a context in which to understand better the management of the budget preparation process. Readers interested in an in-depth knowledge of the technical aspects of budget preparation should go beyond these brief comments to the references provided in the Suggested Readings of Chapters 16 and 17 and Appendix 17. Similarly, readers interested in a more detailed discussion of the behavioral aspects of managing change should refer to the discussion in Chapter 16 (see "Axioms") and the Suggested Readings.

THE PROCESS

Due to both its general complexity and its reiterative nature, the most efficient approach to understanding the organization and management of the budget preparation process is to begin by considering an overview of the entire process. The individual steps involved in preparing a comprehensive budget, as well as the general sequence of effort, are listed in Table 17.1. Each of the identified steps is discussed below.[1]

The discussion of procedural process not only defines the anatomy of budget preparation but also provides the foundation and background for the examination of the related matters of budgetary organization and accountabilities. These topics are addressed in the latter portion of the chapter.

Phases I (corporate strategy development) and II (operational planning) have been addressed in previous chapters. They are mentioned here only to demonstrate the flow of effort and establish a total context.

As has been discussed, phases I and II provide the basis for constructing the hospital's budget. While these phases are the key to the success of the entire budgeting process, their actual accomplishments should not be overestimated. Together they establish the corporate direction and give it quantitative and operational character. They do not, however, answer the basic question of how the institution specifically utilizes its resources to accomplish its operational goals. The answer to this question lies in the completion of phases III through VI. Its implementation lies in phases VII and VIII.

PHASE III

Phase III can be viewed as being principally administrative in character. It is in this phase that the necessary materials (instructions, forms, data) for budget preparation are developed, reviewed, and approved.

---

[1]It should be recognized that, though budget preparation is basically a sequential process, various steps in the process can be accomplished simultaneously. However, for purposes of simplifying the discussion in this chapter, the process is described in a step-by-step fashion.

STEP 1. BUDGET PREPARATION MANUAL REVIEW

Step 1, though the initial component of Phase III, could be accomplished simultaneously with the foregoing phases. Essentially, this step involves the review and, if necessary, the revision of the hospital's budget preparation procedure.

Ideally, the budget preparation process should be set out in a procedure manual that describes the mechanics of preparing the budget. In terms of content, the manual can be viewed as consisting of two basic components: a projection package and an administrative package.

Each of these packages is discussed below. At this point it should suffice to recognize that the projection package is simply a report of projected workloads both for the institution in total and for the volume-dependent responsibility centers.[2] In its final form the projection package loses its independent package identity and is subsumed within the administrative package.[3] The administrative package, in turn, can be viewed as an instruction book that provides the forms, supportive data, and directions necessary for completing the budget.

The purpose of this step is not to examine and approve the materials that are being developed for future use, but to review the previous years' material and process and to identify areas where improvements could be made in terms of clarity, streamlining of the effort, and usefulness of additional information. After their approval, these improvements are then to be incorporated into either the development of the current materials or the operation of the process.

In simplest terms, this step provides the opportunity to learn from previous experience and errors. As such, it is basically an autonomous step that can be accomplished at any point in the budgeting cycle prior to the preparation of the administrative package.

STEP 2. PROJECTION PACKAGE DEVELOPMENT

The concept of packages was first mentioned as part of the discussion of the mechanics of zero base budgeting in Chapter 16. It is a concept that will keep reappearing, for it is an integral component of the budget preparation. In this context, the notion of packages refers to packages of information that are transferred for purposes of communicating either the raw data necessary for decisions or actual decisions between different levels of management (see Figure 16.2).

---

[2] An example of a volume-dependent responsibility center is the inpatient dietary service, for its costs vary with volume; executive management is an example of a volume-independent responsibility center.

[3] It should also be recognized that zero base budgeting decision packages flow from the administrative package.

TABLE 17.1   Sequential Steps: Budget Preparation

Phase	Board	Executive Management	Senior Management	Line Management	Corporate Planning
Phase III*			1. Budget manual review/revision		
				2. Projection package development	
	3. Projection package approval				
				4. Administrative package development	
		5. Administrative package approval			
Phase IV	6. General budget meeting				
				7. Technical budget meeting	
Phase V		8. Administrative meetings			
					9. Decision package development
					10. Administrative meetings, rankings
			11. Revenue budget development		

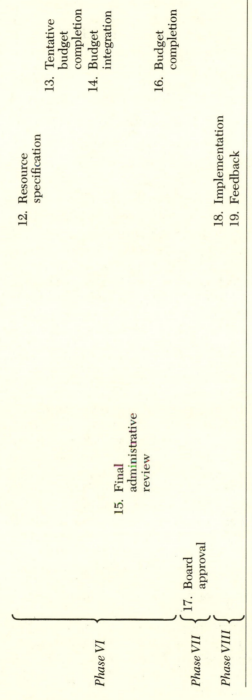

12. Resource specification

13. Tentative budget completion

14. Budget integration

16. Budget completion

15. Final administrative review

17. Board approval

18. Implementation

19. Feedback

Phase VI

Phase VII

Phase VIII

*See Table 16.4 for Phase I and Phase II sequential steps.

The first of these packages is the workload projection package. As was discussed earlier, the genesis of this package lies in the environmental assessment process. The general estimates of future volume, which are contained in the environmental assessment, are refined in this step to provide the specific workload estimates necessary both to develop the details of the operating plan and to calculate resource requirements.

In terms of content, the projection package consists of forecasts of

1. Total admissions and patient days
2. Admissions and patient days per patient care unit
3. Workloads for each of the other volume-dependent responsibility centers

Of these, the admissions and patient day forecasts are perhaps the most critical projections. The admissions and patient day projections represent both an independent estimate of workload and, as Table 17.2 illustrates, the base projections upon which many of the other responsibility center workload forecasts are built.

The forecasting techniques utilized by any particular hospital will vary with that hospital's situation. The management principle is simply to identify a model or technique that consistently produces prediction accuracy, that is, provides a good fit. This can be accomplished by testing alternative forecasting approaches against historical data and evaluating the fit between actual volume and estimated workload. In evaluating fit, the notion of relevant ranges, which was discussed in Chapter 16, should be kept in mind. In this instance the point is simply that if the estimate is consistently within the relevant range of actual, then the fit can be considered acceptable.

Table 17.2 lists, for several major responsibility centers, the workload element to be estimated and possible forecasting techniques. It should be recognized that other techniques, both more or less complicated in nature, can and should be used if they result in an acceptable fit with less effort or produce a better fit for either the same or a justifiable level of additional effort. Also, the role of market research data in adjusting and shaping forecasts should be recognized. Readers interested in additional information on forecasting should refer to the Suggested Readings.

STEP 3. PROJECTION PACKAGE APPROVAL

Before its incorporation into the administrative package, the projection package should be reviewed and approved. The organizational focus for review and approval will be discussed below. At this point, it should be recognized that for purposes of accuracy the volume estimates should be reviewed from the perspective of the impact of such factors as changes in the demographic character of the hospital's service area, technological

TABLE 17.2   Workload Forecasting

Department	Workload Element	Forecasting Technique
1. Total hospital	Total admissions and patient days	Regression analysis Market research
2. Patient care unit	Monthly admissions and patient day projections	Exponential smoothing
3. Dietary	Meals	Meals/patient day x patient days
4. Laundry	Pounds of laundry	Pounds/patient day x patient days
5. Radiology	Relative value units (RVU)	RVU/patient day* x patient days Market research
6. Laboratory	Relative value units (RVU)	RVU/patient day* x patient days Market research
7. Housekeeping	Volume of space	Subjective estimate based on volume and intensity
8. Emergency	Visits	Regression analysis Market research

Note: Readers seeking a more detailed discussion of forecasting techniques should refer to: Lash, Myles P., "Development of An Expense Budgeting Procedure"; Griffith, John R., *Quantitative Techniques for Hospital Planning and Control*; and Wheelwright, Steven C. and Makridakis, Spyros G., *Forecasting Methods for Management*. Readers should also refer to the discussion in Chapter 15 and Appendix 15.

*Relative value units per patient day should be adjusted to reflect changes in medical technology. This can be accomplished either subjectively or through trend analysis techniques.

changes in the practice of medicine, and historical trends. To the extent that such factors are operative, the mathematically forecasted workloads should be subjectively adjusted based on current best estimates.

It should be noted that the projection package can be reviewed and approved together with the other portions of the administrative package. However, a separate review and approval step is suggested both to facilitate budget preparation by allowing activity to take place simultaneously whenever possible and to simplify the review process.

STEP 4. ADMINISTRATIVE PACKAGE DEVELOPMENT

The administrative package is the basic package for communicating budget preparation instructions and information to line management. It includes the data developed in the projection package, tailored to each hospital department. The total patient day forecast is provided to all departments. Specific departmental workload estimates also are provided to those departments having responsibility centers that are volume-dependent. In addition, the following materials should be provided:

1. A cover letter from the chief executive officer or chief operating officer
2. A budget calendar
3. The materials developed in phases I and II
4. Decision package form and instructions
5. Historical volume and cost data
6. Personnel budget detail forms and instructions
7. Current personnel complement, wage, and benefit data
8. Supplies and other expense budget detail forms and instructions
9. Capital budget forms and instructions

Excerpts from a sample administrative package are presented in Appendix 17.

In reviewing Appendix 17 it should be recognized that several departments contributed to the construction of the package. The relative roles and responsibilities of the involved departments are detailed in later sections of this chapter.

STEP 5. ADMINISTRATIVE PACKAGE APPROVAL

This step is the final step before direct line management involvement in budget preparation. Essentially, it is just a "sign off" step wherein the administrative package is reviewed to assure that approved revisions, as identified in Step 1, have been incorporated into the package and that the package is complete.

PHASE IV

Phase IV can be characterized as a communication phase. It consists of two staff meeting steps that interrelate in an additive manner.

STEP 6. GENERAL BUDGET MEETING

The first meeting is an introductory or general meeting that is designed for officially initiating the annual planning and budget preparation process for line management. The meeting should be chaired by the hospital's chief operating or chief executive officer. The agenda should focus on

1. Reviewing and explaining the Phase I and Phase II components of the administrative package
2. Orienting line management to the basic budgeting procedure and process in a general fashion
3. Reemphasizing the value to all levels of management of the budget preparation process and the budget document
4. Making clear the nature and the extent of the budget preparation support and aid that are available to line management upon request

The tone of the meeting should tend toward informality and openness. Expository presentations should be as brief as practicable. Questions from the floor should be encouraged, and sufficient time should be allotted for an extensive question-and-answer period.

STEP 7. TECHNICAL BUDGET MEETING

The second communication meeting is substantially more technical in nature, focusing on the specific mechanics of budget preparation. Operationally, this step may involve either a single meeting or a series of meetings. Moreover, the meeting(s) may be organized on either a total hospital basis or on the basis of program or subprogram areas. The logistics of these meetings should be shaped to complement the history, character, and budgetary sophistication of the hospital's staff. To the extent that operational planning and budget preparation represent a new or complex undertaking, the number of meetings should be increased.

In terms of content, the technical meetings should concentrate on discussing the administrative package. Each section of the package should be reviewed, with particular emphasis placed on

1. Explaining the mechanics, results, and opportunities for revision of the projection package
2. Clarifying the causal relationship of workload projections to personnel and supplies and other expense budgets
3. Making clear the nature and the mechanics of each of the steps involved in preparing decision packages and detailed personnel, supplies and other expenses, and capital budgets
4. Reiterating the importance of meeting the due dates identified in the budget calendar

As was the case with the general meeting, the tone of the technical meeting(s) should lean toward informality and openness. The meeting(s) should be chaired by the director of the fiscal services division, the budget officer, or a designated member of their staffs.

In addition to providing information, the goal of the technical meeting(s) should be to establish or reinforce a feeling of mutual trust and problem solving between line management and the fiscal services division. To assist in accomplishing this, expository presentations should be secondary to answering questions from the floor. Also, the support services that the fiscal services division is ready to provide to line management should be identified clearly, with line management being encouraged to utilize these services whenever possible.

PHASE V

As has been the case in the previous phases, Phase V builds on the foregoing work. This phase, however, differs significantly from the others in two key respects. First, it is an implementation, as opposed to a preparatory, phase. The previous steps have all contributed toward either specifying the design or laying the foundation for the development of the budget. This phase draws together the outputs of these previous efforts and, using line management's imagination and initiative as catalysts, converts them into an initial or tentative budget. The second major distinction is addressed in more detail later in this chapter. At this point, it is sufficient to recognize that it is in Phase V that line management adopts an activist role. The work of Phase III could be accomplished largely apart from day-to-day line operations. Phase IV involves the line manager; however, it is a passive involvement centered on communication. It is not until Phase V that the focus of activity shifts and line management becomes the principal factor in the process.

Phase V is the point in the process at which zero base budgeting (as modified to be pragmatic) takes place. The specific steps that compose this phase are detailed in Table 17.3. This table is an expansion of Table 17.1. Appendix 17, Table 17.4, and Chapter 18 provide insight into the mechanics of each of the involved steps.

The point to be recognized is that the first segment of this phase, steps 8 and 9, produces the project and capital expenditure decision packages (see Table 17.4). These packages are then rank ordered in Step 10. The final output of this phase is a ranked listing, which includes estimated costs of both approved capital expenditure and operating projects. This output, in turn, becomes the input for the next phase of the process.

Before moving ahead to discuss the next phase, it is worthwhile to dwell for a moment on Step 11, revenue budget preparation.

In the conventional business setting, developing the firm's revenue budget is a major and critical management activity. This would also be the case in the hospital setting if it were not for cost-based payment. Cost-based payment creates a situation wherein the expense budget establishes costs

TABLE 17.3   Budget Preparation Process: Phase V Detail

Step 8. Administrative Meetings 1–n: Responsibility Center/Department Level
The goal of these meetings is to translate the department and responsibility center level objectives (see Phase II) into projects and activities at the department and responsibility center level. This translation process may involve a single meeting or a series of meetings. It is completed only when the responsibility center manager and his superior have reached at least general agreement about the nature and direction of the budget period's operations and capital expenditures.

Step 9. Decision Package Development
Based on the decisions reached in Step 8, line management develops decision packages that identify the activity—its benefits, costs, and alternatives. The nature of the activity and its benefits and alternatives should be defined in as much detail as practicable.

The level of programmatic detail should not, however, exceed the informational needs of management. Describing specific tasks and results to the individual project level of detail may be appropriate in certain situations, where management has extensive experience with planning and budgeting and sophisticated costing and financial reporting systems. In other settings, detail to the responsibility center level is all that may be either useful or necessary. With respect to financial detail, at this point the cost of the activity should only be estimated, with detailed costing pending further budgetary approvals.

Decision packages or decision forms should also be prepared for each potential capital expenditure.

Step 10. Administrative Meetings 1–n: Rank Ordering of Decision Packages
This step involves a series of consecutive meetings wherein succeeding levels of management integrate and rank order decision packages prepared in Step 9. It should be noted that, depending upon the budgetary experience of the hospital, this step may be preceded by another set of administrative meetings wherein the decision packages are reviewed for completeness and, if necessary, revised prior to submission.

Capital expenditure decision packages also should be rank ordered at this point. As explained in Chapter 18, the process for ranking these expenditure alternatives may differ somewhat from the project ranking process. For example, the ranking process for small capital items—expenditures of under $X —may involve successive levels of management only up to the program level. Similarly, the ranking process for large items may involve an interdisciplinary committee, successive levels of management, a combination of the two, or some other process.

Step 11. Revenue Budget Development
In conjunction with, but apart from, the above activities, the data from the projection package should be used to calculate the initial revenue budget. This budget is basically the product of the current charge structure, adjusted as appropriate for cost-based payment, multiplied by projected revenue center volumes of service.

TABLE 17.4   Budgeting Decision Package: Form and Instructions

1. Program Area _____ 2. Activity _____
3. Objective _____
_____
_____

4. Activity Description _____
_____
_____

         Starting Date _____ Completion Date _____

5. Activity Benefit/Result   6. Resource Estimates

	Man years	Direct Expense
_____	Mgmt.	Salaries
_____	Super.	Travel
_____	Tech.	Other
	Clerical	
	Total _____	Total _____

7. Alternatives: Alternative Ways of Accomplishing the Same Result

No.	Alternative	Resource Requirement Man years $

8. Alternatives: Alternative Levels of Effort

No.	Alternative	Benefit	Resource Requirement Man years $

9. Ranking

No. Alternative Number Resource Requirement ($) 10. _____

1	_____	Identification of
2	_____	Package Developer
3	_____	
4	_____	
5	_____	Date _____
6	_____	

TABLE 17.4   Continued

Instructions

1. Program Area
   Identification by name of the program area being addressed: for example, Environmental Services, Administration, Outpatient Services.

2. Activity
   Identification of the activity being addressed. In Environmental Services it might be Heating and Cooling Plant; in Outpatient Services it might be Community Mental Health.

3. Objective
   Restatement of the program area's objective or that portion of the objective to which the activity applies. In Outpatient Services, for the Community Mental Health activity, the objective might be to provide the total service area with convenient access to mental health service.

4. Activity Description
   Generic statement of the activity, with starting and completion dates from a process perspective when applicable. For example, under Environmental Services the description of the activities of a heating and cooling plant professional might be the licensed supervision, operation, and minor maintenance of the central heating and cooling system on an around the clock basis. This would be an ongoing activity.

5. Activity Benefit/Result
   Statement in quantified terms of the benefit/result or output of the activity. Result *must* relate to the program area objective and be quantified. For example: Outpatient Services, Community Mental Health—through the use of outreach efforts—provide convenient access to mental health services for the total service area as measured by an increase of 5,000 visits by existing patients and the provision of services to at least 300 new patients.

6. Resource Estimates
   Statement of estimated resource requirements. Expense information should just be direct costs.

7. Alternatives: Alternative Ways of Accomplishing the Same Result
   The purpose of this section is to force consideration of alternatives. In this instance, it is alternative ways of accomplishing the same result.

   The first alternative in this section should be numbered 2 since the alternative indicated in item 4 is number 1. Other alternatives should be ranked sequentially. Under the "Alternative" heading, a different approach to achieving the same end should be identified: hiring a consultant as opposed to doing the job yourself, or purchasing laundry services on a contract basis as opposed to operating the hospital's own laundry, or centralizing OB on a communitywide basis. *If no visible alternative exists, then this section should be left blank.*

   In the "Resource Requirement" section the total man years and direct dollars of expense associated with each alternative should be set out.

Continued

TABLE 17.4   Continued

8. Alternatives: Alternative Levels of Effort.
   The purpose of this section is to focus attention on alternative levels of investment and their resulting benefits. For example: for a $200,000 investment,
   increase patient visits by 3,000 and new patients by 300; for $150,000 invest-
   ment increase patient visits by 3,000 and new patients by 100. This section
   should just address alternatives to the level of activity of choice.

   In the "No." column, the sequential listing of alternatives should be continued
   from the above section. Under "Alternative," the nature of the alternative
   should be briefly stated; for example, 3,000 visits increase, 300 new patients.

   In the "Benefit" column, the benefit obtained from the alternative level of
   effort should be defined: convenient access to only 90% of the total service
   area.

   The "Resource Requirement" column should be completed the same as is the
   case above.

   If the alternative is to forego the activity, then the nature of the lost benefit
   should be set out.

9. Ranking
   The ranking of each of the alternatives should be identified by its sequential
   number.

10. Identification and Date
    Signature of the manager responsible on a day-to-day basis for the operation
    of the activity and the date on which the Decision Package is to be submitted
    for review.

and costs in turn establish, based upon the third party payment contract,
the revenue budget and revenues. Building the expense budget thus results
in simultaneously being able to determine the revenue budget.

This direct linking of hospital expense and revenue budgets is broken
only to the extent that a hospital is able to generate charge-based and non–
patient care revenues. In budgeting these sources of revenue, the traditional
commercial model applies with revenue projections being based on expected volume and price. Figure 17.1 illustrates the linkage between expense and revenue budgets.

PHASE VI

Phase VI represents the detailed costing and financial data integration
segment of the budget preparation process. With the exception of Step 15,
final administrative review, it is basically a computational and clerical phase
wherein the decision packages of Phase V are converted into a traditional
financial budget of the operating budget.

FIGURE 17.1   Hospital Expense/Revenue Budget Linkage

Expense Budget

↓

Total expenses are composed of:

1. Portion of expenses related——►Revenues = Actual allowable
   to patients covered by third   costs (expenses) adjusted
   party payment agreements*   for any plus factor allowed
                                           in the third party contract

2. Portion of expenses related ———►Revenues = (Volume) (Unit Charge)
   to self-pay patients

3 Non–patient care expenses———►Revenues = (Volume) (Unit Charge)

↓

Revenue Budget

*The bulk of hospital expenses relate to patients covered by third party payment contracts, for example, Blue Cross, Medicare, Medicaid. Therefore, the revenue budget, while allowing for management initiative on the margin, is almost entirely a direct distillation of the expense budget.

STEP 12. RESOURCE SPECIFICATION

The initial step of Phase VI involves two components. The first component provides the basis for the metamorphosis of the operating budget into a financial budget by requiring that line management specify the resources needed to carry out approved activity levels and projects. Line management must identify the number, position classification, and, if appropriate, expected hiring date of all personnel (including the number and position classification of any personnel who will receive pay differentials), as well as the nature, timing, and amount of any other expenses—travel, consulting, printing—that are anticipated. In the case of capital expenditure projects, the amount of the expenditure and its timing should be identified.

As discussed earlier, specification of financial detail is deferred to this point to minimize wasted effort and to increase the credibility of the entire budgetary process. If detailed costing were required to take place at an earlier point, line managers would need to invest substantial time and effort in specifying the resource requirements for projects that subsequently might be disapproved. To the extent that this occurred, effort would be wasted and line management's acceptance of the operational planning and budget preparation process would deteriorate. Both of these pitfalls can be avoided by delaying detailed project specification until after the operating plan is complete and initial project and activity level decisions have been made.

The second component of this step is the conversion of line management's detailed resource specifications into actual dollars. This aspect of the process is basically a clerical and computational task and should be carried out primarily by the hospital's fiscal services division. Line management should be consulted, as necessary, to resolve questions and provide any needed additional detail. However, the prime accountability for converting the resource specifications into dollar costs should be the responsibility of the fiscal services division.

STEP 13. TENTATIVE BUDGET COMPLETION

The output of the above conversion process is the input for the generation of the hospital's tentative dollar budget. Organizing and aggregating the data developed in the foregoing step into the tentative budget are also basically clerical and computational tasks. Therefore, the fiscal services division should again have primary accountability for completing this step.

It is important to recognize that the budget that is produced in this step is only a tentative budget. The budget, though consisting of approved activity levels and projects, has not been matched against the revenue budget. If in this matching process an imbalance exists that cannot be resolved through revision of the revenue budget, then obviously either the expense budget, the capital budget, or both must be revised. It is due to the reality of this possibility for adjustment and revision that the budget must still be considered tentative at this point.

Obviously, adjustment to the expense budget at this point will have negative management implications in terms of staff morale and satisfaction with the budgetary process. Often, however, the need for such revisions cannot be avoided. As discussed earlier, the budgetary process should be designed to minimize the need for such decisions by requiring early determination of financial constraints and project approval before detailed costing. Even with a well designed and finely timed process, it is unrealistic to expect that some adjustments might not be required. The best that can be hoped for is that their number and depth can be kept to an understandable level.

STEP 14. BUDGET INTEGRATION

In Step 11, the initial revenue budget was developed. It is identified as initial for it is essentially the product of the current charge structure multiplied by forecasted volume plus projected nonoperating revenues and revenues from cost-based payers. In this step, the revenue budget of Step 11 is integrated with the tentative expense and capital budgets of Step 13.

The integration of these budgets is largely a mechanical task. It is done to determine if the necessary revenue and expense (both total dollar and cash) equalities exist. If they do, the budgets can be completed. However, if, as is more often the case, an imbalance exists, then an additional management judgment step is needed.

STEP 15. FINAL ADMINISTRATIVE REVIEW

Due to the accelerated rates of inflation in hospital costs, it is likely that there will be an imbalance between the initial revenue budget and the tentative expense and capital budgets. When such an imbalance occurs, senior and executive management must make a series of decisions that will bring the two sets of budgets, that is, revenue and expense, into balance on both a total and cash basis.

Generally, the first step in resolving any imbalance is focused on adjusting the revenue budget. If, after adjusting the revenue budget an inequality still exists, then the expense and capital budgets must be revised. In this case, management must return to the rank ordering developed in Phase V and eliminate or defer a sufficient dollar amount of previously approved projects or activities to bring expenses and revenues into equality.

As just discussed, deletion of a project or reduction of an activity level is at this point a painful decision. However, it is a necessary decision if the financial health and perhaps survival of the institution are to be preserved. Therefore, although the decision is necessary and justified, it should be made with line management's full awareness of steps that have been taken to avoid it and the reasons why it is still necessary, even after these measures. It is only with this kind of open communication and full understanding that the demoralizing effects of such decisions can be minimized.

STEP 16. BUDGET COMPLETION

The final step in this phase is generation of the final revenue, expense, and capital budgets, based on the decisions of the previous step. The mechanics and accountabilities of this step are similar to those of Step 13. Also included in this step is the conversion of these primary budgets into the final cash budget. The mechanics of developing a cash budget are discussed in detail in Appendix 13.B.

PHASES VII AND VIII

By this point, the nature of Phases VII and VIII can probably be deduced. Phase VII consists of a single step—board approval of the budget (Step 17). If the above steps have been carefully carried out and the hospital's organizational system of checks and balances has been respected, with approvals being obtained at the necessary and appropriate times, then this step should present little problem, being operationally no more than just a formality. Regardless of whether this step is a formality or a detailed line item review, it is a step that must be completed if the budget is to have the institution's full legal support and commitment.

Phase VIII is shown as consisting of only two steps—implementation

(Step 18) and feedback (Step 19). In theory, this characterization is correct. However, it must be recognized that each of these steps involves a multitude of substeps and tasks.

STEP 18. IMPLEMENTATION

This refers to the operational function of carrying out the decisions made in the budgetary process. Occasionally, effecting these decisions may be a simple—or at least a relatively simple—matter. More often, however, it is a complex problem requiring the expert application of a variety of both general and technical managerial skills. An in-depth discussion of either the mechanics or the application of these skills is beyond the scope of this work. Readers desiring more information in this area should refer to the Suggested Readings.

STEP 19. FEEDBACK

While perhaps not as technically complex as implementation, feedback involves several aspects and subtleties. Moreover, as discussed in Chapter 16, the feedback process is perhaps the most critical contributing factor in realizing the full operational control potential of the budgetary process. Due to the importance of this topic, it is discussed in detail in Chapter 19.

ORGANIZATION STRUCTURE

The foregoing has described the operational steps intrinsic to the development of a hospital's budget. Admittedly, the content of any particular step, as well as the flow of steps, may be revised as the process is tailored to fit a given institution's operating environment and needs. However, as a generalized procedure, the above should serve as a valid baseline for the construction of an individual hospital's unique preparation procedures.

It is important to recognize that procedures, regardless of how well they may have been designed and drafted, are basically impotent. Like a road map, a procedure only identifies the route between points A and B. It does not, however, move one from point A to point B. To traverse the route, a driving force is needed. In the case of operational planning and budget preparation, the force that drives the process and implements the procedure is people.

Clearly, it is impossible to develop and implement effectively an operating plan and budget without the hospital's staff, at all levels, cooperating and actively "working on the problem." Equally obvious is the fact that if the staff is to work efficiently, it must implement the planning and budgeting procedure within the framework of both a tightly designed organization structure and a carefully specified and coordinated set of staff accountabilities.

A well-managed hospital is generally the product of the effort and intellect of a group of individuals who are organized to function in concert toward a common goal. Organization provides the mechanism for allocating responsibilities and channeling efforts so that the objectives of the institution can be efficiently and effectively achieved. Thus, sound organization in all areas of operation is one of the critical elements necessary for successful management.

Sound organization, however, can take a variety of forms. Experience has demonstrated that while there is no single right organization structure that can be recommended universally, certain patterns of organization are generally practicable. Moreover, certain principles can be applied with a high degree of uniformity. Specifically, the organization structure should assist in assuring or providing the structure for

1. A system of management control checks and balances
2. Complete allocation of all requisite duties
3. A clear definition of responsibilities
4. Coordination of responsibilities
5. Operational decision flexibility
6. A systematic policy decision process

Utilizing these concepts, a prototype planning and budgeting organization structure can be defined. Figure 17.2 illustrates this prototype. In considering this example, the reader should be careful to avoid the pitfall of adopting the proposed model as the universal answer to all budgeting organizational questions. It is presented not as an absolute solution but rather as a bench mark or guideline for the tailoring of any particular institution's organization structure.

ACCOUNTABILITIES

The flow of authority is clearly documented in Figure 17.2. A final element, however, is still missing. To give the organization structure dimension and to add the dynamics necessary to convert the process from paper procedure into actions, one must define staff accountabilities and relative roles. This step is needed not only to provide direction and control, but also to provide a check and balance mechanism for assuring the coordination of all efforts.

Table 17.5 describes the accountabilities of the various management levels and/or organizational units in terms of the itemized phases and steps of the process defined in the first part of this chapter.[4] While the table, for

---

[4]Table 17.5 is presented in the same design format as Table 17.1. This was done to allow both the authors and the reader to build upon the earlier material to produce a complete description of the process.

FIGURE 17.2   Prototype: Budgeting Organization Structure

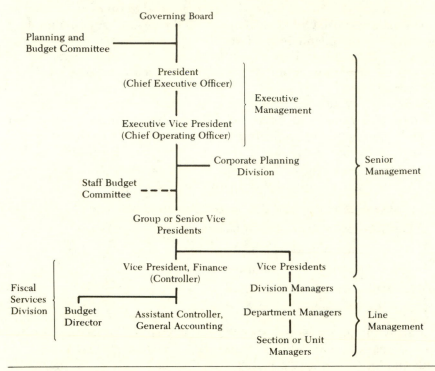

Note: Corporate planning and marketing can be combined into a single division. If the hospital has group and/or senior vice presidents, the chief financial officer (CFO) would typically be at that level.

the most part, is self-explanatory, it may be of value to highlight several points.

GOVERNING BOARD

The hospital's governing board is vested by law with the ultimate authority and responsibility for managing all of the institution's business. Therefore, the governing board is responsible for all phases of hospital operations.

In terms of operational planning and budget preparation, this responsibility, at a minimum, is carried out through the review and approval of the final strategy, operating plan, and budget. In addition, the governing board, given the history and management style of the institution as well as its own prerogatives, may desire and have an ongoing involvement in the development of the plan and budget. From the perspective of obtaining expeditious decisions, increased governing board involvement of a nonoperational, review, and approval nature is desirable.

The organizational mechanics utilized to provide increased governing board involvement will obviously differ from one institution to another. However, as a guideline—if the board is large, meets infrequently, or is uncomfortable or unproductive in dealing at its general meetings with operational details—the device of a budget committee (or a planning and budget committee) may prove to be quite useful. This committee should be board appointed and should consist of a membership that includes, at least, a majority of active board members. Its functions with respect to the budget are[5]

1. Review annual and long-term budgets and determine that forecasts are reasonably and accurately prepared

2. Recommend budgets to the full board (or if appropriate the executive committee of the board) for their approval

3. Periodically review both operating results and, where significant budget variations are found, management's proposal of corrective action

CORPORATE PLANNING

The role of corporate planning can be summarized as consisting of prime staff accountability not only for the preparation of the Phase I, corporate strategy, and Phase II, operating plan, materials, but also for

1. The interface and linkage of the planning process with the budget preparation process; and

2. Performance (program) evaluation with respect to both the operating plan's objectives (Did the hospital do what it planned to do?) and the implications of the environmental assessment (Did the hospital's actions [doing what it planned to do] have the anticipated effect/impact?).

In carrying out these accountabilities, it is vital that corporate planning recognize the necessity of not acting in a vacuum. As discussed in the previous chapters, if the full motivational benefits of the budgetary process are to be obtained, other components of the organization must be involved and contribute in meaningful ways to developing these materials and making the requisite decisions. The points of involvement and the groups to be involved are identified in Tables 16.4 and 17.5.

In large hospitals or in hospitals that are complex business entities, with multiple lines of business, the corporate planning function should ideally be a specific, separate organizational unit. In such cases it should

---

[5]Caruana, Russell A., *A Guide to Organizing the Hospital's Fiscal Services Division*, pp. 12, 13.

TABLE 17.5   Accountabilities: Budget Preparation

Board	Executive Management	Senior Management	Staff Budget Committee	Budget Director	Corporate Planning	Line Management	Fiscal Services
			1. Budget management review/revision	—	—		
				2. Projection package development	—		—
	3. Projection package approval	—					
				4. Administrative package development	—		—
		5. Administrative package approval					
	6. General budget meeting			—	—	—	
				7. Technical budget meeting	—		

Phase III* (items 1–5)

Phase IV (items 6–7)

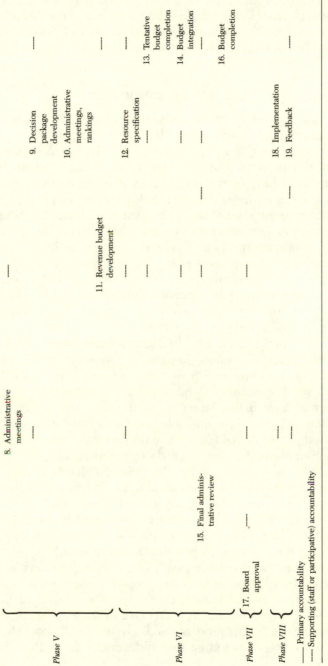

report to either the executive vice president or a group or senior vice president. In smaller hospitals, the corporate planning function can be combined with the functions of the budget director. Even if combined, however, it should be made clear that there are two separate functions involved and that the plan shapes the budget.

STAFF BUDGET COMMITTEE

The creation and use of a staff level budget committee can be considered to be an optional component of the budget preparation organization. It is suggested as part of the prototype, for it both represents a logical extension of the principles of participatory management and provides a vehicle that can yield operational as well as political dividends.

Ideally, the committee should be multidisciplinary in nature, including medical staff representation as well as representation from nursing, administration, and the various general service and patient care departments. The committee's membership should also be designed to reflect a cross section of the institution's organizational hierarchy. Selection of the specific committee members and the chairman should be done by senior management. In making its selections, management should focus on obtaining the involvement of individuals who can and will serve not as parochial delegates, but as representatives of the total institution.

The function of the committee, in addition to reviewing and suggesting revisions to the hospital's budget preparation procedure manual, should be that of serving as an intramural review and advisory group. In this role it can provide useful operational insights into many of the decisions that senior management must make. Moreover, as the surrogate for the total staff, the committee can provide a workable mechanism for increasing staff involvement in the operational planning and budget preparation process and subsequent commitment to the hospital's operating goals.

If increased commitment is actually to be obtained, it should be realized that the committee must be meaningfully involved in the decision process, even if only in an advisory capacity. If the committee even appears to be just "window dressing," its existence may well prove to be counterproductive. Therefore, before creating such a committee, senior management should carefully review its predilections and establish the committee only if it is committed to working with committee members in a participatory manner. In addition to the foregoing, this committee can be of assistance in making capital budget decisions. The nature of the capital investment decision process and the role that a multidisciplinary committee of this type can play in this process are discussed in Chapter 18. The possibility and benefits of including this additional role in the committee's charge should be carefully considered by senior management in determining whether to create such a committee.

LINE MANAGEMENT

All too often, line management bears the brunt of the tedium that is inherent in converting or expressing the operating plan as a budget. As a result, in many instances line management has come to view the planning and budgeting process as a paper exercise wherein clerical skills are of greater importance than either innovative thinking or management judgment.

When this becomes the case, either in reality or in line management's perception of reality, then, as discussed in Chapter 16, the dangers involved in confusing means and ends may well be incurred. The risks in such instances are that the motivational and, to some extent, the control values of the budgetary process may be lost.

Obviously, the operational planning and budget preparation process will always require that line management carry out some clerical tasks. However, to the greatest extent practicable, these tasks should be limited both in scope and content. Line management's role should be primarily that of translating the hospital's strategy and operating plan into successful programs and accomplishments. To the extent that one aspect of this translation process involves the completion of forms, tables, and charts, the responsibility for developing and submitting these materials should lie with line management.

Developing the accounting detail for the financial budget should not be the responsibility of line management. Therefore, the line manager should not be burdened with the clerical tasks related to either this activity or any other activity that involves a process or set of decisions that are beyond his control, for example, preparation of the initial revenue budget. To the extent that these clerical tasks are shifted to the appropriate point in the fiscal services division, not only will the total budgetary process become more efficient, but also, in the larger contexts of total organizational performance and control, management at all levels will be more effective.

In addition to its prime accountability, line management carries several supporting responsibilities. The nature of this staff role is identified in Table 17.5 by dotted lines, as was done in the previous instances. The mechanisms for implementing this role will differ both from one hospital to another and from one task to another. For the sake of simplicity, it may well be most efficient to obtain line management's input to corporate planning and senior management through the vehicle of the staff conferences that should be an ongoing component of any hospital's management control system. Line management's input to the fiscal services division and the budget director should be obtained as needed, through generally less formal mechanisms, for example, telephone calls and scheduled short meetings.

FISCAL SERVICES DIVISION

The fiscal services division's role in the budgetary process has been alluded to. Essentially, it is accountable for the conversion of the planned operating program into dollar cost estimates and the aggregation of the individual cost estimates into a complete, integrated budget package. As such, the division plays a central role in the budgetary process. It is a role that must, however, always be kept in perspective. The operational planning and budget preparation process is neither designed nor intended to function as a service to the financial manager and accountant. Rather, the fiscal services division should and must function as a service and supporting agent to the entire organization and budgetary process.

The fiscal services division contributes in another way to the total process. In addition to its multiple roles as a component of senior and line management, the fiscal services division serves as the staff resource to the total hospital in budget preparation. Typically, the person who can be viewed as the project manager (the budget director) for the entire budget preparation and financial feedback process is organizationally housed in the fiscal services division.

In many hospitals the role of budget director has traditionally been encompassed within the responsibilities of the controller or chief financial officer's office. Often the controller personally developed the hospital's budget. In some instances, this approach may have been and may still be appropriate. However, given the importance of operational planning and budgeting to the financial and functional health of the institution and the resources and time demands of an effective budgetary program, it is questionable if this approach to the allocated responsibilities is still the method of choice. In larger institutions, it clearly is not.

A full-time budget director, who is responsible not only for coordinating the budget preparation process but also for administering the mechanics of the financial feedback process, increasingly is becoming an operational necessity for both large- and medium-sized hospitals. As discussed, the functions of the budget director and corporate planning might, in some instances, be combined. Ideally, however, the two should be separate but coordinated.

The need for a distinct, full-time budget director is particularly acute in those areas where either rate review or prospective payment programs have been implemented. Aside from the demands of the environment, the employment of a full-time budget director is a sound management decision that can produce savings and improvements in staff performance, if properly handled.

The budget director generally reports to the hospital's chief financial officer. His major accountabilities can be summarized as follows:

1. Establish written instructions for a formal budget preparation and management reporting or feedback program
2. Coordinate and provide assistance to activities of all levels of management in the development of their budgets
3. Coordinate the activities of the fiscal services division in both providing support to management in the preparation of the operating plan and in converting the operating plan into a comprehensive financial budget
4. Analyze major variances between actual expenses and budget for management and department heads
5. Establish a procedure for accumulating accurate statistical data, such as patient days, outpatient and emergency room visits, units of service provided by departments[6]
6. Accumulate data for the filing of rate justifications and, if necessary, rate appeals

The task confronting the budget director is, by way of an understatement, an interesting challenge. Not only must he possess technical skills in the areas of finance, accounting, and management, but he also must have sufficient political skill to tread successfully the narrow path between a manager's legitimate, individual prerogatives and the common needs of the institution. Given both the importance and the demands of the job, the budget director, like the controller, must be more than just an accountant. He must have the imagination and drive to breathe life, energy, and priority into a difficult task whose successful performance is beyond his direct control, and the skill to utilize, and help others to utilize, the resulting product as an effective management tool.

CONCLUSION

The foregoing has been an attempt to define the budget preparation process first by identifying the individual steps involved in the process and then by describing the organization structure and accountabilities that provide the process with its driving force. The emphasis has been on providing both an anatomical and a holistic overview of the process.

By design, certain facets of the process have only been touched lightly and certain simplifying assumptions have been made. The first category of decisions reflects an appreciation of the existing literature and an attempt

---

[6]This accountability would apply in those jurisdictions that utilize some form of extramural rate review for purposes of establishing payment levels.

to avoid duplication. An exception to this rule is, perhaps, made in the following chapter, which addresses capital investment decisions and capital budgeting. In this instance, a different type of balance with the existing literature was sought, leaning more toward the analytic and quantitative.

The second category of decisions reflects the fact that for some questions there are no single right answers. In considering the material in the latter portion of the chapter, the reader should always bear in mind the essential principle that there is no universal solution to organizational questions. In the case of the budgetary organization, a variety of structural patterns can be effective if they: (1) allow for a participatory approach to decision making; and (2) allocate responsibility in a manner that enables each participant to feel that the job he is doing—the accountability he is assigned—is worthy of his time and efforts.

SUGGESTED READINGS

Brown, Ray E. *Judgment in Administration.*

Caruana, Russell A. *A Guide to Organizing the Hospital's Fiscal Services Division.*

Dillon, Ray D. *Zero Base Budgeting for Health Care Institutions.*

Esmond, Truman H., Jr. *Budgeting Procedures for Hospitals.*

Greater Detroit Area Hospital Council. *Management Guide to Effective Budgeting.*

Griffith, John R. *Quantitative Techniques for Hospital Planning and Control.*

Grimaldi, Paul L. and Micheletti, Julie A. *Diagnosis Related Groups: A Practitioner's Guide.*

Heckert, J. Brooks and Wilson, James D. *Controllership.*

Lipson, Stephen H. and Hensel, Mary D. *Hospital Manpower Budget Preparation Manual.*

Pyhrr, Peter A. *Zero Base Budgeting.*

Schein, Edgar H. *Organizational Psychology.*

Silvers, J.B. and Prahalad, C.K. *Financial Management of Health Institutions.*

Suver, James D. and Neumann, Bruce R. "Zero Base Budgeting."

Sutermeister, Robert A. (ed.). *People and Productivity.*

Vraciu, Robert A. "Programming, Budgeting, and Control in Health Care Organizations: The State of the Art."

Warner, D. Michael; Holloway, Don C.; and Grazier, Kyle L. *Decision Making and Control for Health Administration.*

APPENDIX 17
EXAMPLE OF AN ADMINISTRATIVE PACKAGE
(EXCERPTS FOLLOW)

INTER-OFFICE MEMORANDUM

TO: *Department Heads*
Management Roundtable

FROM: *Martha Wolfgang, President*

SUBJECT: *Fiscal Year Budget*

Attached for your review and use is the Administrative Package that will be used for the development of the fiscal year operating plan and budget. As in previous years, the forms and instructions contained in this package have been reviewed and approved by the Budget Committee.

Since this package contains both the information needed and the procedures to be used in preparing the hospital's budget, I urge you to review it carefully and to be prepared to raise any questions you might have at either the general or technical budget meetings.

During the coming year, we estimate that our inpatient services and census will remain at about their present level. Occupancy rate, however, will increase due to a reduction in bed capacity. Additional services will be added in the primary care area in order to respond to the current need and future demand in our community. These services can be expected to reduce emergency room visits while simultaneously adding to the laboratory and radiology workload.

You should, as a matter of standard operating procedure, discuss your department's present operations and future plans with those persons who are directly responsible to you. Staff should be briefed on the hospital's financial situation and plans for the year, and their assistance should be solicited. Other department heads whose responsibility centers affect your departmental operations can also be of value in the preparation of your budget. You are urged to consult with them.

To permit time both for consolidation of all budgets and for review of the total budget prior to presentation to the Governing Board, you are requested to begin preparation as soon as possible and to comply with the due dates as set out in the budget calendar.

The Budget Officer and the Division of Fiscal Services are available to provide you with any needed technical support or data. Call upon them whenever they can be of assistance.

ADMINISTRATIVE PACKAGE
BRT GENERAL HOSPITAL

	Budget Calendar
	Budget Calendar
March 20	General Meeting
March 22	Technical Budget Meetings
March 30–April 13	Administrative Meetings—I
April 13	*Decision Packages Due*
April 17–24	Administrative Meeting—II: Rank Orderings
April 25–May 2	Administrative Meeting—III: Rank Orderings
May 4	Final Rank Ordering and Specific Project Funding Decisions
May 11	*Personnel, Supplies and Other Expenses, and Capital Budget Detail Forms Due*
May 23	Initial Integrated Budget Due from Fiscal Services
May 27–June 1	Administrative Meeting—IV: Budget Review and Adjustment
June 6	Budget Completed and Distributed to the Governing Board
June 15	*Board of Governors Review and Approval*

BRT GENERAL HOSPITAL
STATEMENT OF GENERAL OBJECTIVE AND POLICIES[7]

In recognition of both its role as a community resource and its obligation to the community, the governing board of BRT General Hospital commits itself to using the resources entrusted to it:

to deliver needed health services to the community with the primary purposes of improving health status of individuals and continuing to increase the value of the community's health services expenditures.

In order to achieve this purpose, the governing board establishes the following general policies as parameters for purposes of guiding the operation of the corporation:

Operating

1. To the extent of its resources, the hospital will operate for the benefit of those not able to pay.
2. Consistent with the requirements for quality care, the hospital will not restrict the use of its facilities to a particular group of physicians or surgeons.
3. Through the application of sound and imaginative management techniques and leadership, the hospital will not only protect its assets and income against subversion, but also assure that those assets are utilized in a manner that produces the greatest benefit to its service areas.

Financial

1. Inpatient expenses per admission should increase by no more than 4.8%.
2. A positive aggregate operating margin of 6% should be generated.

---

[7]This statement was initially approved by the Governing Board at its May 198W meeting and has been reviewed (as appropriate and as required by the hospital's operating environment), revised, and reaffirmed annually since that date.

BRT GENERAL HOSPITAL
ENVIRONMENTAL ASSESSMENT STATEMENT[8]

The following is an analysis of the hospital's present operating environment. This analysis describes the environment in terms of the strengths and weaknesses of the hospital, the nature of its role within the community, the nature of the population being served, and the general condition of the hospital's operating milieu.

I.   Internal Environment

   A. Physical Plant
      Average age of plant is ten years. Plant is fully air conditioned and meets not only state health and fire codes, but also the Federal Life Safety Code. Maintenance costs are stabilized but can be expected to increase over the next two to five years.
      Plant is presently utilized to capacity; grounds will accommodate additional facilities, but additions to services will require new construction.

   B. Patient Services
      Currently, a full range of inpatient services is provided. Hospital has also been designated as an end stage renal center. Hospital has operating and transfer agreements with the regional medical center and with local skilled nursing facilities and home health programs.
      Ambulatory care program relatively weak, particularly in light of the community's lack of primary care resources.
      Radiology facilities also weak in terms of special procedures capacity and capability.

   C. Organization
      Staff levels, with the exception of the Nursing Services Division, are at 95% of table of organization approved complement.
      Staff turnover stabilizing and a maturing work force developing.
      Medical staff well organized and sensitive to both the hospital's and the community's needs. Open staffing in community has resulted in medical staff size being sufficient to support the hospital's capacity.

   D. Financial
      Net margin has increased slightly over the past three years. As a result, a modest reserve has been generated. However, due to

_____
[8]Excerpts.

cutbacks in the Medicaid program, further increases in net margin will be difficult to obtain.[9]

Internal resources are not yet sufficient to support any large-scale capital expenditure programs. Moreover, though the development program effort has been under way for a year, it is still unclear as to amount—either the number or the magnitude—of gifts that it will generate.

E. Quality of Services

Accreditation and licensure status in good standing.

Continuing medical education program becoming institutionalized with a resultant interlocking relationship developing between Director of Medical Education office and the Credential Committee.

II. External Environment

A. Community

The hospital's primary service area currently has an estimated population of 120,000 persons. This population has remained relatively stable in size. However, it has declined marginally in economic status while sometimes polarizing into two demographic groups: one aging and the other young and relatively unskilled in terms of the labor market.

Health resource in the community has declined in proportion to the community's ability to incur out-of-pocket expenses. This decline has been particularly marked in the primary care area. As a result, community groups are placing increased pressure on the hospital to expand its emergency room and walk-in facilities.

B. General Economics

The overriding economic and social factor for hospitals and for every other sector of the economy, is the federal budget deficit. The top economic priority of the administration will continue to be the battle against the deficit. The programs it develops will directly affect hospitals. Hospitals can expect government resources increasingly to be directed to other sections of the economy with the result that hospitals are likely to be affected severely.

C. Legislation

At the national level, the regulatory changes in the Medicare program have placed and will continue to place increased pres-

---

[9]For some hospitals, the importance of examining the Medicaid and public assistance environments cannot be overemphasized. For hospitals with large patient loads financed by these sources, these factors may be the main environmental detriments. Therefore, such hospitals must plan based on their assessment of what will be happening to Medicaid and public assistance eligibility and payment levels.

sure on the hospital's financial condition. For the present these pressures are being accommodated successfully. However, continued lowering of the prospective payment system's prices may well result in some Medicare costs having to be subsidized.

At the local level, rate review legislation has not been enacted. While evidencing frustration and disappointment with the performance of the state's health care system, the legislature has determined that the prudent course is to wait until experience is gained with the various new federal acts and regulations.

III. Analysis

The hospital is in reasonable operating and financial condition. However, demand for both services and resources is increasing, particularly in terms of the provision of primary care.

The future regulatory picture, however, is uncertain. While for the moment no further major intrusions into management prerogatives are expected, this situation could reverse itself quickly.

ASSUMPTIONS[10]

The following assumptions represent management's best judgment as to the major phenomena that will affect hospital operations. These assumptions should be reviewed carefully and amplified through the projection of more detailed operational assumptions.

I.   National Hospital Industry Assumptions (Excerpts)

    A. General

       1. The Economy

          Most recent economic forecasts confirm continued growth throughout 198X. Unemployment, however, will remain at historically high levels.

       2. Gross National Product

          Real GNP is expected to grow by 2.0% in 198X, after increases of 2.1% and 4.4% in the previous two years, respectively.

       3. Inflation

          Inflation is expected to remain at relatively low levels over the near term. As measured by the CPI, inflation during 198X is expected to be 3.8%.

       4. Employment

          The number of jobs in the economy is expected to increase substantially over the near term. Even so, unemployment will remain at historically high rates (7+%). Employment in the hospital industry can be expected to shrink due to cost containment efforts.

       5. Implications: General

          Given an economic outlook characterized by unacceptably large federal budget deficits, cutbacks in federal programs can be expected. Domestic programs and particularly social welfare programs are most vulnerable.

       6. Implications: Hospital Industry

          If government budgets are contained to slower growth rates, hospitals will face increased economic pressures. Hospital closings are likely, as larger production units will be needed to obtain the necessary economies of scale.

---

[10]Assumptions are defined as statements describing future events or developments that will affect hospital operations but whose occurrence is beyond the direct control of hospital management.

B. The Patient

    1. Assumptions

        a. Future increases in the human life span will occur as the results of changes in social habits, rather than in disease control as has been the case in the past. The major sources of mortality are currently accidents, violence, and chronic illness. As a consequence, personal health habits and environmental factors are the variables that will have to be influenced in the future to produce significant improvements in longevity.

        b. As public interest in and concern about health and health care activities increase, consumers will seek access to additional types and sources of information on these subjects.

        c. Problems of housing for the aged and for psychiatric patients increasingly will become interlocked with the provision of health care services at various levels.

        d. Emphasis on consumer choice of alternative health insurance plans, with varying degrees of financial responsibility beyond basic benefits being optional, will heighten public interest in health insurance coverage and benefit levels.

        e. There will be increased emphasis on preventive care for children, particularly among the poor, coupled with long-term plans to improve health levels and to conserve health care resources.

    2. Implications: Hospital Industry

        a. Hospitals should increase the likelihood that they will be viewed as the most accessible providers of information respecting disease prevention and health promotion.

        b. Particularly important will be the need for hospitals to assess the health care concerns of each age segment of the population, in order to determine the appropriate mix of services in individual hospitals.

C. Financing

    1. Assumptions

        a. Alternatives to traditional forms of payment and financing will continue to be developed and tested in a variety of settings.

        b. There will be an increase in the number of commercial insurers offering to insure smaller markets. Commercial insurance companies are likely to be the source of the most aggressive competition as they seek to expand their share of new markets. Any gains that they achieve will probably be at the expense of the Blue Cross and Blue Shield plans, which currently retain the largest market shares. More precise rating strategies for small markets and the ability of commercials to take advantage of any cost containment measures successfully implemented by the Blue Cross–Blue Shield plans will benefit the commercial insurance companies.

c. Trade-offs will be made by purchasers of insurance between options to increase health benefits for employees or to provide wage gains. Business purchasers of health care insurance increasingly will seek to provide employees a broader, more tailored array of benefits, with employees having an opportunity to select the type and scope of benefits most appropriate for their needs. Additional health care benefits, such as dental insurance, will increase the demand for some types of service that previously were less fully covered. Preventive health services will offer a new field for insured benefits.

d. In order to provide a broader package of benefits, employers will ask employees to choose between carrying a percentage of the health care costs themselves and traditional salary increases or full company coverage with modified wage gains. Purchasers of insurance will demand value for any additional charges.

e. The federal government will continue attempts to restrict the amount and techniques for capital spending by hospitals.

f. Future capital expenditure levels will be determined by the interaction of financial market conditions, inflation in the costs of construction, and regulation of capital expenditures through planning and certificate of need programs. Debt financing is likely to continue to grow as the most important source of capital funding, because it generally will be the most readily available and/or least expensive source of funding, although there are likely to be exceptions in the cases of many individual institutions.

g. Private philanthropy will continue to be one of the voluntary health care industry's greatest strengths and sources of support.

h. The cost of research and teaching conducted at teaching hospitals increasingly will be recognized as a distinct element of the costs incurred by these hospitals. Alternative payment mechanisms will be explored to cover these costs, thus making the cost of patient care at teaching hospitals more readily comparable to costs at nonteaching hospitals.

2. Implications: Hospital Industry

   a. Hospitals can expect to negotiate with several types of third party payer, particularly as alternative care settings increase and the market share held by traditional third party insurers decreases.

   b. Hospitals will be forced to diversify their economic base into nontherapeutic profit-oriented enterprises in order to offset losses in inpatient care.

   c. Increased competition for accounts is likely to spill over into more stringent restrictions on payments to hospitals.

   d. Increased mandated benefits will foster alternatives to inpatient care.

   e. Hospital earnings and equity will remain an important source of capital funding, although accounting for no more than a fifth or a sixth of total funding.

   f. Decisions to purchase capital equipment will depend on the ability of an institution to obtain funds.

   g. The public increasingly will view hospitals as institutions operated on a business basis and, as a result, the impact of the hospital as a philanthropic or charity-type community institution will erode.

II. State and Local Assumptions (Excerpts)

   A. Legislation

      1. Assumption
         State rate review/control is not expected within the next three years.

      2. Implication
         No direct implication as a result of legislative requirements. However, the potential of legislation requires that steps be taken immediately to dampen the possible intrusionary effect of regulation by increasing productivity and controlling costs.

   B. Demands for Services

      1. Assumptions

         a. Demand for inpatient services in the coming fiscal year is expected to remain at about the same level that is currently being experienced.

b. As a result both of the continued shift in the demographic composition of the community and of the decrease in the supply of local physician services, an increased proportion of the hospital's service area will be looking to it as the principal source of primary care.

c. As a result of both technological advances and the increased demand for primary care, routine laboratory and radiology workload can be expected to increase. If channeled properly, the increase in primary care demand will result in a moderate decrease in emergency room visits.

2. Implications: Hospital

a. Inpatient Services

No new implication. Increased attention, however, must be focused on increasing the productivity of the inpatient production function.

b. Primary Care Services

An opportunity will exist to serve the local community better. To capitalize on this opportunity, increased capital and operating resources will have to be devoted to primary care.

c. Ancillary and Emergency Room Services

Plant and equipment capacity in both laboratory and radiology is sufficient to accommodate a moderate to medium increase in workload. In view of the complementary need to increase efficiency, a moderate increase in workload in these areas should be accommodated through increased staff productivity. A medium increase in workload will require an increase in staff.

The decrease in emergency room workload, while significant, will not be sufficient to result in any major staffing pattern changes.

OPERATING POLICY DECISIONS[11]

Program Priorities

Given the general objective of the hospital and management's evaluation of both the environmental statement and the statement of assumptions, program area priorities have been established as follows:

1. Ambulatory care services
2. Inpatient acute services
3. Radiology
4. Ancillary patient services
5. Laboratory
6. Surgical services
7. Environmental services
8. Personnel and education
9. Fiscal services
10. Administrative services

Program Directives

Program Area I—Inpatient Acute Services
Program Directive: Maintain the hospital's traditional standards of patient care services while at the same time reducing bed capacity in order to produce an 87% occupancy rate.

1. Control nursing vacancies to a level equal to no more than 10% of approved professional staff complement.
2. Review procedures and performance re JCAH standards, and implement necessary corrective action prior to accreditation review.

For the coming year, resources should remain at the current budget level.

Program Area II—Ambulatory Care Services
Program Directive: Maintain existing emergency services program. Add outreach programs that will make the hospital's services more conveniently accessible to the community.
Outreach program emphasis should be on

1. Worksite services
2. Services to the aged
3. Pediatric services

For the coming year, resources should expand.

_____
[11]Excerpts.

Program Area III—Environmental Services
Program Directive: Maintain current quality standards while continuing to increase productivity by 15.5%.

For the coming year, resources should be maintained at current services level, adjusted for productivity improvement.

Division Directives[12]

Program Area I—Inpatient Acute Services
Program Directive: Maintain the hospital's traditional standards of patient care services while at the same time reducing staffed bed capacity in order to produce an 87% occupancy rate.

1. Maintain on a continuing basis nursing vacancies at a level equal to no more than 10% of approved professional staff complements.
2. Review procedures and performance re JCAH standards, and implement necessary corrective action prior to next year's accreditation review.

For the coming year, resources should remain at the current services level.

Nursing Services

Maintain current nursing hours and staff mix to patient day ratios. Prior to year-end and in conjunction with Social Services Division, design and implement a discharge planning program. By year-end, close nursing units 3 West and 3 North. Resources should remain at the current services level/patient day. (This, however, should reflect a reduction in total budget as compared to current year.)

Nursing Administration

Implement nurse recruitment program designed to generate in year 1 a net increase in the nursing staff of 35 professional nurses. In year 2 and beyond, the program should generate 25 new nurses.

Implement salary and career ladder program that reduces turnover to 15% in year 1 and maintains it at 10% in year 2 and beyond.

Resources should grow by 5% in year 1 and in year 2 remain at the current services level.

Table 17.4 illustrates how the Projection Package is tailored to the needs of each responsibility center. All responsibility centers would receive the foregoing patient day projections. Those responsibility centers whose workload is volume-dependent would also receive a projection, such as that shown for Hematology, that is unique to their needs. The Administrative

---

[12]Excerpts.

Package would be similarly tailored—in regard to historical cost data and current personnel complement data—to reflect the history and current situation of each particular responsibility center receiving the package.

For further reading on budgeting procedures, review the following resources:

Esmond, Truman H., Jr. *Budgeting Procedures for Hospitals.*
Griffith, John R. *Quantitative Techniques for Hospital Planning and Control.*
Greater Detroit Area Hospital Council. *Management Guide to Effective Budgeting.*
Lash, Myles P. *Development of an Expense Budgeting Procedure.*
Lipson, Stephen H. and Hensel, Mary D. *Hospital Manpower Budget Preparation Manual.*

A sample procedure for preparing the capital budget, including forms and instructions, is presented in Appendix 18.

PROJECTION PACKAGE[13]
TOTAL PATIENT DAY FORECAST[14]

Year	Admissions	Patient Days	Approximate Occupancy, Percent
1	15,494	123,951	75
2	17,516	138,375	80
3	17,336	135,221	78
4	17,923	138,011	80
5	18,244	138,656	80
Projected	18,945	138,300	87

[13]The projection package should be customized for each of the volume-dependent responsibility centers by providing both total patient days and unique workload estimates for the particular responsibility center; for example, for a patient care unit: patient days/that unit; for dietary: projected meals by type of diet.

[14]Excludes nursery days.

TOTAL PATIENT DAYS PER MONTH*

Year	Total	†	July	Aug.	Sept.	Oct.	Nov.	Dec.	Jan.	Feb.	Mar.	Apr.	May	June
1	123,870	3	9,296	10,499	10,535	9,292	8,676	9,916	11,155	12,395	12,312	9,999	9,296	9,296
2	138,373	11	11,051	9,686	11,761	11,089	10,379	11,010	11,071	13,144	13,145	14,529	11,130	10,378
3	135,221	−2	11,494	8,789	13,523	11,493	10,817	9,465	11,495	11,493	10,818	13,524	12,169	10,141
4	139,000	2	11,040	10,331	12,439	11,699	11,761	12,435	11,715	11,985	11,052	11,083	12,395	11,065
5	139,114	0	11,092	10,399	11,788	11,785	11,054	11,764	11,807	11,785	12,464	11,094	12,949	11,133
Proj.	137,605	−1	12,406	10,372	11,796	11,755	11,041	11,064	11,778	11,708	11,777	11,780	12,447	9,681

*Excludes nursery days.
†Percent change from previous year.

WORKLOAD PROJECTIONS: TESTS HEMATOLOGY DEPARTMENT

Year	July	Aug.	Sept.	Oct.	Nov.	Dec.	Jan.	Feb.	Mar.	Apr.	May	June	Total
1	8,367	9,450	9,450	9,482	8,367	7,809	8,925	10,040	11,156	11,081	9,000	8,367	111,494
2	10,388	9,105	11,056	10,424	9,757	10,350	10,407	12,356	12,357	13,658	10,463	9,756	130,077
3	10,920	8,350	12,847	10,919	10,277	8,992	10,921	10,919	10,278	12,848	11,561	9,634	128,466
4	10,488	9,815	11,817	11,114	11,173	11,814	11,130	11,386	10,500	10,529	11,776	10,521	132,063
5	11,425	10,711	12,142	12,139	11,386	12,117	12,162	12,139	12,838	11,427	12,869	11,467	142,822
Proj.*	13,399	11,202	12,740	12,696	11,925	11,950	12,721	12,645	12,720	12,723	13,443	10,456	148,620

*Relative workload value/test in projection year 3.22.

18

Capital Budgeting and Capital Investment Decisions

Brief reference was made in Chapter 17 both to the development of capital expenditure decision packages and to the mechanics of the capital investment rank ordering and decision process.

Essentially, two decisions are required. The first is a capital investment decision, focusing on the intrinsic merits of the investment opportunity. The second is a capital budgeting decision, focusing on which of the investment opportunities have merit, or can be funded. Often, these two decisions become intertwined, as the capital budget preparation process is used as the vehicle for addressing both matters.[1]

The mechanics of addressing the first issue, that is, the decision on the intrinsic merits of an investment opportunity, is generically similar to traditional financial investment analysis. Though similar, the analysis does differ in an important way. In the hospital setting not only do the potential investment's cash flow streams have to be analyzed and discounted, but the expected nonmonetary patient care benefits streams have to be identified and evaluated. The similarity, as well as the distinction, will become more apparent in the following pages.

The mechanics of the capital budget preparation process also differs somewhat from that of preparing the general operating budget. In view of these differences and of the importance of the decisions, the matter of capital decisions is addressed here as a separate chapter. The body of the chapter focuses on the mechanics of the capital investment decision anal-

---

[1]Different terminology is often used to describe these two decisions. For example, "capital rationing" may be used instead of "capital budgeting." Regardless of the labels employed, it should be recognized that the total process involves two separate but linked decisions.

ysis. An appendix addresses itself to capital budget preparation, integrating investment analysis into the funding decision process. A second appendix focuses on sources of capital.

IMPORTANCE

Of the myriad decisions that will confront a hospital manager throughout his professional career, those involving capital investment choices are likely to be the most crucial. Not only might these decisions involve the classic "life and death" trade-offs, but, if an error in judgment is made, the costs of the decision error can be expected to be incurred over a considerable length of time. Given the importance of these decisions, hospital management should utilize carefully structured decision methodologies designed to minimize the probability of decision errors. Unfortunately, this has often not been the case.

Historically, the literature addressing hospital budgeting has been noted primarily for its paucity. Recently, however, the work of several major authors, as well as the demands of the capital markets, have acted to fill many of the previously existing gaps (see the Suggested Readings).

When one considers the nature of a hospital's traditional financial environment, the lack of literature is not surprising. In an environment dominated by cost-based retrospective reimbursement and private philanthropy, it can be easily understood why hospital managers felt little pressure for rigorous investment decision analysis and often opted for the safer, though perhaps more costly, alternative of facilities and services expansion. Private philanthropy was eager to contribute funds and seldom questioned the real need for additional hospital capital. Similarly, cost-based retrospective reimbursement, by paying incurred costs, neither questioned nor provided a braking force on the operating costs associated with unneeded capital expenditures.

The operating situation, however, has changed. The recent implementation of Medicare prospective pricing, combined with the implementation of price-driven private sector payment systems and changes in traditional utilization and practice patterns, has resulted in increased pressures for operating cost control and capital rationing. Reinforcing these pressures have been various federal (and state) statutes requiring more carefully evaluated capital decisions.[2] In response, hospitals have begun to utilize more rigorous capital investment analysis and decision techniques.

---

[2]These statutes include Public Law 92–603 with its section 234 capital budgeting and section 221 capital approval provisions, Public Law 93–641, the National Health Planning and Resource Development Act, Public Law 96–79, the amendments to PL 93–641, and various state certificate of need statutes.

As indicated, the literature of the past several years has begun to provide a sound theoretical and pragmatic foundation for hospital capital budgeting. While a detailed duplication of this literature would serve little value, a conceptual approach complements the previous material and adds to the existing literature and state of the art. The following material utilizes such an approach. It is supplemented by a section focusing on the policy and mechanics of evaluating, quantifying, and ranking the nonfinancial benefits of investment alternatives. Readers interested in a more detailed discussion of the theory or mechanical techniques of capital budgeting should refer to the Suggested Readings at the end of this chapter and to the Bibliography.

PROCESS

To provide the basis for sound decisions, a hospital's capital budgeting system must encompass the following major activities. These activities should be carried out in a sequential flow with all expenditure alternatives progressing through the process as a group.[3] Appendix 18.A illustrates this process from a procedural perspective.

1. PROJECT IDENTIFICATION

The initial step in the process is the identification of all potential expenditure projects. This step should involve not only the formulation of proposals, but also the evaluation of proposals to assure that the potential expenditure is consistent with the community's needs and the hospital's corporate strategy and operational plan (see previous chapters for a discussion of corporate strategy and operational planning).

It is important to note that this evaluation step represents the first decision point in the capital investment decision process. It should be given careful management attention as a device for sifting out inappropriate projects and as a mechanism for increasing the creditability of the entire budgetary process.

2. CASH FLOW IDENTIFICATION

The second step begins to add quantitative definition to project proposals by requiring for each project the specification of all relevant cash flows.

---

[3]This holistic approach to the decision process is necessary in order to reduce the possibility of benefit suboptimization. Presuming limited funds, if projects were considered independently on an "as ready basis," then all available funds might be spent on projects which, while having positive value, do not include alternatives that surface later in the period and possess incremental values greater than those of some of the funded projects. To avoid this pitfall, all expenditure alternatives should be identified and decided upon as a group. In this way the analysis can include an absolute and relative evaluation and can identify the set of projects that will yield the greatest total benefit for the available funds.

Due to the nature of the hospital's business, it may be difficult—if not impossible—to quantify all cash flows definitively. To the extent possible, cash flows should be projected objectively. However, where quantitative objectivity is not practical, cash flows should be estimated on a best judgment basis.

In developing estimates, projections of the magnitude and the relative timing of cash inflows and outflows should be made. These estimates, however, should only include, from all sources, the incremental costs that will be incurred as a result of undertaking the project. Previously incurred costs (sunk costs) and costs that would be incurred regardless of the investment decision (nonincremental costs) should not be included in the cash flow estimates.

Incremental capital and operating costs obviously should be treated as cash outflows. Any revenues, direct or indirect, that the investment is expected to generate plus any anticipated salvage value (discussed in Chapter 4) should be treated as cash inflows. Also, in those instances where the investment will not produce revenue but will result in decrease in operating costs, the expected savings should be viewed, for purposes of later analysis, as being a form of cash inflow.

Partially hidden within the last point is a troublesome inconsistency. In a typical business setting, expected savings can be viewed, for purposes of investment analysis, as being the same as revenues because they result in additional cash being available. Cash that otherwise would have been spent is now, due to the investment, available for other uses. In the hospital setting the situation is somewhat different. Due to third party cost-based payment, "savings" result in a reduction in revenues. This is the case because the savings reduce cost, and revenues are based on cost.

The decision-making implications of this difference should not be lost. An investment opportunity may appear to be sound based on the savings it generates. However, when the potential savings are discounted or lost due to the effects of cost-based payment, the attractiveness of the investment may disappear. Caution must be exercised. Cash inflows due to savings must be identified and evaluated not only as part of the financial analysis discussed below but also separately, as part of the final decision process.

The existence of cost-based payment also has another cash flow implication. For purposes of illustration, if one assumes that all of the hospital's revenues come through cost-based payment and that the payment agreement treats interest and depreciation as allowable costs, then the cash inflows plus anticipated salvage value will equal the cash outflows. This will be true for all investments. Alternative investments have no apparent financial differences or advantages. To the extent that revenues come from sources other than cost-based payers, financial differences will appear. The point, however, is that the existence of cost-based payment can distort the type of financial analysis described below. This fact does not negate either the need for or the desirability of financial analysis. Rather, it is a reality of hospital operations that must be kept in mind.

3. FINANCIAL ANALYSIS

Several alternative techniques are available for evaluating the financial implications of any given investment opportunity. Of the alternatives, net present value and internal rate of return analysis are the more theoretically acceptable approaches. These are preferred because both of these analytical techniques recognize the time value of money; that is, a dollar today, because it can be invested and earn a return (interest), is worth more than the promise of a dollar a year from today. Between the two techniques, net present value is the method of choice, because it avoids the reinvestment bias intrinsic to the internal rate of return approach. (The internal rate of return approach assumes that cash inflows can be reinvested at the discount rate at least. To the extent that cash inflows can only be reinvested at lesser rates, the calculated rate of return is inaccurately inflated.)[4]

A detailed discussion of the underlying theory and the mechanics of calculating a potential expenditure net present value (as well as present value tables for various interest rates) can be found in most general financial management textbooks. For purposes of this text, the example presented in Table 18.1 should provide a sufficient illustration and explanation of the mechanics of net present value analysis.

The calculations in the table are based upon the following formula:

$$PV = \sum_{t=1}^{T} \overbrace{\frac{CI_t}{(1 + I)^t} + \frac{S}{(1 + I)^T}}^{\text{cash inflows}} - \overbrace{\frac{C_t}{(1 + I)^t} + \frac{CO_t}{(1 + I)^t}}^{\text{cash outflows}}$$

where:
PV = present value
t = time period (usually a year)
T = life of investment
CI_t = cash inflow in period t (either revenue or savings)
S = salvage value
C_t = capital cost
CO_t = cash outflow in period t
I = interest rate (discount rate)

The input data for the above formula are obtained for the most part in step 2. The value for the interest or discount rate I is not, however, identified in that step and presents somewhat of a unique quantification problem.

---

[4]Readers seeking a more detailed discussion of this point should refer to Van Horne, J.C., *Financial Management and Policy*, or Horngren, Charles T., *Cost Accounting: A Managerial Emphasis*.

TABLE 18.1 Example: Net Present Value Analysis

The following is an example of the calculation of the net present value for an assumed capital equipment investment. The basic financial facts can be summarized as follows:

PV = present value

T = useful life of 10 years

CI_t = \$15,000/year for years 1 through 5; \$14,000/year for years 6 through 10

S = \$3,000

C_t = \$25,000

CO_t = \$9,000/year for years 1 through 5; \$12,000/year for years 6 through 10

I = 7%

$$PV = \sum_{t=1}^{T} \frac{CI_t}{(1+I)^t} + \frac{S}{(1+I)^T} - \frac{C_t}{(1+I)^t} + \frac{CO_t}{(1+I)^t}$$

$$PV = \sum_{t=1}^{T} \frac{\text{Net Cash Flow*}}{(1+I)^t} + \frac{S}{(1+I)^T} - \frac{C_t}{(1+I)^t}$$

Present Value of Net Cash Flow

Year	CI_t	CO_t	Net Cash Flow $(CI_t\text{-}CO_t)$	Present Value Factor @ 7%†	Present Value
1	\$15,000	\$ 9,000	\$6,000	.934	\$ 5,604
2	15,000	9,000	6,000	.873	5,238
3	15,000	9,000	6,000	.816	4,896
4	15,000	9,000	6,000	.762	4,572
5	15,000	9,000	6,000	.712	4,272
6	14,000	12,000	2,000	.666	1,332
7	14,000	12,000	2,000	.623	1,246
8	14,000	12,000	2,000	.582	1,164
9	14,000	12,000	2,000	.544	1,088
10	14,000	12,000	2,000	.505	1,016
					\$30,428

Present Value of Salvage

Year	S	Present Value Factor @ 7%	Present Value
10	\$3,000	.508	\$1,524

Net Present Value of Investment

PV = Σ(\$30,428 + \$1,524 − \$25,000‡)

PV = \$6,952

---

*Net Cash Flow = CI_t minus CO_t

†Obtained from standard present value tables; see Tables 18.2 and 18.3.

‡Present value is \$25,000 due to the assumption that the expenditure is made in its entirety at the beginning of the period.

TABLE 18.2   Present Value of $1 Received Annually at the End of Each "Year" for "N" Years

Years (N)	1%	2%	4%	6%	8%	10%	12%	14%	15%	16%	18%	20%	22%	24%	25%	26%	28%	30%	35%	40%	45%	50%
1	0.990	0.980	0.962	0.943	0.926	0.909	0.893	0.877	0.870	0.862	0.847	0.833	0.820	0.806	0.800	0.794	0.781	0.769	0.741	0.714	0.690	0.667
2	1.970	1.942	1.886	1.833	1.783	1.736	1.690	1.647	1.626	1.605	1.566	1.528	1.492	1.457	1.440	1.424	1.392	1.361	1.289	1.224	1.165	1.111
3	2.941	2.884	2.775	2.673	2.577	2.487	2.402	2.322	2.283	2.246	2.174	2.106	2.042	1.981	1.952	1.923	1.868	1.816	1.696	1.589	1.493	1.407
4	3.902	3.808	3.630	3.465	3.312	3.170	3.037	2.914	2.855	2.798	2.690	2.589	2.494	2.404	2.362	2.320	2.241	2.166	1.997	1.849	1.720	1.605
5	4.853	4.713	4.452	4.212	3.993	3.791	3.605	3.433	3.352	3.274	3.127	2.991	2.864	2.745	2.689	2.635	2.532	2.436	2.220	2.035	1.876	1.737
6	5.795	5.601	5.242	4.917	4.623	4.355	4.111	3.889	3.784	3.685	3.498	3.326	3.167	3.020	2.951	2.885	2.759	2.643	2.385	2.168	1.983	1.824
7	6.728	6.472	6.002	5.582	5.206	4.868	4.564	4.288	4.160	4.039	3.812	3.605	3.416	3.242	3.161	3.083	2.937	2.802	2.508	2.263	2.057	1.883
8	7.652	7.325	6.733	6.210	5.747	5.335	4.968	4.639	4.487	4.344	4.078	3.837	3.619	3.421	3.329	3.241	3.076	2.925	2.598	2.331	2.108	1.922
9	8.566	8.162	7.435	6.802	6.247	5.759	5.328	4.946	4.772	4.607	4.303	4.031	3.786	3.566	3.463	3.366	3.184	3.019	2.665	2.379	2.144	1.948
10	9.471	8.983	8.111	7.360	6.710	6.145	5.650	5.216	5.019	4.833	4.494	4.192	3.923	3.682	3.571	3.465	3.269	3.092	2.715	2.414	2.168	1.965
11	10.368	9.787	8.760	7.887	7.139	6.495	5.937	5.453	5.234	5.029	4.656	4.327	4.035	3.776	3.656	3.544	3.335	3.147	2.752	2.438	2.185	1.977
12	11.255	10.575	9.385	8.384	7.536	6.814	6.194	5.660	5.421	5.197	4.793	4.439	4.127	3.851	3.725	3.606	3.387	3.190	2.779	2.456	2.196	1.985
13	12.134	11.343	9.986	8.853	7.904	7.103	6.424	5.842	5.583	5.342	4.910	4.533	4.203	3.912	3.780	3.656	3.427	3.223	2.799	2.468	2.204	1.990
14	13.004	12.106	10.563	9.295	8.244	7.367	6.628	6.002	5.724	5.468	5.008	4.611	4.265	3.962	3.824	3.695	3.459	3.249	2.814	2.477	2.210	1.993
15	13.865	12.849	11.118	9.712	8.559	7.606	6.811	6.142	5.847	5.575	5.092	4.675	4.315	4.001	3.859	3.726	3.483	3.268	2.825	2.484	2.214	1.995
16	14.718	13.578	11.652	10.106	8.851	7.824	6.974	6.265	5.954	5.669	5.162	4.730	4.357	4.033	3.887	3.751	3.503	3.283	2.834	2.489	2.216	1.997
17	15.562	14.292	12.166	10.477	9.122	8.022	7.120	6.373	6.047	5.749	5.222	4.775	4.391	4.059	3.910	3.771	3.518	3.295	2.840	2.492	2.218	1.998
18	16.398	14.992	12.659	10.828	9.372	8.201	7.250	6.467	6.128	5.818	5.273	4.812	4.419	4.080	3.928	3.786	3.529	3.304	2.844	2.494	2.219	1.999
19	17.226	15.678	13.134	11.158	9.604	8.365	7.366	6.550	6.198	5.877	5.316	4.844	4.442	4.097	3.942	3.799	3.539	3.311	2.848	2.496	2.220	1.999
20	18.046	16.351	13.590	11.470	9.818	8.514	7.469	6.623	6.259	5.929	5.353	4.870	4.460	4.110	3.954	3.808	3.546	3.316	2.850	2.497	2.221	1.999
21	18.857	17.011	14.029	11.764	10.017	8.649	7.562	6.687	6.312	5.973	5.384	4.891	4.476	4.121	3.963	3.816	3.551	3.320	2.852	2.498	2.221	2.000
22	19.660	17.658	14.451	12.042	10.201	8.772	7.645	6.743	6.359	6.011	5.410	4.909	4.488	4.130	3.970	3.822	3.556	3.323	2.853	2.498	2.222	2.000
23	20.456	18.292	14.857	12.303	10.371	8.883	7.718	6.792	6.399	6.044	5.432	4.925	4.499	4.137	3.976	3.827	3.559	3.325	2.854	2.499	2.222	2.000
24	21.243	18.914	15.247	12.550	10.529	8.985	7.784	6.835	6.434	6.073	5.451	4.937	4.507	4.143	3.981	3.831	3.562	3.327	2.855	2.499	2.222	2.000
25	22.023	19.523	15.622	12.783	10.675	9.077	7.843	6.873	6.464	6.097	5.467	4.948	4.514	4.147	3.985	3.834	3.564	3.329	2.856	2.499	2.222	2.000
26	22.795	20.121	15.983	13.003	10.810	9.161	7.896	6.906	6.491	6.118	5.480	4.956	4.520	4.151	3.988	3.837	3.566	3.330	2.856	2.500	2.222	2.000
27	23.560	20.707	16.330	13.211	10.935	9.237	7.943	6.935	6.514	6.136	5.492	4.964	4.524	4.154	3.990	3.839	3.567	3.331	2.856	2.500	2.222	2.000
28	24.316	21.281	16.663	13.406	11.051	9.307	7.984	6.961	6.534	6.152	5.502	4.970	4.528	4.157	3.992	3.840	3.568	3.331	2.857	2.500	2.222	2.000
29	25.066	21.844	16.984	13.591	11.158	9.370	8.022	6.983	6.551	6.166	5.510	4.975	4.531	4.159	3.994	3.841	3.569	3.332	2.857	2.500	2.222	2.000
30	25.808	22.396	17.292	13.765	11.258	9.427	8.055	7.003	6.566	6.177	5.517	4.979	4.534	4.160	3.995	3.842	3.569	3.332	2.857	2.500	2.222	2.000
40	32.835	27.355	19.793	15.046	11.925	9.779	8.244	7.105	6.642	6.234	5.548	4.997	4.544	4.166	3.999	3.846	3.571	3.333	2.857	2.500	2.222	2.000
50	39.196	31.424	21.482	15.762	12.234	9.915	8.304	7.133	6.661	6.246	5.554	4.999	4.545	4.167	4.000	3.846	3.571	3.333	2.857	2.500	2.222	2.000

Source: From Robert N. Anthony and James S. Reece, *Management Accounting: Text and Cases, Fifth Edition* (Homewood, IL: Richard D. Irwin, Inc., 1975), p. 815. Copyright © 1956, 1984 by the President and Fellows of Harvard College.

TABLE 18.3 Present Value of $1 Received at the End of the "Year"

Years Hence	1%	2%	4%	6%	8%	10%	12%	14%	15%	16%	18%	20%	22%	24%	25%	26%	28%	30%	35%	40%	45%	50%
1	0.990	0.980	0.962	0.943	0.926	0.909	0.893	0.877	0.870	0.862	0.847	0.833	0.820	0.806	0.800	0.794	0.781	0.769	0.741	0.714	0.690	0.667
2	0.980	0.961	0.925	0.890	0.857	0.826	0.797	0.769	0.756	0.743	0.718	0.694	0.672	0.650	0.640	0.630	0.610	0.592	0.549	0.510	0.476	0.444
3	0.971	0.942	0.889	0.840	0.794	0.751	0.712	0.675	0.658	0.641	0.609	0.579	0.551	0.524	0.512	0.500	0.477	0.455	0.406	0.364	0.328	0.296
4	0.961	0.924	0.855	0.792	0.735	0.683	0.636	0.592	0.572	0.552	0.516	0.482	0.451	0.423	0.410	0.397	0.373	0.350	0.301	0.260	0.226	0.198
5	0.951	0.906	0.822	0.747	0.681	0.621	0.567	0.519	0.497	0.476	0.437	0.402	0.370	0.341	0.328	0.315	0.291	0.269	0.223	0.186	0.156	0.132
6	0.942	0.888	0.790	0.705	0.630	0.564	0.507	0.456	0.432	0.410	0.370	0.335	0.303	0.275	0.262	0.250	0.227	0.207	0.165	0.133	0.108	0.088
7	0.933	0.871	0.760	0.665	0.583	0.513	0.452	0.400	0.376	0.354	0.314	0.279	0.249	0.222	0.210	0.198	0.178	0.159	0.122	0.095	0.074	0.059
8	0.923	0.853	0.731	0.627	0.540	0.467	0.404	0.351	0.327	0.305	0.266	0.233	0.204	0.179	0.168	0.157	0.139	0.123	0.091	0.068	0.051	0.039
9	0.914	0.837	0.703	0.592	0.500	0.424	0.361	0.308	0.284	0.263	0.225	0.194	0.167	0.144	0.134	0.125	0.108	0.094	0.067	0.048	0.035	0.026
10	0.905	0.820	0.676	0.558	0.463	0.386	0.322	0.270	0.247	0.227	0.191	0.162	0.137	0.116	0.107	0.099	0.085	0.073	0.050	0.035	0.024	0.017
11	0.896	0.804	0.650	0.527	0.429	0.350	0.287	0.237	0.215	0.195	0.162	0.135	0.112	0.094	0.086	0.079	0.066	0.056	0.037	0.025	0.017	0.012
12	0.887	0.788	0.625	0.497	0.397	0.319	0.257	0.208	0.187	0.168	0.137	0.112	0.092	0.076	0.069	0.062	0.052	0.043	0.027	0.018	0.012	0.008
13	0.879	0.773	0.601	0.469	0.368	0.290	0.229	0.182	0.163	0.145	0.116	0.093	0.075	0.061	0.055	0.050	0.040	0.033	0.020	0.013	0.008	0.005
14	0.870	0.758	0.577	0.442	0.340	0.263	0.205	0.160	0.141	0.125	0.099	0.078	0.062	0.049	0.044	0.039	0.032	0.025	0.015	0.009	0.006	0.003
15	0.861	0.743	0.555	0.417	0.315	0.239	0.183	0.140	0.123	0.108	0.084	0.065	0.051	0.040	0.035	0.031	0.025	0.020	0.011	0.006	0.004	0.002
16	0.853	0.728	0.534	0.394	0.292	0.218	0.163	0.123	0.107	0.093	0.071	0.054	0.042	0.032	0.028	0.025	0.019	0.015	0.008	0.005	0.003	0.002
17	0.844	0.714	0.513	0.371	0.270	0.198	0.146	0.108	0.093	0.080	0.060	0.045	0.034	0.026	0.023	0.020	0.015	0.012	0.006	0.003	0.002	0.001
18	0.836	0.700	0.494	0.350	0.250	0.180	0.130	0.095	0.081	0.069	0.051	0.038	0.028	0.021	0.018	0.016	0.012	0.009	0.005	0.002	0.001	0.001
19	0.828	0.686	0.475	0.331	0.232	0.164	0.116	0.083	0.070	0.060	0.043	0.031	0.023	0.017	0.014	0.012	0.009	0.007	0.003	0.002	0.001	
20	0.820	0.673	0.456	0.312	0.215	0.149	0.104	0.073	0.061	0.051	0.037	0.026	0.019	0.014	0.012	0.010	0.007	0.005	0.002	0.001	0.001	
21	0.811	0.660	0.439	0.294	0.199	0.135	0.093	0.064	0.053	0.044	0.031	0.022	0.015	0.011	0.009	0.008	0.006	0.004	0.002	0.001		
22	0.803	0.647	0.422	0.278	0.184	0.123	0.083	0.056	0.046	0.038	0.026	0.018	0.013	0.009	0.007	0.006	0.004	0.003	0.001	0.001		
23	0.795	0.634	0.406	0.262	0.170	0.112	0.074	0.049	0.040	0.033	0.022	0.015	0.010	0.007	0.006	0.005	0.003	0.002	0.001			
24	0.788	0.622	0.390	0.247	0.158	0.102	0.066	0.043	0.035	0.028	0.019	0.013	0.008	0.006	0.005	0.004	0.003	0.002	0.001			
25	0.780	0.610	0.375	0.233	0.146	0.092	0.059	0.038	0.030	0.024	0.016	0.010	0.007	0.005	0.004	0.003	0.002	0.001	0.001			
26	0.772	0.598	0.361	0.220	0.135	0.084	0.053	0.033	0.026	0.021	0.014	0.009	0.006	0.004	0.003	0.002	0.002	0.001				
27	0.764	0.586	0.347	0.207	0.125	0.076	0.047	0.029	0.023	0.018	0.011	0.007	0.005	0.003	0.002	0.002	0.001	0.001				
28	0.757	0.574	0.333	0.196	0.116	0.069	0.042	0.026	0.020	0.016	0.010	0.006	0.004	0.002	0.002	0.002	0.001	0.001				
29	0.749	0.563	0.321	0.185	0.107	0.063	0.037	0.022	0.017	0.014	0.008	0.005	0.003	0.002	0.002	0.001	0.001					
30	0.742	0.552	0.308	0.174	0.099	0.057	0.033	0.020	0.015	0.012	0.007	0.004	0.003	0.002	0.001	0.001	0.001					
40	0.672	0.453	0.208	0.097	0.046	0.022	0.011	0.005	0.004	0.003	0.001	0.001										
50	0.608	0.372	0.141	0.054	0.021	0.009	0.003	0.001	0.001	0.001												

Source: From Robert N. Anthony and James S. Reece, *Management Accounting: Text and Cases, Fifth Edition* (Homewood, IL: Richard D. Irwin, Inc., 1975), p. 816. Copyright © 1956, 1984 by the President and Fellows of Harvard College.

In the typical commercial setting the quantification of the discount rate factor is relatively straightforward. Traditional theory holds that the discount rate should be equal, at a minimum, to the rate of return that the firm earns on its total assets. If investments are made based on a discount rate that is less than the rate of return on total assets, the effect would be to lower the overall rate of return and consequently reduce the value of the firm to the owners.[5]

In the hospital setting, this approach is of little use. Due to the preponderance of cost-based reimbursement and other intrinsic internal operating factors, hospitals typically have a relatively low operating margin (an average of 2% to 4%). As a result, their rate of return is low, providing an unrealistic bench mark for establishing a discount rate. An alternative approach must, therefore, be used.

In considering its expenditure opportunities an individual hospital might select one of the following three rates:

1. The historic earnings rate on its investment portfolio;
2. The interest rate that it would have to pay if it borrowed funds; or
3. The rate of return allowed under Medicare for investor-owned hospitals.

The hospital might also select a rate somewhere between these alternatives. Unfortunately, no fixed decision rules are available. The specific discount rate chosen by a particular hospital must be a subjective decision. The rate will generally fall between the extremes represented by the above listing, with the interest rate on borrowed funds serving as the discount rate floor. However, in selecting its discount rate, a hospital not only should evaluate its credit and general financial condition, but also should seek expert financial advice as to both the condition of the capital market and the capital market's appraisal of an acceptable discount rate.

BENEFIT ANALYSIS

4. BENEFIT IDENTIFICATION

The previous steps have concentrated exclusively on the financial aspects of capital decisions. Due to the nature of a hospital's business, analysis of only financial data is inadequate. If sound decisions are to be made, the

---

[5]The discount rate is essentially the long-run cost of capital to the firm. That is, it is the amount that the firm has to, or would have to, pay—in the market—to attract risk funds. That amount, or rate of return, must be commensurate with the long-run returns on investments in other enterprises with corresponding risks. Thus, the discount rate is a reflection of both the firm's long-run earning power, from the perspective of the current owners and their unwillingness to dilute their rate of profitability, and the rate set in the market, based on risk, capital structure, and the return being paid on other investments of a similar nature.

financial evaluation must be complemented by the examination of the intangible factors, that is, the patient care and services, or benefits that a particular investment will produce. The first step in this benefit evaluation is the identification of the benefits that accrue to any particular project.

Essentially, benefits must be identified in terms of both their qualitative and quantitative aspects. The quantitative aspect of expected benefits refers to the volume of service anticipated from a particular project: the number of persons who will benefit. The qualitative aspect refers to the nature of the service that will be provided: lifesaving with full recovery, lifesaving with partial recovery, age of persons benefiting, disease prevention.

Exhibit I describes a technique that can be used to categorize the nature and extent of a project's benefits. Readers should refer to this exhibit for a detailed discussion of benefit identification.

5. BENEFIT EVALUATION

Benefit evaluation centers on the matter of converting, through the application of a systematic process, the data developed in the previous step into useful decision-making information. In principle, this step is similar to step 3. However, in terms of mechanics it differs markedly.

The mechanics of benefit evaluation is addressed in Exhibit II. The material in the exhibit is presented as an example of a pragmatic benefit evaluation technique. It is not presented as the definitive answer to the benefit evaluation problem. Rather, it is shown as an alternative to less structured approaches and as a stimulus to the development of more effective techniques.

6. MERGER OF FINANCIAL AND BENEFIT EVALUATION DATA

As the final step before decision, the output of the financial and benefit evaluation steps must be merged into one or more unified measures. Unified measures should be statistics that integrate cost and benefit data into a single index that can be used for the initial rank ordering of projects.

Utilizing the methodology described in Exhibits I and II and net present value analysis, examples of the type of measure that can be developed are illustrated in the statistics that follow:

$$\text{Cost/Benefit Index} = \frac{\text{Net Present Value}}{\substack{\text{Present Value of} \\ \text{Capital Costs}}} (\text{Lifetime Benefit Value})$$

$$\text{Benefit/Capital Cost Index} = \frac{\text{Lifetime Benefit Value}}{\text{Capital Costs}}$$

$$\text{Operating Cost Index} = \frac{\text{Annual Benefit Value}}{\text{Annual Operating Costs}}$$

EXHIBIT I   Benefit Analysis: Benefit Identification

The benefits expected to be derived from any given investment project generally can be viewed as being both qualitative and quantitative in nature. The quantitative aspect of expected benefits refers to the volume of service that is anticipated. The qualitative aspect refers to the nature of the service that will be produced. For purposes of analysis, both of these aspects can be considered through the use of the following benefit categories:

A. Utilization
B. Service availability
C. Nature of expected benefits
    1. Degree to which patients benefit, for example,
    2. Lifesaving
        a. Full recovery
        b. Disability
    3. Nonlifesaving
        a. Health restoration—full
        b. Health restoration—partial
        c. Fatal disease prevention
        d. Nonfatal disease prevention
        e. Increased patient convenience or improved operations
        f. Number of patients who will benefit
        g. Characteristics of patients who will benefit

Given these benefit categories, each proposed project must be evaluated in terms of its expected performance with respect to each category. That is, the expected benefits must be identified and measured relative to each category of benefit. Thus, for example, the type and quantity of benefits for an ambulatory care facility might be as follows:

A. Utilization—36%
B. Service availability—service presently not available in sufficient quantity
C. Nature of expected benefits
    1. Degree to which patients will benefit—benefits in all nonlifesaving areas, though approximately half of the patients are expected to benefit in regard to both categories of health restoration
    2. Number of patients who will benefit—20,000

Note: This material, or a variant of it, would generally be included in the Budget Officer's Budget Support and Analysis Preparation Manual but would not be provided to all staff as part of the Administrative Package.

The material is presented here as an example of a technique that can aid in the evaluation of the service and patient care benefits of alternative capital expenditures. Such evaluation obviously is needed if sound capital budget decisions are to be made.

The methodology is not presented as the definitive answer to the benefit evaluation problem. Rather, it is presented as an alternative to less structured approaches and as a stimulus to the development of more accurate techniques.

EXHIBIT II   Benefit Analysis: Benefit Evaluation

The second step in the benefit analysis process is subjectively—but systematically—to assign numerical weights or values to each category of benefit (see Exhibit I for discussion of benefit categories). The schedule of benefit weights should be determined—if the staff budget committee approach discussed in the chapter is not utilized—by senior management. The weighting schedule should be reviewed annually, prior to initiation of the budget preparation process, to assure that it adequately reflects the hospital's and the community's current attitudes and priorities. A sample benefit weighting schedule is presented below:

Sample Benefit Weighting Schedule*

Benefit Category	Weight
Utilization	1 unit
Service availability	2 units
Nature of expected benefit	
1. Lifesaving	
a. Full recovery	10 units
b. Disability	8 units
2. Nonlifesaving	
a. Health restoration—full	6 units
b. Health restoration—partial	5 units
c. Fatal disease prevention	4 units
d. Nonfatal disease prevention	3 units
e. Increased patient convenience or improved operations	1 unit

In addition to specifying the benefit weighting schedule, the relationship between the quantity of benefits and the value of weight assigned to each benefit category must be determined. This step is necessary, for in order to use the foregoing weighting schedule the weights must be expressed in terms of weighted unit per some given quantity of benefit. Thus, the hospital must determine a common denominator for each category of benefits, that is, what percentage of utilization is equal to one unit, how many lives saved equals ten units, and so forth. A sample relationship schedule is presented below.

Sample Benefit-Weighting Relationship Schedule†

Benefit Category	Weight	Benefit Quantity–Weight Relationship
Utilization	1 unit	Percent actually utilized
Service availability	2 units	Full value of services are presently not available in sufficient quantity; zero value if they are available

EXHIBIT II   Continued

Nature of expected benefit
1. Lifesaving
   a. Full recovery   10 units   10 units per each life saved
2. Nonlifesaving
   a. Health restoration—
       full   6 units   6 units per each 5,000 patients treated
   b. Health restoration—
       partial   5 units   5 units per each 5,000 patients treated
   c. Fatal disease
       prevention   4 units   4 units per each 5,000 patients treated
   d. Increased patient
       convenience or im-
       proved operations   1 unit   1 unit per each 5,000 patients treated

It should be noted that the above weighting and relationship schedules are presented only as illustrations and should not be capriciously adopted. The hospital should consider the implication of several feasible schedules and determine independently the one that most appropriately reflects the community's needs and philosophies. A technique known as sensitivity analysis may be quite useful in regard to this task. In simplest terms, sensitivity analysis involves experimenting with several possible schedules and comparing the results that are obtained under each schedule. In this way, alternative schedules can be evaluated and a determination can be made as to which weighting system is the most appropriate.

Using the weighting and relationship schedules and information about the nature of specific project benefits, the next step is to calculate the benefit value for each project under consideration. This process can be explained most easily through the use of the following examples (see Tables A and B), which rely on both the above material and the material presented in Exhibit I.

As can be seen by these examples, the total (lifetime) project benefit value is the sum of the benefit values for each benefit category multiplied by the useful life of the investment. Benefit values, by category, are determined by multiplying the benefit weight by the (according to the relationship schedule) quantity of benefits. Thus, the benefit value calculation can be summarized as follows:

Lifetime Benefit = (Investment's Useful Life) (Annual Benefit Value)

    Utilization Benefit Factor [that is, (percent utilization) (benefit weight)]
+ Service Availability Factor
+ Nature of Benefit Factor [that is, (benefit quantity by nature of benefit)
                             (benefit weight)]
_____
    Annual Benefit Value

The above technique provides a unique value for the annual and total useful life benefit of each investment alternative. These data can be merged, in a variety of ways, with financial data; for example,

Continued

EXHIBIT II   Continued

$$\frac{\text{Net Present Value}}{\text{Present Value of}} \text{ (Lifetime Benefit Value)} = \text{Cost/Benefit Index}$$
Capital Costs

$$\frac{\text{Lifetime Benefit Value}}{\text{Capital Costs}} = \text{Benefit/Capital Cost Index}$$

$$\frac{\text{Annual Benefit Value}}{\text{Annual Operating Costs}} = \text{Operating Cost Index}$$

to provide a set of relative indexes that can be used for purposes of establishing project priority rankings.

It should be noted, however, that the index values should be mechanically applied—with a rank order listing being an automatic byproduct of the evaluation technique. Project rankings should be established based on management's judgment as to the total evaluation and importance of the project. The benefit indexes should only serve as an input to this judgment.‡

Note: This material, or a variant of it, would generally be included in the Budget Officer's Budget Support and Analysis Preparation Manual but would not be provided to all staff as part of the Administrative Package.

The material is presented here as an example of a technique that can aid in the evaluation of the service and patient care benefits of alternative capital expenditures. Such evaluation obviously is needed if sound capital budget decisions are to be made.

The methodology is not presented as the definitive answer to the benefit evaluation problem. Rather, it is presented as an alternative to less structured approaches and as a stimulus to the development of more accurate techniques.

These weights are not suggested weights. The committee should thoroughly discuss and develop its own understanding of each benefit component so as to be able subjectively to assign weights that it feels are appropriate to local needs and values.

†For purposes of this sample, pediatric benefits are assumed to be weighted double, for example, 20 units per each life saved.

‡The scope of the foregoing weighting schedule is only illustrative. For initial use, a hospital may wish to utilize only two or three benefit categories and then, as it becomes more experienced with this technique, phase in a more lengthy and comprehensive listing. This phasing approach will simplify implementation of the benefit analysis procedure and should be considered.

These measures provide an indexing statistic that defines benefits in terms of the investment (cost) required to obtain the benefits. Of the above examples, the cost/benefit index is the most comprehensive single statistic, including both capital and operating cost factors as well as the ratio of these factors to capital costs and the relationship of all financial factors to total benefits.

For projects with positive net present values and equal lifetime benefit values, the larger the cost/benefit index number the better the project's value; that is, a project with an index of 500 is generally more desirable than a project with an index of 60. This is the case for, presuming benefits are held constant, the larger the numerator the better the financial aspects

EXHIBIT II—TABLE A   Benefit Analysis Calculation, Example I, Ambulatory Care Unit

(1) Benefit Category	(2) Benefit Quantity	(3) Benefit Weight	(4) Relationship	(5) Benefit Value (Col. 2 × Col. 3)
Utilization	.36	1	percent utilized	.36
Service availability	present service insufficient	2	sufficient; insufficient $\dfrac{\text{Col. 2}}{\text{Col. 4}}$ Col. 3	2.00
Nature of expected benefit				
1. Health restoration—full	10,000 patients (7,500 adults; 2,500 peds.)	6	5,000 pts. = 6	
2. Health restoration—partial		5 5.5* 5.5	5,000 pts. = 5	Adults = 8.25† Peds. = 5.50
3. Fatal disease prevention	10,000 patients (7,500 adults; 2,500 peds.)	4	5,000 pts. = 4	
4. Nonfatal disease prevention		3	5,000 pts. = 3	
5. Increased patient convenience or improved operations		1 2.67* 2.67	5,000 pts. = 1	Adults = 4.01† Peds. = 2.67
			Total Annual Benefit Value	22.79
			Useful Life	30 years
			Lifetime Benefit Value (22.79 × 30)	683.70

*These weightings, once established, do not change from project to project. However, due to the benefit quantity distribution, it is necessary to determine the average benefit weight. Therefore, since 10,000 patients will benefit in the first two categories, the average benefit weight is 5.5. Ten thousand patients will also benefit in the last three areas. Thus, the average benefit weight for these categories is 2.67.

†Since the adult population is 7,500 patients, the benefit value, given the relationship schedule, is equal to (1.5) (average benefit weight). In the case of pediatrics, the benefit value, given the relationship schedule and the double pediatrics weighting, is equal to (.5) (average benefit weight) (2).

EXHIBIT II—TABLE B Benefit Analysis Calculation, Example II, Kidney Dialysis Unit

(1) Benefit Category	(2) Benefit Quantity	(3) Benefit Weight	(4) Relationship	(5) Benefit Value (Col. 2 x Col. 3)
Utilization	.05	1	percent utilized	.05
Service availability	present service insufficient	2	sufficient; insufficient $\dfrac{\text{Col. 2}}{\text{Col. 4}}$ Col. 3	2.00
Nature of expected benefit				
1. Lifesaving				
a. Full recovery	8	10	1 life = 10	80.00
b. Disability	2	8	1 life = 8	16.00
			Total Annual Benefit Value	98.05
			Useful Life	6 years
			Lifetime Benefit Value (98.05) (6) =	588.30

of the investment and the larger the final quotient. Therefore, assuming two projects with similar benefit values, the project with the better financial implications, that is, the greater ratio of net cash inflows to capital costs, is, generally, the project of choice.

In the case of projects with negative net present values, the mechanics of calculating the index numbers is the same. However, due to the reversal of numerical signs (negative numbers are being calculated), the smaller the absolute index number, the more desirable (typically) is the project.

DECISIONS

Application of the foregoing steps will produce a set of statistics that can be used to rank order alternative projects. The resulting listing does not, however, automatically dictate investment decisions for the hospital as it might for a commercial firm.

In the case of a commercial firm, unless external factors reverse the general decision rules, only projects with positive net present values would be considered as realistic investment alternatives. Unfortunately, this kind of simple decision rule is not applicable in the hospital setting.

Due to both the hospital's community resource character and its complex objective function, hospital management must consider projects with either positive or negative net present values as realistic alternatives. Moreover, because of the predominance of cost-based reimbursement, the funding decision is further compounded by the need to distinguish between projects that generate a positive net present value due to revenues and those that produce a positive value due to savings.[6]

Appendix 18.A illustrates one approach to the decision process. It should be recognized that the committee mechanism described in the appendix is just one of a variety of alternative organization structures that can be used for making these types of decision. The committee approach, while having certain advantages due to its interdisciplinary structure, should not be slavishly imposed. As is the case with regard to other complex organizational questions, no single correct answer exists. Each institution must structure its own solution in light of its own history, character, environment, and goals.

CAPITAL FINANCING

Appendix 18.A also briefly references the role that debt (borrowing) can play in making investment decisions. Appendix 18.B addresses this

---

[6]This is necessary because, by definition, cost-based reimbursement will absorb the savings and not generate funds to meet the incremental capital costs. Therefore, these projects, though having a positive net present value, have financial implications similar to projects with negative present values. If financial stability is to be provided, the hybrid nature of these projects must be identified and accounted for in the decision process.

issue in a bit more detail.[7] It is important to recognize, however, that an in-depth understanding of capital financing, including the role that leasing can play, is beyond both the capability of a single text and the operational needs of most hospital managers.

Typically, it will be when large sums are needed to finance an approved renovation, expansion, or rebuilding project that a voluntary not-for-profit hospital will need to enter the capital market.[8] In those instances, however, when a hospital must enter the capital market, management should immediately obtain the advice and assistance of an expert capital market consultant.[9]

The capital market is a highly segmented, complex, and volatile market. Its equity component is distinct from its debt component. Moreover, each is lined with potential pitfalls that can inadvertently increase either funds acquisition costs or carrying costs. Compounding the matter are the unique operating character and regulatory environment of hospitals.

Cost-based payment, for example, can positively or negatively affect a hospital's debt capacity. To the extent that bad debts or free service costs are not allowed as reimbursable costs, debt capacity is limited. However, to the extent that interest costs and depreciation expenses are allowed, debt capacity—if debt repayment and depreciation schedules are synchronized—is expanded. In this latter instance, if a large proportion of a hospital's patients are covered by cost-based payers, who pay their full economic costs or financial requirements, debt capacity can easily exceed the traditional industrial guidelines, becoming a function more of the third party payer's financial condition and abilities than of the condition of the hospital.

Regulatory sanctions, requiring planning agency approval of proposed projects, also affect debt capacity as well as the basic financial viability, if not legality, of a proposed investment.

In view of these complexities, it is foolhardy for a hospital to attempt to decipher or conquer the capital market on its own. The most valuable general rules that can be set out at this point are that

---

[7]The purpose of Appendix 18.B is to provide an introduction to capital financing alternatives. Readers interested in more information should refer to the references in the Suggested Readings. Also, readers should seek out the advice of an investment banker; for example, Goldman Sacks and Co.; Blyth Eastman Paine Webber, Inc.; Smith Barney Harris Upham & Co., Inc.; Wertheim & Co., Inc. At least a general level of advice can be provided at a firm's local office.

[8]Investor-owned (proprietary or for-profit) hospitals make much greater use of capital markets, obtaining their basic financing from the equity component of the market.

[9]The distinction between capital and money markets should be noted. Money markets supply short-term (working capital) funds. In contrast, capital markets are the source of long-term funds, for example, stock, long-term debt. Hospitals, as discussed in Chapter 14, may make frequent use of the money market.

1. Financial considerations should be included as part of the initial planning of any large-scale project that might require use of the capital market for obtaining funds.

2. It is generally financially sound to use debt to finance projects having revenue-generated positive net present values.

3. Before debt is used to finance any capital expenditure, expert advice should be obtained not only to discover the least cost source of capital but also to assure that the debt will not seriously impair the institution's financial position.

DIVESTITURE

Before concluding, an additional consideration should be raised. The foregoing has viewed investment analysis and decision making from the perspective of acquiring additional assets. The same analytical framework can be used to examine divestiture opportunities.

It has been said that the ability and willingness to divest activities are the key to innovative management. While the complete accuracy of this statement might be debatable, its essential message has merit. Little if anything is to be gained by continuing to provide the community with services that it does not feel it needs. Similarly, the hospital's total value to its community is lessened if it continues to provide a service of marginal value, as opposed to one of greater need, simply because it has provided that particular service in the past.

To sort through these choices is admittedly a difficult task. However, by: identifying services, even if subjectively, whose value is questionable; evaluating the costs and benefits of these services through the techniques discussed above; and comparing that evaluation to similar evaluations of new opportunities, a hospital may not only find capital to support new ventures, but also the drive to remain a dynamic force within its community.

CONCLUSION

The preceding has attempted to describe in a cogent fashion the nature of the capital decision process. Particular emphasis has been placed upon bringing a systematic, though admittedly to some extent subjective, approach to the making of capital investment decisions.

In view of the importance of these decisions, such an approach represents perhaps only a minimal level of decision rigor. Certainly, additional research and pragmatic experimentation are needed to refine the decision process further. However, while this work is proceeding, the historical void should be filled through the implementation—on a phased basis if necessary—of budgeting and financing processes similar to that described above and in the accompanying appendices.

SUGGESTED READINGS

American Hospital Association. *Capital Financing for Hospitals.*

Arbel, Avner and Grier, Paul. "Investment Generation Process in Hospital Facilities: The Response of Supply to Capacity Utilization Measures."

Cleverley, William O. *Financial Management of Health Care Facilities,* Chapter 11.

Cohodes, Donald R. "Hospital Capital Formation in the 1980s: Is There a Crisis?"

Dittman, David A. and Smith, Kenneth R. "Consideration of Benefits and Costs: A Conceptual Framework of the Health Planner."

Esmond, Truman H., Jr. *Budgeting Procedures for Hospitals.*

Griffith, John R. *Quantitative Techniques for Hospital Planning and Control,* Chapter 9.

Lindsay, J. Robert and Sametz, Arnold W. *Financial Management: An Analytical Approach.*

Long, Hugh W. "Asset Choice and Program Selection in a Competitive Environment."

Robinson, Roland I. *Money and Capital Markets,* Chapters 1, 9-13.

Silvers, J.B. and Prahalad, C.K. *Financial Management of Health Institutions,* Chapters 5, 6, and 7.

Suver, James D. and Neumann, Bruce R. "Cost of Capital."

Topics in Health Care Financing. "Capital Financing," Fall 1978.

Topics in Health Care Financing. "Capital Projects," Winter 1975.

Van Arsdell, Paul M. "Considerations Underlying Cost of Capital."

Vraciu, Robert A. "Decision Models for Capital Investment and Financing Decisions in Hospitals."

APPENDIX 18.A[10]
CAPITAL BUDGETING

A hospital's plant and equipment investment program can be viewed as consisting of two basic components: a long-term planning or major acquisitions component and a short-term budgeting component. The major acquisitions segment of the program focuses on new program and construction opportunities. Decisions as to which projects should be undertaken should be made only after a thorough cost-benefit analysis of each of the available opportunities. Financing for projects of this type is generally beyond a single year's internal capabilities. However, if these projects are to be funded either partially or totally from internal sources, then decisions

---

[10]Appendix 18.A is excerpted from the budgeting procedure designed for a 300-bed community general hospital. The organizational control relationships described in the procedure reflect the organization structure of the particular hospital. In a different institution, the details of the process may have to be revised; for example, more meeting and decision steps may need to be built into the procedure to accommodate properly the different organization structure. Also, in different institutions, the titles of the forms may have to be changed to reflect the particular institution's nomenclature.

as to whether or not a project is undertaken should be part of the regular annual capital budgeting process. The forms used for capital budget decision making, as well as the instructions for completing the forms and an explanation of the decision process, are presented below.

CAPITAL BUDGETING FORMS AND INSTRUCTIONS

Step 1. Initial Budget Meeting. Department supervisors should meet with the administrator for their department and discuss all potential capital investment expenditures for the coming fiscal year.

1. To avoid wasting the department supervisor's time in preparing detailed proposals for all potential expenditures, tentative agreement should be reached at this point as to which projects or items will be requested for the coming fiscal year.

2. Each administrator should also review with his department supervisors the mechanics of both the Plant and Equipment Budget Request Form and the Small Item Plant and Equipment Budget Request Form so that each department supervisor will know when to use each form, how to complete each form, and the nature of the supporting material that should be provided for each item listed on the Plant and Equipment Budget Request Form.

Step 2. Small Item Budget Form. Based on the tentative agreements reached in the preceding step, the department supervisor should complete the Small Item Plant and Equipment Budget Request Form for all expenditure requests of $500 and under (see Form I).

Example Form Entries:

1. Description of Request—brief statement of the item being requested, for example, electric typewriter.

2. Quantity—indication of the number of items requested.

3. Nature—indication as to whether the request is for the replacement of obsolete or worn-out equipment, renovation of obsolete or insufficient facilities, or the addition of new equipment or facilities.

4. Estimate of Cost—indication of unit and total purchase cost (including installation costs).

5. Purchase Date Requested—indication of when the expenditure will be made. This information is needed for purposes of preparing the cash budget.

6. Justification of Request—an explanation of why the item should be purchased, for example, needed for the new secretary who is to be hired.

Department _____

SMALL ITEM PLANT AND EQUIPMENT
BUDGET REQUEST FORM

Form I

| Description of Request | Quantity | Nature | | | Estimate of Cost | | Purchase Date | Justification of Request | Decision | |
		Replace.	Renova.	Addition	Total	Each			App.	Class.

7. Decision—this column should be completed by the assistant administrator responsible for the department.

Step 3. Plant and Equipment Budget Form.   Based on the tentative agreements reached in Step 1, the department supervisor should complete the Plant and Equipment Budget Request Form for all expenditure requests of over $500 (see Form II).

Example Form Entries:

1. Description of Request—brief statement of the item, work, or program being requested, for example, cardiac defibrillator.

2. Quantity—indication of the number of items desired.

3. Nature—indication as to whether the request is for the replacement of obsolete or worn-out equipment, renovation of obsolete or inefficient facilities, or the addition of new equipment or facilities.

4. Estimate of Cost—indication of unit and total purchase cost (including installation costs).

5. Purchase Date Requested—indication of when the expenditure should be made. If the expenditure will be over a number of months, the amount by month should be indicated. This information is necessary for cash budgeting purposes.

6. Reason for Request—a brief statement of why the request is being made; for example, presently, one of the hospital's three defibrillators is nonoperative and cost of repair exceeds cost of replacement.

7. Classification—indication of the urgency or need for the expenditure. Classification A should be given to those expenditures necessary for continuing or maintaining present services, including new equipment needed to meet volume growth. Classification B should be given to those expenditures whose principal benefit will be either a cost savings or profit within the present scope of services. Classification C should be given to those expenditures whose principal benefit will be an increase in quality and or effectiveness of present services. Classification D should be given to those expenditures whose principal benefit will be an expansion of present services through new programs.

8. Department Supervisor's Recommended Priority Ranking—a numerical indication of the relative importance of each of the requested items.

Step 4. Small Items Decisions.   Department supervisors should review both budget request forms with the assistant administrator responsible for their departments.

Form II

Department _____

(DEPARTMENTAL)
PLANT AND EQUIPMENT BUDGET
REQUEST FORM

| Description of Request | Quantity | Nature | | | Estimate of Cost | | Purchase Date | Reason for Request (brief statement) | Classi. | Priority Rank |
		Addition	Renova.	Replace.	Total	Each				

1. The assistant administrator should examine each of the items listed on the Small Item Request Form and come to final agreement with the department supervisor as to whether or not the requested item should be approved and, if approved, which of the above classifications, that is, A, B, C, or D, should be assigned to it. The decision in regard to each item should be indicated in the "Decision" column of the Small Item Request Form. The approved Small Item Request Form should then be forwarded to the budget officer for inclusion in the final Plant and Equipment Budget. (It should be noted that the budgeting process for these requests is completed at this point. Therefore, care must be exercised to assure that all requests are valid and necessary.)

2. The assistant administrator should examine each item listed on the Plant and Equipment Request Form and come to a final agreement with the department supervisor as to which items will be included in the request and the classification of each included item.

Step 5. Plant and Equipment Request Support Documentation. Department supervisors should prepare supporting material for each item listed in the Plant and Equipment Budget Request Form.

1. Nature of the supporting material
   In support of each expenditure request, the department supervisor should prepare an expenditure proposal that indicates in detail
   a. The task for which the facility or equipment is to be used
   b. The necessity and importance of the task
   c. The expected utilization of the facility or equipment (seven days/week; 24 hours/day = 100% utilization)
   d. The extent of the current availability of the same or similar services from other sources
   e. The nature of expected service and patient care benefits
      1) The degree to which patients benefit, for example, lifesaving, health restoration, disease prevention, increased patient convenience
      2) The number of patients who will benefit, and the characteristics of the patients who will benefit, for example, age, sex
   f. The expected life of the facility or equipment
   g. The capital costs of the facility or equipment (including acquisition costs, installation costs, and major maintenance costs; and the year or years in which these costs can be expected to be incurred)

h. The operating costs of the facility or equipment—by year of operation

i. The savings or profits (if any)—by year—that can be expected if the expenditure is made

2. Cooperation

In preparing the above supporting documentation, department supervisors should, as needed, call upon the purchasing department, the budget officer, the controller's office, and administration for assistance.

Step 6. Request Package Review. To assure that all necessary data have been provided and that there is agreement as to the items requested, department supervisors should review the Plant and Equipment Budget Request Form and all the required supporting documentation with the assistant administrator responsible for their departments. Following this review and agreement, the request form and the supporting materials should be forwarded to the budget officer for analysis and presentation to the Plant and Equipment Budget Committee.

CAPITAL BUDGETING DECISION PROCESS

Step 1. Budget Office Receipt of Requests. The budget officer should receive all departmental budget request forms and supporting materials. Additionally, he should receive from administration the Plant and Equipment Budget Request Forms and the appropriate supporting documentation for all facility or equipment expenditures that administration wishes to initiate. (The forms and the required supporting materials are identical to those previously described.)

Step 2. Budget Office Analysis and Summary. The budget officer should analyze the information provided in the request forms and supporting documentation and prepare summary budget request forms for presentation to the Plant and Equipment Budget Committee (see Forms III, IV, V, and VI).

1. The budget officer should review each Classification A request and if the request is for current operational needs, he should summarize it on Form III. Those requests that do not appear to meet the Classification A definition should be returned to the issuing department supervisor for clarification or change of classification and priority.

2. The budget officer should compute the internal rate of return for each Classification B item that is expected to generate a profit and summarize each of the requests on Form IV-A. Net present value

Form III

SUMMARY
PLANT AND EQUIPMENT BUDGET REQUESTS
CLASSIFICATION A ITEMS

Description of Request	Dept	Quantity	Total Capital Cost	Summary of Supporting Materials	Dept Prior Rec.	Committee Action Dec.	Rk. Order

Form IV-A

SUMMARY
PLANT AND EQUIPMENT BUDGET REQUESTS
CLASSIFICATION B ITEMS: INTERNAL RATE OF RETURN

Description of Request	Dept.	Quantity	Capital Costs by Year	Summary of Supporting Documentation: Benefits	Dept. Prior. Rec.	Internal Rate of Return	Committee Action	
							Dec.	Rk. Order

Form IV-B

SUMMARY
PLANT AND EQUIPMENT BUDGET REQUESTS
CLASSIFICATION B ITEMS

| Description of Request | Dept. | Quantity | Cost by Year | | Net Present Value | Summary of Supporting Documentation: Benefits | Dept. Prior Rec. | Comm. Action | |
			Capital	Oper.				Dec.	Rank Ord.

Form V

SUMMARY
PLANT AND EQUIPMENT BUDGET REQUESTS
CLASSIFICATION "C" ITEMS

Description of Request	Dept.	Quantity	Cost by Year		Net Present Value	Summary of Supporting Documentation: Benefits	Dept. Prior Rec.	Comm. Action	
			Capital	Oper.				Dec.	Rank Ord.

Form VI

SUMMARY
PLANT AND EQUIPMENT BUDGET REQUESTS
CLASSIFICATION D ITEMS

| Description of Request | Dept. | Quantity | Cost by Year | | Net Present Value | Summary of Supporting Documentation: Benefits | Dept. Prior. Rec. | Comm. Action | |
			Capital	Oper.				Dec.	Rank Ord.

should be computed for each Classification B item that is expected to produce a savings relative to the current level of operations, and each of the requests should be summarized on Form IV-B. Those requests that do not meet the Classification B definition should be returned to the proper department supervisor for clarification or change of classification and priority.

3. The budget officer should compute the net present value of each Classification C item and summarize the costs and service and patient care benefits of each of the requests on Form V.[11] Those requests that do not meet the Classification C definition should be returned to the proper department supervisor for clarification or change of classification and priority.

4. The budget officer should compute the present value of the total cost of each Classification D item and summarize the costs and service and patient care benefits of each of the requests on Form VI.[11] Those requests that do not meet the Classification D definition should be returned to the proper department supervisor for clarification or change of classification and priority.

Step 3. Plant and Equipment Budget Committee. The summary forms should be presented to the Plant and Equipment Budget Committee (this can be the staff budget committee described in the chapter) for action.

1. Due to the interdepartmental nature of the Plant and Equipment Budget, a representative committee, including at least administration, nursing, the medical staff, and the various general service and patient care departments, should be used to review and evaluate all expenditure requests. The chairman of the committee should be appointed by the director of the hospital.

---

[11]Note to the reader. The matter of categorizing and quantifying benefits has long been an issue of controversy. A variety of techniques ranging from a subjective approach, wherein the relative value of alternative benefits is intuitively appraised, to an objective econometric technique, wherein an attempt is made to calculate the specific dollar impact of a particular set of benefits, can be used to attempt to quantify benefits. Given the current state of the art, the econometric approach, while theoretically attractive, is encumbered with methodological and pragmatic problems that significantly impair its efficacy. Similarly, the completely subjective approach is open to criticism in that basic values are never explicitly defined or tested.

An alternative technique that attempts to recognize the deficiencies of the above approaches by adding quantified definition to subjectively established values is presented in Exhibits I and II of this chapter. It should be noted that the material illustrated in the exhibits would generally not be included as part of the forms and instructions provided in the Administrative Package. Moreover, it should be recognized that the approach presented is not the definitive answer. Rather, it is an intermediate step toward a more effective decision process. It is presented here both as an alternative to less structured approaches and as a stimulus to the development of more accurate techniques.

2. The Plant and Equipment Budget Committee should review all requests by classification category and recommend whether or not a request should be approved.

3. Also, the committee should rank order—in terms of priority for funding—all requests that it recommends should be approved.

   a. The rank ordering of Classification A items should be based on a subjective evaluation of the need for each item.

   b. The rank ordering of Classification B items should be based largely on the internal rate of return that each project will generate. That is, generally the project with the highest rate of return should be ranked first. Projects producing savings should be ranked subsequent to expenditures producing a profit. Generally, the project with the largest ratio of net present value to initial capital costs should be ranked first.

   c. The rank ordering of Classification C items should be based on a subjective evaluation of the costs and benefits expected from each item.

   d. The rank ordering of Classification D items should be based on a subjective evaluation of the costs and benefits expected from each item.

4. Additionally, the committee should indicate any exceptions that it feels should be made in the general order of funding items. That is, generally, all Classification A items should be funded before any Classification B items are funded. However, if the committee feels, for example, that item D-1 should be funded prior to item C-3, it should indicate this change in general priority.

Step 4. Committee Recommendations. The recommendations of the Plant and Equipment Budget Committee should be forwarded to the director of the hospital for consideration in determining the plant and equipment budget funding decisions.

Step 5. Funding Decisions. Given the committee's recommendations, the next issue is that of determining the total amount of funds available for plant and equipment expenditures. This determination should be made by the controller and the director of the hospital after a review of the revenue, expense, and cash budgets and the forecasted margin. Once this amount is determined, the completion of the plant and equipment budget is a relatively simple matter.

Based on the quantity of available funds, the final budget should be prepared by funding, in the appropriate order, items approved through the small item budgeting mechanism and then by funding, in the appropriate order, other approved items until the entire amount of funds is appropriated.[12] Thus, the general funding order, unless either the Plant and Equipment Budget Committee recommends exceptions or the director of the hospital resets the priority of specific items, would be:

Order	Classification	Item
1	A	Small Item Requests
2	A	Plant and Equipment Requests
3	B	Small Item Requests
4	B	Plant and Equipment Requests
5	C	Small Item Requests
6	C	Plant and Equipment Requests
7	D	Small Item Requests
8	D	Plant and Equipment Requests

APPENDIX 18.B[13]
CAPITAL FINANCING

Historically, hospitals have had little interaction with the private capital markets. Prior to World War II, hospital capital needs were met primarily through retained earnings and philanthropy. After World War II, these traditional sources were supplemented by federal government funds provided through the Hill-Burton program.

Since the mid-1960s, however, the situation for the nonprofit hospital has changed markedly. For a variety of economic, reimbursement, and tax reasons, philanthropy has not been able to keep up with the accelerating pace of hospital capital needs. As a result, hospitals have had to look increasingly to private capital markets, that is, principally debt, since nonprofit hospitals have not raised equity. This reliance on the private capital markets has been increased further with the emergence and growth of the investor-owned hospital chains. In entering the private capital markets, the hospital is trying to obtain funds at the most attractive possible terms and appropriate risk. The intensifying complexity of the capital markets has created opportunities and risks that are likely to make an ongoing comprehensive capital management program a necessity for all hospitals. Manag-

---

[12]It should be noted that at times it may be necessary to revise the revenue budget or to borrow in order to obtain sufficient monies to fund all necessary expenditures. The necessity of this action will depend on the size of the recommended expenditures list and on the amount of funds available. Also, at times, funds may be borrowed to finance Classification B projects that have a profit potential and an internal rate of return greater than the interest rate.

[13]The original material for Appendix 18.B was excerpted from various documents prepared by R. Neal Gilbert, including: "Capital Financing," *Topics in Health Care Financing*, Vol. 5, No. 1, Fall 1978. Reprinted with permission of Aspen Publishers, Inc. Special thanks and appreciation are also due to Mary Alice Lightle and Stephen Wood for their work in updating and revising this appendix.

ing the acquisition capital and maintaining a capital portfolio involve a several step process. This process includes an inventory of capital requirements, review of the existing capital position, assessment of the debt capacity of the hospital, identification of potential sources of capital, evaluation of alternatives, and a sensitivity analysis to identify future risks.

A capital financing strategy should seek to balance a desired level of risk with desired interest cost saving. The goal is to achieve the maximum interest cost savings given prudent management of risk. Capital financing approaches vary from low risk conventional, essentially project-based financing to extremely aggressive approaches that attempt to position the hospital to take advantage of lowest possible interest rates. A balanced strategy finances long-term fixed assets with long-term debt and shorter-term assets with lower cost short-term debt. Equity is reserved for business opportunities that may require cash investments.

The new environment requires that the institution must not only select the optimum method of financing, but also must structure the terms and conditions of loans in a way that is most economically beneficial to it. This latter task is a complex problem that cannot be undertaken without expert financial assistance. With respect to the method of financing, there are several major alternatives. Each of these is discussed below.

TAX-EXEMPT REVENUE BONDS

This type of financing vehicle is by far the most popular and has retained a great deal of popularity in recent years. More than 70% of all hospital long-term debt financing is now tax-exempt. Because the interest earned on these bonds is exempt from federal income taxes, investors have been willing to receive up to 2.5% lower return on their investment than they would on taxable issues of similar quality. Bonds may be issued by a state or municipal hospital authority, by a county or city, or directly by the nonprofit corporation under current IRS guidelines if a beneficial interest in the facility is given to a municipality.

If the bonds are issued through an authority, title to the hospital may remain with the authority until the bonds are retired, at which time it is reconveyed to the hospital. In other cases, loan agreements, lease-leasebacks, or mortgage loans may be used. Bonds are usually secured by a pledge of the revenues of the hospital being financed. The credit behind them is generally not the credit of the authority or municipality, but rather the present and future financial strength of the hospital.

Tax-exempt revenue bonds allow for the highest ratio of financing to project cost or total assets of any method. Many facilities can finance up to 100% of their project costs plus financing expenses, interest during construction, and refinancing of existing debt. This is because tax-exempt creditworthiness is based more on revenue-generating capability and cash flow than on property value, which is more important to investors in taxable hospital financings. In addition, this method allows for the longest maturity, which reduces annual debt service.

Advantages[14]

1. Interest costs are usually 1.5% to 2.5% lower than other methods of financing.

2. The term of the loan can be 35 years, reducing annual debt service requirements.

3. Since the loan amount is determined by the ability of the facility to generate revenue, up to 100% of total project costs might be financed.

4. Interest payments can be capitalized during construction.

5. Tax-exempt bond issues are usually structured with open-ended provisions allowing for issuance of additional bonds or alternative indebtedness, provided certain levels of financial performance are maintained.

6. Existing debt can usually be refinanced.

7. "Fast track" construction is possible; that is, financing can often be arranged before final plans and specifications for construction are complete.

8. A borrower's creditworthiness can be reflected in a better rating, more flexible terms, and a lower interest cost.

9. Public offering through an underwriting group taps both regional and national sources of capital among institutional and individual investors.

10. Bonds can sometimes be privately placed.

Disadvantages[14]

1. In some cases, title to the facility may be transferred to the authority during the life of the issue.

2. Financing expenses, including the underwriting discount, feasibility study, bond counsel, other legal fees, and printing costs, are generally higher than in some other methods of financing.

3. A debt service reserve fund, usually equaling one year's average principal and interest payment, is generally required. The reserve fund, however, is used to pay off the last maturing bond principal and is usually reinvested in securities earning enough to pay the cost of interest on the reserve fund.

4. Bonds sold to the public require disclosure of the hospital's operating and financial history.

---

[14]Since all segments of the capital markets are in a constant state of change, this summary and the other summaries should be viewed as only general guidelines.

SHORT-TERM TAX-EXEMPT BONDS

The tax-exempt bond market has been changing for hospitals in very recent years. High interest rates, combined with uncertainty generated by changes in forms of health care delivery and payment mechanisms, have led to financing techniques in the 1980s that are quite different from prior periods. Specifically in the 1980s hospitals have increasingly used short-term tax-exempt financing vehicles that place a premium on lower interest cost and flexibility in terms of maintenance covenants, ability to prepay, and general ability to adapt to a changing environment.

Several different financing vehicles have been developed for hospitals that address the need for flexibility in the capital financing process. Tax-exempt commercial paper, variable-rate demand bonds, short-term fixed rate bonds, and pooled debt programs enable hospitals to choose the best suited financing vehicle for a particular situation. In combination with more conventional long-term debt instruments, these financing vehicles can enable a hospital to manage its capital acquisition program more effectively.

Many of the new financing vehicles are considered short-term debt. Short-term financing vehicles usually require credit support instruments such as a bank line of credit or letter of credit, bond insurance, or liquid equity in the form of cash or short-term securities. As various financing vehicles are increasingly used, credit support instruments have become more popular. By 1984 about 40% of all publicly offered tax-exempt hospital bonds were insured. In addition, many of the remaining tax-exempt bonds carried letter of credit bank support in 1984.

Advantages and disadvantages are associated with each type of financing vehicle. Deciding which strategy to adopt is a complex process requiring the expert advice of experienced bankers, underwriters, and legal counsel. Factors to consider in the decision range from interest cost differentials to placement costs and put features. However, some general guidelines do apply to all types of short-term debt when compared to long-term debt. It is usually unwise to finance long-term assets with short-term debt. Thus, while the appeal of less expensive short-term debt is strong, its use is usually limited to the construction phase of a project, or as a tool to time entry into the long-term debt market.

Advantages	*Disadvantages*
1. Often, interest costs are the lowest of any form of hospital debt financing.	1. Often, bank letter of credit or line of credit, or insurance is needed.
2. Easy to prepay variable-rate demand bonds or discontinue commercial paper programs.	2. Risk that bondholders will "put" or investors not purchase reissued paper must be carefully analyzed.

3. Under certain circumstances, can be used to generate significant arbitrage earnings.

4. Can be quickly implemented.

3. Reissuance costs are incurred each time investors exercise put options or commercial paper is rolled over.

4. Credit quality of the hospital could be adversely affected, raising the cost of all future debt.

CONVENTIONAL MORTGAGES OR TAXABLE BONDS

This health care financing alternative covers all taxable nongovernment guaranteed financing vehicles that utilize private institutional lenders as the source of funds. This includes mortgages, notes on either a secured or unsecured basis, term loans with commercial banks, and interim construction loans. Institutional lenders include private and public pension funds, mutual savings banks, insurance companies, savings and loan associations, and real estate investment trusts.

This method of financing can be tailored to meet the particular financial priorities of the hospital, although this flexibility is limited to the parameters of any particular lender's requirements. Negotiating privately with one sophisticated lender can avoid costs and delays that can occur in methods involving governmental approval or a public offering of securities.

A disadvantage of the private placement technique is that the percentage of total project cost that can be raised through this method is generally lower than the percentage that can be raised through other financing techniques such as the government insured or guaranteed programs. This lower loan-to-value ratio dictates that a greater percentage of project cost be raised by the hospital or that the hospital be in a very strong capital position to begin with.

The hospital should be very careful in negotiating the covenants of the loan agreement. Private placements can be very restrictive with regard to prepayment provisions and additional financing. A typical loan might be noncallable for ten years and then only at a gradually declining premium. Additional financing might only be allowed if a certain loan-to-value ratio is not exceeded.

In understanding private placements, one must keep in mind the differences between institutional lenders. Their attitudes, lending policies, and interest charges will vary dramatically depending on money market conditions, the makeup of their loan portfolio, lending criteria, interest requirements, cash flow, fiduciary responsibility, and the personalities involved. What holds true for one lender may be totally inappropriate for another, and what was true one time may be wrong a few months later.

These points emphasize the general need to utilize a capable investment banker in executing this method of financing. An investment banker who is thoroughly familiar with the market and is in constant contact with a large cross section of institutional lenders will be able to identify the best lenders for a particular situation. This capability will usually save the hospital time and money. In addition, an experienced investment banker will guide the hospital through the complicated negotiating process and obtain the most favorable available terms.

Advantages

1. This method of financing allows the hospital to structure a financing package most suitable to its financial priorities through negotiations with one lender.

2. The hospital does not have to conform to HHS/FHA construction standards.[15]

3. There are no discount points required, since interest rates are freely negotiated.

4. Since the interest rate can be negotiated well before closing, the hospital can more accurately predict total costs and debt service requirements.

5. A feasibility study is frequently not required; printing expenses are reduced or avoided; and legal fees are usually less expensive than with other alternatives, particularly those involving public sale.

Disadvantages

1. The interest rate will be higher than in tax-exempt or FHA/GNMA financings.[15]

2. The loan-to-value ratio rarely exceeds 70%. Therefore, the hospital may have to contribute a higher percentage of equity to use this method of financing.

3. The loan term may be shorter than the alternative methods of financing: 20 to 25 years compared with 25 to 30.

4. The loan covenants are usually more restrictive than in other methods.

5. Funds may be difficult to obtain when money markets are tight if the hospital is located in an unattractive area or if elements of speculation exist.

THE FHA-242

FHA-insured hospital mortgages were made possible in 1968 by Section 242 of Title II to the National Housing and Urban Development Act. The section authorized the commissioner of the Federal Housing Administration (FHA) to insure mortgage loans used to finance the construction or rehabilitation of not-for-profit hospitals and the purchase of major movable equipment for such institutions. Amendments in 1970 and 1983 added eligibility for proprietary hospitals and public hospitals.

Hospitals utilizing the FHA-242 program may borrow up to 90% of the replacement value of the facility for a term of up to 25 years plus the period of construction. For hospitals with sufficient equity in the form of existing property, plant, and equipment, the financing program may be used to finance 100% of eligible project costs.

The process by which hospitals obtain an FHA commitment is to file

---

[15]Health and Human Services (HHS); Federal Housing Administration (FHA); Government National Mortgage Association (GNMA).

a loan application with the Department of Health and Human Services (HHS). Under an agreement between the Department of Health, Education, and Welfare and FHA, HHS has the responsibility for evaluating and passing on its project approval to FHA. The evaluation process is conducted in three principal areas: financial feasibility, architectural and engineering conformance to federal guidelines, and service program need. In most instances, an independent feasibility study supports the basic application documentation. Notwithstanding a favorable evaluation by HHS, the project application is then analyzed by the multifamily mortgage credit section of FHA for conformance with numerous other financing guidelines. Furthermore, all projects must have federally recognized certificates of need.

Advantages

1. Loan-to-replacement value ratio can be as high as 90%.

2. The value of the land, existing buildings, and major movable equipment may satisfy hospital's equity requirement.

3. Most preparation and application costs can be included in eligible costs.

4. The United States government's full faith and credit guarantee allows the hospital to secure an attractive interest rate.

5. If the hospital is undergoing an expansion or modernization program, eligible debt can include refinancing of existing debt.

6. The term of the loan can be as much as 25 years after completion of construction.

7. Prepayment of 15% of the original principal amount is permitted in a calendar year without penalty. In addition, the loan can be structured to allow for prepayment in excess of this amount at any time for a negotiated penalty.

8. FHA financing is extremely compatible with other government programs.

Disadvantages

1. Processing of the FHA application can be time-consuming.

2. Construction must conform to FHA/HHS standards.

3. Construction labor costs can be higher than with other methods of financing because of strict government regulations.

4. Additional borrowing to finance subsequent payments is severely restricted.

5. If the FHA coupon rate is below current money market rates, the hospital must pay front-end discount points to bring the yield to the investor up to market levels.

6. The hospital must pay an annual mortgage insurance premium of 0.5% of the unamortized principal amount.

7. The hospital must pay front-end inspection and filing fees totaling 0.8% of the principal amount.

FARMERS HOME ADMINISTRATION (FmHA) GUARANTEE
AND DIRECT LOAN PROGRAMS OF HOSPITALS

The Rural Development Act of 1972 authorized Farmers Home Administration (FmHA) to fund essential community facilities including hospitals, clinics, and other health related facilities. Credit is provided for the construction or renovation of these health facilities through two of the FmHA programs: the Community Facilities Program and the Business and Industrial Loan Program. Both programs also provide funds to non–health related community facilities and have policies stating which types of facility have priority over others for receipt of credit assistance.

Each program is allocated a certain amount of credit yearly on a national level which is then distributed to the states and eligible territories based on population and income figures. Within these geographic areas, each program can extend credit only up to its budgeted amount each year, with priority given to those individual applicants whose projects fall within the highest priority FmHA categories of project type. Historically, the demand for assistance under both these programs has exceeded the yearly budget allocations, resulting in many lower priority projects being turned down, thus not being constructed at all or being forced to rely on conventional sources of funds.

To be eligible for assistance under either program, a proposed health care project must meet certain standard criteria and provide certain assurances, including

1. Coordination with state, areawide, and local planning programs

2. Possession of a certificate of need

3. Demonstration of financial ability to repay loan

4. Compliance with state and local building and zoning ordinances

5. Possession of clear title to the project's assets

6. Provision of nondiscrimination and equal employment opportunity assurances

THE COMMUNITY FACILITIES LOAN PROGRAM (CFL PROGRAM)

Credit assistance under the CFL Program is available to all political subdivisions of a state and other organizations operated on a nonprofit basis, such as districts, authorities, corporations, associations, and cooperatives. The purpose of the program is to provide funds for the construction and equipping of essential facilities to serve the community where located which cannot obtain commercial credit on "reasonable terms or at reasonable rates." In determining that commercial credit is not available on these terms FmHA will examine only private market sources, not the terms available under other government programs for hospital financing such as FHA-242 insured mortgages. In determining the "reasonableness" of private market terms FmHA will consider front-end costs as well as interest rate and the project's ability to pay debt service under those conditions.

In addition to the nonavailability of credit criteria, eligibility for the CFL Program is subject to the following conditions:

1. The proposed project must be located in a rural area of under 20,000 population.

2. Applicant must show legal authority to construct, operate, and maintain the proposed facility.

3. Private nonprofit sponsors must show significant community ties as evidenced by community control of the governing board or substantial public funding via taxes or philanthropy.

If an applicant and proposed project are found eligible for direct FmHA loan assistance, there are a number of requirements that must be met prior to loan closing and during and after construction.

THE BUSINESS AND INDUSTRIAL LOAN PROGRAM (B & I PROGRAM)

Assistance under the B&I Program is available to any legal entity, public or private, for-profit or nonprofit, that proposes to finance a project that will improve the economic or environmental climate of a rural area, with priority given to projects that save existing jobs or create the highest number of new permanent employment opportunities. To be eligible for assistance, the proposed project must be in any area outside the boundary of a city of 50,000 or more population or outside a city's adjacent areas with population density exceeding 100 persons per square mile. Priority is given to those projects in areas of population of 25,000 or less.

The assistance provided is in the form of an FmHA loan guarantee, where the loan is arranged with, made, and serviced by a private lender who is indemnified by FmHA for a certain percentage of his losses should a default occur. FmHA can provide a guarantee of up to 90% of the principal and interest on the loan to the private lender. In return for this guarantee, the applicant must pay FmHA a fee equal to 1% of the guaranteed principal amount at loan closing.

The benefit of the FmHA guarantee to the lender is not primarily to strengthen the financial credit of a proposed project to give it access to private lenders, but to provide the lender with a federal government guarantee so that he can provide funds to certain project types in excess of that amount allowed for these projects without the guarantee. As the projects receiving the FmHA guarantee must be good credit risks to qualify for assistance, receipt of the guarantee plus the payment of the 1% fee by the applicant will generally result in financing whose cost is not appreciably lower than that normally associated with conventional sources.

EQUITY

Equity is the owner's paid-in capital. In a for-profit business, the owner's equity arises from the sale of stock or partnership interests. In a nonprofit firm, equity is provided from gifts and grants by both private and public (government) sources and cash equity.

As a source of capital, equity is fundamentally different from debt. Debt is a contractual obligation between borrower and lender. By contrast, equity is a residual interest.

The difference between the equity of a for-profit organization and that of a nonprofit organization is established by the Internal Revenue Code and state corporation laws. The principal characteristic of a nonprofit organization is that no part of its profits or assets can inure to any private person. For this reason, nonprofit corporations do not pay dividends. The terms of some gifts and grants may provide for the gift to revert to the donor if certain conditions are not met. For example, land may be deeded to a hospital with the stipulation that it be used only as the site of the hospital. If the hospital is closed or relocated, the land reverts to the donor. Except for such cases, any assets in a nonprofit corporation remaining after satisfaction of liabilities must be transferred to another nonprofit entity.

Equity in a for-profit enterprise may take the form of stock in a corporation or an interest in a partnership. Recently, not-for-profit hospitals have begun to participate in for-profit joint ventures through subsidiary corporations. The primary difference between a corporation and a partnership is that revenues and expenses of a partnership flow through to the partners and are not taxed in the partnership. Also, the liability of stockholders is limited to their initial investment. In partnership arrangements, general partners are personally liable for all liabilities. All partnerships have at least one general partner. In a limited partnership, limited partners' liability is limited to the amount of their investment.

Offerings of stock or partnership interests made to the general public are subject to registration requirements under the Securities Act of 1933 and state securities laws. In general, private placements are exempt from these requirements (or subject only to the perfection of an exemption) if only a few offers are made and offers are made to financially sophisticated investors.

There are no legal limits on how much equity a corporation must have. Some state for-profit corporation laws require a nominal initial equity investment of $1,000 as a condition of incorporation. Sometimes, lenders will require an equity contribution to a financing, but this often can be met with equity accumulated in the corporation rather than the issuance of stock or solicitation of new contributions.

There are two important pragmatic considerations, however, in choosing between debt and equity capital sources. First, higher leverage (or the greater the share of assets financed with debt) leads to greater financial risk within the corporation. When larger portions of cash flows are committed to the repayment of indebtedness, adverse operating variances are likely to impair the corporation's ability to meet its obligations to lenders. Second, the uncertain regulatory environment has increased hospitals' need to raise equity capital. Increased competition among providers of health care services and pressures from business and government to reduce their outlays for hospital expenditures may result in reduced utilization or payment for services. These developments may also make it more difficult to repay debt. As a matter of prudence, corporations should maintain a balance of debt and equity in their capital structures.

A NOTE OF CAUTION

In addition to the foregoing, some of the financing alternatives can be combined, in some cases resulting in an optimal financing package. The financing techniques vary in time requirements, processing procedures, total cost, flexibility, interest rates, and impact on cash flow. Each alternative requires professional financial expertise to insure proper execution, and each has advantages and disadvantages that must be carefully evaluated before one approach is selected.

19

Implementation

The previous chapters have attempted first to lay out a conceptual foundation for planning and budgeting and then to build on that foundation by constructing a general process to be used for developing a hospital's strategy, plan, and budget. Such a framework is useful. However, unless theory can be turned into practice, unless the foregoing can be implemented successfully, no management or operational progress can be achieved. Therefore, the focus of this chapter is on implementing the planning and budgeting processes.

It is important to recognize that implementing any planning and budgeting process is fundamentally an exercise in the management of change. An extensive body of literature is available that addresses the theory as well as the practice of managing change. Little is to be gained by trying to summarize here what has been set out elsewhere. Additionally, though significant progress has been made, the state of the art still has not reached the point where there is either a definitive set of principles or a universal approach to managing the implementation of change successfully. In the face of these realities, this chapter will limit its focus to attempting only to identify a set of pragmatic implementation bench marks or rules of thumb for management to consider in implementing a hospital's planning and budgeting process.

While some repetition is both necessary and helpful, this chapter has attempted to avoid the comments made in previous chapters. Therefore, the reader is urged to refer to earlier chapters, particularly Chapter 16.

CHANGE

Implementing change is and always has been difficult. Even as more is learned and the state of the art advances, it is likely that implementing new ways of conducting business, new approaches to day-to-day activities, new ideas, and any other changes from the status quo will continue to be one of management's greatest and most difficult challenges. However, if an organization is to remain viable, change cannot be avoided. In fact, controlled change must be sought.

The central reason behind the difficulty in implementing change lies in the fact that all change affects people in some way. The effect will vary from individual to individual as it operates through the individual's perceptions of his environment, the nature of the change being made, and the resulting effects of the proposed change of his environment. Because of the differences not only in people and their perceptions but also in their level of information and degree of understanding, the resulting attitudes about any proposed change will vary in explicable as well as seemingly inexplicable ways. However, as a general rule, it is likely, unless a situation has reached a commonly recognized level of intolerability, that an individual's initial reaction to a proposed change will be that of resistance.

The factors that produce the resistance reaction are several. Depending upon the individual and the particular situation, these factors may act singly or in combination. For purposes of discussion, they can be grouped around three generic themes.

UNCERTAINTY

Uncertainty is the most obvious cause and usually is suggested as the major source of resistance attitudes. People are generally comfortable with the status quo. Change disturbs the status quo and thus brings with it the uncertainty inherent in a new situation and the concomitant fear of the unknown. To minimize, if not eliminate, this fear, change is resisted.

In the same vein, to the extent that there is inadequate information about a proposed change, all relevant parties have not been involved in the change decision process, and/or there is a lack of confidence and trust in management, change will be resisted. The reasons for this lie in the fact that everyone has some level of insecurity. To the extent that one's pocket of insecurity is penetrated due to confusion, lack of involvement, or distrust, the natural, nearly automatic, reaction is to resist the perceived threat, that is, the proposed change.

ECONOMIC AND PSYCHOSOCIAL

A very practical reason for resisting change is concern over possible economic loss; for example, having laboratory technician jobs automated out of existence. Short of eliminating jobs, change still raises the possibility of economic loss due to reduced earnings, caused, for example, by the loss of overtime, or of the same earnings but increased production requirements.

The same notion of losses carries over into the area of social and job satisfaction losses. The mere fact that a change is being imposed is evidence of the autocracy of management and the limits of employee independence. Also, change involves the restructuring of formal and informal relationships. Such restructuring not only produces an initial void but also may result in the loss of organizational status; new relationships that are not as rich and rewarding as the old; or an increased isolation of the employee from his colleagues.

These are all losses that, from the employee's perspective, are to be avoided. The first line of defense for accomplishing this is resisting the proposed change.

ENVIRONMENTAL CONSTRAINTS

The history of the organization and its past experience with change, the ripple of change on the various components of the organization, and the existence of unions are all examples of potential phenomena operating in a hospital's environment that can act to produce resistance to change. For example, if past change has been handled badly, a negative predisposition to future change will exist. Similarly, if a change in one department affects its relationship with other departments, the reaction of the secondarily affected departments may produce resistance sufficient to stop implementation of the first department's proposed change. Finally, the existence of a union, because of the general role that its membership might expect it to play, may be an a priori source of resistance, regardless of the merits of the proposed change.

Given the resistance reaction, if management is successfully to implement a planning and budgeting process, it must convert resistance into acceptance or, better yet, support. The first step in doing this is to recognize the natural tendency to resist change. The second step is to build this recognition into an explicit, carefully designed plan for implementing change.

It is an unrealistic management expectation to assume that a process as complex and a change as threatening as planning and budgeting can be implemented successfully on an ad hoc, randomly coordinated basis. If implementation is to succeed, it must be guided by a well conceived, integrated course of development. In essence, a planning and budgeting process is not only a prerequisite but also a necessity.

In developing a planning and budgeting process, the most critical point to appreciate is that there are no single right answers. Each hospital's plan must reflect its history, experience, managerial sophistication, and external

environmental demands, as well as its ability to accept, adapt to, and insti-
tutionalize change. Even though no one right approach exists for hospitals,
there are several general principles that, though they may not apply universally, are worthy of consideration in all instances.

PLANNING TO PLAN: PRINCIPLES

In designing its plan, management must address two sets of issues.
The first centers on the matter of implementation style. The second focuses
on defining the timing and design of the change.

IMPLEMENTATION STYLE

At its core, implementing change relies on one's having the managerial
power to control events, that is, to make something happen. Operationally,
the power to effect change can be exercised or utilized in two basic ways:
unilaterally or shared.

Unilateral power is reflected in one-way communication, wherein management directly imposes the proposed change on the organization. Im-
position or, more politely, implementation, is carried out by fiat. In contrast,
shared power involves participation in the proposed change by those who
will be affected. Power can be shared by involving others in the change
decision processes or by delegating to others either the identification of the
need for, the design of, or the installation of the proposed change.

Successful implementation of change typically involves a blend of these
two approaches to applying power. The reasons for this should be clear.

A primary goal of the implementation process is to convert resistance
into a more positive attitude, that is, support. Shared power provides a
vehicle for increasing the general level of understanding of the need for a
potential change; perhaps even more important, it also provides a device
for allowing those who will be affected by the change to work through
alternative solutions and to adopt the proposed change as their own approach. As is the case with management by objectives, to the extent that a
proposed change is understood and internalized as one's own idea, commitment to it and to its potential for success increases.

In counterpoint to the benefits of shared power and participative decisions is the need to balance corporate democracy with a mechanism that:
sets parameters; keeps the shared power process from becoming unduly
mired; ratifies the proposed solution; and commits the hospital's resources
to effecting the accepted change. This need is met through the productive
application of unilateral power. Unilateral power in effect becomes the driving force behind shared power.

Functionally, the two are inextricably intertwined in a mutually reinforcing relationship. Unilateral power provides the impetus to remain on course while moving toward problem resolution. Shared power obtains its authority from unilateral power. It provides the means for moving forward in a manner that co-opts, or at least minimizes, resistance.

The lacing together of these two approaches to utilizing power is a delicate task. Mechanically, the kinds of thing that must be done to bring the two together include

1. Making as certain as possible that everyone who is or will be involved in the change understands the situation that makes the change necessary. The goal is to produce a common level of understanding and a general level of concurrence on the need for change. This component of implementation is initially unilateral in character, evolving to a shared recognition of the problem and, ultimately, of the proposed solution.

2. Involving meaningful participation in the entire change process. On a step-by-step basis the change process can be viewed as consisting of the following elements:

    a. *Creation of the climate for change*

    This step involves establishing both an operating environment that is willing to carry out meaningful change and a generally understood recognition of the need for a specific change. The key variable for accomplishing this is management leadership.

    Management must create a fertile environment for change by convincing the key parties that change is important to the continued vitality and success of the hospital. With respect to a specified change, management must, as described above, present the facts of the situation in a manner that produces a common level of understanding among all the concerned parties as to the need for change. In carrying out both these tasks, management must use individual meetings and small group meetings as well as committees and working groups to create a common base and level of knowledge. Combined committees are particularly useful in working with the board and medical staff in addressing changes like planning and budgeting, which affect the total hospital.

    This step, as described above, is initially unilateral in character.

    b. *Identification of the problem and alternative solutions*

    The key to this step is to differentiate between symptoms and causes, focusing on causes in order to identify the range of alternative courses of corrective action or improvement. This step should be participative in character, reflecting shared power.

c. *Decisions as to which alternative is to be pursued, that is, selection of the change to be implemented*

This step can be a mixture of shared and unilateral power.
Shared power can be used to narrow the choice of alternatives
and even to make specific recommendations. Unilateral power,
however, must be used to make or ratify the final choice.

d. *Implementation of the selected course of action, that is, the proposed change*

Like the above, this step is also a mixture of shared and unilateral
power. However, in contrast to the above, this step does not stand
alone. Successful implementation is dependent not only on what
is done in this step, but also on each of the preceding steps as
well as the following step.

This step should be participative, reflecting shared power. Importantly, participation must be at a meaningful level. Meaningful participation will contribute to reducing potential resistance
while, at the same time, garnering support for the proposed
change. Participation that is perceived as being a sham will obviously have the opposite result, increasing resistance as employee distrust and insecurity are heightened.

With respect to planning and budgeting, an oversight committee can be a useful initial means for providing meaningful participation. Such a committee should be authorized by the board
and should be multidisciplinary in membership, including members of the board. As the planning and budgeting processes proceed, other committees at the operating level can also be
established. These latter committees can be used for designing
or reviewing procedures and forms, reviewing plans and budgets, and so forth.

The importance of thoroughly involving senior management
and the board cannot be overstressed. Their involvement, however, should be focused, emphasizing only critical decision points.

e. *Modification of the change based on experience*

As discussed below, the change process is evolutionary in nature. It can be characterized as a reiterative process that circulates
within itself at the same time as it moves forward (see Figure
19.1).

This step is also a mixture of unilateral and shared power.
Feedback on the operational effect of the change and the possibilities for further improvement should be obtained on a participative basis. Unilateral power, however, must make or ratify the
decision as to whether to continue to modify the current approach, that is, to recycle the change process.

3. Providing a safe means for venting the tensions produced by implementation of the proposed change. The implementation of change, regardless of either the merits of the change or how carefully the implementation is planned, will generally result in some employee tension. Management should not meet this tension with hostility. Rather, it should provide a safe tension release mechanism through which employees can vent their pent-up feelings and concerns without endangering either their own job security or the performance of the hospital. Once this venting has been accomplished, the barriers to acceptance may be reduced. Unilateral power must be used to provide the mechanism for releasing tension.

Prescribing style is a difficult task. How management ultimately brings together these two approaches to applying power into a single implementation style will vary with the character of the organization and the nature of the change to be implemented. Perhaps the best that can be said is that management should proceed with a recognition of, and a sensitivity to, the effects of change on both physicians and staff. The incorporation of this sensitivity into an implementation plan and a style for managing change should reflect the foregoing principles. However, application of these principles must be shaped to the unique circumstances of the hospital.

TIMING AND DESIGN

Part of the key to successful management of change is limiting the change to what is practicable and doable. Structuring the timing and design of a proposed change to reflect what is within the art of the possible is a major check or control point in the change process. Often, this safety valve is seemingly forgotten as management, as well as the staff involved in the change, becomes caught up in enthusiasm for the proposed change. Such

FIGURE 19.1   Evolution of Change

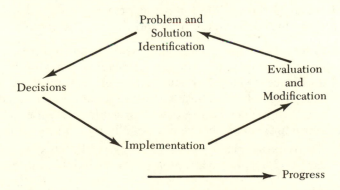

enthusiasm, while desirable, should not be allowed to mask the dangers inherent in trying to accomplish too much at once.

The fundamental point to be kept in mind is that change is evolutionary in nature. The significance of this point cuts in two ways. First, it argues that there is no need to attempt everything at once. Second, it highlights the fact that change can be accomplished in stages, with one stage setting the necessary conditions for moving to the next. The operating implication of this principle is that implementation should only move forward in manageable bites, with the scope of the intended change being limited to what the organization can productively absorb. Depending on the nature of a particular change, the implementation plan might thus encompass several years of work.

Given the complexity of the planning and budgeting process, it is not unreasonable that full implementation might encompass a number of stages or phases and several years of work. In fact, due to the dynamic nature of planning and budgeting, it is a fundamental mistake for management to attempt to implement its program too quickly. Rather, management should capitalize on the evolutionary nature of change. To do this, implementation should proceed in a manner that

1. Allows for time to modify the process as it moves forward, increasing in sophistication and comprehensiveness

2. Reduces resistance to change by allowing future stages to appear as adjustments to the existing system.

The key is thus not the speed of the implementation, but rather the design of an implementation approach that builds on itself; that is, an approach that reinforces what has been done while at the same time both moving ahead and setting the stage—preparing the organization for the next phase of implementation. The construction of such an implementation plan requires careful thought, for each phase must be meshed with both preceding and succeeding steps. It is only through this kind of careful planning, however, that complex changes can be implemented successfully.

In addition to evolution, the following principles should be kept in mind with respect to shaping the timing and design of a potential change:

1. Disturb as little as possible of the existing informal relationships. Informal relationships are a powerful factor in contributing to successful organizational performance. Therefore, only those relationships that absolutely must be affected by the proposed change should be altered. Moreover, to the extent possible, the informal organization structure should be used as an ally by management.

2. Keep the proposed change as simple as possible. This is particularly important with respect to a complex process like planning and bud-

geting. In the case of planning and budgeting, the process should be sufficiently simple so that the average manager can use it despite the pressures of his job, the lack of intensive training, and the fact that he really does not want to plan. If it is unduly complicated, planning is apt to become a bureaucratic ritual, rather than an exercise in creative and vigorous thinking.[1] Several mechanical devices that can be useful in helping to assure simplicity are

a. Keeping the planning and budgeting staff as small as possible

b. Writing a mission statement for the planning and budgeting function that circumscribes its purview

c. Designing forms that are simple to complete and to review

d. Keeping the generation and distribution of paper to a minimum

3. Shape the change to recognize that the entire organization does not always have to do exactly the same thing. With respect to planning and budgeting, recognize that there are a set of core activities that all hospital departments must do, as well as a set of secondary activities that are only relevant to selected departments. By tailoring the process to require that the various departments only do relevant planning and budgeting, management can make the entire process more efficient while at the same time reducing management frustration and dissatisfaction.

PERSEVERANCE

The chapters of Part IV have covered a wide range of material on planning, budgeting, and control. The reader should not, however, be overawed by the scope or paralyzed into inactivity by the magnitude of the tasks. Pursuit of perfection is an endless task. Management, therefore, should not be trapped into waiting for the perfect process before proceeding. Instead, it must assume the calculated risk. The initial planning and budgeting process can always be revised and adjusted to reflect the hospital's actual experience.

Excellence in management takes time, sensitivity, common sense, perseverance, and leadership. Excellence in planning, because it is a basic part of management, requires the same.

The key to the entire process, therefore, is the management leadership to begin and the management perseverance to follow through in a sensitive way.

---

[1] The Conference Board, *Planning and the Corporate Planning Director*, Chapter 8.

SUGGESTED READINGS

The Conference Board. *Planning and the Corporate Planning Director.*
Flippo, Edwin B. *Management: A Behavioral Approach.*
Greiner, Larry E. "Patterns of Organization Change."
Lewin, Kurt. "Group Decision and Social Change."
Longest, Beaufort B., Jr. *Management Practices for the Health Professional.*
Peters, Joseph P. *A Strategic Planning Process for Hospitals.*

Control and Analysis

Success rests on a clear vision,
a humane touch and an inflexible commitment
to quality and services

R. Brumlik

20

Management Reporting

An outstanding feature of a hospital budget system should now be apparent: effective budgeting requires group participation by personnel from responsibility centers upward to the administrative offices. That participation should not be a token partnership, but an active one in which the employee involved feels input from his level is important in planning and in accomplishing objectives.

Budgeting should be a living process with a reasonable degree of flexibility, fluidity, and mobility to meet changing conditions and unforeseen exigencies. Conditions can change within a budget period or, more likely, within the time span leading to the projected planning horizon.

If the position is taken that budgeting is a dynamic rather than a static process, one must be prepared to adjust to changes in demand for services, changes in the costs of services or supplies, and changes in a variety of other conditions that force adjustments in budgetary projections.

The next logical thought is: If a hospital's manager and its governing board are to retain their managerial perspective and administrative balance by keeping the budget process adaptable to change and flexible in response to changing needs, they must be kept informed.

Plans are good only as road maps. Operations people must read the signposts and change routes when necessary to reach objectives, if the first route or plan proves unworkable or ineffective.

(The authors digress a moment to make an important point by analogy: Think of a hospital in terms of a commercial venture. Most administrators realize what a precarious situation a supermarket chain is in when it attempts to operate on a net profit of 1% or 2%. Executives in that kind of operation are walking forever on the brink of disaster. However, they do have some capability to adjust prices and to change marketing emphasis within a competitive framework in an attempt to retain profitability. Hospitals also often operate on less than a 2% margin, but they have very limited maneuverability in changing operating conditions to avoid deficits or even disaster. This digression, it must be evident, was made to emphasize the great need of keeping "on top of things" to maintain the solvency of a hospital. That means accurate, relevant information must be available when needed.)

INFORMATION FLOW

If management is to have access to relevant, accurate information, it must plan a flow of information on the basis of daily, monthly, and, possibly, quarterly inputs so that comparisons with planned results as well as with previous periods can be charted and trends can be projected. This flow of information can come up the organization's "stairway" by the same route as did the original planning information. Later in this chapter this stairway concept will be considered not only in the sense of information flowing upward, but also in the context of the downward flow of performance data.

Ideally, the budget officer, through the hospital's chief financial officer, should direct the financial and performance reporting system. This system should provide for the exchange of actual performance and corrective action information between persons in charge of the various cost centers, departments, divisions, and programs of the hospital. Reports of financial and work performance will enable managers at the various levels to measure the performance of their responsibility centers in terms of the objectives set for the budget period. Since each person in charge of a responsibility center or group of responsibility centers participates in the planning and budgeting process, each manager should expect, in turn, to receive reports that can be used to monitor and to evaluate performance.

To return to the information stairway concept, data are input at the various organizational levels (cost centers, departments, divisions) and moved through the organizational hierarchy to the fiscal services division. The fiscal services office collects the responsibility center data inputs, adds financial data, collates them, and prepares reports that portray actual performance. These reports should, at a minimum, compare actual performance with that anticipated in the budget projections, usually on a monthly or quarterly basis, and summarize performance to date with budget projection to date for the budget year.

To complete the up and down of the information flow concept, the fiscal services division must prepare reports that interpret the operations and budget information for the responsibility center managers and send the reports down to them so they can evaluate performance in budget terms. This concept is shown in Figure 20.1.

FIGURE 20.1   Organizational Information Stairway

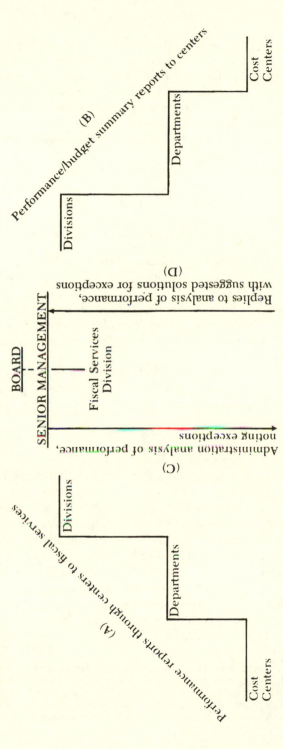

Legend: (A) indicates the upward movement of monthly reports of manhours registered, work units performed, and patients served from the various centers and divisions to the fiscal services office. (The fiscal services office collects data from all necessary sources and prepares summary reports of hospital performance as related to budget projections. Complete summaries are sent to senior management.) (B) indicates movement of departmental performance/budget projection summaries from the fiscal services office to the various departments or centers. (C) marks the movement of memoranda on analyses of performance/budget projections with notations on exceptions from the senior administrator to divisional offices and down to all centers. (D) marks the movement of replies to memoranda of (C), with suggested remedies for the exceptions.

A word of warning must be repeated. The authors realize that it is impossible to design a budget system that will fit the needs of every hospital in every detail. However, the basic principles and objectives of a performance reporting system can be identified and can serve as general guidelines. In the pages that follow, several examples of reports will be given which may not fit the particular needs of some institutions precisely. Nevertheless, it is believed that the principles being described can be adapted to most situations.

To put the reporting mechanism into proper perspective, it should be remembered that the discussion will be focused on expense and capital budgets principally, and on the revenue budget to a lesser degree.[1]

STATISTICAL REPORTS

As stated earlier, the fiscal services division is responsible for collecting data input, for generating financial statistics, and for obtaining any other information needed to compile reports for the comparison of the hospital's performance to the budget projections. This information can come from many sources so that the fiscal services division can fulfill its clearinghouse function of collecting data and preparing budget reports for management to interpret and act upon.

A brief examination of the reporting activities of a nursing department may illustrate how one department might feed information into the system. The fiscal services division would then assimilate these data for reports to the various levels of management.

NURSING

The nursing department is the largest in terms of personnel in the hospital. Furthermore, all inpatients are statistics in the various units of the department. Two types of information about nursing which need to be gathered are patient population and nurse staffing. Most hospitals collect patient information in a midnight census. This is a convenient method and time for determining what beds are occupied and by whom. This census can be used for daily room charge billings and for calculating official occupancy rates. The data on a patient's status at midnight on any given day should include, as a minimum: room number; bed number (if not a private room); and name, age, and sex the patient. The percentage of the total beds that are occupied will give the occupancy rate.

---

[1]Revenue is beyond the control of line management because prices or fees are set by senior management. Volume of services rendered also is largely beyond the control of line management. Therefore, it is unreasonable either to expect line managers to be accountable for revenue performance or to hold them accountable. Since they should not be held accountable, it is generally not necessary to report revenue to line management.

The authors do not wish to make a point as to how the information should be collected. This could be done by either manual or automated methods. The basic information can be assembled on a worksheet. For example, a nursing unit might be considered a responsibility center; the total inpatient nursing department might be a cost center. For an example we have selected a single nursing unit, Second Floor North, a 20-bed surgical nursing unit. A worksheet for the midnight census of June 14, 1986 for the responsibility center known as Second Floor North (2N) could contain the necessary patient statistics as shown in Figure 20.2.

If the total inpatient nursing department is considered a cost center, it seems likely the worksheets of all the inpatient nursing units for June 14, 1986 would be summarized for nursing administration in a form similar to that shown in Figure 20.3. It will be noted that this sheet gives occupancy and occupancy percentages for each unit and for the total hospital for that day.

Another element that is useful in performance evaluation is a work measurement statistic. One of the most common measurements used in nursing departments is the ratio of hours of nursing per patient day. A worksheet for 2N for June 14, 1986 might show the roster of the nursing staff of that unit for three shifts as described in Figure 20.4. From this roster worksheet the total nursing hours can be divided by the number of patients to determine the nursing hours/patient ratio. (Note that in the example no recording was made of the time worked by the supervisor, by clinical nursing specialists, or by therapists giving direct care. A hospital designing a work measurement formula might wish to prorate some of the work statistics to units served by these special staff members or might wish to charge these personnel to nursing administration.)

Still another possibility to be considered by those who wish to inject an element of quality of care into the work measurement statistic would be to weight the work of the nursing staff. An example is given in Figure 20.5. In this example the basis of weighting was the relationship of salary rates to position, taking the staff nurse's rate as 1.00. Under this rating scale, the head nurse was weighted as 1.25 times the hours she worked; staff nurse 1.00; licensed practical nurse 0.75; and aide or orderly 0.50. Other values for weighting could be used for assessing quality of care. According to a weighting plan, as can be seen, two rosters of the same number of nursing employees with different distributions of professional training could show quite different values on a quality of nursing scale.

In the examples given of data collection in the nursing department, statistics have been gathered daily, at the unit level, on patient census and nursing work hours. Generally, these data would be transmitted to nursing administration, where they would be summarized each month. A monthly report would be sent through the divisional office to the fiscal office for the

FIGURE 20.2   Midnight Census Worksheet

Unit 2N   Date June 14, 1986

Room	Bed	Patient	Sex	Age
2N1	A	Aaron Unger	M	32
	B	D. C. Anders	M	59
2N2	A			
	B			
2N3	A	D. Dillon	F	26
	B	Alissa Havens	F	29
2N4	A	J. Havens	M	62
	B	Jamie Berman	M	66
2N5	A	Gene Sibery	M	45
	B			
2N6	A	Amy Friedman	F	65
	B			
2N7	A	T. Dillon	M	37
	B	Tim Tuller	M	32
2N8	A	Lindsay Dale	F	18
	B	S. M. Eide	F	23
2N9	A	B. McPherson	M	47
	B	Brian Blitz	M	55
2N10	A	M. Friedman	F	42
	B	K. Blitz	F	22

Bed Complement	20
Patients	16
Occupancy rate	80%
Patients 65 or older	2

final compilation of the monthly hospital performance/budget projection
reports for four levels of management. An example of a nursing department
monthly census and work hours summary prepared for the fiscal office is
given in Figure 20.6.

FIGURE 20.3   Midnight Census, Summary Sheet

Date   June 14, 1986

Unit	Beds	Occupied	Percentage
2N	20	16	80
2S	20	12	60
2E	20	18	90
2W	20	14	70
3N	20	16	80
3S	20	14	70
3E	20	12	60
3W	20	20	100
4N	20	20	100
4S	20	18	90
4E	20	15	75
4W	20	20	100
ICU	10	5	50
CCU	5	2	40
OB	15	5	33.3
PED	10	5	50
Long-term	20	18	90
	300	230	
Nursery	10	6	60

Average occupancy, excluding nursery, 76.7%

OTHER RESPONSIBILITY AND COST CENTERS

All departments will not have the same data to collect although they will be similar, for staffing and work units will be the basic considerations. Radiology and clinical laboratory both must consider the ratio of weighted work units to staffing. They also are concerned with work scheduling to meet service demands. Physical therapy may have a weighted treatment modal system as a work measurement; dietary may report in number of meals served, the laundry in pounds of linen washed—whatever the unit of measurement, the senior administrator finally receives a performance report, against which he can match the projections for the budget period.

In a responsibility center, as shown in Figure 20.7, the principal items to be covered would be

1. Personnel costs
2. Work units performed (where applicable)

FIGURE 20.4   Worksheet: Nursing Staff Schedule

Unit 2N   Date June 14, 1986

Position	Morning	Hours Worked	Afternoon	Hours Worked	Evening	Hours Worked
Head nurse	Mackis Berman	8				
RN	E. Killingsworth	8	D. Cohn	8	G.L. Warden	8
LPN	S. Holloway	8	R. Snyder	8		
Aide	E. Tuller	8	G.S. Eide	8	R. Klein	8
	Hours per shift	32		24		16

Total hours, all shifts   72
Total patients on census   16
Average hours per patient   4.5

3. Occupancy rates (where applicable)
4. Revenue (where applicable)[2]
5. Capital expenditures (where applicable)[3]
6. Other expenditures (for example, supplies)

FINANCIAL AND PERFORMANCE REPORTS

The point was made in the information flow illustration that information moves two ways. First, reports are sent up to the fiscal services division. In addition to the data from cost centers, the fiscal services division collects data from other sources as needed to compile performance reports. Second, the fiscal services division sends performance reports, designed for the pertinent level of operation, back to management. This series of reports allows each level of management to review performance against budget projections.

A performance report for a responsibility center called nursing unit 2N is shown in Figure 20.7. The operations items can be compared with budget projections. The format of the report and the manner in which it is compiled will vary among hospitals. The reports, however designed, should show

---

[2]Although revenue is beyond the control of line management, revenue figures can be used comparatively with expenses to determine operation realities.

[3]Depending on the level of activity, capital expenditures may need a separate report.

FIGURE 20.5   Worksheet: Nursing Staff Schedule Weighted for
                Quality of Care

Unit _2N_   Date_June 14, 1986_

Morning shift		
1 Head nurse	8h. x 1.25	10
1 RN	8h. x 1.00	8
1 LPN	8h. x .75	6
1 Aide	8h. x .50	4
Afternoon shift		
Head nurse	x 1.25	
1 RN	8h. x 1.00	8
1 LPN	8h. x .75	6
1 Aide	8h. x .50	4
Night shift		
Head nurse	x 1.25	
1 RN	8h. x 1.00	8
LPN	x .75	
1 Aide	8h. x .50	4
	Weighted hour values	58

Total weighted hour values	58
Total patients on census	16
Average weighted hour values per patient	3.625

deviations (exceptions) from the performances projected in the budget. The exceptions should be studied by the manager and his superior to review the factors affecting operations: workload/revenue ratios; salary adjustments; unforeseen expenses; and even unrealistic projections.

Department or multiple cost center supervisors should also receive summary reports each month. These reports should compare actual expenses and work performance for the month and for the budget year to date with budget projections for all the cost centers for which the manager is accountable. An example is shown in Figure 20.8.

In the same manner, divisional and succeeding levels of management should receive monthly summary reports of expenses and performances for all departments or cost centers reporting to them. An example of a program level report, one for the patient service program, is given in Figure 20.9.

Finally, a monthly summary report that compares actual expenses and work performance for the whole hospital with budget projections should

FIGURE 20.6   Nursing Department Monthly Census and
                Work Hours Summary, June 1986 (30 days)

Unit	Beds per Unit	Mo. Bed Complement (beds x days)	Patient Days per Unit for Month	Occupancy Percent per Unit	Nursing Hours for Month	Average Nursing Hours per Patient Day
2N	20	600	480	80	2,160	4.5
2S	20	600	360	60	1,800	5.0
2E	20	600	540	90	2,160	4.0
2W	20	600	438	73	1,971	4.5
3N	20	600	420	70	2,016	4.8
3S	20	600	510	85	2,142	4.2
3E	20	600	402	67	2,010	5.0
3W	20	600	570	95	2,166	3.8
4N	20	600	402	67	2,010	5.0
4S	20	600	492	82	2,214	4.5
4E	20	600	450	75	2,025	4.5
4W	20	600	420	70	1,932	4.6
ICU	10	300	180	60	1,080	6.0
CCU	5	150	75	50	600	8.0
OB	15	450	225	50	900	4.0
PED	20	600	288	48	1,152	4.0
Long-term	20	600	540	90	1,890	3.5
	310	9,300	6,792		30,228	

Percentage occupancy = $\dfrac{6,792}{9,300}$ = 73.03%

Average nursing hours per patient day = $\dfrac{30,228}{6.792}$ = 4.45 h.p.p.d.

be prepared by the fiscal services division for senior management. An example is given in Figure 20.10.

In addition, the fiscal services division should be asked to prepare a variance report for the senior administrator. This report should identify any significant variances or exceptions from budget projections. This itemized list can be a valuable worksheet on which to focus suggestions for solutions to exceptions to the budget. (See Figure 20.11.)

Suggested solutions to exceptions to budget projections should be sought from line management. This statement is posited on the same thinking that concluded that line management involvement was basic to budget planning. The line manager is at the point of performance in the operation of a health facility. He should have excellent insight into the problems and needs to be faced in effecting good management and in meeting budget projections.

FIGURE 20.7 Monthly Budget Report, June 1986

Nursing Unit 2N

	Month		Year to Date	
Item	Budget	Actual	Budget	Actual
Personnel costs	$9,500.00	$10,200.40*	$60,000.00	$62,000.20
Work units per patient day	4 hours	4.5 hours*	4 hours	4.2 hours*
Occupancy rate	83%	80%	82%	81%
Supplies	$4,000.00	$3,920.00	$24,000.00	$22,400.00*

*A 5% variance figure is used to illustrate the principle of exceptions—an automatic signal that administration should investigate the deviation from the budget projection. Any percentage or degree of deviation can be used, but it should be agreed upon by administration and line managers on a mutual basis at the beginning of the budget period.

FIGURE 20.8 Departmental Monthly Expense Report

Center_____   Month_____

	Month		Budget Year to Date	
Unit	Actual	Budget	Actual	Budget
2N	$	$	$	$
2S				
2E				
2W				
3N				
3S				
3E				
3W				
4N				
4S				
4E				
4W				
ICU				
CCU				
OB				
PED				
L-T	_____	_____	_____	_____
Total				

FIGURE 20.9   Patient Service Program Expense Summary
Report

Centers	Month			Year to Date		
	Actual	*Budget*	*Variance*	*Actual*	*Budget*	*Variance*
Nursing						
Pharmacy						
Physical therapy						
Inhalation therapy						
Medical records						
Medical secretaries						

Source: Adapted from Berman and Bash, "Operational Budgeting Systems," with permission.

Note: This report is designed for the associate administrator or other head of a hospital division.

Consequently, each manager should be required to file a report on each significant budget exception in his area of responsibility. The form can be quite simple: identification of the unit and the exception; and statement of the proposed solution of the exception. An example is given in Figure 20.12.

The method of discussion of exceptions and proposed solutions, and the manner in which steps are taken to correct the exceptions, will vary from hospital to hospital and from exception to exception. Generally stated, communication will take place at the several levels of management as necessary. Input should be possible at any level from the lowest to the highest whenever any of the management personnel can contribute to the solution of a problem.

It should be recognized, however, that despite the fact that an exception is identified, corrective action may not be either necessary or appropriate. The budget should be examined for acceptability *prior* to taking corrective action. Situations where signals of exceptions might call for budget changes as opposed to corrective action are

1. Change of environment might call for budget revision.

2. The assumptions on which the dollar budget was developed may not have been valid.

3. Furthermore, year to date figures should be looked at warily so new monthly budget needs are not penalized to make up for previous exceptions. Also, management should keep in tune with external

FIGURE 20.10   Summary Budget Report, Expenditures

June 1986

	Current Month		Year to Date	
	Actual	Budget	Actual	Budget
Category				
Personnel				
(list various centers)				
Supplies				
(can be detailed as needed)				
Maintenance				
(can be detailed as needed)				
Other expenses				
(can be detailed as needed)				
Revenues				
Category				
(List all revenue centers)				
Capital Expenditures				
Category				
(List projects)				

*Asterisk indicates items that are above or below the percentage allowed for exceptions.

FIGURE 20.11   Expense Summary Report of Significant
                Budget Variances

	Month		Year to Date	
Cost Centers	Actual	Budget	Actual	Budget

Source: Adapted from Berman and Bash, "Operational Budgeting Systems," with permission.
Note: This report is designed for the chief administrative officer of the hospital.

FIGURE 20.12   Budget Variance Report, RC Supervisor's
                Follow-Up

Month_____   Year_____

RC_____

Variances:

Cause:

Solution:

Source: Adapted from Berman and Bash, "Operational Budgeting Systems," with permission.

indicators to ensure that there is a realistic climate for budget consideration. Those external indicators should include complaints of patients' families and of nurses, findings of the utilization review committee and other committees, as well as all indications of community health care needs.

The art of administration becomes a necessary element in budget/performance reconciliation. Assuming that budget construction has been done with realistic guidelines, the problem of coping with exceptions and deviations is not insurmountable if it can be accomplished at regular intervals.

ANNUAL REPORTS

Annual summary reports will evolve from the monthly, quarterly, and semiannual reports. The annual reports will show performance expressed in actual expenses, revenues, capital spending, and work output correlated with projected figures. These reports along with the balance sheet of assets and liabilities are the basic data on which management policy decisions—financial and otherwise—can be made.

PUBLIC ACCOUNTABILITY

A practice that is becoming more common each year is for the hospital to make an annual public accounting to its community. These reports are similar to those made by commercial corporations to their stockholders. The documents tell what the financial condition of the hospital is: what the flow of revenues and expenses has been and what changes have occurred in the capital account. An annual report gives the hospital an excellent opportunity to tell its community what it has done to supply good health care to persons in its service area. Some hospitals develop a narrative style that adds a human interest element to the story. The specialized treatment centers are described, educational divisions are photographed, personnel and their contributions to good care are talked about, and the medical staff are listed by name and specialty. Quite often statistics are listed that are believed to be of interest to the public, such as: number of patients admitted and discharged; surgery performed; therapy treatments given; laboratory tests performed; and activities of volunteer groups. Babies born, average census, and average length of stay are statistics commonly quoted as are the number of anesthetics administered, meals served, prescriptions filled, X rays taken, pounds of laundry processed, social service cases handled, and EEGs and ECGs performed. Some hospitals show a distribution of patients by sex, age, point of origin, or classification of payment. Others show how the patient dollar is spent: how many cents for nursing, housekeeping, dietary, ancillary services, administration, maintenance. (See Figures 20.13, 20.14, and 20.15.)

FIGURE 20.13 Financial Summary

	June 1986		June 1985	
Operating revenue from service to patients		$28,448,118		$24,883,320
Deduction from revenue	*1986*		*1985*	
Contractual adjustments Medicare, Medicaid	$ 1,765,469		$ 1,622,199	
Provision for uncollectible accounts and charity	711,558	2,477,027	395,732	2,017,931
Net patient revenue		25,971,091		22,865,389
Other operating revenue		806,987		555,995
Net operating revenue		$26,778,078		$23,421,384
Operating expenses	*1986*		*1985*	
Salaries and wages	$13,174,950		$11,356,158	
Fringe benefits	2,001,155		1,871,825	
Contractual service	2,749,817		2,540,656	
Supplies	3,771,832		3,067,630	
Depreciation	810,028		784,700	
Other expenses	2,272,416		1,949,727	
Total operating expenses		$24,780,198		$21,570,696
Income from operations		$ 1,997,880		$ 1,850,688
Nonoperating revenue		490,701		366,920
Revenue over expenses		$ 2,488,581		$ 2,217,608
Equipment purchased for facilities		670,737		400,966
Debt retirement interest, funds for building and equipment replacement		$ 1,817,844		$ 1,816,642
Balance		-0-		-0-

FIGURE 20.14   Statistics from Community Hospital for 1985 and 1986

	1985	1986
Admissions	16,196	16,249
Births	1,574	1,691
Average daily census	307.1	315.5
Average LOS (adults & peds.), days	6.9	7.1
Percentage occupancy	76.02	78.32
Patient days	112,094	115,486
Newborn nursing days	6,275	6,656
Anesthetics	7,101	7,210
Central supply requisitions	260,455	274,158
Emergency room visits	35,180	35,501
Laboratory tests	224,642	228,718
EEG examinations	1,961	1,996
ECG examinations	10,281	10,566
Meals served	563,798	565,155
Surgical procedures	7,807	8,134
Pharmacy prescriptions*	801,763	881,389
Physical therapy treatments	20,599	21,768
Respiratory therapy treatments	131,302	156,361
Radiological procedures	66,751	68,452
Social service cases	2,559	2,970
Laundry (pounds)	1,764,812	1,844,370
Recovery room patients	5,897	6,002

*The unit dose system is used in this hospital.

These annual reports to the public tend to humanize the hospital image, particularly in the case of the larger institutions. The physicians, nurses, and other staff members who are described tend to become warm human beings rather than figures in starched white uniforms. Even the balance sheet shows how closely expenditures for giving good care come to consuming all the hospital's revenues.

Some hospitals tell their story in well-designed brochures similar to corporation reports to stockholders. These can be mailed to friends and employees of the hospital and can be used to inform prospective donors. The story also can be told by buying advertising space in the local newspaper in the same way any public agency does that must make a formal report of its activities to the community. Whatever means is used, the objective should be to tell as much as possible to as wide a segment of the public as can be reached about what the hospital is doing to serve its community and how it is spending its money to do the job.

FIGURE 20.15   Community Hospital Patient Dollar
Distribution, 1986

Nursing services	$ .21
Surgical services	.09
Emergency and clinic services	.05
Laboratory services	.09
Radiology services	.09
Pharmacy services	.03
Central supplies	.02
Administration and fiscal services	.08
Patient record administration	.05
Plant operations	.06
Housekeeping services	.03
Laundry and linen services	.01
Dietary services	.06
Employee benefits	.08
Other services (Delivery room, physical therapy, pulmonary medicine, EEG, ECG, alcoholism treatment)	.05
	$1.00

Several years ago the American Hospital Association issued a statement about disclosure of information which is applicable today. The AHA statement is discussed in the following paragraphs.

DISCLOSURE OF FINANCIAL AND OPERATING INFORMATION

In recognition of the need for disclosure of financial and operating information at times, the American Hospital Association issued a "Guidelines" under that general title in 1979.

Financial information is important for public knowledge about the operation of health care institutions, understanding, accountability, making public policy affecting those institutions, and establishing financial credibility in the money market. In fact, AHA has listed as potential users of this information: investors and creditors; resource providers; oversight bodies; constituents; third party payers; and regulatory bodies and commissions.

It is the ultimate responsibility of the board of trustees of an institution to make financial disclosures. These should be based on accepted accounting procedures. The AHA suggests several types of financial disclosure report: financial statements, annual reports, special purpose reports, and forecast reports.

According to the AHA, an annual financial statement (audited by independent CPAs) should include: a balance sheet; a statement of revenues and expenses; a statement of changes in equity or fund balance; a statement of change in financial position; notes explaining the accounting principles being followed; and other necessary information.

Annual reports are basically for the purpose of relating the financial condition of the institution to its purpose and goals. Annual reports might also be designed to describe the institution's services and the patient population it serves. There might be included statistical data on the medical staff, on employees, and on contributors. There could be special reports on the educational and research activities of the institution. The chairman of the board could report on the present and future operational objectives. Special reports may be necessary from time to time to satisfy regulatory bodies or to use in the application for grants for special purposes, and so forth. Some of the reports will by necessity contain elements of forecasting to comply with the aforementioned regulatory and grant purposes. The public relations office of the hospital or other health care institution will be able to compile the annual reports in an attractive and easily read form.

INFORMATION SYSTEMS AND REPORTING

Up to this point in the chapter, the discussion of management reporting has been from the standpoint of the information to be generated and the flow of that information within the hierarchy. It was stated that individual hospitals have different needs for information and have different facilities and capabilities for collecting and disseminating it. At one end of that facilities spectrum could be a primitive, manual method using simply a pencil and paper, at the other a sophisticated computer system.

Computerized information systems for health care facilities can be classified into two general categories. They are the administrative information system (AIS), which is the widest application of the art, and the clinical information system (CIS), the nomenclature used by Charles J. Austin and others. (CIS is sometimes called medical information system (MIS), the title used in the El Camino Hospital project in Mountainview, California, and by others.)

AIS collects and uses data from and for

1. Admissions, discharges, census
2. Facilities utilization and scheduling
3. Accounting
4. Materials handling
5. Payroll
6. Personnel
7. Budgeting
8. Financial planning and modeling

The CIS and MIS, as the titles indicate, are focused on the clinical care of patients and are likely to include information from or for

1. Medical records
2. Physicians' orders
3. Clinical laboratory
4. Radiology
5. EKG and EEG
6. Pharmacy

THE ADMINISTRATIVE INFORMATION SYSTEM

The administrative information system is easier to implement and operate because the data handled are more likely to be factual rather than judgmental, fewer employees are involved, and training is less difficult because of the predominantly factual aspects.

Admissions, discharges, preadmission appointments, and bed census information, when put into a computer system and programmed to give desired summaries in printouts, can be of great value in the management reporting process.

Facilities utilization and scheduling input can be very useful not only for efficient operation, but also as basic information for planning and budgeting.

Accounting is a key source of information for the management reporting process. Accounting can include not only general ledger accounting, accounts receivable and payable, and patient billings, but also budget monitoring, cost analysis, allocation of costs of nonrevenue departments to revenue cost centers, third party billings and reports, and generation of varied financial information as an input to the reporting system.

Materials handling can include purchasing (and relate it to the monies available under the budget), inventory control (which strangely enough seems to be a weak point in many hospitals), and inventory value adjustments.

Payroll management was one of the first computer applications in hospitals and came into being via bookkeeping machines and other mechanical devices. Most hospitals have some kind of electronic data processing payroll application. Of that number, many have contracted with outside sources. Payroll information can be coupled with personnel data to furnish basic material for cost projections and management planning.

Personnel data systems can generate information about the staff which can be useful for reporting and planning. These data can summarize turnover and absenteeism, employee characteristics, employment trends, and departmental incidents to help with cost projections and departmental planning. Some hospitals have used employee profiles developed on computers to indicate abilities and capabilities in addition to those necessary for the job assigned. In case of emergency, the employee may be shifted to cover possible staff shortages. This can be an important factor in planning for emergencies.

Budgeting is of central importance in any kind of hospital information system, manual or computerized. In any effective system, information on costs, revenues, personnel, utilization, scheduling, purchasing and inventories, construction, planning, and institutional needs and activities is channeled to administration and the budget officer.

Financial planning and modeling can be done effectively only on valid information. The computer, properly programmed, can supply a means of information output, assimilation, and plan or model design far superior to any manual operation.

THE CLINICAL INFORMATION SYSTEM (CIS) (MIS)

The clinical information system collects data about physicians' orders, nurses' notes, any nursing plan, medications, therapies, laboratory services, radiology, EKG, EEG, and the use of special units such as the emergency room, the delivery room, the operating rooms, the intensive care unit, cardiac care, outpatient clinic, and other special services for patients.

One of the latest uses of an information system is to aid in coding cases according to diagnosis-related groups (DRGs). This is a serious undertaking because accurately coding diagnoses into 470 categories for Medicare patients and some others is a true test for a hospital.

A CIS is much more difficult to implement because of judgmental elements affecting the information put into the system and because of the greater number of persons involved. However, information can be generated in the CIS that would be useful in financial planning. This information could be composed of data on facilities and equipment use and scheduling, on quality of care indexes, profiles of ancillary services, drug distribution and pharmacy costs, and any other needed information that could be programmed.

Many variations of information systems are evolving. It is to be hoped that they are being tailored to the needs of the individual institution, rather than being purchased as a packaged deal from a commercial supplier. In differing degrees, departments or sectors in information systems are being integrated or designed in parallel or tandem so that necessary information can be retrieved at different levels. All this is working toward a total hospital information system (THIS). A group at Yale has designed a regional information system. This regional effort, however, must be based on uniformity of reporting and recording of information, if there is to be a workable exchange of data.

The human element seems to be the weakest point. First, there is a lack of knowledge at the administrative level about what information is important to put into the system, and how to implement the system. (The so-called information explosion of the past generation was cursed before computers became so common. Then, we complained about all the unnecessary paper work we had to do. With computers, we marveled at how much information we could put into the monster. Now, we are beginning to realize that we have to be selective: what do we *need* to know?)

The second human element is the persons who are responsible for input and output. After the system has been designed in a suitable manner for processing the desired kind of information, how can the physicians, nurses, and others on the staff be trained to use the system and be convinced it is worth all the effort? Without full and proper participation by these key people, the system does not operate up to potential.

The final word is, of course, that financial officers, administrators, and planners should use whatever information is available to the best possible advantage in the reporting process.

HOSPITAL ADMINISTRATIVE SERVICES

More than 600 hospitals—running the whole gamut of bed size, kinds of services offered, and teaching activity—use the Hospital Administrative Services (HAS) of the American Hospital Association as an adjunct to any internal reporting system or other statistical collection from hospital records. The HAS data bank offers profiles of departmental costs and revenues, employee productivity, utilization of services and units of care, and man-hours per patient day or service modality.

Hospitals that subscribe to the HAS have the ability to know not only their own performance, but also their performance relative to that of other institutions of like size, and to others in all of the nine census regions of the country. Monthly, quarterly, and six-month national data reports not only enable financial officers to compare the hospital's productivity, costs and revenues, and utilization of inhospital departments, outpatient clinics, and extended care units to those of other institutions, but also to chart the trends in these activities. HAS is a tool for financial managers and administrators.

PERORATION

A program of good planning and budgeting is one of the principal tools of the financial management of hospitals. In like manner, accurate, timely, and two-way reporting is one of the important elements of an effective, comprehensive planning and budgeting system. Given the general guidelines described in this chapter, the authors believe it is possible for a hospital financial team to design a performance reporting system that will fit the particular needs of their institution.

SUGGESTED READINGS

Austin, Charles J. *Information Systems for Hospital Administration.*

Austin, Charles J. and Greene, Barry R. "Hospital Information Systems: A Current Perspective."

Berman, Howard J. and Bash, Paul L. "Operational Budgeting Systems: Hackley Hospital, Muskegon, Michigan."

Esmond, Truman H., Jr. *Budgeting Procedures for Hospitals.*

Falcon, William D. (ed). *Reporting Financial Data to Management.*

Cost Accounting

Chapters 4, 5, and 20 have described aspects of cost finding, cost analysis, and budgeting. The present chapter describes cost accounting as a tool to be used by managers for assessment of profit and loss, for monitoring budget performance, and for fiscal planning—department by department.

Just a short time ago reimbursement to hospitals by third parties was based predominantly on cost or cost plus. This was the source of as much as 90% of the revenue of many hospitals. Change has been coming rapidly. Instead of paying cost per hospital stay, for example, Medicare is paying on the basis of a predetermined amount per diagnosis-related group (DRG). Other third parties, particularly some of the Blue Cross plans, are experimenting with the DRG concept for all their subscribers, irrespective of age. Another growing reimbursement plan is that of insurers' contracting with providers on a capitation basis. The HMO idea has been marketed widely in the United States. The insurer may own its hospital facilities or contract for hospital beds and services. Likewise, physician services can be contracted for from individual doctors or from groups of doctors associated in some kind of partnership or professional corporation.

Whatever the method of payment, cost still is a basic factor in management decisions. These new developments in Medicare, and among other insurers, can be based only on accurate information about costs and utilization. Competition is increasing, and contracts are squeezing profit factors to a point that survival for hospitals and other providers can be dependent on well-structured cost data and imaginative analysis of those data.

This chapter has been adapted and compiled, with permission, from *Cost Accounting and Financial Analysis for the Hospital Administrator*, by Steven F. Kukla, copyright 1986 by American Hospital Publishing, Inc. All rights reserved.

The hospital administrator must be knowledgeable about cost information to make decisions or to advise his board on fiscal policies. To be informed, the administrator must obtain reliable information from systematically related sources. In many institutions, the most common sources include existing financial reporting systems, newly installed cost accounting systems, budgets, and departmental productivity reports. Yet, all too often, these exist as separate systems, utilized for narrowly defined, highly specialized functions that offer little management access.

Perhaps because cost-based reimbursement did not emphasize the allocation of limited resource inputs, a strong centralized information system and strong organizational goals were not mandatory. However, the payment systems now being adopted require the provider to have a better understanding of the total price and the cost inputs for the services rendered. This brings with it the need for increasingly integrated information systems to facilitate effective decision making. Management must now have information that effectively relates cost to price and relates the activities of the hospital's production system to the hospital's overall organizational objectives.

The need for an integrated information system crosses both the responsibility and the functional areas of the hospital. Executive management must have information on clinical management, capital investment, and operational efficiency. Department managers need information on the demand for their services, departmental efficiency, and contribution margins. Physicians need information on their clinical practices by patient and in total.

This chapter describes the methods for identifying the individual sources of data, the methods of integration, and their value to the administrator. It is not intended to provide a detailed implementation plan for an individual hospital. This is neither possible nor desirable, as the operational systems and characteristics of each hospital are different. Management will individually analyze the hospital's own situation and then add to the structural approaches discussed here.

METHODS OF ASSEMBLING COST ACCOUNTING INFORMATION

As a major financial information system for management analysis and decision making, the hospital's cost accounting system provides

1. Internal reporting to managers for use in the planning and control of routine operations
2. Internal reporting to managers for use in making nonroutine decisions and in formulating major policies and plans for future activities
3. External reporting to stockholders, government agencies, and creditors[1]

---

[1]Horngren, Charles T., *Cost Accounting: A Managerial Emphasis*, 1977.

The planning and control functions are foremost among the activities supported by the cost accounting system. In planning, managers select performance objectives or desirable goals for the organization and identify the actions necessary for goal achievement. The control function provides subsequent monitoring to ensure operational conformity to the plan. Furthermore, cost accounting is recognized as the principal tool available to management in planning and controlling the operations of the hospital's individual products and programs.

The initial step in the implementation of a cost accounting system is to assemble revenues, costs, and standard performance criteria by individual product definition. Once all pertinent data are collected, cost accounting is used to analyze and interpret them. This requires actual performance data, standard (anticipated) performance data, and the correlation of each type of data to the other.

Table 21.1 lists three basic methods of assembling cost accounting data: responsibility costing, full costing, and differential costing. Each has specific strengths and weaknesses, and all apply to the assembly of related revenues to costs and related budgets to performance. Each method can stand on its own merits. Yet, because of their individual attributes, their usefulness is maximized if the hospital uses all three to augment one another.

Responsibility costing traces the costs of the individual organizational units called responsibility centers. Estimates of future responsibility center costs are established initially during the hospital's budgeting process. A historical accounting of the actual costs incurred in a responsibility center is used during the hospital's fiscal year to measure the performance of the responsibility center and to analyze deviations from the approved budget. Responsibility center reports are extremely useful for organizational control and objective setting because they present both the goals a manager has

TABLE 21.1   Methods of Assembling Cost Accounting Data and Their Uses

Method of Assembly	Uses	
	Historical Data	*Future Projections*
1. Responsibility	Financial reporting and performance analysis Management control	Planning and budgeting
2. Full	Financial reporting and performance analysis Product costing	Planning and budgeting Pricing decisions
3. Differential	N/A	Alternative investment analysis

set for the specific production functions for which he is responsible and his responsibility center's performance relative to those goals. Reported variances make it clear which individuals need to consider implementing corrective action.

Full costing, of goods manufactured or services produced, sums the direct costs related to the production process plus a fair share of the indirect costs that the organization incurs as overhead. Full costing is used most in evaluating contribution margins on a product basis. Full costing must, therefore, begin with some product or program definition that collects and aggregates costs separately from traditional responsibility center costing.

Differential costing estimates how the costs and revenues in one situation will differ in alternative situations. It, therefore, focuses management's analysis on the incremental costs that come with adding or deleting products or programs.

RESPONSIBILITY COSTING

Systems of responsibility costing are widely used by hospitals both for internal performance reporting and for meeting the cost reporting requirements of third party payers. Responsibility costing structures data and performance along the organizational lines drawn by management for supervisory purposes. In addition, overhead costs are allocated to the revenue-producing departments because executive management may desire the managers of those departments to be concerned with the level of overhead costs and to convey that concern to the managers of the overhead departments. Such cost assignment provides executive management with indirect influence on the level of overhead costs that the hospital incurs and a means of tying the performance of the overhead departments into the organization's overall financial structure. Responsibility costing has a natural appeal in that it specifies a boundary of authority, assigns control to an identifiable individual, and distinguishes between the manager's controllable and uncontrollable costs.

Table 21.2 represents the designated reporting and responsibility relationships. The managers of each responsibility center report directly to the individual above them.

Each manager is held responsible for the costs related to the operation and production functions of his responsibility center:

—*Direct Materials.* All nonlabor costs that can be controlled by the responsibility center manager.

—*Direct Labor.* Total labor costs (salaries and fringe benefits) for those individual employees within the responsibility center coming under the manager's supervisory control.

TABLE 21.2   Hospital Organization Structure by Responsibility
                Center

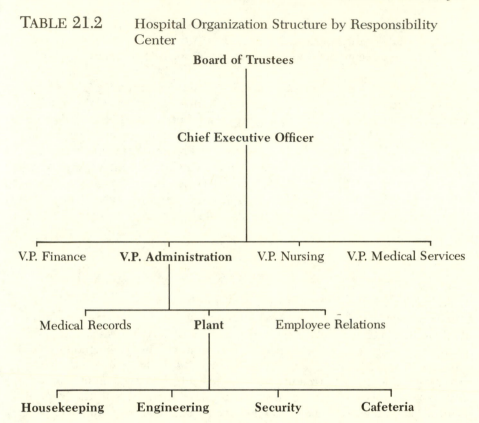

—*Hospital Overhead.* Overhead departments are nonrevenue-producing departments such as housekeeping, laundry, plant operations,
maintenance, purchasing. In cost analysis, revenue-producing departments are charged with a share of the cost of overhead
(nonrevenue-producing) departments. (See Chapter 5.) The manager
of a revenue-producing department may have little control of overhead costs, but overhead (as previously mentioned) is apportioned
to his center basically for recovering overhead costs through an aggregated billing of *all* costs to the patient or third-party payer.

Responsibility center performance reports should include information
on current period and year to date financial performance. They must also
include information on both the actual and budgeted performance of the
department. Management uses this comparison of the actual costs incurred
in the operation of the department to the approved operating budget for the
period to identify deviations either in the costs incurred or in the level of
production experienced. Scanning the responsibility center performance

reports for material deviations focuses management's attention on areas that require further analysis or corrective action.

Responsibility costing may be expanded to provide the department manager with greater detail. The primary means of improving the communication quality of a responsibility costing system is to increase the amount or specificity of data reported.

Financial data should be accompanied by statistical performance information; in its simplest form, this may simply be a reflection of the responsibility center's unit cost. The unit cost is derived by dividing the responsibility center's total budgeted and actual expenses by the applicable units of service for the period. Figure 21.1 illustrates a sample responsibility center performance report for an intensive care unit.

Responsibility center reports should be tailored to the needs and organization of the individual hospital. Within reasonable limits, each department should be allowed to determine the extent of the detailed information provided to it on its performance reports. The more detail and the more specific to the department, the better the translation of departmental and managerial performance. Managers should receive performance information for wages and fringe benefits, perhaps by wage class of employee, principal supply items, other direct costs, and the allocated overhead. Preferably, controllable and uncontrollable items should be separated and subtotaled. This allows the manager to concentrate on the items subject to his influence. Finally, the budget data should be flexible. Approved deviations from performance should be subsequently reflected in an adjusted budget to prevent repeated reports of the same performance deviation.

Responsibility costing is not useful when the hospital attempts analysis of diagnosis-related groups (DRGs) or another form of product line analysis. Line expenses incurred in the payment of salaries or supplies cannot be coded to the product at the same time they are accounted for in the hospital's responsibility accounting records. Product outcome data do not exist in a readily available form in the hospital's responsibility center cost accounting system and are therefore beyond the capabilities of this method of costing.

FULL COSTING AND DIFFERENTIAL COSTING

Both full costing and differential costing are methods of performing product line analysis. Whereas responsibility costing is the most effective means of organizing costs by control areas, product line analysis is an effective method of relating expenses to revenues on a product or program basis. Product line analysis requires a specific definition of the costs to be accumulated, a specific set of product definitions, and a cost accounting system for capturing the financial and clinical performance of the hospital's products.

FIGURE 21.1 St. Christopher Hospital ICU—Sample Responsibility Center Performance Report for the Period Ending July 31, 1984

	Current Month			YTD			
	Actual	*Budgeted*	*Variance Fav. (Unfav.)*	*Actual*	*Budgeted*	*Variance Fav. (Unfav.)*	*Total Budget for Year*
Direct Costs							
Salaries and wages	$47,500	$50,000	$2,500	$295,000	$350,000	$55,000	$500,000
Medical supplies	12,000	11,000	(1,000)	80,000	80,000	—	125,000
Temporary clerical labor	1,500	2,000	500	3,500	5,000	1,500	6,000
Office supplies	300	200	(100)	2,400	2,000	(400)	5,000
Total direct costs	$61,300	$63,200	$1,900	$380,900	$437,000	$56,100	$636,000
Allocated Costs							
Building operations	$10,000	$10,000	—	$76,000	$70,000	($6,000)	$120,000
Depreciation on equipment	2,000	2,000	—	14,000	14,000	—	21,000
General and admin. expense	5,000	4,500	(500)	33,000	31,500	(1,500)	54,000
Total allocated costs	$17,000	$16,500	($ 500)	$123,000	$115,500	(7,500)	$195,000
Total costs	$78,300	$79,700	$1,400	$503,900	$552,500	$48,600	$831,000
Responsibility Center Statistics							
Patient days	1,000	1,000	—	6,200	6,200	—	12,000
Nursing hours	1,160	1,200	40	7,192	7,440	248	14,400
Average cost per patient day	$78.4	$79.7	$1.3	$81.3	$90.7	$9.4	$69.5
Average cost per nursing hour	$67.5	$66.4	$1.1	$70.1	$75.6	$5.5	$57.9

Definition of Cost. The full cost of a product is the sum of its direct costs plus a fair share of the indirect or overhead costs. Direct costs are costs that are specifically traceable to or that directly cause the production of a product or service. Indirect costs are costs that are associated with the operation of the organization, but that are not directly traceable to any of the individually produced products. It is not possible, or at least not feasible, to measure directly how much of these costs are attributable to a single product. Normally, some related production statistic is utilized to allocate indirect costs among products.

In identifying direct and indirect costs, it is appropriate to rely initially on the hospital's traditional distinction between revenue-producing departments and nonrevenue-producing departments. Costs assigned to revenue-producing departments are classified as direct costs, and hospital expenses recorded in nonrevenue-producing departments are indirect costs. Periodically, reporting efficiency can be improved by a reassessment of the individual line items of expense in each department according to their direct or indirect relationship to the hospital's production process. Once the hospital has made a decision on the nature of each line expense, the placement of the line item into a department whose status in the costing process results in direct charging or in allocation will assure the proper treatment of the expense in the development of the full cost definition.

Differential costs are costs that are incremental under projected conditions. The term can refer both to the elements of cost and to the amounts of cost. For example, in most situations, direct labor is a differential cost because additional production capacity or product lines require more labor inputs. Additionally, the amount of cost that is incremental (either positive or negative change) is said to be the amount of the differential cost. Table 21.3 illustrates a differential costing analysis.

Three important differences between full cost and differential cost can be identified.

The full cost of a product is the sum of its direct cost plus a fair share of applicable indirect cost. Differential cost includes only those elements of direct cost that differ in the conditions under consideration. Per-case cost can be determined by appropriately allocating direct and indirect costs on either a full cost or a differential cost basis. Under full costing, all hospital expenses, including fixed costs, are apportioned to the individual cases. Under differential costing, only direct costs are allocated. Thus, full costing provides a measure of average cost, and differential costing provides an estimate of the incremental resources needed for additional products, patients, or management ventures. The choice of full versus differential costing can have a significant impact on cost estimates and, ultimately, on the conclusions drawn. Because of the significance of average versus marginal cost, care must be exercised in interpreting the results and impact of either the full or the differential method.

TABLE 21.3   Differential Costing Analysis of Option to Purchase
                     Laboratory Services

Revenue		
Revenue received from operating laboratory		$2,500,000
Revenue received from purchasing laboratory services		2,000,000
Net loss of revenue from purchasing laboratory services		$ 500,000
Expenses		
Costs saved by eliminating laboratory		
Direct labor	$575,000	
Direct materials	80,000	
Lease costs	40,000	
Other costs	155,000	
Total costs eliminated		850,000
Cost of purchasing laboratory services		400,000
Net reduction in costs of purchasing laboratory services		450,000
Net disadvantage in purchasing laboratory services		$ 50,000

Information on full cost can be obtained directly from a hospital's routine accounting system. Accounting systems record the expenses that make up full cost on a regular basis and routinely report these expenses to management in prescribed responsibility formats. To yield the full cost of the products and services offered, the responsibility information is rearranged along products and product lines. There is no comparable system for routinely collecting differential cost. The appropriate items that constitute differential cost are assembled to meet the requirements of the specific problem, and each problem is different. Some of the data used to construct differential cost may come from the responsibility accounting system and the hospital's full cost accounting system, but other data must come from nonroutine, and sometimes nonfinancial, sources.

The full cost accounting system collects costs on a historical basis: it measures costs as they are reported in the hospital's general ledger. However, in developing differential cost, more care is required because less evident future circumstances may need to be considered. Differential costing is intended to show what the effect on cost would be if a certain course of action were adopted.

Product Definitions. The traditional definition of hospital products has been patient days and ancillary procedures. These service measures have historically been the basis for both charge- and cost-based reimbursement. Under per-case payment systems, the unit of payment does not correspond to these output measures, but to a more inclusive per-case definition of the units of service, that is, discharges, admissions, visits, incidents. Therefore, the hospital's collection of costs and revenue must be redefined in terms of a unit of service that facilitates the matching of consumed resources and per-case payment.

In recent years, patient classification systems have been developed that use more aggregate definitions of hospital services as the unit of payment. These systems provide a way to define a hospital's product using a combination of the patient's diagnoses, the procedures consumed, the severity of the patient's condition, and various other patient characteristics, such as age and sex. DRGs are the most commonly chosen product definition.

Hospitals should not, however, allow third party methodologies to determine internal management reporting systems. For internal management purposes, other more aggregate product definitions may provide more pertinent and usable management information. Among the available alternatives are major diagnostic categories (MDCs), physician specialties, hospital lines of business, or a partial costing based on those DRGs for which the hospital experiences significant volume. The choice of a particular definitional scheme for product line accounting inevitably requires a trade-off between the sensitivity of the data and the manageability of the data.

Four factors should be considered in choosing a product definition:

—Product lines should be defined as broadly as possible. As the number of products increases, the cost of analysis also increases. Analyzing 5,000 cases classified into 467 DRGs is generally more costly than analyzing the same cases classified by major diagnostic category or physician specialty, primarily due to the review of additional data and output. Important relationships may also be lost due to product fragmentation into small nonsignificant groups.

—Product definitions should be medically meaningful for integration into the hospital planning process and to ensure physician understanding and support. Many middle managers and physicians are cautious of DRGs as performance measures because of their lack of severity identifying capability and their relatively new application as a product classification methodology.

—Product lines should be selected so that resource use is relatively homogeneous across cases. It is very critical that the hospital's product definition group like products. Homogeneity can be measured in a particular sample by studying the coefficient of variation on per-case costs. In a general sense, the coefficient of variation measures how closely individual cases are clustered around the average value for the grouping. The lower the coefficient, the more tightly clustered the cases and the greater the homogeneity of the items. Conversely, the higher the number, the greater the variation in the individual items being grouped. Less confidence is placed in an analysis in which resource use varies widely among cases in a product line for valid reasons. Recent data on DRGs indicate that many of the current DRGs have high coefficient of variation values.

—The amount of homogeneity is affected by the available sample size. The number of cases in any product line must provide statistical confidence. Because of the variation in patients not accounted for by many product line definitions and because cost and volume estimates are imprecise, valid conclusions can only be drawn from large groupings, when the size of the group compensates for the individual uniqueness of each case.[2]

Systems for Cost Accumulation. Product line analysis requires an information system that reformats and refines the already available clinical and financial data (see Figure 21.2). For the most part, the data are extracted from medical record abstracts, patient bills, cost allocation sheets, the general ledger, and the payroll ledger. From these sources come data on the types of patient admitted to the hospital, the types of services provided, and the costs of those services.

Medical records list reasons for hospitalization, surgical and other procedures provided during the hospital stay, and patient demographic characteristics. Patient bills detail the volume of service rendered and types of service used by each patient during the hospital stay. The general ledger provides cost information on elements of services used by patients. This leaves the question of how to allocate and aggregate financial data into the hospital's definition of a product.

ACCOUNTING SYSTEMS FOR PRODUCT COSTING

Full costing and differential costing are methods for arriving at cost estimates. Each requires a cost accounting system to accumulate the relevant costs of the products produced. A cost accounting system is a particular method of collecting costs and assigning them to the products that have been identified. For product costing, there are two types of cost accounting system: job order costing and process costing. A job order cost system individually collects costs for a physically distinct collection of work (a job) as it moves through the hospital. A process cost system collects the costs for all the products as they are produced by a defined production area during a given accounting period, and determines unit cost by dividing total cost by total number of units.

JOB ORDER COSTING

The "job" in a job order cost system may consist of a single unit (for example, a patient or a procedure), or it may consist of all units of identical or similar characteristics covered by the single job or production order (for

---

[2]Chadwick, Edward, "Special Report #5, Product Line Analysis," American Hospital Association, Chicago, IL, 1983. Reprinted with the permission of the American Hospital Association, copyright 1983.

FIGURE 21.2   Flowsheet of Hospital Information Systems

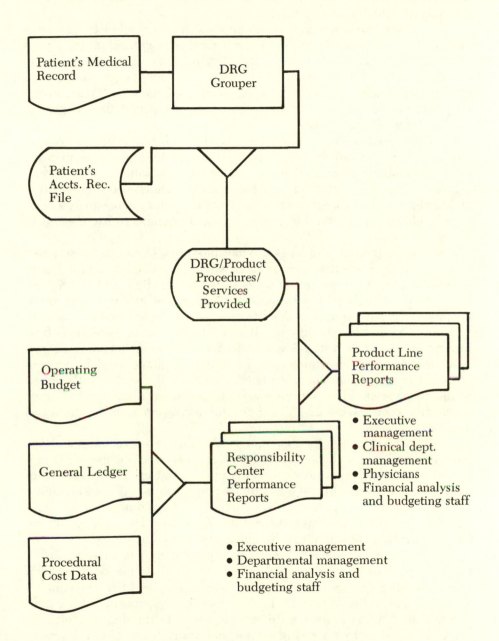

example, a batch of laboratory tests, a group of patients). Usually each job is given an identification number, and its costs are collected on a separate cost record, called a job order ticket.

In the hospital, each patient can be viewed as a single job. The associated costs or charges for the service provided are collected on the equivalent of the patient's job order ticket—the patient's accounts receivable record. Traditionally, charges are recorded on the patient's accounts receivable record as the patient moves through the various departments in the hospital receiving services. When the patient is discharged, the charges are totaled to find the total charge of the job.

Patient identification initially lends itself to job order costing because patients are easily and discretely identifiable and hospitals have in place readily available data collection procedures that use patient specific identification. However, individual patients must ultimately be grouped into appropriate product categories that are large enough to make analysis cost beneficial and meaningful before management attempts to use these data for decision making.

When the patient is used as the job definition, costs can be assigned to the individual job tickets in several ways. The simplest method is to develop average cost per unit of service, that is, per diem and per chargeable activity. This begins with the full allocation of indirect costs to the hospital's revenue-producing departments, using departmental allocation statistics. Overhead costs may be allocated to the patient care areas by a direct allocation or by a step-down method to arrive at the total cost in each revenue-producing department. Per diem costs and ancillary department cost-to-charge ratios are then calculated from the full cost data and applied to the case specific days and ancillary charges on each patient's accounts receivable record. Table 21.4 illustrates the development of per diem and ancillary costs.

Table 21.5 estimates the total cost attributable to a particular job. Each patient service has a charge that is recorded to each job as the job is processed. Upon discharge the job ticket is pulled, and the charges are summarized and converted to cost estimates. Per diem routine costs and ancillary services cost-to-charge ratios are multiplied by the number of days and ancillary services charges, respectively, for each case. The total cost of the job is determined by summing the individual cost components.

This costing process is known as the "ratio of costs to charges" (RCC) method and is utilized by the majority of the currently marketed hospital cost accounting systems. Critics of this methodology feel that inaccuracies occur because of differences in the cost-to-charge relationship of the individual departmental procedures in a revenue-producing department. This can be adjusted for by reviewing the hospital charge records, deriving more detailed cost-to-charge ratios for departmental services, and substituting

TABLE 21.4 Development of Per Diem and Ancillary Costs

	Routine Services		Ancillary Services				
	Adults and Peds.	Spec. Care	Radiology	Laboratory	PT/OT	Pharmacy	Other
Direct costs	$11,006,224	$ 672,679	$1,734,345	$2,029,110	$467,869	$2,029,110	$10,499,281
Indirect costs							
Capital related costs	518,880	45,972	96,462	183,321	19,796	16,257	179,362
Employee benefits	986,244	141,275	158,192	174,774	57,462	87,727	381,740
Administration and general	649,937	38,214	144,324	178,314	58,985	182,761	373,954
Operation of plant; maintenance	590,766	96,694	142,878	105,414	17,336	29,889	354,875
Laundry	384,371	40,247	5,471	—	—	—	75,712
Housekeeping	357,429	25,777	37,142	45,765	3,192	2,735	71,686
Dietary	972,883	46,243	—	—	—	—	—
Nursing administration	274,834	21,729	—	—	—	—	279,480
Central service and supply	—	—	—	—	—	—	—
Pharmacy	8,648	570	8,491	2,941	972	376,396	5,627
Medical records and library	192,873	6,417	—	—	—	—	—
Social services	97,412	8,166	—	—	—	—	—
Cafeteria	452,648	48,700	—	—	—	—	—
Interns and residents	196,457	27,758	9,473	54,121	9,484	—	28,767
Subtotal: Indirect costs	5,683,382	547,762	602,433	744,650	167,227	695,765	1,751,203
Total cost	$16,689,606	$1,220,441	$2,336,778	$2,773,760	$ 635,096	$2,724,875	$12,250,484
Routine service statistics							
Inpatient days	91,884	4,980					
Routine cost per diem	$181.64	$245.07					
Ancillary service statistics							
Total charges			$2,927,658	$4,627,737	$1,327,870	$4,074,907	$18,898,770
Ratio of costs to charges			.798173	.593377	.478282	.668696	.648216

TABLE 21.5 Development of Product Cost by DRG for DRG 134: Hypertension

	Routine Services		Ancillary Services					Total Cost
	Adults and Peds.	Spec. Care	Radiology	Laboratory	PT/OT	Pharmacy	Other	
Per diem	$181.64	$245.07						
Ratio of costs to charges			.798173	.599377	.478282	.668721	.648216	
No. Patient name and I.D.								
1 Boston, J. 71-734								
Days/charges	10	1	$700.00	$985.00	0	$515.00	$1,200.00	
Cost	$1,816.40	$245.07	$558.72	$590.39	0	$344.39	$ 777.86	$4,332.83
2 Otto, T. 73-440								
Days/charges	11	0	$715.00	$1,000.00	0	$515.00	$1,100.00	
Cost	$1,998.04	0	$570.70	$599.38	0	$344.39	$ 713.04	$4,225.55
3 Clary, M. 74-970								
Days/charges	12	2	$685.00	$1,015.00	0	$500.00	$1,585.00	
Cost	$2,179.68	$490.14	$546.75	$608.37	0	$334.36	$1,027.42	$5,186.72
54 Terry S. 79-342								
Days/charges	10	0	$685.00	$985.00	0	$515.00	$1,150.00	
Cost	$1,816.40	0	$546.75	$590.39	0	$344.39	$ 745.45	$4,043.38
Totals								
Days/charges	540	15	$37,825.00	$53,210.00	$1,800.00	$27,275.00	$58,735.00	
Cost	$98,085.60	$3,676.05	$30,190.89	$31,892.85	$ 860.91	$18,239.37	$38,072.97	$221,018.64
Average per patient case								
Days/charges	10	0	$700.00	$985.00	$33	$505.00	$1,088.00	
Cost	$1,816.00	0	$559.00	$591.00	$16	$338.00	$ 705.00	$4,025.00

relative value units that are specific to procedures for the more aggregate departmental RCC. This simple step effectively transforms the hospital's price list into a relative value scale that is sensitive to the cost-to-charge relationship of specific hospital procedures. The next section of this chapter provides further discussion of relative value units.

Other techniques for determining specific costs are industrial engineering, time studies, and statistical analysis. These techniques are used to identify the cost components of the hospital's individual procedures and services. For example, the cost of a chest X ray could be determined by estimating film and supply costs as well as the associated direct labor and expenses. Fixed cost is still assigned on the basis of allocation statistics. While these approaches give a more accurate estimate of the true average cost of a procedure, the analysis of all hospital procedures utilizing industrial engineering, time studies, and statistical techniques is both costly and time-consuming.

A reasonable compromise to increase the accuracy of cost estimates is to combine the two approaches: identifying major procedures within hospital departments and utilizing a method of process costing and engineering analysis to arrive at relative values for the individual procedures within the revenue-producing departments. These relative values are then used to compute estimates of procedure cost in conjunction with the average unit cost within the department in future operating periods. For the remaining procedures, the hospital's charge records and departmental RCC are retained as a meaningful estimate of resource consumption. Over time, the industrial engineering studies can be shifted to review additional areas, until a substantial portion of the hospital's charge master has been verified.

PROCESS COSTING

In a process cost system, all costs for an accounting period, such as a month, quarter, or year, are collected in a single ledger account. These costs are not identified with specific units or products either as the accounting transactions are processed or at the time services are provided. A record of the number of units produced during the period, however, is maintained. By dividing total cost by the total units, an average cost per unit is derived. The result is an averaging of all costs over all the products of the individual cost center without differentiating the effort and resources utilized on an individual procedural basis.

Process costing is most effective at the department level for determining a unit cost for the individual services. A hospital process costing system begins with the accumulation of costs and procedures by department. The costs of all the resources used to produce the services of the department are accumulated and are averaged over the department's total output. A patient utilizing the services of the department is charged with one share of the department's cost for each unit of service received. The total of unit costs for the services utilized is the total cost of the patient's care. The finer the costing units established within each department, the more procedure specific the averages developed and the more accurate the assignment of costs to products.

Relative value units may also be used to allocate costs more accurately among specific services provided within each department. In Table 21.6, all laboratory tests are classified into ten subgroups. The subgrouping of a department's procedures is based upon similar consumption patterns of departmental labor and nonlabor costs. The average cost of all laboratory tests is used to derive a relative value index. During future periods, the relative value index for each subgroup is used to adjust the average laboratory cost of that production period to a unit cost estimate for each subgroup. This does not account for varying resource efficiency in the production of individual services. However, these differences are not considered material and, as a standard costing procedure, waste is spread across the actual units produced by a uniform weighting factor.

Optimally, both job order and process costing are utilized simultaneously. Process costs may be used to accumulate the costs at the department level and to develop departmental performance standards, relative value indexes, and individual procedure costs. The process costs can then be used in the hospital's job order costing on a per procedure basis to replace or enhance the ratio of cost to charges method.

STANDARD COST

The basic objective of the systems outlined thus far is to charge units of a product with a fair share of the actual costs incurred in making the product. To evaluate the performance of the hospital, the cost accounting system must also have a bench mark for comparing the actual costs and actual units produced to projected values, that is, the costs that should have been incurred on those products rather than the costs that actually were incurred. Such a system is called a standard cost system. Standard cost can be established for either a job order cost system or a process cost system. Both require a heavy managerial commitment to the establishment of performance standards by product line.

Because the standard cost is dependent upon the departmental resources used to provide patient services, the development of the standard must begin at the department level. Using information from physicians and department managers, hospital service volumes are budgeted by number of patients and by type of product. Given a patient volume budget by product, the department manager budgets the operating expenses of the department based on the anticipated demand for departmental services (for

TABLE 21.6   Development of Departmental Relative Value Units: Hospital Laboratory

Development of RVU using direct labor hours as proxy (sample period)

Category of Lab Procedure	Direct Labor Hours/Procedure		Average Direct Labor/Procedure Category		Relative Value/Procedure Category
1	.10	÷	.10	=	1.0
2	.05		.10		.5
3	.05		.10		.5
4	.15		.10		1.5
5	.10		.10		1.0
6	.10		.10		1.0
7	.15		.10		1.5
8	.15		.10		1.5
9	.05		.10		.5
10	.10		.10		1.0

$$1.00$$
$$\div\ 10 \quad \text{Categories of procedure}$$
$$.10 \quad \text{Average direct labor per procedure category}$$

Development of Adjusted Number of Procedures Performed (current operating period)

Category of Lab Procedure	Number of Procedures Performed	Relative Value/ Procedure Category	Adjusted Number of Procedures Performed
1	4,000	1.0	4,000
2	3,500	.5	1,750
3	2,000	.5	1,000
4	4,000	1.5	6,000
5	4,500	1.0	4,500
6	6,000	1.0	6,000
7	2,200	1.5	3,300
8	1,800	1.5	2,700
9	4,000	.5	2,000
10	3,000	1.0	3,000
	35,000		34,250

Weighted Average Cost per Procedure (current operating period)

Total cost of operating laboratory during period	$753,500
Adjusted number of procedures performed	÷ 34,250
Weighted average cost per procedure	$ 22.00

RVU Cost per Procedure (current operating period)

Category of Lab Procedure	Weighted Average Cost/ Procedure	Relative Value/ Procedure Category	Adjusted Cost/ Procedure	Number of Procedures Performed	Allocated Cost
1	$22.00	1.0	$22.00	4,000	$ 88,000
2	22.00	.5	11.00	3,500	38,500
3	22.00	.5	11.00	2,000	22,000
4	22.00	1.5	33.00	4,000	132,000
5	22.00	1.0	22.00	4,500	99,000
6	22.00	1.0	22.00	6,000	132,000
7	22.00	1.5	33.00	2,200	72,600
8	22.00	1.5	33.00	1,800	59,400
9	22.00	.5	11.00	4,000	44,000
10	22.00	1.0	22.00	3,000	66,000
				35,000	$753,500

example, patient days, X rays, laboratory tests). A profile for the previous year's service volume by product category is provided to the department manager so that hospital inpatient and outpatient volume is related to the demand for departmental services. When a standard cost system is linked to the hospital's budget process, each unit of a product is given a standard direct material cost, a standard direct labor cost, and a standard overhead cost. The standard costs are developed by running the hospital's approved budget by responsibility center through the same product line cost accounting system used for processing the hospital's financial performance data during the operating year. The total standard cost is obtained by multiplying the standard unit cost per product by the number of units budgeted or the number of units produced during the period.

ANALYZING AND REPORTING PERFORMANCE

In most situations, actual revenues and costs will not correspond to planned revenues and costs. Management needs to know what the differences between actual and planned results are and, more important, why they occurred. Analytical techniques that divide the total difference between actual and planned performance into several elements may identify the causes of the difference as

1. Gross margin variance
2. Selling price variance
3. Sales volume variance
4. Gross margin mix variance
5. Quantity (usage) variance
6. Price (rate) variance

The gross margin, selling price, sales volume, and gross margin mix variances apply at the product level. Quantity and price variances apply at the product and department levels. Once it has identified how much of the total difference is attributable to each type of variance, management is in a position to fix responsibility, to ask relevant questions, and to take corrective action.

Individual organizations develop guidelines for determining which variances will be investigated. Common criteria include

1. All variances that exceed a specific dollar threshold
2. All variances that exceed budgeted levels by a fixed percentage
3. All unfavorable variances

The criteria chosen in any given organization depend on management's judgment and experience and the level of detail reported. The general rule for analysis also applies to investigations of variance; that is, any technique for developing information should provide information that is worth more than the costs of developing the information.

VARIABLE AND FIXED COSTS

Another method of defining costs is to examine their fixed and variable characteristics. There are three basic types of cost: variable, fixed (nonvariable), and semivariable (partly variable). In accounting, variability relates both to changes in the amount of the costs experienced over time and to changes in the level of costs based upon the level of activity that is taking place in the production of goods and services.

Variable costs are items of cost that vary directly and proportionately with production volume. If the total amount of cost increases as volume increases, the item is a variable cost. Figure 21.3 shows this relationship. Additionally, the percentage of the cost increase or decrease that results is proportionate to the percentage change in the volume of production. For example, if volume increases by 10%, the total amount of cost should also increase by 10%. Direct labor, direct material, and indirect cost all have components of variable cost. Each should be individually analyzed to ascertain its variable elements.

Fixed costs do not vary with changes in production volume. Fixed costs, in aggregate, will remain the same even though increases or decreases of production volume may occur. Building depreciation, taxes, supervisory salaries, and utilities (heat and light) are examples of expenses that behave in a fixed manner.

Semivariable costs are costs that vary with changes in volume, but the increase or decrease in the percentage of change in cost is not the same as the increase or decrease in production capacity. The change is, of course, always in the same direction and is normally lower than the percentage change in production. For example, if volume increases by 10%, the total amount of semivariable costs will increase, but by some amount less than 10%. Semivariable costs increase in block steps as production increases. As capacity increases and additional plant or equipment is required, all costs eventually take on semivariable characteristics. For example, salary cost for nursing supervision is generally unaffected by the level of activity within the nursing unit until capacity reaches a level when an additional supervisor is needed to maintain efficient operations. One way of viewing semivariable costs is that they are fixed costs that increase sharply because of the extent of production range being analyzed. Examples of semivariable costs include indirect labor, maintenance, equipment, and clerical costs.

FIGURE 21.3   Diagram of Fixed and Variable Cost Elements

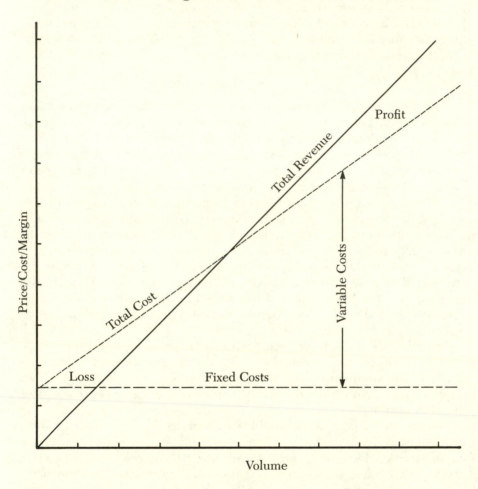

UNIT COSTS

The three types of cost—variable, fixed, and semivariable—are normally expressed in terms of the total costs for a particular product or period. However, a useful way of viewing these characteristics of cost is in the form of unit costs. In unit cost terms, the description of variable and fixed costs reverses.

Variable cost per unit of production is a constant; by definition, it does not change as volume changes.

Fixed cost per unit changes with changes in volume. As volume increases, fixed cost per unit decreases proportionately; as volume decreases, fixed cost per unit increases proportionately. This is an important factor to take into consideration in a payment situation involving fixed price per unit of service. Because fixed cost per unit of production decreases, the profit margin per unit of production increases with each additional unit provided.

Semivariable cost per unit also changes with changes in volume, but just as in the case of total semivariable costs, the percentage of change is not proportionate to the percentage of volume change.

The relationship of variable, fixed, and semivariable unit costs is illustrated in Table 21.7.

BREAK-EVEN ANALYSIS

The sales volume at which sales revenues equal the costs of making and selling the products is of prime interest to management. Another tool available for departmental performance evaluation and planning is break-even analysis. In break-even analysis, fixed cost is spread across the anticipated profit margin.

$$\text{Break-even Point (in units)} = \frac{\text{Total Fixed Cost}}{\text{Sales Price per Unit} - \text{Variable Cost per Unit}}$$

$$\text{Break-even Point (in dollars)} = \frac{\text{Total Fixed Cost}}{\text{Contribution Margin Percentage}}$$

Break-even analysis computes the units or dollars of production necessary to cover the full cost of production. It is useful in both pricing and efficiency analysis to focus management's attention on the computation of profit margin per unit and on the residual contribution of a product or product line to the hospital's operations.

The relationship of variable and fixed costs can be integrated with the application of break-even analysis. The relationship of cost to volume to profit suggests that a useful way of viewing the basic profit characteristics of a business is to focus on the total fixed cost of production and the contribution margin from each additional unit sold. There are essentially four ways in which the profits of a product may be increased:

—Increase the selling price of each unit and thereby increase the contribution margin per unit.

—Decrease the variable costs per unit and thereby increase the contribution margin per unit.

—Decrease the fixed cost and thereby decrease the number of units required to effect fixed cost coverage.

TABLE 21.7   Analysis of Unit Costs

| | Volume (units) | | |
	100 units	125 units	150 units
Total Cost			
Variable costs	$300	$375	$450
Fixed cost	600	600	600
Semivariable costs	600	625	650
Unit Cost			
Variable cost	$3.00	$3.00	$3.00
Fixed cost	6.00	4.80	4.00
Semivariable cost	6.00	5.00	4.34

Note: As volume increases by 50% (that is, from 100 to 150 units),
  —Total variable costs increase by 50%.
  —Total fixed cost remains unchanged.
  —Total semivariable costs increase but by less than 50%.
  —Variable cost per unit remain unchanged.
  —Fixed cost per unit decreases.
  —Semivariable cost per unit decrease, but not by as much as the decline in
    fixed cost per unit.

Source: Adapted from Anthony, Robert N. and Reese, James S. *Management Accounting,*
5th Edition. Homewood, IL: Richard D. Irwin, Inc. 1975. Reprinted by permission of the
publisher.

  —Increase the volume of goods or services to increase the number of
    units that earn a contribution margin in excess of the number re-
    quired to cover fixed cost.

Table 21.8 illustrates these four ways of increasing profits.

CONCLUSION

It is not unusual today to read that hospital management is concerned
with the amount of cost accounting information that is available and the
accuracy of the available data in portraying the "true" cost of producing the
hospital's services. Since the adoption of inclusive fixed price methodologies of payment, hospital management has attempted to reorganize and,
sometimes, reorient the existing hospital cost accounting system to model
more closely those systems used traditionally in non–health care industries.

This is appropriate to a degree. Management now needs more service
specific revenue and cost information. Management also needs organizational revenue and cost information to maintain the hospital's production
functions.

Hospital management must be aware of the trade-off between more

TABLE 21.8   Effects of Changing Price and Cost Factors

Fixed cost = $1,000
Selling price = $10.00
Variable cost = $5.00
Contribution margin in dollars = Selling price − Variable costs = $5.00

Contribution margin in percent = $\dfrac{\text{Selling price} - \text{Variable costs}}{\text{Selling Price}}$ = 50%

Increase Selling Price per Unit
Selling price = $12.00
Increase of $2.00 per unit
Additional $2.00 per unit contribution margin × 200 units = additional
  $400 profit

Decrease Variable Cost per Unit
Variable cost = $3.00
Decrease of $2.00 per unit
Additional $2.00 per unit contribution margin × 200 units = additional
  $400 profit

Decrease Fixed Cost
Fixed cost = $800
Decrease of $200
Contribution margin per unit remains $5.00, but fixed cost per unit declines
  from $5.00 per unit to $4.00 per unit.
Decline of $1.00 × 200 units = additional $200 profit

Increase Volume
Sales volume = 300 units
Because fixed costs are covered by the first 200 units sold, each additional unit
  generates an additional profit equal to the fixed cost per unit at the break-even
  point.
100 additional units × $5.00 per unit revised contribution margin = $500
  additional profit

perfect cost information and the potential risks of imperfect decisions. Hospital management also must become more familiar with the cost accounting approaches of other industries before attempting to adapt them to the hospital environment. For example, the question of product definition provides a very difficult problem. Generally, a hospital produces more distinct products than its manufacturing counterpart. This single difference between the health care and non–health care industries requires the hospital cost accounting system to consider more accurate data collection procedures and finer definitions of the components of the hospital's product line. More important, hospital management must become familiar with using the cost accounting data that are available, making assumptions, assessing investment risk, and taking action. No amount of information guarantees perfect decision making.

SUGGESTED READINGS

Anthony, Robert N. and Reese, James S. *Management Accounting.*

Burik, David and Duvall, Paul J. "Hospital Cost Accounting."

Chadwick, Edward G. "Special Report #5, Product Line Analysis."

de Mars Martin, Pamela and Boyer, Frank J. "Developing a Consistent Method for Costing Hospital Services."

Esmond, Truman H., Jr. *Budgeting Procedures for Hospitals,* Chapters 2, 3, and 4.

Horngren, Charles T. *Cost Accounting: A Managerial Emphasis.*

Nackel, John G. and Barnard, Cynthia. "Special Report #10, Evaluating Case Mix Reporting Systems."

22

Financial Analysis

The foregoing chapters have discussed the financial environment of hospitals as well as the financial management techniques needed for efficient hospital operations and effective use of capital. The results of the application of these and the other management techniques and initiatives are ultimately all displayed in the hospital's financial and operating reports. Chapters 14 and 20 have described these reports. This chapter addresses the techniques for analyzing the data in the hospital's two principal financial reports—the balance sheet (position statement) and the income statement (operating statement).

In the narrowest sense, financial analysis is the set of mathematical and comparative techniques used to interpret a firm's financial and operating data in order to assess its performance and financial position. This view, while correct, is sterile. It conceives of financial analysis as an end unto itself rather than as a means to an end.

A more useful perspective is to view financial analysis as an aid to management decision making. It is the set of concepts and analytical techniques that helps management to evaluate past—and to plan for future—investment, operating, and financing decisions. The usefulness of financial analysis, however, extends beyond just the examination of resource deployment decisions. It is also valuable as a systematic means for evaluating management's own performance. It is in this larger and more dynamic sense that financial analysis is discussed in this chapter.

ESTABLISHING THE FACTS

In simplest terms financial analysis consists of a three-step process. The first step involves establishing an accurate fact base. The second is arithmetic, focusing on the development of comparisons and the calculation of various indexes that can be measured against past performance and against normative as well as objective standards. The final step is perhaps the most difficult. It involves the application of perspective and judgment to the data generated in step two in order to draw conclusions as to the effectiveness of resource allocation decisions, management performance, and financial status.

The starting point in establishing the fact base is typically the hospital's audited financial statements.[1] Given that these statements have been prepared and certified by an independent auditor, the obvious question is why can't they be accepted as the fact base—"as is"? The answer has nothing to do with the accuracy of the statements. They can be assumed, within the context of their purpose, to be accurate. Rather, the answer lies in the perspective that is being taken and the fact that the financial analyst's perspective is different than that of the accountant and auditor.

As discussed in Chapter 3, the auditor's unqualified opinion evidences that the hospital's financial statements have been prepared in accord with generally accepted accounting practices and that within the context of those practices the statements fairly portray the financial position of the hospital. Generally accepted accounting practices, however, allow for considerable flexibility in stating results. Moreover, they allow for variation—between firms—in the accounting treatment of various business transactions. Both factors make the direct comparison of "raw" financial statement data inappropriate for purposes of financial analysis.

To be useful for financial analysis the audited statements have to be reconstructed so that they portray the monetary—as contrasted with the accounting—results of the hospital's business transactions and resource commitments. The reconstruction process is accomplished through a series of adjustments to the accounting statements. These adjustments have the effect of recasting the financial statements so that they show actual, normal operating results on a consistent—year to year—basis. That is, operating results exclusive of items like: nonrecurrent transactions, transactions involving deductions or credits due to the use of contingency or other arbitrary reserves, year to year changes in the accounting treatment of items such as depreciation and inventories, and accounting conventions that miscategorize the monetary effects of resource allocation decisions, for exam-

---

[1]Financial analysis can for internal management purposes be done more frequently than annually. Obviously, unaudited data would be the basis of such analysis. In determining the frequency of analysis, management should recognize both the variability of month to month data and their potential for distortion of results as well as the fact that some data, for example, capital structure, change infrequently. A common middle ground is quarterly analysis for internal management purposes and annual analysis for external purposes.

ple, recognizing the reality that cash segregated for plant additions is really part of the hospital's current assets.[2]

The adjustment process obviously can become quite involved. Regardless of the number or the complexity of the adjustments the goal is always the same: to reconstruct the financial statements so that they portray on a consistent basis the monetary effects of the decisions that management has made. Figure 22.1 illustrates a typical set of hospital financial statements as provided by an independent auditor. These statements have been prepared in accord with generally accepted accounting practices and originally were accompanied by an unqualified opinion. Figure 22.2 shows the same statements for the same period—after adjustments. For purposes of financial analysis, the statements presented in Figure 22.2 are the fact base. Tables 22.1 and 22.2 explain the adjustments.

The data in Figures 22.1 and 22.2 are provided to illustrate, and to give the reader a feel for, the adjustment process. Readers interested in a more detailed discussion of the theory or mechanics of financial analysis adjustments should see the references in the Suggested Readings at the end of this chapter.

COMPARISONS AND INDEXES

The next step in the financial analysis process is to convert the fact base into a set of quantitative measures that can be used to develop judgments about the hospital's financial status and operating performance. The level of analysis can vary from straightforward comparisons to detailed specialized studies of assets (for example, cash forecasts) or of operations (for example, break-even analysis, variations in margin). The time perspective of the analysis can also vary from historical to projected. Prospective or projected analysis is done through use of budget information and the translation of those data into adjusted, estimated financial statements. Historical analysis is done through the use of the hospital's audited financial statements, adjusted as discussed above.

The most direct approach to financial analysis is comparative analysis using historical statements. Mechanically, it is done by presenting similar financial statements on a side by side basis and then examining the changes that have occurred from year to year on an item by item basis. Figures 14.1 and 14.2 in Chapter 14 illustrate comparative statements.

The value of comparative statement analysis lies in its usefulness in identifying trends. Examination of comparative statements can reveal the direction, pace, and size of changes in operating performance and financial

---

[2]In the case of for-profit hospitals, adjustments might also be needed to reflect taxes in relation to earnings.

FIGURE 22.1   Financial Statements: St. Christopher Hospital Balance Sheet, June 30, 198X

UNRESTRICTED FUNDS

Assets

Current		
Cash		$ 103,000
Temporary investments		2,600,000
Accounts receivable, patients	$11,500,000	
Allowances		
Contractual adjustments	$ 200,000	
Uncollectibility	4,140,000	
	4,340,000	7,160,000
Accounts receivable, other		108,000
Due from other funds		90,000
Inventories		575,000
Prepaid expenses		2,670,000
		$13,306,000

Property and Equipment	Cost	Accumulated Depreciation	Net
Grounds	$ 1,300,000		$ 1,300,000
Buildings	33,700,000	$ 8,600,000	25,100,000
Equipment	17,500,000	7,500,000	10,000,000
	$52,500,000	$16,100,000	$36,400,000

Liabilities

Current		
Current installment of long-term debt		$ 525,000
Accounts payable		
Trade	$1,100,000	
Cost report settlements	825,000	
		1,925,000
Accrued compensation		360,000
Accrued other exp.		1,400,000
		$ 4,210,000

Long-Term Debt	
Note payable, $9,450,000 less current maturity of $525,000	8,925,000

Assets		Fund Balance	
Other			
Investments in cash equivalents at cost			39,626,000
Debt service reserve			
(Market value, $862,000)	805,000		
Board designated funds			
(Market value, $2,000,000)	2,250,000		
	$52,761,000		$52,761,000

RESTRICTED FUNDS

Assets		Liabilities	
		Expansion Fund	
Expansion Fund		Fund balance	$642,000
Investments in treasury obligations			
(Market value, $708,000)	$642,000		
	$642,000		$642,000
		Specific Trust Funds	
Specific Trust Funds		Due to other funds	$ 21,000
Cash	$ 25,000	Fund balance	683,000
Certificate of deposit	660,000		
Due from other funds	19,000		
	$704,000		$704,000

Continued

FIGURE 22.1   Continued: St. Christopher Hospital Statement of Revenues and Expenses, Year Ended June 30, 198X

Revenue from services to patients			
Inpatients			$57,425,000
Outpatients			6,525,000
Outpatients			$63,950,000
Deductions from patient revenues			
Contractual allowances		$ 2,600,000	
Charity allowances		850,000	
Uncollectible receivables		1,900,000	5,350,000
Net revenue from services to patients			$58,600,000
Other operating revenue			
Cafeteria sales		$ 712,000	
Gift shop sales		200,000	
Anesthesiologists		450,000	
Medical education program		138,000	
Other		520,000	2,020,000
Total operating revenue			$60,620,000

Operating expenses		
Salaries and wages	$31,900,000	
Fringe benefits	5,900,000	
Depreciation	3,260,000	
Interest	700,000	
Insurance	400,000	
Other expenses	17,840,000	60,000,000
Net revenue from operations		$ 620,000
Nonoperating revenue		
Income from endowment	$ 350,000	
Interest income		
Debt service reserve	90,000	
Temporary investment	102,000	
Board designated funds	625,000	
Loss on sale of equipment	(150,000)	
		$ 1,017,000
Excess of revenue over expenses		$ 1,637,000

FIGURE 22.2 Adjusted Financial Statements: St. Christopher Hospital Balance Sheet, June 30, 198X

Assets

*Current**
Cash[1]		$ 128,000
Marketable securities[2]		708,000
Accounts receivable, patients[3]	$11,300,000	
Allowance for uncollectibles	4,140,000	
		7,160,000
Accounts receivable, other		108,000
Inventories		575,000
Prepaid expenses		300,000
		$ 8,979,000

Property and Equipment
Grounds	$ 1,300,000	
Building (net of depreciation)	25,100,000	
Equipment (net of depreciation)	10,000,000	
		36,400,000

Other Assets
Investments for debt service reserve[4]	862,000	
Certificate of deposit[5]	3,260,000	
Board designated funds[6]	2,000,000	
		6,122,000

Deferred Charges[7]
	2,370,000
Total assets	$53,871,000

Liabilities

Current
Current installment of long-term debt		$ 525,000
Accounts payable		
Trade	$1,100,000	
Cost report settlements	825,000	
		1,925,000
Accrued compensation		360,000
Accrued other expenses		1,400,000
		$ 4,210,000

Long-Term Debt
Note payable, $9,450,000	
less current maturity of $525,000	8,925,000

Equity
Unrestricted	$37,343,000	
Restricted		
Board[8]	2,708,000	
Other[9]	685,000	
		40,736,000
Total liabilities and equity		$53,871,000

Revenue from services to patients		
Inpatients[1]	$54,825,000	
Outpatients	6,525,000	
		$61,350,000
Allowances and uncollectibles[2]		
Uncollectibles	1,900,000	
Charity/free service	850,000	
Allowance		2,750,000
Net revenue from services to patients		$58,600,000
Other operating revenue[3]		
Programs and services		
Cafeteria sales	712,000	
Gift shop sales	200,000	
Anesthesiologists	450,000	
Medical education program	138,000	
Other recurring operations	520,000	
Total other operating revenue		2,020,000
Total operating revenue		60,620,000

Continued

FIGURE 22.2   Continued

Assets		Liabilities	

Investment revenue
Income from endowment   350,000
Income from investments[4]   817,000
                                                      1,167,000

    Total revenue $61,787,000

Expenses[5]
Salaries and wages   31,900,000
Fringe benefits   5,900,000
Depreciation   3,260,000
Interest   700,000
Insurance   400,000
Other   17,840,000
                                                      60,000,000

    Excess of revenue over expenses $ 1,787,000

*Amounts due from or to other funds are eliminated as they are interfund transactions that are absorbed in the consolidation of funds.

TABLE 22.1   Adjustment Entries: St. Christopher Hospital Balance
Sheet, June 30, 198X

[1]Cash—consolidation of cash in the unrestricted fund of $103,000 and cash in the
Specific Trust Fund of $25,000. These two accounts are consolidated because
they both involve cash assets under the control of management that can be
used at the discretion of management to meet the hospital's needs.

[2]Marketable Securities—US Treasury obligations in the Expansion Fund at market
value of $708,000. Market value is used because it reflects the assets available
to the hospital.

[3]Accounts Receivable—reduced by contractual allowances as these are amounts
that are not actually an obligation to the hospital.

[4]Other Assets—investments for Debt Service Reserve are required by the bond
indenture and are therefore not available for other purposes. These resources
are shown at market value.

[5]Other Assets—certificates of deposit can only be liquidated prior to maturity at
a penalty. Therefore, they are shown as "Other Assets" as opposed to a "Current Asset."

[6]Other Assets—Board Designated Funds are shown at market value. Arguably,
these assets could be shown as current assets. However, because it is the
board's intention to hold these assets for the long term they have been shown
here.

[7]Deferred Charges—the bulk of prepaid expenses have been placed here to reflect
the particular "near" expense nature of these assets and to distinguish them
from current assets that can be readily converted into cash. Note that $300,000,
for insurance premiums, remains as a prepaid expense.

[8]Equity—Board Restricted Equity reflects assets set aside by decision of the board.
The $2,708,000 is composed of "Other Assets" of $2,000,000 and "Marketable
Securities" of $708,000.

[9]Equity—Other Restricted Equity represents donor restricted assets, equivalent
to the monetary assets in the Specific Trust Fund of $685,000.

status data. The identification of trends, however, does not necessarily provide management with answers. Rather, it yields clues as to where further
analysis might be useful. For example, the simple fact that accounts receivable increased from year to year by 8%, in and of itself, is of limited use.
However, an 8% increase in accounts receivable when combined with a
10% increase in patient billings begins to portray a pattern. Yes, accounts
receivable increased but they did not increase as much as "sales" increased.
Therefore, assuming the payer mix remained unchanged, the credit and
collection operation is improving its performance. Comparative analysis
pointed out the change in accounts receivable. Further analysis was required to interpret what, in a managerial sense, the change meant.

Contrasting one year to the next and identifying the absolute dollar
amounts of change is the most basic form of comparative analysis. The

TABLE 22.2   Adjustment Entries: St. Christopher Hospital
              Statement of Revenue and Expenses,
              Year Ended June 30, 198X

[1]Revenues—figures shown are net of Medicare and Medicaid contractual allowances. These allowances are "netted out" and sales revenues are overstated by these amounts, which by contract are not part of the payer's obligation.

[2]Allowances and Uncollectibles—these are reductions from revenues due to bad debts and free care.

[3]Other Operating Revenue—includes revenues both from nonclinical services and ongoing operations. Revenues from ongoing nonclinical operations are included because they are a regular source of income to the hospital—which can be used to meet operating expenses. Anesthesiologist revenue reflects the business billing arrangement that the hospital has with its anesthesiologists.

[4]Income from Investments—revenues reflect an ongoing stream of income. Nonrecurrent items should be eliminated from a single year analysis. However, they should be included in any long-term analysis. Thus, if the sale of equipment were a unique event the loss on the sale would not be taken into consideration in evaluating performance for 198X. If equipment sales were made every year, then the loss should be taken into account in a single year analysis. In this instance the sale is assumed to be a nonrecurrent event.

[5]Expenses—expense data could be provided in more detail either by natural account or by functional area and responsibility center. The degree of detail provided should match the depth of the analysis. Additional detail, as well as previous year's information for purposes of comparative analysis, can be provided as needed through supplemental schedules. Again, as was noted above, nonrecurrent events should be eliminated from a single year analysis.

analysis can be enhanced by showing not only absolute dollar changes but also, percentage changes. (See example in Figure 22.3). Both measures are useful because they give insight into the relative magnitude of any changes that are taking place. That is, a 20% change on a base figure of $10,000 is not as significant as a 20% change on a base figure of $100,000; alternatively a $100,000, 1% change is not as significant as $30,000, 30% change.

In comparing more than two or three years of data, the year to year approach such as that illustrated in Figure 22.3 can become unwieldly. A technique for avoiding this is to convert annual data into a series of index numbers. Index numbers are calculated by establishing a particular year as a base year. The data for all items in the base year are given an index value

FIGURE 22.3   St. Christopher Hospital Comparative Financial
Statement As of June 30, 198X

	198W	198X	Change $	%
Cash	$ 120,000	$ 128,000	$ 8,000	7
Marketable securities	3,750,000	708,000	(3,042,000)	(81)
Accounts receivable (net)—patients	5,600,000	7,160,000	1,560,000	28
Accounts receivable (net)—other	105,000	108,000	3,000	3
Inventories	419,000	575,000	156,000	37
Prepaid expenses	100,000	300,000	200,000	200
Total	$10,094,000	$8,979,000	$(1,115,000)	

of 100. The index values for all subsequent years are calculated by reference to the base year. Thus, for example, if the hospital had inventories of $1,500,000 in 198X, the base year, $1,500,000 would have an index value of 100. If four years later (198X+4) the value of inventories was $1,800,000 then the index value for 198X+4 would be 120. If the value of inventories had been $1,000,000 then, the index value would have been 67.[3]

Index value trend analysis is useful for providing a common denominator for the examination of large masses of data and for beginning the analysis of time series changes in the composition of groups of accounts, such as working capital. It also, however, has limits. Index value data for instance, because of its arithmetic construction of calculating values as a percentage of differing base items, does not provide information that is as useful for evaluating matters like financial condition as that produced by other analytic techniques.

Another mechanism for establishing a common denominator is to construct common size financial statements. As discussed in Chapter 14 (see Figure 14.1), common size comparative reports differ from direct comparative statements in that the data for each line item are presented in terms of a percentage of the total instead of in absolute dollars.

Common size reports are useful for both vertical and horizontal analysis. Like the above approaches to presenting financial data, comparative common size reports are an aid to trend or horizontal analysis because they can portray relative changes in line items over time. Common size reports also provide a tool for examining the internal structure and composition of

---

[3]Index values are calculated as follows:

$$\frac{\text{(Balance in Current Year)}}{\text{(Balance in Base Year)}} \times 100 = \text{Index Value}$$

data within a section of a financial statement. This analysis of structure and distribution is known as vertical analysis. Figure 22.4 presents an excerpt from a common size financial statement. The data in Figure 22.4 are derived from the information in Figure 22.3.

As noted common size statements are valuable to managers in that they show proportions as well as changes in proportions of components within groups of assets, liabilities, and costs. The changes in proportions provide insight into the monetary effects of individual decisions on both a specific item and on the relation of that item to other elements in the financial statement. For example, as illustrated in Figures 22.3 and 22.4, the decision with respect to marketable securities not only reduces the absolute amount of marketable securities but also increases the relative proportion of accounts receivable as an element of current assets. The proportionate increase in accounts receivable is greater than its absolute increase, that is, accounts receivable represent 79.7% of the total whereas they would represent only 70.9% if the total amount of current assets had not decreased. The net 'effect of this is a change (a decrease) in the relative liquidity of the hospital.'

The ability of common size statements to portray proportions is also helpful for interhospital comparisons. Once financial statements are translated into a common size format, the financial data of a number of hospitals can be presented (regardless of the absolute amounts of the individual accounts being compared) in a uniform and comparable manner. Examination of such data across hospitals or against composite industry statistics can then be used to flag variations in capital structure or cost distribution that merit further management investigation.

RATIO ANALYSIS

A more popular technique for interhospital comparisons as well as for structural analysis of a hospital's own financial statements is ratio analysis. Ratio analysis is probably the most widely used of all financial analysis

FIGURE 22.4   St. Christopher Hospital Common Size
Financial Statement As of June 30, 198X

	198W	198X
Cash	1.2%	1.4%
Marketable securities	37.2	7.9
Accounts receivable (net)—patients	55.5	79.7
Accounts receivable (net)—other	1.0	1.2
Inventories	4.2	6.4
Prepaid expenses	1.0	3.3

techniques. As such it is a valuable tool. However, it is also a technique that is subject to misuse and misinterpretation.

A ratio expresses the mathematical relationship between two quantities. Thus for example, the ratio of 90 to 30 is expressed as 3 to 1 or, more simply, as 3. It is the ease of calculating ratios and the simplicity of expressing the results that are both the great value of ratios and their potential limit. Any two quantities can be drawn together to calculate a ratio. As a result, hundreds of ratios can be developed. The sheer mass of data, if not controlled, not only can make the conversion of data into information an arduous task but also can obstruct any useful analysis and evaluation.

To be useful, ratios must not only express a mathematical relationship but, more important, must express a relationship that has management significance. For example, there is a clear and direct relationship between cash income (net income plus depreciation) and debt service costs (principal and interest payments) in terms of the security of the debt and the hospital's ability to repay the debt. Thus, the relationship of income to debt service costs is significant. The ratio expressing this relationship is useful to both managers and creditors. In contrast the comparison of inventories to allowances for uncollectibles does not represent an understandable direct relationship. While the ratio of these two quantities is calculable, it has no significance and, therefore, has no analytical usefulness.

The danger to be avoided is clear. The goal of ratio analysis must not be to process and "crunch" as many numbers as possible. Rather, it must be to summarize key financial data in a format that makes it easier to (1) translate financial and operating data into information, and (2) understand and evaluate the information that has been developed.

For any particular hospital, a degree of imagination and flexibility should be allowed in selecting the specific ratios to be examined. This flexibility is needed to adjust the analysis to the hospital's environment as well as to the interests and concerns of its management and board. Table 22.3 summarizes and defines commonly used ratios. These ratios are grouped into four major categories: liquidity, capital structure, activity, and operating margin. These categories are used to provide a basic structure for analysis, encompassing both the balance sheet and income statement.

Liquidity refers to the ability of a hospital to meet its short-term obligations such as accounts payable, the current portion of long-term debt, and federal withholding taxes. Highly liquid resources are assets such as cash and near cash investments (for example, short-term certificates of deposit, money market funds, and short-term marketable securities). Other current assets (for example, accounts receivable and inventories) are also considered to be liquid resources but, as compared to cash, to a lesser degree. This is the case because these assets must first be converted into cash before they can be used to meet obligations. If the conversion process

TABLE 22.3   Ratio Analysis

Liquidity Measures

$$\text{Current Ratio} = \frac{\text{Current Assets}}{\text{Current Liabilities}}$$

Ratio of current assets to current liabilities. It is used as the basic index of financial liquidity. The higher the ratio value, the better the hospital's ability to meet its obligations.

$$\text{Acid Test Ratio} = \frac{\text{Cash + Marketable Securities}}{\text{Current Liabilities}}$$

Ratio of the sum of cash and marketable securities to current liabilities. It is the most rigorous test of liquidity, taking into account the composition of current assets and recognizing that accounts receivable and inventories—while current assets— are not cash. The higher the ratio value, the better the hospital's ability to meet its obligations.

$$\text{Collection Period} = \frac{\text{Net Accounts Receivable}}{\text{Average Daily Operating Revenue}}$$

Ratio of accounts receivable net of uncollectibles to daily operating revenue (total revenue divided by 365 days). It is a measure of the length of time accounts receivable are outstanding. Increasing values for this measure indicate a lengthening of the collection period and can signal future liquidity problems. The collection period should also be kept in balance with a similar ratio measuring payment period. Separate collection period ratios can be calculated for patient care and non–patient care accounts receivable as well as for accounts receivable by class of payer.

Capital Structure

$$\text{Long-Term Debt to Fixed Assets} = \frac{\text{Long-Term Debt}}{\text{Net Fixed Assets}}$$

Ratio of the proportion of fixed assets that have been financed through long-term debt. The higher the ratio the less relative security perceived by a lender and the more difficult it will be for the hospital to secure future loans. Also, as the ratio increases the hospital should examine its profitability position so that it is better able to support existing debt and flexible enough to acquire additional debt. This examination should include not only operating efficiency considerations but also rate structure matters.

$$\text{Long-Term Debt to Equity} = \frac{\text{Long-Term Debt}}{\text{Unrestricted and Board Restricted Equity}}$$

Ratio of the two long-term sources of the hospital's financing. As this ratio increases the hospital becomes more highly "leveraged" and its ability to acquire future debt financing is reduced.

$$\text{Debt Service} = \frac{\text{Net Income + Depreciation}}{\text{Debt Principal Payment + Interest}}$$

Ratio that measures the ability of the hospital to pay its debt, both principal and interest. The higher this ratio the more secure the lender and the greater the hospital's future debt capacity. This ratio identifies the relationship of debt capacity to earnings and cash flow. Commonly used variations of this ratio are:

TABLE 22.3   Continued

$$\frac{\text{Net Income} + \text{Depreciation}}{\text{Interest}} \quad \text{and} \quad \frac{\text{Net Income} + \text{Depreciation}}{\text{Total Liabilities}}$$

The first is the measure of the ability to pay interest expenses and the second is an indicator of the cash available to meet all obligations.

Activity

$$\text{Total Asset Turnover} = \frac{\text{Total Revenue}}{\text{Total Assets}}$$

Ratio that is used to indicate the relative efficiency of the use of assets. Typically, high values for this measure are viewed as indicating higher levels of performance. The denominator of this ratio should be net of depreciation. Variations of this ratio include fixed asset turnover and current asset turnover. While these activity ratios can be used as surrogate measures of efficiency, other indexes and factors must also be considered, for example, occupancy rates, plant age and design, payer mix.

$$\text{Inventory Turnover} = \frac{\text{Total Operating Revenue}}{\text{Inventory}}$$

Ratio that measures the hospital's investment in inventories. Low values typically imply overstocking—an excess investment in inventories and an inappropriate use of assets.

Operating Margin

$$\text{Operating Margin} = \frac{\text{Total Revenue} - \text{Total Expenses}}{\text{Total Revenue}}$$

Ratio of net income to total revenue. It is a measure of profitability. Operating margin can be calculated in aggregate as well as for patient care services and non–patient care services (nonoperating revenues). In calculating this measure the revenue figures should reflect net revenue, that is, revenues less contractual adjustments.

$$\text{Return on Assets} = \frac{\text{Income} + \text{Interest Expense}}{\text{Total Assets}}$$

Ratio of net income to total investment in the hospital. It is a measure of the relationship of operating margin (total revenue − total expense) to the assets, that is, the investment, in the hospital. Interest expense is added back to eliminate bias due to the method of financing the assets. The ratio can also be calculated net of interest expense.

$$\text{Nonoperating Income Contribution} = \frac{\text{Nonoperating Net Income}}{\text{Net Income}}$$

Ratio of nonpatient care services (nonoperating) net income to total net income. It provides a measure of the importance of nonoperating revenues to the hospital's overall financial status.

---

must be done quickly, there is some risk that a loss in asset value might be incurred, thereby reducing the liquidity value of such assets. For obvious reasons, liquidity is particularly important from a creditor's perspective.

Capital structure ratios are also of particular interest to creditors. Capital structure refers to the mix of financing (equity and debt) used by the hospital to support its assets. The less the relative level of debt the more secure, at least psychologically, the creditors are likely to feel. Conversely, the more heavily "leveraged" the hospital, that is, the greater the proportion of capital structure supplied by debt, the less willing creditors will be to provide additional debt. The status of the hospital's capital structure thus directly affects the amount of financing available to it and, as a result, the hospital's ability to grow.

Capital structure status and liquidity are also related. The greater the proportion of a hospital's capital financed through debt, the greater the debt service expenses. As debt service expenses increase, liquid assets must also increase—if the hospital's overall liquidity position is not to be reduced.

Activity ratios address the relationship of assets and revenues. They are intended to provide an indicator of efficiency. Mechanically, they draw data from both the balance sheet and the income statement, integrating them to demonstrate how assets (inputs) finance various activities (outputs). Outputs are measured in terms of revenues, which are a substitute for direct measures of production.

Operating margin ratios are the hospital analogy to the profitability ratios of the commercial enterprise. The data for these measures are also drawn from both the income statement and the balance sheet. The purpose of operating margin ratios is to provide an indication of how effectively the hospital is making resource deployment decisions. Operating margin ratios are also related to liquidity and the hospital's ability to attract and service debt (capital structure), in that as profitability increases so can liquidity and debt capacity. Conversely, as profitability erodes so do liquidity and resulting debt service capacity. Figure 22.5 illustrates the ratios of Table 22.3, using data drawn from Figure 22.2.

In addition to the foregoing general financial analysis tools, there are a variety of special purpose analytical techniques. These techniques focus on specific financial statements or segments of statements (for example, sources and uses of funds statements, cash flow projections, break-even analysis) or on the operating conditions of a particular industry (for example, occupancy rates, operating margin by class or payer, philanthropy studies). Readers interested in more information about these tools and techniques should see the Suggested Readings at the end of this chapter.

PERSPECTIVE AND JUDGMENT

The final step in the financial analysis process is the most difficult. It involves bringing together the data developed in the first two steps to provide the basis for making an appraisal of the financial performance and status of the organization. In this step, judgment replaces mechanical manipulation of data as the key ingredient.

There is little that is magic about judgment. It is the result of hard

FIGURE 22.5   Ratio Analysis: St. Christopher Hospital As of
               June 30, 198X

Liquidity	
Current ratio	2.1
Acid test ratio	.2
Collection period	43 days
Capital Structure	
Long-term debt to fixed assets	.25
Long-term debt to equity	.22
Debt service coverage	4.1
Activity	
Total asset turnover	1.15
Inventory turnover	105
Operating Margin	
Aggregate operating margin	3%
Patient care operating margin	1%
Return on assets	5%
Nonoperating income contribution	65%

Analysis
Capital structure is strong with little debt. Liquidity, however, is weaker than expected due to the high level of current assets being held as accounts receivable. The combination of the liquidity position and the low operating margin from patient care and related services limits immediate additional debt capacity. Profitability needs to be examined with a goal of increasing operating revenues. In particular, the charge structure should be reviewed.

work, experience, and investigative curiosity. There is no simple formula that can be suggested for this step, but there are several bench marks that can be useful.

First, the analyst must adopt a specific perspective or point of view. That is, he must determine what he is looking for and how he wants to look for it. Without establishing the objectives of the analysis, almost any data and any evaluation technique can suffice. The temptation will be to "run all the numbers" and make all the comparisons, without differentation. The result is not an in-depth analysis, but rather no analysis.

While establishing a point of view is important, it must be recognized that different points of view are not mutually exclusive. The difference is more one of focus than of basic direction. For example, lenders are primarily concerned about the security of their investment and protection against risk. Owners in the commercial setting are most concerned about profitability and the increasing value of their investment. In the nonprofit hospital setting, owners or the community are interested in the efficiency of operations and the amount of services provided to the community. The driving force underlying all of these concerns and interests is the effectiveness with which assets have been obtained, deployed, and utilized. This last matter is the primary concern of management and encapsulates all others. Therefore, as at least a starting place, it is suggested that a management point of view be adopted.

Second, the hospital's financial statistics standing alone have relatively little meaning. To have value and usefulness there must be some measure to which individual hospital data can be compared. At a minimum, the hospital can measure itself against itself, comparing current data to data of the previous year or years. If management knows or can establish the direction in which the statistics should move to show progress or improvement, then this approach provides a useful relative indicator of performance. Its obvious shortfall is that because it is a self-measure it does not provide an indication of absolute performance.

Generally, two approaches are used for measuring performance on an absolute basis. Both approaches use "financial ratio standards"; they differ simply in the source of the standards. In one instance the standards, often called norms, are composite figures representing data from many hospitals in a metropolitan area, a state, or the nation. The notion is that if an individual hospital's data or ratios compare well to the composite statistics, then it can be presumed that the hospital is performing well. The composite statistics are assumed to be objective standards. Examples of conventionally accepted composite financial ratio standards are shown in Table 22.4.

Whether or not the composite data are absolute standards can be argued. They are certainly more rigorous indexes than the relative measure of the year to year comparison of the hospital to itself. However, the composite data, by virtue of their aggregate character, reflect common practice rather than optimum performance. To this extent, they can be viewed as somewhat relative measures.

The second approach to developing standards attempts to correct for this weakness. In this instance the norms are tailored to the individual hospital, reflecting the unique characteristics of its external operating environment. Given the constraints of the hospital's external operating environment, ratio standards can be developed using the techniques discussed in the previous chapters to calculate the optimum amounts of the various components of working capital. These data can then be combined with various industry composite data on capital structure, activity, and operating margin to yield a set of statistical norms that can be a useful tool to management.

This approach while having benefit for internal management purposes also has a significant limitation. Because the standards are tailored to the individual hospital's external operating environment, they result in measures that may not be commonly recognized or accepted by outside interests such as investors or lenders. The solution is obvious. Both approaches should

TABLE 22.4 Example: Composite Standard Financial Ratio Values

	Composite Ratio Value
Liquidity	
Current ratio	2.25
Acid test ratio	.4
Collection period	64 days
Capital Structure	
Long-term debt to fixed assets	.5
Long-term debt to equity	1.5
Debt service coverage	1.5
Times interest earned	1.5
Activity	
Total asset turnover	1.2
Inventory turnover	2.5
Operating Margin	
Aggregate operating margin	6%
Patient care operating margin	6.2

Note: It should be noted that if the composite data are based on state or metropolitan area aggregations then, because the external environment is more homogeneous, the measures move closer to being absolute standards. The examples in this table have been derived from state and national empirical data and subjective estimates reflecting the conventional wisdom.

be used: the first to satisfy external audiences and the second to focus management on reaching optimum performance results.

CAVEATS

Perhaps the greatest hidden danger inherent in financial analysis lies in management being lulled into the trap of quantitative analysis and an unquestioning belief in the numbers. The most that financial analysis can provide, regardless of the method or approach used, is a signal, an indicator of performance, not a true and definitive measure of performance. To grant it any more value is a mistake.

Even so, from some perspectives and to some audiences, the signals are important. To the lender for example, performance and financial status as measured by the hospital's ratios are vital factors in considering a loan. Lenders are typically risk avoiders; making loans to hospitals with "good numbers," that is, ratios that match or exceed the composite industry figures, is prima facie evidence of prudence on the part of lenders. Therefore, while financial analysis might only provide signals, it is important that the signals be good ones.

Similarly, prudent management should also be looking for and heeding the signals of financial analysis. Management should be regularly conducting its own financial analysis, examining the hospital's ratios to understand why they are what they are and what continuing steps can be taken to maintain them or as necessary improve them.

Financial analysis while imperfect is a useful and important management tool. It provides the hospital, particularly the nonprofit hospital, with a quantitative means of assessing its performance and financial status. While it is not a perfect analogy to the "bottom line" measure of the commercial corporation, it can—along with other data and analysis of services (see Chapter 20)—provide some quantitative objectivity to the fundamental need of a hospital to evaluate its operations and return to its community. Within a recognition of its limits, hospital managers should therefore at least annually utilize financial analysis to bring a degree of measurability to performance assessment.

SUGGESTED READINGS

Bernstein, Leopold A. *The Analysis of Financial Statements.*

Caruana, Russell A. and McHugh, E. Thomas. "Comparing Ratios Shows Fiscal Trends."

Cleverley, William O. "Financial Ratios: Summary Indicators for Management Decision Making."

Cleverley, William O. and Nilsen, Karen. "Assessing Financial Position with 29 Key Ratios."

Graham, Benjamin; Dodd, David L.; and Cottle, Sidney. *Security Analysis.*

Helfert, Erich A. *Techniques of Financial Analysis.*

PART
VI

The Future

Future Trends

Looking into the future is to a certain extent peering through a cloudy lens with a limited range of visibility. However, some trends are self-evident and, at least for the short term, are fairly certain to take place.

FUTURIST STUDIES

Futurists use many tools in making their predictions. They examine and analyze financial, political, social, and experiential data as background. Two well-structured futurist studies have been conducted by Delphi or semi-Delphi methodology using outstanding authorities as respondents. One study was done by Arthur Andersen & Co. in conjunction with the American College of Healthcare Executives. It was published in 1984 under the title *Health Care in the 1990s: Trends and Strategies*. The other study was done by Arthur D. Little, Inc. for the Health Insurance Association of America. This was published in 1985 with the title *The Health Care System in the Mid-1990s*.

The authors of the present book have not attempted to summarize or copy from either of the studies, but refer readers to the studies as outstanding examples of current works of futurism as related to American health care of the next decade.

BACKGROUND FOR THE FUTURE

Some of the serious general problems and conditions that will affect the health care system in the future have been with us, and growing, for some time: steady population growth which creates need for more services;

shift in employment from heavy industries to service industries, to high technology, to white collar work in general. Unemployment is too high, but many of the younger unemployed lack skills for any work except jobs at minimum wages. The unemployed from heavy industry likewise lack skills for other types of employment but may be more able to be retrained, if retraining is available, than the younger unemployed.

We, as a people, are growing older. A steady percentage increase is evident in the number of persons over 65 years of age, and particularly in the number over 75. This aging of the population is going to lay an additional burden on the provision of health and social services.

The nation is facing a sinister danger from within, a quisling, a terrifying growth in the use of narcotics and other habit-forming drugs, as well as the misuse of alcohol and tobacco. Another shadow over the land which may endanger many thousands is the spread of AIDS.

Out of all this comes a surge of violent crime, such as has never been seen before. Americans may have to reassess their lifestyle, their priorities, their "freedoms," their attitudes toward the laws of the land and take their responsibilities into account.

Fiscal matters also will affect individuals, hospitals and other providers, commercial corporations, and governments as the nation tries to maintain fiscal integrity in face of deficit financing, defaults by foreign nations, and a sharp rise in consumer credit with the attendant drop in individual savings. Foreign investments by Americans, to a certain degree, will be at the mercy of those nations. In addition we have not seen all the implications of the recent plunge in the price of crude oil.

PROBLEMS OF THE FUTURE

An encyclopedic format has been followed here to make the text more usable as reference. It should be understood that this account does not purport to be all-inclusive or to be entirely data-based. After all, a look into the future must have elements of speculation.

ACCESS TO CARE

Some years ago it was promulgated that the access to health care was not a privilege but a right for all. Not many would quarrel with the statement that all ill persons should be able to receive adequate and good quality care without regard to ability to pay. Somewhere in the process, ability to pay must be considered.

Most Americans have some health insurance, or benefits under Medicare or Medicaid. However, some of the insurance may not be full coverage so there may be a sizable balance after insurance. The problem of the future will be how to pay for the uninsured or the underinsured.

At present there are horror stories of seriously ill patients being refused by the community hospital and being shipped in dangerous condition to a county hospital that has to accept charity patients.

An idea whose fruition is possible in the future is that of a safety net fund to be available to pay for care of the needy. The promoters of the idea say that the fund could be built up from taxes collected and administered by the states.

ADVERTISING

Some leading metropolitan hospitals are advertising on television that they are centers of great scientific and technical activity and imply that in a short time ahead their researchers are likely to have a breakthrough in the treatment of some life-threatening disorder. To whom does the advertising appeal? As institutional advertising, it is a good image builder for the hospitals. Is the appeal to potential hospital patients? Patients seldom have a chance to choose a hospital unless their doctor has staff privileges in more than one hospital. If not associated with the advertised hospital, will a doctor apply for admission to the staff?

Is such advertising an allowable cost? With hospital costs as high as they are, this kind of advertising may not be considered an allowable cost item.

AGED

As previously mentioned, the elderly are increasing as a percentage of the total population, with the over-75 age group increasing proportionally more than the 65-to-75 age group. This increase in the number of the elderly means an increase in health care needs, particularly in nursing home care of the domiciliary type.

Nursing home care under Medicare is limited to skilled nursing facilities, but the major demand is for facilities offering domiciliary care. The financial reserves of a nursing home patient can be exhausted in a short time; then the patient must turn to Medicaid for service under state rules.

One of the big health care problems of the future will be to build sufficient nursing home beds, to assure that there is quality of care in the homes, and to devise a method for financing this care.

Not all the elderly are poor. Probably as a class they are not too unlike the other adult population in financial means, only the elderly have more health care expenditures. Many of the aged purchase medigap insurance to cover Medicare copayments and deductibles, or are now looking at Medicare-HMO combinations as the way to go in the future.

AMBULATORY CARE

With the general shift of care from inpatient to outpatient or ambulatory care for cost savings and convenience, it is not expected the trend will change.

Outpatient departments, walk-in clinics, surgicenters, and other forms of ambulatory care facilities will continue to thrive. Some of the investor-owned groups are beginning to move into the field. It would seem possible that some of the units now operating independently would be absorbed by other care groups.

CAPITAL FORMATION

The opinion has been expressed that capital formation for construction of hospitals and other facilities will be no problem because sufficient funds will be available through the sale of tax exempt bonds.

The cloud in the sky is that personal savings are declining, which reduces somewhat the market for bonds. Also, unless the federal fiscal situation gets better, the government may compete for those funds. Capital formation may not be as easy to accomplish in the future as some individuals think.

CATASTROPHIC INSURANCE

At the time this is being written, President Reagan is voicing support for a national catastrophic insurance program. The new secretary of HHS, Dr. Otis Bowen, also is speaking in favor of the idea. Specifics of the program have not yet been outlined, but it would seem a popular move if means of financing it could be developed.

COALITIONS

A new term has been added to the health care vocabulary: "coalitions." In this case coalitions are community groups made up of employers, professional individuals, financial experts, and other community leaders. Their purpose is to analyze the costs and conditions of medical and hospital care in order to find options for providing good quality care at the lowest possible price. Coalitions in the future will have increasing influence on the health care of their communities.

DRGS AND BEYOND

The use of diagnosis-related groups (DRGs) as a yardstick for reimbursement in Medicare has been a recent step in trying to control hospital stay and payment within diagnostic experiential averages.

The immediate problem seems to be coding properly from nearly 500 diagnostic categories. Fortunately, most cases fall within one or two scores of classification. Miscoding eventually becomes a burden on fiscal intermediaries and carriers to correct with as little delay as possible. This increases administrative overhead.

There is a movement for the DRG system to be extended from Medicare alone to Blue Cross–Blue Shield plans and other insurance companies for subscribers of less than Medicare age.

Already there is conversation about what comes after DRGs. There is some suggestion that an improved capitation system will replace DRGs. Without being cynical, it might be good to look at the future and ask about what will follow capitation. Change is in the air.

FEDERAL GOVERNMENT: POST-MEDICARE TRENDS

Presently the federal government is trying desperately to balance its budget. This is placing pressures on Medicare reimbursements, copayments, and deductibles.

The costs of Medicare have been a problem since the inception of the program. Government pressures on Medicare, Medicaid, and other health programs are not likely to abate in the future. It is not going to be any easier to "do business" with the federal government in the future.

FEE-FOR-SERVICE

The percentage of physicians working on a fee-for-service basis has declined in the past few years, with more doctors working either for a salary or in a partnership in a capitation plan. The trend will continue, especially as the ratio of physicians to population continues to grow.

HEALTH ADMINISTRATION EXECUTIVES SUPPLY

There is wide discussion about the coming oversupply of physicians, but little attention has been paid to the possible oversupply of health administration executives.

Since Michael Davis started the graduate program in hospital administration at the University of Chicago in 1934, both graduate and undergraduate programs in health administration have proliferated. In the early days of health administration education, placement of graduates was no problem because hospitals alone could absorb all of the students. Before the demands for employees by hospitals were met, the job opportunities were appearing in Blue Cross–Blue Shield, commercial insurance companies, state and federal government agencies, university teaching programs, and other related operations.

No estimates are available as to the oversupply, if any, of health administration graduates.

HEALTH COSTS AND THE GNP

One comparison that illustrates the rapid rise in health care costs is that of the costs and the gross national product. In pre-Medicare days (the

1950s), health care costs represented about 4.4% of the GNP. In 1967, after a full year of Medicare and Medicaid, the rate was 6.4%. Thereafter the rate rose rapidly, reaching 10.5% in 1982. Panelists in the Arthur Andersen–ACHE study predicted a leveling off at about 12% in the period from 1990 to 1995.

Another measurement is the relationship between the rise in health care costs and the rise in the consumer price index. For many years health care costs have been rising faster than the CPI. Respondents look for a narrowing of the difference but expect health care costs to continue rising faster.

HMOS AND OTHER COMPETITIVE MEDICAL PLANS

There are over 400 HMOs in the United States with a variety of operating plans, but basically they are capitation plans for hospital and medical care. The growth in new plans has been phenomenal in the past few years, and they have become highly competitive. Growth is likely to continue at a slower rate.

There can be an analogy drawn for the present HMO growth and competition with that of the American automobile industry early in this century. At that time there were 300 to 400 automobile manufacturers, many with imperfect products, some precariously underfinanced, with poor facilities and inexperienced management. By the time the Ford Model T was introduced in 1908, many companies had closed up shop because they were not strong enough to compete. Hundreds of companies were started, but only the Big Four survived.

Many HMOs, PPOs, IPAs, and other competitive medical plans are going to find it impossible to cope with such competitors as Blue Cross–Blue Shield, Kaiser-Permanente, large insurance companies, investor-owned chains, and intrenched and well-financed independents. Those insurers are going to make it difficult for newcomers to enter or for small, underfinanced, and poorly managed plans to survive.

Thus, the authors predict a shakedown in the capitation insurance business. The surviving companies will need to offer national insurance coverage to satisfy the national corporations that have employees across the country.

Already Blue Cross–Blue Shield is building a national network, with over 30 HMOs at present and with PPOs being formed in addition. Blue Cross–Blue Shield has tried to operate on a local community service basis. This community tie may be to the advantage of the Blues in developing standard and alternative plans.

Kaiser-Permanente is no longer solely a California or Pacific Coast operation. It is growing and spreading in the Southwest, in the mountain states, in the Midwest, in New England, and it is moving into cities along the eastern seaboard.

Investor-owned hospital corporations have widespread hospital management-ownership systems that could develop into national networks. Some of the large insurance companies have extensive experience in health insurance and have national insurance systems plus large, available financial assets.

A shakedown is imminent. It seems likely that merger and purchase will be the methods of network building more than elimination of competition through bankruptcy or discontinuance. The surviving form no doubt will be a capitation plan or plans under which groups and individuals can be enrolled for a premium of "so much a head" to cover complete hospital and medical care. National groups may be organized in a number of regional subdivisions for adjustments in rates to accommodate differences in regional costs and patient mix.

The optimal health insurance plan will be a system (or systems) that offers coverage anywhere in the nation and has arrangements with federal and state governments for the inclusion of Medicare and Medicaid enrollees. This optimal plan will be the goal, will be pluralistic, and will be within the private sector.

Hospitals are not likely to continue, as some do now, to operate in or own capitation plans. The present hospital plans are more likely to contract with large, surviving capitation plans, sell their plants to those plans, or merge into larger hospital complexes.

Physicians will adjust to the optimal goal by sharing in the capitation plan on either a salary or a partnership basis. Physicians will have better hours of work and freedom from most paper work and insurance reports— with the added benefit of malpractice insurance coverage.

The shakedown and the movement toward merger of insurance plans are inevitable. How many survivors there will be is unknown, but they will be competitive and will offer national coverage with regional adjustment.

The capitation concept will prevail until a better idea comes along— which is likely in the future.

HOME CARE

The practice of visiting public health nurses delivering home care is not new. For many years there have been published accounts of frontier nurses on horseback in Appalachia making nursing care visits to patients in remote areas. Nearly 25 years ago, Blue Cross of Michigan approved a benefit for home care nursing, hospital-based, in a rural county in Michigan, and since that time home care including nursing, homemaking, and physical therapy has become quite common in city and rural settings.

Home care can be delivered at a lower cost than inpatient service and with more satisfaction, generally, to the patient and family. Home care is a growth project for the future.

HOSPICE SERVICE

Nursing service and personal care for the terminally ill with a projected life of six months or less will be extended and refined in the coming years. The basic appeal of hospice service is that patients can spend their last days at home with their families, supported by nursing and therapy care from the hospice headquarters. Provision is made for trips by the patient to the hospital for short stays for inpatient care or during a respite for the person in the home caring for the patient.

Hospices have originated both from hospitals and from independent entities. It is expected that continued growth for hospice service will occur at both sources.

HOSPITAL SUBSIDIARIES

Hospitals will continue to develop new subsidiaries for the purpose of generating profits outside the hospital proper. Many hospitals have built professional office buildings, public restaurants, adjoining motel-like facilities for visitors and patients' families. Some hospitals have sold contract services to other facilities such as purchasing, laundry, therapy, mobile imaging, personnel management, data processing, billing, and insurance processing. These have been set up as subsidiary operations. This will be a growth activity.

HOSPITAL TRUSTEES

Precarious times can be ahead when strategic planning, financial expertise, and management experience make necessary an examination of the quality of hospital trustees.

There is no uniform method of selection of trustees, but appointments should be based on ability to contribute strength and knowledge to the board. The hospital in turn should offer continuing education about hospital operation to both new and long-serving trustees.

Some observers seem to think trustees of investor-owned hospitals might have more expertise and might be more willing to contribute time and effort to board and committee meetings. Trustees should be selected with as much care as corporate executives are. It has been advocated by some who are knowledgeable of hospital affairs that hospital trustees should be paid honoraria for their services as other corporate board members are. In the future, whatever the method or terms of serving, trustees should be chosen for ability rather than popularity in the community.

INFORMATION RESOURCE CENTER

The American Hospital Association has developed a Resource Center combining an unusual library book collection, a hospital historical book and photograph collection (with the collaboration of the American College of Healthcare Executives), the beginnings of an archival repository of papers and memorabilia, plus a data bank of the hospital field, and a 51-volume oral history collection of interviews with persons who helped shape the present health care system.

The Resource Center also offers a bibliographical search service (with connections to the National Library of Medicine). Services are available to clients, as well as an interlibrary loan system for books and documents. The Resource Center will continue in development in future years.

INFORMATION SYSTEMS

Information systems are still in the early stages of development. Any system of future decades is likely to surpass any that is commonly imagined today. The computer invasion is far from complete but promises greater access to internal and external data.

INSURANCE GOOD RISKS

Special health insurance has been designed to reward persons considered good risks with lower rates or refunds. Good risks could be nonsmokers, nondrinkers, persons with blood pressure in a normal range. Monitoring the performance of the good risks might pose a problem; they might have to be monitored after the fact.

In the future, if the plan tends to make individuals live more sensibly, then it will be worthwhile.

INVESTOR-OWNED

The share of hospital beds in investor-owned hospitals in the United States will continue to enlarge in the short-term future but probably at a much slower rate than during the first five years of the 1980s. There will be a trend toward management contracts between investor-owned corporations and large teaching hospitals including university medical centers and specialized institutions such as psychiatric hospitals.

The investor-owned corporations will continue to diversify within the field. Emphasis will be put on widening HMO operations and health insurance activity generally. The broad need for nursing home beds will be addressed, particularly as financing for domiciliary care can be found either through insurance or state or federal aid.

Another attractive opportunity for the investor-owned will be housing for retired persons which offers pleasant living accommodations and health care service on the site. There are many affluent seniors who can afford a monthly fee. Two or three levels of care can be offered through which a guest can move as he advances in age and declines physically—from free movement and ambulatory care to bed care.

Investor-owned health corporations will continue to expand by acquiring supply companies such as hospital supply companies and drug wholesalers and manufacturers which are important to the corporations' operations. operations.

In many states investor-owned or investor-operated facilities are clustered close enough for regional operations within the corporation. This will make possible regional technology centers where expensive equipment can be shared or from which mobile units can operate. Shared services will be refined, and exchange of personnel in sharing operations will also be strengthened.

Investor-owned corporations will be so diversified and programmed that they will be able to shift and move with health care delivery changes under the pressures of demand and rising costs.

JOINT COMMISSION ON ACCREDITATION
OF HOSPITALS

For over 40 years the JCAH has monitored hospitals and hospital activities with significant success. In the past decade the Joint Commission has been working closely with long-term facilities, psychiatric units, and institutions for the retarded. Now in the future possibly the JCAH could look into some problems that seem related to its present work. Is the Commission considering nursing homes and ambulatory units not connected with an approved hospital? Can the JCAH supplement the AMA's efforts to oversee the credentialing of physicians?

It has been suggested that the Commission should look at quality of care in terms of "outcome quality." Would this complement PRO activities? Is there a possibility of the JCAH entering the PRO field?

The JCAH has served as an accrediting body that has satisfied federal and state governments in most incidents. It would seem likely that the Commission would try to cover in an examination of an institution all conditions of interest to the various government bodies so that "policing" could be in the private sector.

MALPRACTICE INSURANCE

One of the largest overhead expenses for a physician is malpractice insurance. Premium rates to cover malpractice have risen so rapidly in the past few years that some specialists (OB-GYNs and neurosurgeons particularly) in metropolitan areas pay premiums of $100,000 or more annually. This is true if the physician can find an insurer, for some companies are discontinuing insurance to cover malpractice.

Physicians will have to find a new source for malpractice insurance if commercial firms withdraw. Some groups, such as the Hospital Association of Pennsylvania, have formed insurance companies to protect member hospitals and their staffs. Some of the multihospital systems can pool insurance funds and self-insure. Some of the larger investor-owned chains have their own insurance facilities. Other capitation plans, Kaiser-Permanente for example, can offer insurance protection to the physicians in their groups.

Many attorneys take malpractice cases with the understanding that a legal fee is payable only on the winning of an award, in or out of court. This so-called contingency fee usually is based on a fairly high percentage of any award. Some observers believe the contingency fee encourages patients to sue greedily. Some persons believe juries are likely to make large awards to plaintiffs because the award money is coming from an impersonal, faceless, rich insurance corporation, and thus no individual is being harmed.

The contingency fee arrangement is not used in the same manner in Canada. There, malpractice suits are less numerous and awards are smaller than in the United States.

Several suggestions have been offered to reduce huge malpractice awards: have malpractice cases heard before a panel of judges; have recommendations made by a commission of experts; eliminate or reduce the contingency fee; set up a strict policy of credentialing and oversight of physicians by the American Medical Association.

A balance is needed to assure integrity on the part of practitioners and institutions, but with protection of the welfare of the patient.

MEANS TEST

A means test for participating in health care and other social programs is an anathema to liberals who look upon social programs as being available to all regardless of level of income. A means test, under any euphemism, will become more common as health care costs continue to rise. Persons who have adequate income will be expected to pay a portion of the costs of care above the deductibles and copayments that all have to pay (in Medicare, for instance). There has been a means test in Medicaid since it became operative in 1966.

The Internal Revenue Service started collecting income tax in 1984 on Social Security payments from those whose incomes were in the higher brackets. This may be a means test in reverse, but the principle is the same: those who have the means will have to help pay their way for health and social services in the future.

MEDICAID GATEKEEPER

Some infringements of rules have been observed among Medicaid beneficiaries particularly in metropolitan areas. Some of these individuals have been going to more than one physician and have been receiving medications through more than one doctor.

Under the gatekeeper principle the beneficiary is assigned to a primary doctor who treats the patient as needed and refers the patient to a specialist as needed. It is believed that the gatekeeper will reduce, if not eliminate, duplication of service.

MEDICAL EDUCATION—TEACHING HOSPITALS

The teaching hospital is placed in a noncompetitive position in situations where other hospitals are giving discount contracts to HMOs and other capitation plans. Teaching hospitals are more costly to operate.

One offsetting feature is that teaching hospitals treat serious and unusual cases that cannot be treated suitably in less specialized treatment centers.

Medical education costs both in the medical school and in the teaching hospital have been a perennial problem for which there seems to be no easy solution.

MEDICARE

Medicare copayments and deductibles are rising so fast that the time will come soon when a means test, direct or indirect,[1] will have to be used. Those who can afford to pay part or all of the costs of Medicare will be able to do it directly, through a special insurance, or through a tax on Social Security payments.

MULTIHOSPITAL SYSTEMS

In many parts of the country, groups of hospitals have associated under a corporate umbrella or under a contract arrangement. The "multis" sometimes are chains of hospitals under one ownership or one management. Some of the groups are church affiliated, some are nonchurch and not-for-profit, others are investor-owned and investor-managed.

Still another approach is for a large hospital to build a satellite system with a group of smaller hospitals owned or operated by the parent hospital.

Such multihospital systems can benefit from the use of shared services such as purchasing, accounting and auditing services, personnel department expertise, diagnostic and therapeutic technology, data processing,

---

[1]The plan started in 1984 of levying income tax on Social Security payments of the affluent may set the pattern for an indirect means test.

administrative pools, specialized medical service referral, financial management, and access to capital. The advantages to group pooling are self-evident and will be developed still further in the future.

NATIONAL HEALTH INSURANCE

For the short-term future, national health insurance does not appear to be a strong issue. The Medicare experience shows that a way has not been found to control health care costs. National health insurance would probably aggravate the problem.

NURSING

The nurse will continue to grow professionally, will be better educated, and will be better recompensed. The long-term goals of nursing leaders are a baccalaureate degree in nursing as a minimum, greater professional responsibility in carrying out prescribed nursing plans, and financial recognition of the professional contributions of nurses.

ORGAN TRANSPLANTS

Organ transplantation has captured the imagination of the public as death-defying surgery with the possible dramatic saving of a patient from an early death.

Problems with transplantations must be solved in the near future: the identification and registering of possible donors; and the training of physicians and technicians in the handling and preservation of donor organs. Organ banks must be operated on a nonprofit basis and offer fair access. Present registry and matching of donors and receivers will be improved.

Not every organ can be transplanted with the same chance of success. There has been more success, for example, in transplanting kidneys than in transplanting livers.

Another factor in transplantation is the approval of third parties on the site and surgical teams for each kind of transplant. For example, a medical center might be approved to do a kidney transplant but not a liver transplant.

The costs for this type of surgery are very high, in some cases exceeding $100,000. However, the cost of insurance coverage is usually only a few dollars a month. The low cost of insurance can be explained because the incidence of the procedure is rare when considered in the population as a whole.

Organ transplantation and artificial organ implantation will continue to be experimental, and one hopes that the rate and length of survival will increase.

OVERCAPACITY

There have been at least two major causes of overbedding or excess capacity in hospitals: overconstruction, and reduced utilization due particularly to change in reimbursement methods which reduced hospital admissions. The present bed supply in the United States is about 4.6 per 1,000 population. In contrast to this, the Kaiser-Permanente Health Plan has set a standard of 1.1 beds per 1,000 subscribers and finds it works well.

The result of overbedding is that many hospitals are operating at 60% of capacity or less. Low occupancy levels are uneconomic and costly. It is expected that some of the hospitals operating at low levels will be forced to close or to change to another type of operation such as long-term care or intermediate care (nursing home care).

PHYSICIAN OVERSUPPLY

The American Medical Association Master File listed over 500,000 medical doctors in the United States in the early 1980s. With American medical schools graduating 15,000 to 16,000 new physicians a year, there will be an oversupply of doctors before the year 2000. There have been various estimates of the oversupply by the end of the century, ranging from a low of 30,000 to a high of 144,000.

The oversupply has come about because of a fear in the 1950s and 1960s that there would be a severe shortage of physicians. This fear led to the establishment of a number of new American medical schools. The rise in the number of graduates of American medical schools, plus an influx of graduates of foreign medical schools, is causing what some have labeled a physician "glut."

One result of the large increase of medical doctors will be that some of the new doctors will tend to locate in medically underserved areas: rural areas and innercity neighborhoods of the big cities. Another result may be that new doctors will seek salaried jobs in HMOs and in government posts.

Questions come to mind. How will medical practices be affected? Will doctors have fewer patients? Will doctors schedule more appointments with their patients than they have in the past? Will doctors' incomes be affected? Will doctors with established practices be less likely to be seriously affected than new doctors?

Doctors will suffer somewhat in income. There will be fewer patients per doctor. Overhead and insurance will be higher in proportion to gross income. More frequent patient visits will not be called for, because patient visits have risen in the past decade or so from two or three visits to a doctor per year to over five at the present time.

No doubt medical schools, particularly the newer ones, will be forced by circumstances to reduce class size to prevent the oversupply from worsening.

PLANNING AND CERTIFICATE OF NEED

Planning for health care delivery must be done expertly and, one hopes, through a supervisory body that has authority to approve or disapprove large construction plans or major equipment purchase; otherwise the system could be costly and inefficient.

A recent incident in one of the larger states illustrates a way that even planning authority can be circumvented. According to a newspaper account, state authorities decided that three of the new lithotriptors for breaking up kidney and ureteral stones and calculi by extracorporeal shock waves would be sufficient to serve the state and adjoining areas. The three largest general hospitals in the state applied for permission to purchase the machines, which with installation and site construction would cost about two million dollars each. The three hospitals did not wait for approval to purchase but bought and installed the equipment and trained staffs. Some patients were alleged to have been treated without cost while the hospitals waited for approval.

On the face of it this would seem to be a status struggle to maintain leadership in services over competing hospitals. Unfortunately for patients, all three hospitals are in the largest metropolitan area of the state, which is at the extreme end of one of the longest states. The big city will probably be overserved while the rest of the state, with medical centers, will go unserved, at least conveniently. This condition of ignoring approval processes should be corrected.

PREVENTIVE MEDICINE

Before World War II, many advances in health care came through public health oriented preventive medicine. There was widespread immunization for diseases for which biologicals had been found. In fact, it was the age of biologicals in which it seemed that vaccines, immunogens, or serums might be found to prevent or treat most infectious diseases.

During wartime, a dramatic therapeutic change took place. Penicillin, streptomycin, and sulfa drugs came into use to treat many difficult or previously untreatable diseases. A great search began for other antibiotics, other forms of sulfa, other synthetic drugs. Research was supported both by commercial drug firms and by the federal government.

Since World War II, knowledge in most facets of medical care and technology has blossomed. However, now the nation is faced with other public health needs. New educational efforts are needed to convince Americans to live healthful lives, reducing the use of tobacco and alcohol, and refusing to become part of the drug culture. The spread of AIDS must be stopped before it becomes epidemic.

REPRESENTATION

There is no longer a single focus of representation for American hospitals at local, state, and national levels. At the present time and for the foreseeable future, the American Hospital Association has more members, more staff, more extensive information facilities, and more political influence than any other hospital group.

However, the Federation of American Health Systems represents investor-owned hospitals, Voluntary Hospitals of America is a bloc of not-for-profit institutions, and Associated Hospital Systems speaks for a group of multihospital organizations on a national basis. Also but smaller in membership, many church hospital groups—Catholic, Protestant, Lutheran, Methodist—have organizations to represent them.

There are many metropolitan and regional hospital groups that work within their areas of interest and lobby and work with the national hospital associations.

There are many other health professional groups particularly among health care executives in the United States that need representation but do not have the necessary power alone to make a desired impression on government and community. There is a beginning movement for an umbrella organization that not only will represent several groups but also will offer educational programs to elevate members of those professions. The movement is headed by the American College of Healthcare Executives (formerly the American College of Hospital Administrators). ACHE is offering its considerable strength in organization and continuing education to draw many of the smaller professional groups under its umbrella. It would seem that the ACHE umbrella organization in the future would stress continuing education and work closely with the American Hospital Association and others in national representation.

RIGHT TO DIE

At a time when definitions of life and death have not been determined fully under law, Americans are frustrated in trying to cope with "the right to die."

The media often give coverage to the "heroic measures" taken to sustain breathing in patients who are in a suspended state, and who, no doubt, would stop breathing if artificial aids were discontinued.

Until a resolution is made, the right to die is a problem that will be faced by the courts, physicians, clergy, health institutions, Medicare, and insurance companies. Many individuals in soundness of mind want to make a will empowering their executors to order the end of any efforts to prolong breathing when medical experts attest recovery from a vegetative state is hopeless.

RIGHT TO LIFE

The subject of abortion has created great controversy ranging from moral and religious arguments to the biological question of when life begins. It does not seem at present with the intense feelings among members of both sides of the argument—antiabortion and proabortion—that a resolution can be found that generally will be acceptable.

TAX ON HEALTH BENEFITS

Some action was taking place in early 1986 in Congress to tax health fringe benefits paid by employers. There does not seem much chance of this being enacted. A better argument will be made to tax any bonuses received by employees from employers or insurance companies for low use or nonuse of health care for any set period.

TECHNOLOGY

The key to the future of health care may lie in the rapid change in medical technology. When one looks backward a generation and sees the great changes in the care of the ill just during that period, through newly developed technology and advances in clinical practice resulting from that technology, one can only attempt to imagine what the state of the art will be in 2000 A.D.

UNEMPLOYED

During the 1970s a downturn in business in the heavy industries took place which caused the layoff of thousands of workers. There were provisions made by a few employers to continue health insurance for a few months of unemployment. Unfortunately, many other workers were left with no insurance coverage.

Proposals for including health insurance with unemployment benefits have been made. Whether health insurance would be extended to coincide with unemployment benefits is not clear. Also it is not certain if the expense of such a program could be funded by an addition to the employers' expense of unemployment insurance. Whatever the course of events, this is another health problem that must be acted on in the near term.

WELLNESS AND LIFESTYLE

One tragedy of life is that Americans do not live as sensibly as they know how to. Many overeat, do not get enough exercise, smoke too much, and do not get enough rest.

In a more serious vein, alcohol consumption is high, and the use of hard drugs is increasing rapidly. In fact, the country is spending billions of dollars a year to thwart the insidious habit of using hard drugs. It seems unbelievable that educated, intelligent, white collar people with better than average income are using drugs as part of a lifestyle. Those addicts who do not have sufficient income to support a habit often must resort to crime for needed money. These are problems health care must face: how to break the addiction of these unfortunate persons and how to educate the population as to the perils of drug use.

WOMEN IN THE HEALTH PROFESSIONS

At the present time admissions of women to health profession schools are increasing greatly. Many medical schools, particularly the newer ones, have beginning enrollments of women of nearly 50%. Pharmacy schools and health administration programs likewise have heavy enrollments of women. The effect this increased enrollment of women will have is unknown. The patterns of women's medical specializations are not fully formed either. Will women in medicine seek to specialize in internal medicine, OB-GYN, pediatrics, or will women follow a specialty distribution similar to males? Will women medical graduates follow the predominant pattern of nurses: work the first few years of practice, then take time out to raise a family, and later return to practice?

Whatever the future holds, women in medicine will tend to be a positive and lasting influence.

POSTSCRIPT

There will be many problems in health care delivery in the closing years of the century. Some of the problems have been outlined above.

In spite of the cost of care, uncertainty about reimbursement, worry over the federal government as third party and regulator, the authors are optimistic. Progress will be made in spite of problems. Health care will be widespread, and technological and clinical advances in treatment of illness will move the art of medicine closer to scientific certainty.

Glossary

Accelerated Depreciation.   Depreciation methods that write off the cost of an asset at a faster rate than the write-off under the straight-line method. The two principal methods of accelerated depreciation are (1) sum-of-years digits and (2) double declining balance.

Accounting.   The art of recording, classifying, and summarizing in a significant manner and in terms of money transactions which are, at least in part, of a financial character—and interpreting the results thereof.

Accounting Costs.   All tangible costs that can be measured in terms of release of value.

Accounts Receivable.   Amounts due from patients for services rendered to them.

Accrual-Basis Accounting.   An accounting system wherein revenue is recorded in the accounting period in which it is earned, whether or not cash has been received, and expenses are recorded in the accounting period in which they are used or consumed in producing revenue, whether or not cash is disbursed in the payment of those expenses.

Accruals.   Continually recurring short-term liabilities. Examples are accrued wages, accrued taxes, and accrued interest.

Accrued Interest.   Interest earned on a bond issue from the dated date to the date of delivery. Accrued interest is credited to the issuer at delivery.

Aging Schedule.   A report showing how long accounts receivable have been outstanding. It gives the percent of receivables not past due and the percent past due by, for example, one month, two months, or other periods.

Algebraic Method.   A cost finding technique involving the simultaneous distribution of general service cost center costs to both general service and final cost centers.

Amortize.   To liquidate on an installment basis; an amortized loan is one in which the principal amount of the loan is repaid in installments during the life of the loan.

Asked Price.   The price at which bonds are offered to potential buyers.

Assignment.   A relatively inexpensive way of liquidating a failing firm that does not involve going through the courts.

Authority.   A municipal or state entity formed through a special legislative act to perform the specific function of distribution of bonds.

Bad Debt.   An account that is charged off due to the fact that it is unpaid, although the patient has the ability to pay.

Balloon Payment.   When a debt is not fully amortized, the final payment is larger than the preceding payments and is called a balloon payment.

Bank Line.   The funds that a bank keeps available to a borrower, which can use some or all of its line at any time.

Bankruptcy.   A legal procedure for formally liquidating a business, carried out under the jurisdiction of a court of law.

Basis Point.   One basis point is equal to one one-hundredth of one percent or .01%.

Benefit.   A payment or service provided under an insurance policy or prepayment plan. In the case of Blue Cross, payment is made directly to the hospital on behalf of all patients who are covered. Commercial insurers make payment either to the hospital or to the patient.

Best Efforts Underwriting.   A relationship in which the underwriter acts as agent for the issuer and there is no commitment to purchase any of the bonds. If the underwriter has given a firm commitment, he is acting as principal and has agreed to buy the entire issue.

Bid.   The price a buyer offers to pay for bonds; the price at which the seller may dispose of them.

Bond.   A long-term debt instrument.

Bond Discount (or Debt Discount).   Amount by which the selling (or purchase) price is less than the face value of a bond or other form of indebtedness.

Bond Premium (or Debt Premium).   Amount by which the selling (or purchase) price exceeds the face value of a bond or other form of indebtedness.

Book Value.   The value of an asset as shown in the accounting records of a firm.

Capital.   The capital of a hospital includes the long-term debt (including current portion of long-term debt and capital equipment leases), capitalized leases, and both restricted and unrestricted fund balances. Pro forma capitalization reflects these categories after giving effect to proposal financing.

Capital Asset.   An asset with a life of more than one year that is not bought and sold in the ordinary course of business.

Capital Budgeting.   The process of planning expenditures on assets whose returns are expected to extend beyond one year.

Capital Rationing.   A situation in which a constraint is placed on the total size of the capital investment during a particular period.

Capital Structure.   The permanent long-term financing of the firm. Capital structure is distinguished from *financial structure*, which includes short-term debt plus all reserve accounts.

Capitalization Rate.　A discount rate used to find the present value of a series of future cash receipts; sometimes called *discount rate*.

Cash Budget.　A schedule showing cash flows (receipts, disbursements, and net cash) for a firm over a specified period.

Cash Cycle.　The length of time between the purchase of raw materials and the receipt of the cash generated by the sale of the final product.

Cash Inflows.　Revenues actually received by the hospital.

Cash Outflows.　Expenses actually paid by the hospital.

Certificate of Need (CON).　A confirmation, usually legal in nature, by an approved agency that a proposal for establishing a program or constructing a facility meets an estimated unmet need in a defined service area.

Chart of Accounts.　A listing of accounts and titles, with numerical symbols, employed in a compilation of financial data concerning the assets, liabilities, capital, revenues, and expenses of an enterprise.

Chattel Mortgage.　A mortgage on personal property (not real estate). A mortgage on equipment would be a chattel mortgage.

Collateral.　Assets that are used to secure a loan.

Commercial Paper.　Unsecured, short-term promissory notes of large firms, usually issued in denominations of $1 million or more. The rate of interest on commercial paper is typically somewhat below the prime rate of interest.

Compensating Balances.　Cash deposits required by a bank as partial compensation for lending and other services that it provides to a hospital.

Compound Interest.　An interest rate that is applicable when interest in succeeding periods is earned not only on the initial principal, but also on the accumulated interest of prior periods. Compound interest is contrasted to *simple interest,* in which returns are not earned on interest received.

Compounding.　The arithmetic process of determining the final value of a payment or a series of payments when compound interest is applied.

Conditional Sales Contract.　A method of financing new equipment by paying it off in installments over a one- to five-year period. The seller retains title to the equipment until payment has been completed.

Continuous Compounding (Discounting).　As opposed to discrete compounding, interest is added continuously rather than at discrete points in time.

Corporate Strategy.　The hospital's mission statement, or statement of purpose, and the program directives that flow from and are held together by the mission statement. Included within the corporate strategy are also overall financial guidelines and financial guidelines for each program directive.

Cost.　The monetary valuation applied to an asset or service that has been obtained by an expenditure of cash or by a commitment to make a future expenditure.

Cost-Based Reimbursement.　The reimbursement approach sometimes used by third party payers. Under this approach, the third party pays the hospital for the care received by covered patients at cost, with the expense elements included and excluded from cost determined by the third party.

Cost Finding. The process of apportioning or allocating the costs of the non-revenue-producing cost centers to each other and to the revenue-producing cost centers on the basis of the statistical data that measure the amount of service rendered by each center to the other centers.

Cost of Capital. The discount rate that should be used in the capital budgeting process.

Cost-Plus Contract. A type of agreement widely used in construction, in which the owner agrees to pay for all costs incurred by the contractor in executing the plans and specifications, plus an additional amount (fixed sum, percentage, or other arrangement) as fee or profit.

Coupon Rate. The stated annual rate of interest that the borrower promised to pay to the bond holder.

Current Yield. The percent relation of the annual interest received to the price of the bond.

Debenture. A long-term debt instrument that is not secured by a mortgage on specific property.

Default. The failure to fulfill a contract. Generally, default refers to the failure to pay interest or principal on debt obligations.

Depreciation. The annual estimated cost of expired services of fixed assets.

Direct Distribution. A cost finding technique involving the distribution of general service cost center costs directly to final cost centers.

Discounting. The process of finding the present value of a series of future cash flows. Discounting is the reverse of compounding.

Discounting of Accounts Receivable. Short-term financing arrangement in which accounts receivable are used to secure the loan. The lender *does not* buy the accounts receivable, but simply uses them as collateral for the loan. Also called *pledging of accounts receivable.*

Division Directive. The "linking pin" between program directives and operating objectives. It is a specific, measurable, or verifiable statement of desired results or accomplishments for a program area subunit, that is, a division.

Double Distribution. A cost finding technique involving the distribution of general service cost center costs first to the appropriate general service centers and then to final cost centers.

Economic Cost. The full cost of operations. It includes both tangible and intangible costs.

Economic Order Quantity (EOQ). The optimum (least cost) quantity of merchandise that should be purchased in any single order.

Endowment Fund. The account group used to record transactions arising from funds that have been given to the hospital and for which a moral and legal responsibility exists to comply with the terms of the endowment.

Equity. The net worth of an enterprise.

Expected Return. The rate of return a firm expects to realize from an investment. The expected return is the mean value of the probability distribution of possible returns.

Expenses. Costs that have been used or consumed in carrying on some activity and from which no measurable benefit will extend beyond the present. In the broadest sense, expense includes all expired costs.

Factoring. A method of financing accounts receivable in which a firm sells its accounts receivable (generally without recourse) to a financial institution (the *factor*).

Federal National Mortgage Association (FNMA) (Fannie Mae). A federal agency that purchases FHA insured mortages to assure a wider secondary market for such securities.

Financial Structure. The entire right-hand side of the balance sheet—the way in which a firm is financed.

Fixed Assets. Assets of a relatively permanent nature held for continuous use in hospital operations and not intended to be converted into cash through sale.

Fixed Charges. Costs that do not vary with the level of output.

Full Financial Requirements. Those resources that are not only necessary to meet current operating needs, but also sufficient to permit replacement of the physical plant when appropriate and to allow for changing community health and patient needs, education and research, and all other factors necessary to the institutional provision of health care services that must be recognized and supported by all purchasers of care.

Fund Accounting. A system of accounting wherein the hospital's resources, obligations, and capital balances are segregated into logical account groups according to legal restrictions and administrative requirements. Each account group, or fund, constitutes a subordinate accounting entity, created and maintained for a particular purpose.

Funded Debt. Long-term debt.

General Fund. The account group used to record transactions arising out of the general operations and the regular day-to-day operations of the hospital.

General Obligation. A bond secured by pledge of the issuer's full faith, credit, and taxing power.

Goals. The general ends or directions that are established for the hospital, the attainment of which will help to further the hospital's mission. Goals are designed to identify end states that are desired over a period of years and are likely to be altered less often than objectives, but more often than the hospital's mission.

Goodwill. Intangible assets of a firm established by the excess of the price paid for the going concern over its book value.

Government National Mortgage Association (GNMA) (Ginnie Mae). A federal agency that issues its own securities on the open market, backed by the yields on federally insured mortgages.

Health Care Institution. An establishment with permanent facilities and with medical services for patients; the forms of such an establishment include inpatient care institutions, outpatient care institutions with organized medical staffs, and home care institutions.

Indenture. A formal agreement between the issuer of a bond and the bond holders.

Insolvency.   The inability to meet mature or due obligations.

Internal Control.   The plan of organization of all the coordinated methods and measures adopted within a business to safeguard its assets, check the accuracy and reliability of its accounting data, promote operating efficiency, and encourage a change to prescribed managerial policies.

Internal Rate of Return (IRR).   The rate of return on an asset investment. The internal rate of return is calculated by finding the discount rate that equates the present value of future cash flows to the cost of the investment.

Investment Banker.   Also known as an underwriter, is the middleman between the issuer and the public market. The investment banker usually functions as principal rather than agent and initially purchases all of the bonds from the issuer.

Line of Credit.   An arrangement whereby a financial institution commits itself to lend up to a specified maximum amount of funds during a specified period.

Liquid.   Refers to the ability to sell marketable securities rapidly, without a loss in principal.

Liquidity.   Refers to a firm's cash position and its ability to meet maturing obligations.

Lock-Box Plan.   A procedure used to speed up collections and to reduce float.

Major Third Party Payers.   Organized groups or government programs that usually pay hospitals directly for the hospital services provided to group members or program beneficiaries.

Marginal Cost.   The cost of an additional unit. The *marginal cost of capital* is the cost of an additional dollar of new funds.

Market Research.   The techniques for learning the needs and wants of people, their preferences as to how they wish to satisfy those desires, and their attitude toward the organization and its services. The aim of market research activities is to provide the hospital with information that will help it to make decisions which result in its being able to deliver greater satisfaction to its target markets or community.

Marketable Security.   Short-term financial instrument that can be bought or sold readily, without a loss in principal. Often used as a short-term investment alternative for temporary surplus cash balances.

Marketing.   The applied science concerned with the successful management of exchange relationships and transactions between and among significant groups both inside and outside the hospital. An exchange relationship is the offering of something of value to someone in exchange for something of value. In the eyes of each party to the exchange transaction, what is given up is of less value than what is received. Included in the marketing discipline are such activities as: market research; product development (product design and testing); promotion (advertising, sales, pricing); distribution; communications.

Mission.   A broad, general conception, defining the scope of the hospital's role. Equivalent to *purpose*.

Mission Statement.   A formal document presenting the hospital's mission in language developed for both internal and external audiences (also referred to as *statement of purpose*).

Money Market. Financial market in which funds are borrowed or loaned for short periods. (The money market is distinguished from the capital market, which is the market for long-term funds.)

Mortgage. A pledge of designated property as security for a loan.

Municipal Bond. A bond issued by a state or a political subdivision, such as a county, city, or village. The term also refers to bonds issued by state agencies and authorities. Generally, interest paid on municipal bonds is exempt from federal income taxes. The term municipal bond is usually synonymous with *tax-exempt bond.*

Negotiated Underwriting. A private sale of bonds by the issuer as contrasted to an advertisement for public bids. Most hospital bond underwritings are negotiated due to special marketing considerations.

Net Worth. The capital and surplus of a firm.

Objective. Specific end representing measurable results that are to be achieved at a specific time. Objectives are designed to contribute directly to the attainment of goals. Objectives may be altered frequently.

Objective Probability Distributions. Probability distributions determined by statistical procedures.

Opportunity Cost. The rate of return on the best *alternative* investment that is available. It is the highest return that will *not* be earned if the funds are invested in a particular project.

Overstocked. A condition wherein inventory stocks exceed demand.

Par Value. The face amount of the bond. The amount of money due at maturity—usually $1,000.

Plant Fund. Account group used to record the transactions involving the hospital's investment in land, buildings, and equipment.

Pledging of Accounts Receivable. Short-term borrowing from financial institutions when the loan is secured by accounts receivable. The lender may physically take the accounts receivable but typically has recourse to the borrower; also called *discounting of accounts receivable.*

Points. The same as *percentage.* In the case of a bond, a point means $10 since a bond is quoted as a percentage of $1,000. A bond or bond issue that is discounted two points is quoted at 98% of its par value.

Prepayment Provision. The provision in the bond or mortgage indenture that specifies at what time and on what terms repayment of principal amount may be made prior to maturity.

Present Value (PV). The value today of a future payment, or stream of payments, discounted at the appropriate discount rate.

Prime Rate. The rate of interest commercial banks charge very large, strong corporations.

Private Placement. The placement of an issue in the private (that is, nonpublic) money market. This private market comprises different types of financial institution (banks, life insurance companies, pension funds, real estate investment trusts).

Program Area. The group of activities all directed toward the same goal or end result.

Program Directive.   The specific desired results and constraints established for each program area. Program directives define the hospital's operational direction and provide an initial framework for operational planning and budgeting decision making.

Prospectus.   Commonly, a written document conforming to state and federal regulations containing disclosures about a business entity that is seeking additional debt or equity financing, together with information about the terms and purposes of the financing.

Rate of Return.   The internal rate of return on an investment.

Recourse Arrangement.   A term used in connection with accounts receivable financing. If a firm sells its accounts receivable to a financial institution under a recourse agreement, then if an account receivable cannot be collected, the selling firm must repurchase the account from the financial institution.

Redemption Provision.   A provision allowing the issuer, at its option, to call the bonds at fixed price after a certain date.

Refunding.   New securities are sold by the issuer, and the proceeds are used to retire outstanding securities. The object may be to save interest cost, to extend the maturity of the debt, or to relax certain existing restrictive covenants.

Registered Bonds.   Bonds registered with the bond trustee, which designates ownership. Transfer of ownership of the bonds must be registered with the bond trustee so that new bond holders continue to receive principal and interest.

Regression Analysis.   A statistical procedure for predicting the value of one variable (dependent variable) on the basis of knowledge about one or more other variables (independent variables).

Relative Value.   Index number assigned to a procedure based upon the relative amount of labor, supplies, and capital needed to perform the procedure.

Responsibility Accounting.   An accounting system that accumulates and communicates historical and projected monetary and statistical data relating to revenues and controllable expenses, classified according to the organizational units producing the revenues and responsible for incurring the expenses.

Revenue Bond.   A bond payable solely from the revenue generated from the operation of the project being financed. In the case of hospital revenue bond financing, the bond is typically payable from the gross receipts of the hospital.

Salvage Value.   The value of a capital asset at the end of a specified period. It is the current market price of an asset being considered for replacement in a capital budgeting problem.

Self-Responsible Patient.   A patient who pays either all or part of his hospital bill from his own funds as opposed to third party funds.

Serial Bonds.   Not a distinct class of bonds but rather an issue of bonds with different maturities, as distinguished from an issue in which all the bonds have identical maturities (term bonds). Serial bonds are usually retired either in equal annual amounts or on a level debt service basis.

Series Bonds.   Secured by the same assets or revenue, but issued at intervals with different dates. They may or may not mature at the same time.

"63-20" Financing. A type of tax-exempt hospital financing requiring a special ruling from the Internal Revenue Service based upon a 1963 Ruling (#20). The bonds are issued by the hospital and, when they are fully retired, title is tendered to a municipality or other public body.

Step-Down. A cost finding technique involving a single distribution of general service cost centers to both general service and final cost centers.

Stock-Out. A condition wherein demand exists for an inventory item but none is available.

Subjective Probability Distributions. Probability distributions determined through subjective procedures without the use of objective data.

Subordinated Debenture. A bond having a claim on assets only after the senior debt has been paid off in the event of liquidation.

Tangible Assets. Physical assets as opposed to such intangible assets as goodwill and the stated value of patients.

Tax-Exempt Bond. A bond upon which the interest is exempt from federal income taxes.

Term Loan. A loan generally obtained from a bank or insurance company with a maturity greater than one year. Term loans are generally amortized.

Third Party Payer. An agency such as Blue Cross or the Medicare program which contracts with hospitals and patients to pay for the care of covered patients.

Trade Credit. Interfirm debt arising through credit sales and recorded as an account payable by the buyer.

Underwriter. Generally, one or more investment bankers who, for a fee, undertake to market a debt or equity security issue for the issuing entity or, in the case of a secondary offering, for the selling shareholders.

Working Capital. Refers to a firm's investment in short-term assets—cash, short-term securities, accounts receivable, and inventories. *Gross working capital* is defined as a firm's total current assets. *Net working capital* is defined as current assets minus current liabilities.

Wraparound Mortgage. A mortgage loan in which the lender takes a junior lien position, but undertakes to make the payments on the prior lien, usually without assuming any legal obligation to pay it. This device is used to leverage an additional loan by charging a higher rate of interest on both old and new balances, while paying only the lower prior rate.

Yield. The rate of return on an investment. Also called *internal rate of return.*

SOURCES

Segments of the glossary were adapted from the following sources:

Hay, Leon E. *Budgeting and Cost Analysis for Hospital Management.*

Lindsay, J. Robert and Sametz, Arnold W. *Financial Management: An Analytical Approach.*

Moyer, C.A. and Mautz, R.K. *Intermediate Accounting: A Functional Approach.*

Seawell, L. Vann. *Hospital Accounting and Financial Management.*
Seawell, L. Vann. *Principles of Hospital Accounting.*
Taylor, Philip J. and Nelson, Benjamin O. *Management Accounting for Hospitals.*
Topics in Health Care Financing. "Capital Financing," Fall 1978.
Weston, J. Fred and Brigham, Eugene F. *Managerial Finance.*

Bibliography

PART A

Abernethy, David S. and Pearson, David A. *Regulating Hospital Costs: The Development of Public Policy.* Ann Arbor, MI: Health Administration Press, 1979.

Aday, Lu Ann and Andersen, Ronald. *Development of Indices of Access to Medical Care.* Ann Arbor, MI: Health Administration Press, 1974.

Aday, Lu Ann; Andersen, Ronald; Loevy, Sara Segal; and Kremer, Barbara. *Hospital-Physician Sponsored Primary Care: Marketing and Impact.* Ann Arbor, MI: Health Administration Press, 1985.

Allcorn, Seth. *Internal Auditing for Hospitals.* Gaithersburg, MD: Aspen Systems, 1979.

Altmeyer, Arthur J. *The Formative Years of Social Security.* Madison, WI: University of Wisconsin Press, 1968.

American Hospital Association. *Capital Financing for Hospitals,* Chicago: The Association, 1974.

American Hospital Association. *Chart of Accounts for Hospitals.* Chicago: The Association, 1976.

American Hospital Association. *Cost Finding and Rate Setting for Hospitals.* Chicago: The Association, 1968.

American Hospital Association. Diagnosis Related Groups. Special Report #7. Chicago: The Association, 1983.

American Hospital Association. *Environmental Assessment of the Hospital Industry.* Chicago: The Association, 1979.

American Hospital Association. *Managerial Cost Accounting.* Chicago: The Association, 1980.

American Hospital Association. *Managing Under Medicare Prospective Pricing.* Chicago: The Association, 1983.

American Hospital Association. The Medicare Case Mix Index. Special Report #4. Chicago: The Association, 1983.

American Hospital Association. Medicare Payment: Cost Per Case Management. Special Report #1, Special Report #2. Chicago: The Association, August and October 1982.

American Hospital Association. Medicare Prospective Pricing. Summary of Regulations. Special Report #6. Chicago: The Association, 1983.

American Hospital Association. "Principles of Payment for Hospital Care." Chicago: The Association, 1963.

American Hospital Association. *Report of a Special Committee on the Provision of Health Services*. Chicago: The Association, 1970.

American Hospital Association. *Report of the Task Force on Principles of Payment for Hospital Care*. Chicago: The Association, 1963.

American Hospital Association. *Statement on the Financial Requirements of Health Care Institutions and Services*. Chicago: The Association, 1969, 1977, 1979.

American Hospital Association. Third-Party Audits of Hospital Bills. Technical Advisory Bulletin. Chicago: The Association, 1984.

American Hospital Association. Office of Public Policy Analysis. Hospital Economic Performance: 1981. Policy Brief #42. Chicago: The Association.

American Institute of Certified Public Accountants. *Hospital Audit Guide*. New York: The Institute, 1972.

Andersen, Ronald and Anderson, Odin W. *A Decade of Health Services*. Chicago: The University of Chicago Press, 1967.

Anderson, Odin W. *Blue Cross Since 1929: Accountability and Public Trust*. Cambridge, MA: Ballinger, 1975.

Anderson, Odin W. *Health Services in the United States: A Growth Enterprise Since 1875*. Ann Arbor, MI: Health Administration Press, 1985.

Anderson, Odin W. *The Uneasy Equilibrium*. New Haven, CT: College & University Press, 1968.

Anthony, Robert N. *Management Accounting*. Homewood, IL: Irwin, 1975.

Anthony, Robert N. and Herzlinger, Regina E. *Management Control in Nonprofit Organizations*. Homewood, IL: Irwin, 1975.

Anthony, Robert N. and Reese, James S. *Management Accounting, Sixth Edition*. Homewood, IL: Irwin, 1979.

Arbel, Avner and Grier, Paul. "Investment Generation Process in Hospital Facilities: The Response of Supply to Capacity Utilization Measures." *Health Services Research*, Fall 1979.

Archer, Stephen H. and D'Ambrosio, Charles A. *The Theory of Business Finance*. New York: Macmillan, 1967.

Association of University Programs in Health Administration. *Financial Management of Health Care Organizations: A Referenced Outline and Annotated Bibliography*. Washington, DC: The Association, 1978.

Austin, Charles J. *Information Systems for Hospital Administration, Second Edition*. Ann Arbor, MI: Health Administration Press, 1983.

Austin, Charles J. *The Politics of National Health Insurance*. San Antonio, TX: Trinity University Press, 1975.

Austin, Charles J. and Greene, Barry R. "Hospital Information Systems: A Current Perspective." *Inquiry,* June 1978.

Ball, Robert M. *Social Security: Today and Tomorrow.* New York: Columbia University Press, 1978.

Baumol, William J. "The Transactions Demand for Cash: An Inventory Theoretic Approach." *Quarterly Journal of Economics*, November 1952.

Beranek, William. *Analysis for Financial Decision.* Homewood, IL: Irwin, 1963.

Beranek, William. *Working Capital Management.* Belmont, CA: Wadsworth, 1966.

Berki, Sylvester E. *Hospital Economics.* Lexington, MA: Heath, 1972.

Berman, Howard J. "Financial Management: Necessity or Nicety?" *Hospital Administration*, Summer 1970.

Bernstein, Leopold A. *The Analysis of Financial Statements.* Homewood, IL: Dow Jones–Irwin, 1984.

Bisbee, Gerald E. and McCarthy, Margaret M. "Planning, Budgeting, and Cost Control in HMOs." *Inquiry*, Spring 1979.

Blue Cross Association–American Hospital Association. *Financing Health Care of the Aged:* Parts 1 and 2. Chicago: The Association, 1962.

The Boston Consulting Group, Inc. *Reimbursing Hospitals on Inclusive Rates.* Rockville, MD: The National Center for Health Services Research and Development, Department of Health, Education, and Welfare, 1971.

Bower, James B.; Connors, Edward J.; Mosher, John E.; and Rowley, Clyde S. *Hospital Income Flow: A Study of the Effects of Source of Pay on Hospital Income.* Madison, WI: Mimir Publishers, Inc. for The University of Wisconsin Graduate School of Business, 1970.

Brook, Robert H. *Quality of Care Assessment: A Comparison of Five Methods of Peer Review.* Washington, DC: Department of Health, Education, and Welfare, Pub. No. HRA-74-3100, 1973.

Brown, James K. and O'Connor, Rochelle. *Planning and the Corporate Planning Director.* New York: The Conference Board, 1974.

Brown, Ray E. *Judgment in Administration.* Hightstown, NJ: McGraw-Hill, 1966.

Bulletin of the Operations Research Society, Spring 1974.

Bureau of Public Health Economics and Department of Economics, The University of Michigan. *The Economics of Health and Medical Care.* Ann Arbor, MI: The Bureau, 1964.

Burik, David and Duvall, Paul J. "Hospital Cost Accounting." *Healthcare Financial Management*, February-April 1985.

Bursk, Edward C. and Chapman, John F. (eds.). *New Decision-Making Tools for Managers.* Cambridge, MA: Harvard University Press, 1971.

Calman, R.F. *Linear Programming and Cash Management: Cash ALPHA.* Cambridge, MA: The MIT Press, 1968.

Campion, Frank D. *The AMA and U.S. Health Policy Since 1940.* Chicago: Chicago Review Press, 1984.

Cannedy, Lloyd L. "How Hospitals Use Money Market Instruments." *Hospital Financial Management*, November 1969.

Carter, Eugene and DeKoff, Newton, "Health Insurance for the Aged: Number of Hospital and Extended Care Facility Admissions by State." *Research and Statistics Notes*, October 15, 1940.

Caruana, Russell A. *A Guide to Organizing the Hospital's Fiscal Services Division.* Chicago: Hospital Financial Management Association, 1974.

Caruana, Russell A. and McHugh, E. Thomas. "Comparing Ratios Shows Fiscal Trends." *Healthcare Financial Management*, Special Issue, 1981.

Chadwick, Edward G. "Special Report #5, Product Line Analysis." Chicago: American Hospital Association, 1983.

Choate, G. Marc. "Financial Ratio Analysis." *Hospital Progress*, January 1974.

Christie, A.C. *Economic Problems of Medicine*. New York: MacMillan, 1935.

Cleverley, William O. *Financial Management of Health Care Facilities*, Germantown, MD: Aspen Systems, 1975.

Cleverley, William O. "Financial Ratios: Summary Indicators for Management Decision Making." *Hospital and Health Services Administration*, Special Issue, 1981.

Cleverley, William O. and Nilsen, Karen. "Assessing Financial Position with 29 Key Ratios." *Healthcare Financial Management*, January 1980.

Cohodes, Donald R. "Hospital Capital Formation in the 1980s: Is There a Crisis?" *Journal of Health Policy and Law*, Spring 1983.

Coleman, John R.; Kaminsky, Frank C.; and McGee, Frank. "The State of the Art in Financial Modeling." *Hospital and Health Services Administration*, Spring 1980.

Commission on Professional and Hospital Activities. *International Classification of Diseases, 9th Revision, Clinical Modification (ICD–9–CM)*. Ann Arbor, MI: CPHA, 1979.

The Committee for National Health Insurance. *Facts of Life: Health and Health Insurance*. Washington, DC: The Committee, 1969.

Committee on Finance, United States Senate. *Medicare and Medicaid: Problems, Issues, and Alternatives*. Washington, DC: U.S. Government Printing Office, 1970.

The Conference Board. *Planning and the Corporate Planning Director*. New York: The Board, no date.

Corning, Peter A. *The Evolution of Medicare*. Washington, DC: Social Security Administration Research Report No. 29, 1969.

Cunningham, Robert M., Jr. *Governing Hospitals: Trustees and the New Accountabilities*. Chicago: American Hospital Association, 1976.

Cunningham, Robert M., Jr. "Notes on the Birth of the Blues." *Hospitals*. April 16, 1979.

Davidson, Sidney; Schindler, James S.; and Weil, Roman L. *Fundamentals of Accounting*. Hinsdale, IL: Dryden Press, 1975.

Davis, Karen. "Economic Theories of Behavior in Nonprofit, Private Hospitals." *Economic and Business Bulletin*, Winter 1972.

Deegan, Arthur. *Management by Objectives for Hospitals*. Germantown, MD: Aspen Systems, 1977.

de Mars Martin, Pamela and Boyer, Frank J. "Developing a Consistent Method for Costing Hospital Services." *Healthcare Financial Management*, February 1985.

Dewing, Arthur S. *The Financial Policy of Corporations, Fifth Edition*. New York: Ronald Press, 1953.

Dillon, Ray D. *Zero Base Budgeting for Health Care Institutions*. Germantown, MD: Aspen Systems, 1979.

Dittman, David A. and Smith, Kenneth R. "Consideration of Benefits and Costs: A Conceptual Framework of the Health Planner." *Health Care Management Review,* Fall 1979.

Donabedian, Avedis. *Aspects of Medical Care Administration.* Cambridge, MA: Harvard University Press, 1973.

Donabedian, Avedis. *The Definition of Quality and Approaches to its Assessment.* Ann Arbor, MI: Health Administration Press, 1980.

Doyle, Owen; Austin, Charles J.; and Tucker, Stephen L. *Analysis Manual for Hospital Information Systems.* Ann Arbor, MI: AUPHA Press, 1980.

Durbin, Richard L. and Springall, W. Herbert. *Organization and Administration of Health Care.* Saint Louis: Mosby, 1969.

Earhart, Charles H. "An Analysis and Development of Standards for Selected Financial Ratios in Voluntary Non-Profit General Hospitals." University of Iowa master's thesis, 1971.

Ehrenreich, Barbara and Ehrenreich, John. *The American Health Empire: Power, Profits, Politics.* New York: Random House, 1970.

Eilers, Robert D. "Postpayment Medical Expense Coverage." *Blue Cross Reports,* September 1969.

Ernst & Whinney. *The Tax Equity and Fiscal Responsibility Act of 1982: Provisions Affecting Medicare and Medicaid Programs.* Cleveland: Ernst & Whinney, 1982.

Esmond, Truman H., Jr. *Budgeting Procedures for Hospitals, Third Edition.* Chicago: American Hospital Association, 1982.

Falcon, William D. (ed.). *Reporting Financial Data to Management.* New York: American Management Association, 1965.

Feder, Judith; Holahan, John; and Marmor, Theodore (eds.). *National Health Insurance.* Washington, DC: The Urban Institute, 1980.

Federal Register. September 1, 1983 and January 3, 1984. Washington, DC: U.S. Government Printing Office.

Feldstein, Martin. *The Rising Cost of Hospital Care.* Washington, DC: Information Resources Press, 1971.

Financial Accounting Standards Board. Statements of Financial Accounting Concepts, Nos. 1, 3, and 4. New York: McGraw-Hill, no date.

Flippo, Edwin B. *Management: A Behavioral Approach.* Boston: Allyn & Bacon, 1970.

Flook, E. Evelyn and Sanazaro, Paul J. (eds.). *Health Services Research and R&D in Perspective.* Ann Arbor, MI: Health Administration Press, 1973.

Fox, Peter D.; Goldbeck, Willis B.; and Spies, Jacob J. *Health Care Cost Management: Private Sector Initiatives.* Ann Arbor, MI: Health Administration Press, 1984.

Foyle, William R. "Merge the Plant and General Funds—Why Not?" *Hospital Accounting,* June 1965.

Frank, C.W. *Maximizing Hospital Cash Resources.* Germantown, MD: Aspen Systems, 1978.

Freeman, Gary and Allcorn, Seth. "Examine the Balance Fraction Method: Improving Receivables Management." *Healthcare Financial Management,* May 1984.

Friedman, Emily and Wendorf, Carl. "Medicaid." *Hospitals,* August 16, 1977; September 1, 1977; September 16, 1977; October 1, 1977; November 1, 1977.

Fritz, Michael H. "Collection Techniques." Ann Arbor, MI: University Microfilms, item AC3003, 1964.

Ginzberg, Eli. *The Limits of Health Reform: The Search for Realism.* New York: Basic Books, Inc., 1977.

Graham, Benjamin; Dodd, David L.; and Cottle, Sidney. *Security Analysis.* New York: McGraw-Hill, 1962.

Greater Detroit Area Hospital Council. *Management Guide to Effective Budgeting.* Detroit: The Council, 1978.

Greiner, Larry E. "Patterns of Organization Change." *Harvard Business Review,* May–June 1967.

Griffith, John R. *Measuring Hospital Performance.* Chicago: Blue Cross Association, 1978.

Griffith, John R. *Quantitative Techniques for Hospital Planning and Control.* Lexington, MA: D.C. Heath, 1972.

Griffith, John R.; Hancock, Walton M.; and Munson, Fred C. (eds.). *Cost Control in Hospitals.* Ann Arbor, MI: Health Administration Press, 1976.

Grimaldi, Paul L. and Micheletti, Julie A. *Diagnosis Related Groups: A Practitioner's Guide.* Chicago: Pluribus Press, 1983.

Gross, Malvern J. and Warshauser, William, Jr. *Financial and Accounting Guide for Nonprofit Organizations.* New York: Wiley, 1983.

Halse, David L. "Electronic Order Entry in Hospital Purchasing." *Hospital Purchasing Management,* April 1983.

Hauser, Richard. "How to Build and Use a Flexible Budget." *Financial Management,* August 1974.

Hay, Leon E. *Accounting for Government and Nonprofit Entities, Sixth Edition.* Homewood, IL: Richard D. Irwin, 1980.

Hay, Leon E. *Budgeting and Cost Analysis for Hospital Management.* Bloomington, IN: University Publications, 1958.

Healy, Sister Mary Immaculate. "An Analysis of Accounts Receivable with Emphasis on Factoring." Ann Arbor, MI: University Microfilms, item AC 3008, 1961.

Heaney, Charles T. and Riedel, Donald C. "From Indemnity to Full Coverage: Changes in Hospital Utilization." *Blue Cross Reports,* October 1970.

Heckert, J. Brooks and Willson, James D. *Controllership.* New York: Ronald, 1963.

Helfert, Erich A. *Techniques of Financial Analysis, Fifth Edition.* Homewood, IL: Irwin, 1982.

Herkimer, Allen G. *Patient Account Management.* Rockville, MD: Aspen Systems, 1983.

Herkimer, Allen G. *Understanding Hospital Financial Management.* Germantown, MD: Aspen Systems, 1978.

Hillier, Frederick S. and Lieberman, Gerald J. *Introduction to Operations Research, Second Edition.* San Francisco: Holden-Day, 1974.

Hodge, Melville H. *Medical Information System: A Resource for Hospitals.* Germantown, MD: Aspen Systems, 1977.

Hofer, Charles W. and Sahendel, Dan. *Strategy Formulation: Analytical Concepts.* Saint Paul: West Publishing Co., 1978.

Holahan, John. *Financing Health Care for the Poor: The Medicaid Experience.* Lexington, MA: D.C. Heath, 1975.

Holahan, John. *Physician Supply, Peer Review and Use of Health Services in Medicaid.* Washington, DC: The Urban Institute, 1976.

Holahan, John; Scanlon, William; and Spitz, Bruce. *Restructuring Federal Medicaid Controls and Incentives.* Washington, DC: The Urban Institute, 1977.

Holahan, John; Spitz, Bruce; Pollak, William; and Feder, Judith. *Altering Medicaid Reimbursement Methods.* Washington, DC: The Urban Institute, 1977.

Holahan, John and Stuart, Bruce. *Controlling Medicaid Utilization Patterns.* Washington, DC: The Urban Institute, 1977.

Hopp, Michael. "Purchasing and Accounting Information System." Ann Arbor, MI: Community Systems Foundation, 1966.

Horngren, Charles T. *Cost Accounting: A Managerial Emphasis.* Englewood Cliffs, NJ: Prentice-Hall, 1977.

Hospital Financial Management Association. *Managing the Patient Account.* Chicago: The Association, 1970.

Hospital Financial Management Association. *Planning the Hospital's Financial Operations.* Chicago: The Association, 1972.

Hospital Financial Management Association. *Safeguarding the Hospital's Assets.* Chicago: The Association, 1971.

Hospital Financial Management Association. *The State of Information Processing in the Health Care Industry.* Chicago: The Association, 1976.

Hospital Planning Council of Metropolitan Chicago. "Capital Financing of Voluntary Hospitals: The Role of Contributions." Chicago: The Council, 1971.

Hospital Planning Council of Metropolitan Chicago. "Capital Financing of Voluntary Hospitals: The Role of Debt Funds." Chicago: The Council, 1971.

Hospital Planning Council of Metropolitan Chicago. "Capital Financing of Voluntary Hospitals: The Role of Government Assistance." Chicago: The Council, 1971.

Hospital Planning Council of Metropolitan Chicago. "Capital Financing of Voluntary Hospitals: The Role of Internal Funds." Chicago: The Council, 1971.

Hospital Week. September 24, 1982 to January 14, 1983.

Hospitals. October 1, 1982 to January 1, 1983.

Hunt, Andrew D. and Weeks, Lewis E. (eds.). *Medical Education Since 1960: Marching to a Different Drummer.* East Lansing, MI: Michigan State University Foundation, 1979.

Indiana University Graduate School of Business. *Third Party Reimbursement for Hospitals.* Bloomington, IN: The School, 1965.

Knight, W.D. "Working Capital Management—Satisficing Versus Optimization." *Financial Management,* Spring 1972.

Kotler, Philip and Murray, Michael. "Third Sector Management: The Role of Marketing." *Public Administration Review.* September-October 1975.

Kovner, Anthony R. and Neuhauser, Duncan (eds.). *Health Services Management: Readings and Commentary.* Ann Arbor, MI: Health Administration Press, 1978.

Kowalski, James C. "Strategic Planning for Hospital Materials Management." *Hospital Purchasing Management,* August 1984.

Krizay, John and Wilson, Andrew A. *The Patient as Consumer: Health Care Financing in the United States.* Lexington, MA: D.C. Heath, 1974.

Kukla, Steven J. *Cost Accounting and Financial Analysis for the Hospital Administrator*. Chicago: American Hospital Association, 1986.

Latham, G.P. and Yukl, G.A. "A Review of Research on the Application of Goal Setting in Organizations." *Academy of Management Journal*, Vol. 18, 1975.

Law, Sylvia A. *Blue Cross: What Went Wrong?* New Haven, CT: Yale University Press, 1974.

Lerner, Monroe and Anderson, Odin W. *Health Progress in the United States: 1900–1960*. Chicago: The University of Chicago Press, 1963.

Lewin, Kurt. "Group Decision and Social Change." In *Readings in Social Psychology*. T. Newcomb and E. Hartley (eds.). New York: Holt, Rinehart & Winston, 1947.

Lindsay, Franklin A. *New Techniques for Management Decision-Making*. Hightstown, NJ: McGraw-Hill, 1963.

Lindsay, J. Robert and Sametz, Arnold W. *Financial Management: An Analytical Approach*. Homewood, IL: Irwin, 1967.

Linklater, R. Bruce. *Internal Control of Hospital Finances: A Guide for Management*. Chicago: American Hospital Association, 1983.

Lippold, Ronald C. *Hospital Credit Training Manual*. Saint Louis: The Catholic Hospital Association, 1970.

Lipson, Stephen H. and Hensel, Mary D. *Hospital Manpower Budget Preparation Manual*.Ann Arbor, MI: Health Administration Press, 1975.

Loebs, Stephen F. "Medicaid: A Survey of Indicators and Issues." *Hospital and Health Services Administration*, Fall 1977.

Loebs, Stephen F. *Variations Among States in Selected Optional Decisions in the Medicaid Program*. University of Michigan doctoral dissertation. Ann Arbor, MI: University Microfilms, 1974.

Long, Hugh W. "Asset Choice and Program Selection in a Competitive Environment." *Hospital Financial Management*, July-August 1982.

Longest, Beaufort B., Jr. *Management Practices for the Health Professional*. Reston, VA: Reston Publishing Co., 1980.

Lorange, Peter and Vancil, Richard F. *Strategic Planning Systems*. Englewood Cliffs, NJ: Prentice-Hall, 1977.

Luke, Roice. "Dimensions in Hospital Case Mix Measurement." *Inquiry*, Spring 1979.

MacLeod, Roderick K. "Program Budgeting Works in Nonprofit Institutions." *Harvard Business Review*, September-October 1971.

MacStravic, Robin E. *Determining Health Needs*. Ann Arbor, MI: Health Administration Press, 1978.

MacStravic, Robin E. *Marketing Health Care*. Rockville, MD: Aspen Systems, 1977.

McConkey, Dale D. *MBO for Nonprofit Organizations*. New York: Amacom, 1975.

McGregor, D. "An Uneasy Look at Performance Appraisal." *Harvard Business Review*, May-June 1957.

McNerney, Walter et al. *Hospital and Medical Economics*, 2 vols. Chicago: Hospital Research and Educational Trust, 1962.

Magee, John R. and Boodman, D.M. *Production Planning and Inventory Control*. Hightstown, NJ: McGraw-Hill, 1967.

Manney, James D. *Aging in American Society.* Ann Arbor, MI: The Institute of Gerontology, 1975.

Mannix, John R. "Blue Cross Reimbursement of Hospitals." Paper presented at Hospital Summer Management Course, Center for Continuing Education, The University of Michigan, 1969.

Markstein, David L. "How to Make Short-Term Cash Work at Full-Time Rates." *Modern Hospital,* January 1970.

Markstein, David L. "The Pros and Cons of Credit Cards for the Hospital Field." *Modern Hospital,* June 1970.

Martin, George. *Madam Secretary: Frances Perkins.* Boston: Houghton, Mifflin, 1976.

Martin, Glenn J. "What Experiments in Prospective Reimbursement are Teaching Providers, Agencies, Third Parties." *Hospital Financial Management,* November 1970.

Martin, Lawrence E. "Reimbursements by All Inclusive Rates." *HSRD Briefs.* National Center for Health Services Research and Development, Dept. HEW, 5600 Fishers Lane, Rockville, MD, Summer 1970.

Massachusetts Hospital Association. "Follow Up Analysis: Methods and Procedure for Minimizing Financial Loss Risk and Accounts Receivable." Boston: The Association, no date.

Medical Care. Special Issue, February 1980.

Michigan Task Force on Medicaid and Health Care Costs. *Report of the Michigan Task Force on Medicaid and Health Care Costs.* Ann Arbor, MI: The Task Force, January 1979.

Miller, Merton H. and Orr, Daniel. "An Application of Control Limit Models to the Management of Corporate Cash Balances." In *Proceedings of the Conference on Financial Research and Its Implications for Management, Stanford University.* Robichek, Alexander A. (ed.). New York: Wiley, 1967.

Miller, Merton H. and Orr, Daniel. "Model for the Demand for Money by Firms." *Quarterly Journal of Economics,* August 1966.

Mintzberg, Henry. "Planning on the Left Side and Managing on the Right." *Harvard Business Review,* July-August 1976.

Moyer, C.A. and Mautz, R.K. *Intermediate Accounting: A Functional Approach.* New York: Wiley, 1967.

Mulroy, Thomas R. *Hospital Liability Revisited: How Governing Boards Can Protect Themselves and Improve Patient Care.* Chicago: Blue Cross Association, 1980.

Murphy, Thomas. "The Hospital Treasurer and Controller: Duties and Responsibilities." *Hospital Financial Management,* April 1970.

Myers, Robert J. *Medicare.* Homewood, IL: Irwin, 1970.

Nackel, John G. and Barnard, Cynthia. "Special Report #10, Evaluating Case Mix Reporting Systems." Chicago: American Hospital Association.

Novick, David. *Program Budgeting: Program Analysis and the Federal Budget, Second Edition.* Cambridge, MA: Harvard University Press, 1967.

Odiorne, George. *Management by Objectives.* New York: Pittman Publishing Co., 1965.

Odiorne, George. *Planning the Hospital's Financial Operations.* Chicago: Hospital Financial Management Association, 1972.

O'Donoghue, Patrick. *Evidence about the Effects of Health Care Regulation*. Denver: Spectrum Research, 1974.

Orgler, Yair E. *Cash Management: Methods and Models*. Belmont, CA: Wadsworth, 1970.

Perlman, Mark; Adams, Jeffrey; Wolfe, Harvey; and Shuman, Larry. *Methods for Distributing the Costs on Non–Revenue Producing Centers*. Ann Arbor, MI: University Microfilms Hospital Abstract 10600AC, 1972.

Peters, Joseph P. *A Strategic Planning Process for Hospitals*. Chicago: American Hospital Association, 1985.

Peters, Thomas J. and Waterman, Robert H., Jr. *In Search of Excellence*. New York: Harper & Row, 1982.

Ploman, Marilyn Peacock. *Case Mix Classification Systems: Development, Description, and Testing*. Chicago: Hospital Research and Educational Trust, 1982.

Price Waterhouse. *The Challenge of Prospective Payment*. New York: The Company, 1983.

Pyhrr, Peter A. *Zero Base Budgeting*. New York: Wiley, 1973.

Quirin, G. David. *The Capital Expenditure Decision*. Homewood, IL: Irwin, 1967.

Raitz, Robert E. "The Effect of Using an Economic Order Quantity Formula and Exponential Smoothing to Reduce Hospital Purchasing Costs." University of Minnesota master's thesis, 1964.

Reed, Louis S. and Carr, Willine. *The Benefit Structure of Private Health Insurance, 1968*. Washington, DC: Social Security Administration, Office of Research and Statistics, Research Report No. 32, 1970.

Reed, Louis S. and Dwyer, Maureen. *Health Insurance Plans Other than Blue Cross or Blue Shield Plans or Insurance Companies*. Washington, DC: Social Security Administration, Office of Research and Statistics, Research Report No. 35, 1971.

Riedel, Donald C.; Walden, Daniel C.; Singsen, Antone G.; Meyers, Samuel; Krantz, Goldie; and Henderson, Marie. *Federal Employees Health Benefits Program Utilization Study*. Washington, DC: Department HEW, 1975.

Robinson, Roland I. *Money and Capital Markets*. New York: McGraw-Hill, 1974.

Roemer, Milton I. *National Strategies for Health Care Organization: A World Overview*. Ann Arbor, MI: Health Administration Press, 1985.

Roemer, Milton I.; Dubois, Donald M.; and Rich, Shirley W. (eds.). *Health Insurance Plans: Studies in Organizational Diversity*. Los Angeles, CA: University of Calfornia, 1970.

Rorem, C. Rufus. *Origins of Blue Cross*. Privately published, 1971.

Rorem, C. Rufus. *Private Group Clinics*. Chicago: The University of Chicago Press, 1931.

Rorem, C. Rufus. *A Quest for Certainty: Essays on Health Care Economics, 1930–1970*. Ann Arbor, MI: Health Administration Press, 1982.

Ruchlin, Hirsch S. and Roger, Harry M. "Short-Run Hospital Responses to Reimbursement Rate Changes." *Inquiry*, Spring 1980.

Russell, Louise B. *Technology in Hospitals*. Washington, DC: The Brookings Institution, 1979.

Salling, Raymond C. "Can Your Inventory Control Be Scientific?" *Modern Hospital*. October 1964.

Schein, Edgar H. *Organizational Psychology*. Englewood Cliffs, NJ: Prentice-Hall, 1972.

Seawell, L. Vann. *External and Internal Reporting by Hospitals*. Oak Brook, IL: Healthcare Financial Management Association, 1984.

Seawell, L. Vann. *Hospital Accounting and Financial Management*. Berwyn, IL: Physicians' Record Co., 1964.

Seawell, L. Vann. *Hospital Financial Accounting: Theory and Practice*. Chicago: Hospital Financial Management Association, 1975.

Seawell, L. Vann. *Introduction to Hospital Accounting*. Chicago: Hospital Financial Management Association, 1964.

Seawell, L. Vann. *Principles of Hospital Accounting*. Berwyn, IL: Physicians' Record Co., 1960.

Selznick, Phillip. *Leadership in Administration*. Evanston, IL: Row, Peterson, 1957.

Shelton, Robert M. "The Hospital Financial Manager Today." *Hospital Financial Management*, April 1970.

Silvers, J.B. "Identity Crisis: Financial Management in Health Care." *Health Care Management Review*, Fall 1976.

Silvers, J.B. and Prahalad, C.K. *Financial Management of Health Institutions*. New York: Spectrum Publications, 1974.

Silvers, J.B.; Zelman, William; Kahn, Charles N. III (eds.). *Health Care Financial Management in the 1980s: Time of Transition*. Ann Arbor, MI: AUPHA Press, 1983.

Skolnik, Alfred M. and Dales, Sophie R. "Social Welfare Expenditures in Fiscal Year 1970." *Research and Statistics Notes*, November 30, 1970.

Smalley, Harold E. and Freeman, John R. *Hospital Industrial Engineering*. New York: Reinhold, 1966.

Social Security Administration. *Medicare, the First Nine Months*. Washington, DC: U.S. Government Printing Office, 1967.

Social Security Administration. *Medicare, 1972: Enrollment*. Washington, DC: U.S. Government Printing Office, 1975.

Social Security Administration. *Medicare, 1972: Reimbursement by State and County*. Washington, DC: U.S. Government Printing Office, 1975.

Somers, Anne R. and Somers, Herman M. *Health and Health Care: Policies in Perspective*. Germantown, MD: Aspen Systems, 1977.

Somers, Herman M. and Somers, Anne R. *Doctors, Patients and Health Insurance*. New York: Doubleday Anchor Books, 1962.

Somers, Herman M. and Somers, Anne R. "Major Issues in National Health Insurance." *Milbank Memorial Fund Quarterly*, Part I, April 1972.

Somers, Herman M. and Somers, Anne R. *Medicare and the Hospitals: Issues and Prospects*. Washington, DC: The Brookings Institution, 1968.

Southwick, Arthur F. *The Law of Hospital and Health Care Administration*. Ann Arbor, MI: Health Administration Press, 1978.

Spiegel, Allen D. and Podair, Simon (eds.). *Medicaid: Lessons for National Health Insurance*. Rockville, MD: Aspen Systems, 1975.

Starr, Paul. *The Social Transformation of American Medicine*. New York: Basic Books, 1982.

Steiner, George A. *Strategic Planning*. New York: The Free Press, 1979.

Stevens, Robert and Stevens, Rosemary. *Welfare Medicine in America: A Case Study of Medicaid.* New York: The Free Press, 1974.

Stone, Bernell K. "The Use of Forecasts and Smoothing in Control-Limit Models for Cash Management." *Financial Management,* Spring 1972.

Stuart, Bruce C. and Bair, Lee A. *Health Care and Income: The Distributional Impacts of Medicaid and Medicare Nationally and in the State of Michigan.* Lansing, MI: State of Michigan Department of Social Services, 1971.

Stuart, Bruce C. and Spitz, Bruce. *Rising Medical Costs in Michigan.* Lansing, MI: State of Michigan Department of Social Services, 1973.

Sutermeister, Robert A. (ed.). *People and Productivity, Third Edition.* New York: McGraw-Hill, 1976.

Suver, James D.; Kahn, Charles N. III; and Clement, Jan P. *Cases in Health Care Financial Management.* Ann Arbor, MI: AUPHA Press, 1984.

Suver, James D. and Neumann, Bruce R. "Cost of Capital." *Hospital Financial Management,* Fall 1978.

Suver, James D. and Neumann, Bruce R. "Zero Base Budgeting." *Hospital and Health Services Administration,* Spring 1979.

Symonds, Curtis W. *Basic Financial Management.* New York: American Management Association, 1969.

Taylor, Philip J. and Nelson, Benjamin O. *Management Accounting for Hospitals.* Philadelphia: W.B. Saunders Co., 1964.

Thompson, John D.; Averill, Richard F.; and Fetter, Robert B. "Planning, Budgeting, and Controlling—One Look at the Future: Case Mix Cost Accounting." *Health Services Research,* Summer 1979.

Thompson, John D.; Mross, C.D.; and Fetter, Robert B. "Case Mix and Resource Use." *Inquiry,* December 1975.

Tibbits, Samuel J. and Manzano, Allen J. *PROs, Preferred Provider Organizations: An Executive's Guide.* Chicago: Pluribus Press, 1984.

Tonkin, G.W. "The Controller's Role on the Management Team." *Hospital Financial Management,* April 1970.

Topics in Health Care Financing. "Capital Financing," Fall 1978.

Topics in Health Care Financing. "Capital Projects," Winter 1975.

Topics in Health Care Financing. "Rate Regulation," Fall 1979.

Topics in Health Care Financing. Special Issue, "Financial Management Under Third Party Reimbursement," Fall 1976.

Topics in Health Care Financing. Spring 1979.

Tuller, Edwin and Kozak, David. "Logical Thought Process Key to Corporate Plan." *Hospitals,* September 1, 1979.

Tunley, Roul. *The American Health Scandal.* New York: Dell, 1966.

U.S. Department of Health, Education, and Welfare. *Health: United States, 1978.* Washington, DC: U.S. Government Printing Office, DHEW Publication No. (PHS) 78–1232, 1978.

U.S. Department of Health, Education, and Welfare. *Recommendations of the Task Force on Medicaid and Related Programs.* Washington, DC: U.S. Government Printing Office, November 1969.

Van Arsdell, Paul M. "Considerations Underlying Cost of Capital." *Financial Analysts Journal,* November–December 1963.

Van Arsdell, Paul M. *Corporate Finance: Policy, Planning, Administration.* New York: Ronald, 1968.

Van Horne, James C. *Financial Management and Policy.* Englewood Cliffs, NJ: Prentice-Hall, 1977.

Van Horne, James C. *Financial Management and Policy.* Englewood Cliffs, NJ: Prentice-Hall, 1980.

Van Horne, James C. *Financial Management and Policy, Part II.* Englewood Cliffs, NJ: Prentice-Hall, 1969.

Vraciu, Robert A. "Decision Models for Capital Investment and Financing Decisions in Hospitals. *Health Services Research,* Spring 1980.

Vraciu, Robert A. "Programming, Budgeting, and Control in Health Care Organizations: The State of the Art." *Health Services Research,* Summer 1979.

Wacht, Richard F. "Toward Rationality in the Allocation of Hospital Resources." *Financial Management,* Spring 1972.

Waldman, Saul and Peel, Evelyn. "National Health Insurance: A Comparison of Five Proposals." *The Journal of the American Osteopathic Association,* December 1970.

Walls, Edward L., Jr. "Hospital Dependency on Long-Term Debt." *Financial Management,* Spring 1972.

Warner, D. Michael and Holloway, Don C. *Decision Making and Control for Health Administration.* Ann Arbor, MI: Health Administration Press, 1978.

Warner, D. Michael; Holloway, Don C.; and Grazier, Kyle L. *Decision Making and Control for Health Administration: The Management of Quantitative Analysis, Second Edition.* Ann Arbor, MI: Health Administration Press, 1984.

Warner, Kenneth E. and Luce, Bryan R. *Cost-Benefit and Cost-Effectiveness Analysis in Health Care: Principles, Practice, and Potential.* Ann Arbor, MI: Health Administration Press, 1982.

Warren, David G. *Problems in Hospital Law, Third Edition.* Germantown, MD: Aspen Systems, 1978.

Wath, Jacquelyn J. "Health Insurance for the Aged: Participating Health Facilities, July 1970." *Health Insurance Statistics,* January 15, 1971.

Weeks, Lewis E. (ed.). *Education of a Hospital Trustee: Changing Roles for Changing Times.* Battle Creek, MI: W.K. Kellogg Foundation, 1977.

Weeks, Lewis E. (ed.). *Hospital Administration Oral History Collection.* Chicago: American Hospital Association, 1983–.

Weeks, Lewis E. and Berman, Howard J. (eds.). *Economics in Health Care.* Germantown, MD: Aspen Systems, 1977.

Weeks, Lewis E. and Berman, Howard J. *Shapers of U.S. Health Policy: An Oral History.* Ann Arbor, MI: Health Administration Press, 1985.

Weeks, Lewis E.; Berman, Howard J; and Bisbee, Gerald E., Jr. (eds.). *Financing of Health Care.* Ann Arbor, MI: Health Administration Press, 1979.

Weston, J. Fred and Brigham, Eugene F. *Managerial Finance, Fifth Edition.* Hinsdale, IL: The Dryden Press, 1975.

Wheelwright, Steven C. and Makridakis, Spyos G. *Forecasting Methods for Management.* New York: Wiley, 1973.

Williams, John Daniel and Rakich, Jonathan S. "Investment Evaluation in Hospitals." *Financial Management,* Summer 1973.

Williams, William J. "A Report on Insurance and Prepayment for Medical Care." Xavier University master's thesis. Ann Arbor, MI: University Microfilms, item IN2026, 1964.

Wilson, Florence A. and Neuhauser, Duncan. *Health Services in the United States.* Cambridge, MA: Ballinger, 1974.

Witte, Edwin E. *The Development of the Social Security Act.* Madison, WI: University of Wisconsin Press, 1963.

Wren, George R. *Modern Health Administration.* Athens, GA: University of Georgia Press, 1974.

Young, D.E. "Effective Presentation of Reports: Information for Understanding." In *Reporting Financial Data to Management.* William D. Falcon (ed.). New York: American Management Association, 1965.

Zuckerman, Howard S. *Multi-Institutional Hospital Systems.* Chicago: Hospital Research and Educational Trust/W.K. Kellogg Foundation, 1979.

PART B

This part consists of abstracts adapted from *Abstracts of Health Care Management Studies* and is used with permission.

The full text of each abstracted document is available as indicated. Those marked "Available from University Microfilms" can be obtained for a fee from that company at 300 North Zeeb Road, Ann Arbor, Michigan 48106, when ordered by the number of the abstract from *Abstracts of Health Care Management Studies* (AHCMS).

Adair, Jerry D.
A Feasibility Study of an All-Inclusive Rate Structure for Today's Hospitals
Duke University, Durham, NC, 1970, 52 pp.
Available from University Microfilms

An evaluation of the inclusive rate system and a comparison with the itemized charge system.

AHCMS AC2–5830

Aday, Lu Ann and Andersen, Ronald
Who Are the Uninsured?
Center for Health Administration Studies, University of Chicago, Chicago, IL

This paper presents data from a national survey of the United States population concerning the demographic characteristics, employment status, health levels, access to and satisfaction with care of persons with no form of privately or publicly financed health insurance coverage.

AHCMS 20288 IN

Adkins, Loraine
Business and Health: Basic and Supplemental Readings
Institute for Health Planning, Madison, WI, 1981

In response to rising health care costs, business has developed strategies, including health maintenance organizations, coalitions, and health promotion/fitness programs, for containing these costs. The 49 basic and 20 supplemental readings cited in this bibliography relate directly to these cost containment efforts, especially those involving business and health coalitions. Journal articles, books, government documents, and technical reports are referenced.

AHCMS 24351 HC

Ament, Richard P.; Kobrinski, Edward J.; and Wood, Walter R.
Case Mix Complexity Differences Between Teaching and Nonteaching Hospitals
Journal of Medical Education, 56:11, 1981, pp. 894–903.

Several studies have concluded that patient mix is an important determinant of hospital costs, and in a limited number diagnostic case mix variables have been explicitly introduced to explain variation in costs. But the literature provides little information on the case mix component of cost differentials between teaching and nonteaching hospitals. Case complexity was measured in a sample of 200 short-stay general hospitals by the Resource Need Index (RNI), using a cross-classification of 3,490 case types with weights compiled from patient charges. Median RNI values were moderately higher for teaching than for nonteaching hospitals, both for the hospital as a whole and for each clinical service except obstetrics-gynecology. The most resource-intensive case types were relatively more frequent in the teaching hospitals, but the least resource-intensive types were of about equal relative frequency in the two hospital groups. The results show that teaching hospitals could be expected to cost somewhat more per patient even if case mix were the only factor.

AHCMS 26385 HC

American Association of Medical Clinics
An Administrative Information System for a Group Practice Developing a Pre-paid Health Plan
The Association, Alexandria, VA, c. 1975, 45 pp.

Report describes an administrative information system that was developed for prepaid health plans.

AHCMS 13162 IN

American Association of Medical Clinics
A Financial Evaluation System for a Group Practice Developing a Prepaid Health Plan
The Association, Alexandria, VA, 1973, 47 pp.

Purpose of this study is to present an approach to evaluating the financial success of a prepaid health plan; to offer an overview of how information generated by this financial evaluation system supports this approach; and to explain the methodology required for gathering and developing the necessary input data for group practices developing a prepaid health plan.

AHCMS 13158 IN

American Health Planning Association
Report of the Commission on Capital Policy
The Association, Washington, DC, 1984

The Commission on Capital Policy (established by the American Health Planning Association) presents an overview of the evolution of capital payment policy in the United States and describes the payment options considered along with issues relating to their impact on a variety of economic and societal variables.

AHCMS 28411 FM

American Hospital Association
Ameriplan: A Proposal for the Delivery and Financing of Health Services in the United States
The Association, Chicago, IL, 1970, 99 pp.

Monograph describes Ameriplan, the proposal of the AHA's Special Committee on the Provision of Health Services to restructure and finance a delivery system of health care that is considered more accessible, comprehensive, and relevant to the needs of the community. Ameriplan involves the formation of health care corporations at the community level, composed of existing health care provider organizations. The health care corporation would have a primary geographic assignment established by a state health commission; more than one health care corporation may be assigned to the same area, however. Its primary responsibility is the provision of health care services to its registrants. It would also act as a fiscal agency, receiving and disbursing money for the payment of health services. A national health commission would be the primary agency responsible for the continuing assessment of the effectiveness of Ameriplan. It would be responsible for adopting regulations to create uniform benefit packages and state scope, standards of quality, and comprehensiveness of health services. Federal and state legislation is needed to implement the proposal and create the state and national health commissions. The financing system recommended would utilize all existing sources of funds and be based on each citizen's ability to pay, except for the aged for whom coverage would be prepaid.

AHCMS IN3–6696

American Medical Association
Report of the National Commission on the Cost of Medical Care, 1976–1977. Vols. 1, 2, 3
The Association, Chicago, IL, 1978

A three-volume report by the National Commission on the Cost of Medical Care established by the American Medical Association and charged with "delivering innovative solutions to health care cost problems."

AHCMS 21601 HC

Anderson, Odin W. and May, J. Joel
The Federal Employees Health Benefits Program, 1961–1968: A Model for National Health Insurance?
Center for Health Administration Studies, University of Chicago, Chicago, IL, 1971, 60 pp.

An evaluation of the Federal Employees Health Benefits Program as a model for national health insurance in the U.S. Legislative history of the program, its scope and administration are discussed. Data collected by the Civil Service Commission on cost, use, and enrollment are analyzed. The FEHB Program is described as one that was acceptable at the time of its adoption to all groups at interest (government, employees, providers, and insurance agencies) and would be feasible as a national program. A two-class system of medical care could be avoided by allowing low-income individuals a choice of coverage under governmental subsidization.

AHCMS IN4–7739

Arnould, Richard J.; Debrock, Lawrence W.; and Pollard, John W.
Do HMOS Produce Specific Services More Efficiently?

Inquiry, 21:3, 1984, pp. 243–53.

Previous research on the effects of HMOs on health care costs has concentrated on aggregate costs and resource use and has shown that HMOs result in lower costs. The only consistent sources of the cost savings are the lower hospital admission rates and shorter lengths of stay for HMO enrollees. This article contains the results of an investigation of whether HMOs can more efficiently produce a given service. Four common inpatient procedures were analyzed to determine whether there were any differences in resource consumption and overall costs for HMO patients versus fee-for-service patients. Although significant levels of resource savings were found for various procedures for HMO enrollees, these savings did not always result in lower overall costs.

AHCMS 28166 HC

Association of American Medical Colleges
Price Competition in the Health Care Marketplace: Issues for Teaching Hospitals
The Association, Washington, DC, 1981

This document reviews the potential impacts of price competition on teaching hospitals. It is not a policy statement, but a document intended to stimulate further discussion of price competition which will result in constructive, sound recommendations to those responsible for charting the future course of the health care system.

AHCMS 24112 HC

Banta, H. David and Luce, Bryan R.
Assessing the Cost-Effectiveness of Prevention
Journal of Community Health, 9:2, 1983, pp. 145–65.

In an era of limited resources, cost-effectiveness analysis and cost-benefit analysis (CEA/CBA) can be significant policy-making aids. The authors surveyed about 250 CEA/CBA articles concerning prevention to examine whether prevention is cost-effective, and found that few authors have followed generally accepted methodological standards, which raised questions concerning the validity of their findings and conclusions. In addition, prevention itself is a problem in CEA/CBA because of such factors as the long intervals between interventions and outcomes, problems which have rarely been considered in the CEA/CBA prevention literature. At the same time, a number of high quality studies concerning prevention indicate that United States policy-makers have not aggressively pursued significant opportunities to improve health through prevention, for example, by immunizing the elderly and by screening for and treating hypertension.

AHCMS 27812 HC

Bauer, Katharine G.
Containing Costs of Health Services Through Incentive Reimbursement
Cases in Health Services, Series No. 4, December 1973, 293 pp.

Report presents 13 case studies of approaches taken by various third party sponsors, including Medicare and Medicaid programs and Blue Cross plans to contain medical costs by control incentives linked to reimbursement. Each of the case reports describes the plan's sponsorship and stated purposes, types of performance sponsor seeks to encourage, methods for measuring performance, incentives offered and formulae for their calculations. Where available, results are also presented.

AHCMS 12135 IN

Bauer, Katharine G.
Improving Information for Hospital Rate Setting
Harvard Center for Community Health and Medical Care, Boston, MA, 1976, 272 pp.

Based on the findings of a series of working papers on the use of data in hospital rate setting, recommendations are offered for federal and state officials charged with developing guidelines or regulations concerning information for hospital rate setting.

AHCMS 17761 AC

Bays, Carson W.
Case-Mix Differences Between Nonprofit and For-Profit Hospitals
Inquiry, 14:1, 1977, pp. 17–21.

This article tested the proposition that for-profit hospitals specialize in producing only the most profitable types of patient care. Data were collected on differences in case mix within a sample of 41 short-term general hospitals composed of both for-profit and nonprofit types. A univariate one-way analysis of variance of case-mix variables was used for two pairs of hospital types: nonprofit compared to profit, and chain for-profit compared to nonchain for-profit. Results show that the for-profit hospitals have a distinctly different case mix and generally specialize in less complicated cases.

AHCMS 20916 HC

Beck, Richard H.
A Guideline for Financial Ratio Analysis of Publicly Owned Nursing Home and Extended Care Facility Corporations
University of Iowa, Iowa City, IA, 1971, 136 pp.
Available from University Microfilms

Paper discusses the need for responsible financial management of publicly owned nursing homes and extended care facilities. Suggestions are made for establishing a framework for a system of financial ratio analysis, using 12 ratios considered applicable to the nursing home industry.

AHCMS AC1–7016

Berki, S. E.
The Design of Case-Based Payment Systems
Medical Care, 21:1, 1983, pp. 1–13.

Reimbursing hospitals on the basis of treated cases, as in the New Jersey diagnosis-related groups (DRG) experiment, is equivalent to a centrally set pricing scheme, with all of its inherent difficulties. In addition to the problems of appropriate case definition, it is not obvious how hospitals should be classified to form reference groups for cost determination. Empirically derived cost schedules are based on the observed appropriateness, quality, and resource use efficiency that characterize the system from which the data are drawn. If case-based schemes are to incorporate desirable performance incentives, they must be much better specified and take into account the complexity of hospital behavior. This article identifies the basic components of case-based systems of hospital reimbursement and discusses the analytic and empiric problems involved in their design.

AHCMS 26786 HC

Berman, Howard J.
  Debt: How Much Is Too Much?
Hospital Financial Management, 23:11, 1969, pp. 12–13
    Description of a quantitative technique (probabilistic cash forecasting) for
determining debt capacity. The author describes and illustrates with an example
how a hospital can determine the amount of debt that it can safely hold.
                                                                                    AHCMS AC0032

Berman, Howard J.
  Ratio Analysis: A Technique for Financial Management in Hospitals
The University of Michigan, Ann Arbor, MI, 1968, 49 pp.
Available from University Microfilms
    Study develops ratio values for hospitals to use in estimating financial effi-
ciency which are based on a normal financial plan. A comparison of actual ratios
to normal values shows an estimated relative financial efficiency of a particular
hospital. Study includes discussion of hospital debt capacity and working papers
that explain how each figure in the normal financial plan was derived.
                                                                                    AHCMS AC1051

Berman, Howard J. and Bash, Paul L.
  Capital Investment Decisions
The University of Michigan, Ann. Arbor, MI, 1971, 98 pp.
Available from University Microfilms
    This report, designed to provide a practical procedure for evaluating and se-
lecting capital investment opportunities, comprises two sections, each intended as
a separate manual. Section 1 is the Project Application Manual. Section 2 is the
Investment Decision Manual and provides a detailed explanation of the mechanics
of evaluating and rank ordering proposed investments.
                                                                                    AHCMS AC3–6960

Berman, Howard J. and Bash, Paul L.
  Operational Budgeting Systems: Hackley Hospital, Muskegon, Michigan
The University of Michigan, Ann Arbor, MI, 1970, 151 pp.
Available from University Microfilms
    A report on the budgeting practices and procedures of a 400-bed voluntary,
nonprofit hospital. Authors examine the budgeting procedures and present recommendations as to how the existing system can be improved to provide a budgeting process that facilitates management by objectives and responsibility
accounting.
                                                                                    AHCMS AC–6152

Berry, Ralph E., Jr.
  Prospective Reimbursement in New York
Inquiry, 13:4, 1976, pp. 288–301.
    Medicare and Medicaid, national wage and price control, and New York's
prospective reimbursement program are analyzed to determine if hospital cost
inflation is of the "demand-pull" nature. Results indicated that is probably the
case.
                                                                                    AHCMS 19124 IN

Berry, Robert
Analysis of the Medicare Economic Index
Teknekron Research, Inc., Energy and Environmental Systems Division, Berkeley, CA, 1982
Available from National Technical Information Service (PB83-161349)

This report examines the variation in practice costs and fees across physician specialties, relying on data from the Physician Practice Cost Surveys, 1976–78. Results from the analysis indicate that significant differences do exist across specialties in the principal cost shares of rent, supplies, overhead, salaries, auto expenses, malpractice premiums, and net income. These cost shares also vary significantly across region and population groupings, although with the regions disaggregated into states the number of significant findings is fewer. Aggregate cost indexes do not show substantial interregional or interspecialty differences.

AHCMS 26557 HC

Bible, Ronald L.
Using a Labor Management Report to Prepare a Budget
Center for Hospital Management Engineering, American Hospital Association, Chicago, IL, 1984

The forecasting portion of preparing a budget—trying to quantify the future—usually causes the most difficulty. The paper shows how the labor management report or labor productivity report can help in preparing labor costs for a budget.

AHCMS 28225 FM

Birnbaum, Howard; Bishop, Christine; Lee, A. James; and Jensen, Gail
Why Do Nursing Home Costs Vary? The Determinants of Nursing Home Costs
Medical Care, 19:11, 1981, pp. 1095–1107.

Since nursing home care is a major component of the rapidly rising cost of health care, it is appropriate to base public policy discussions about cost containment on the determinants of nursing home costs. This article investigates the determinants of nursing home operating costs and reviews the results of 11 related econometric cost analyses conducted by the authors. Single-equation cost analyses are developed for nursing homes in three states and in the nation. The cost results of a multiequation model of nursing home behavior are also reviewed. The analyses indicate that facility size and occupancy rate are minimally important in determining cost variation. Facility characteristics, particularly type of facility and ownership, are important variables. Nonprofit facilities consistently had higher costs than for-profit facilities, after controlling for patient mix and service differences, and, in one analysis, for a measure of quality.

AHCMS 24809 HC

Bisbee, Gerald E. and Vraciu, Robert A. (eds.).
Managing the Finances of Health Care Organizations
Health Administration Press, Ann Arbor, MI, 1980

This book is a collection of readings about issues related to both financial management and health care financing, published during the period 1972–80. The primary purpose is to help health care administrators understand current issues and techniques. The book is divided into the following sections: (1) payments to health care institutions; (2) planning, budgeting, and controlling; (3) management of current operations and working capital (discusses planning and controlling short-term cash flows); (4) the investment decision (long-run allocation of resources); and (5) sources of financing.

AHCMS 24971 FM

Blair, Roger D.; Ginsburg, Paul B.; and Vogel, Ronald J.
  Blue Cross–Blue Shield Administration Costs: A Study of Non-Profit Health Insurers
Economic Inquiry 13:2, 1975, pp. 237–51.

Administrative costs are examined for Blue Cross and Blue Shield for 1975. Two aspects of the Blue Cross and Blue Shield programs are examined in depth: (1) the costs incurred by each as an intermediary or a carrier for the Medicare program: and (2) the potential efficiencies of merging Blue Cross and Blue Shield when the two plans operate separately in a single area. Analysis of 1971 and 1972 cost data leads to the conclusion that the Blue Cross and Blue Shield programs evidence substantial managerial slack. Variance in costs is much smaller for those costs associated with Medicare administration than for those associated with the direct business of Blue Cross and Blue Shield. Although cost advantages can be demonstrated for a merged organizational form, this form is not prevalent. The evidence suggests that Blue Cross and Blue Shield have not taken advantage of potential economies of scale to reduce the cost of health insurance, but have instead dissipated the potential savings in increased administrative costs.

AHCMS 17772 IN

Blankinship, Richard T.; Kirby, Liane; and Montague, Cynthia
  Total Capital Equipment Programs: A New Direction for Group Purchasing
Hospital Material Management Quarterly, 3:3, 1982, pp. 7–11.

Active involvement in group purchasing and shared service programs has saved considerable money for hospitals, but many shared service groups are now looking for new avenues of cost containment. The program with the greatest potential of all of the applications developed to date is capital equipment budget development analysis and procurement.

AHCMS 28007 EN

Blendon, Robert J. and Altman, Drew E.
  Public Attitudes about Health-Care Costs: A Lesson in National Schizophrenia
New England Journal of Medicine, 311:9, 1984, pp. 613–16.

It is suggested that the ambivalent attitudes of the public about controlling health care costs even though these costs continue to escalate have been critical in preventing any single, sweeping solution from being adopted. The article analyzes data from 15 national public opinion polls on this issue. Major findings are: (1) While the public and elected officials see rising costs as the number one health care problem, this issue is not ranked high on a list of the most important problems facing the nation. (2) While Americans are disturbed by sharply rising costs of health care in general, they are not troubled by the growing share of the nation's economy devoted to health care and most believe society spends too little rather than too much for these services. (3) Although most feel that the present health care arrangements are not satisfactory, they do not want to change the way they currently receive medical care. (4) Because most Americans are satisfied with the medical care they personally receive, they tend to support only the cost-containment proposals that leave their present personal health care arrangements intact and oppose solutions involving any major reorganization of the health care system. (5) Physicians' views on proposals for change are more influential with the public than those of government officials, and business and labor leaders. Long- and short-term solutions to rising health care costs are then assessed in terms of public support. While the public supports research and changes in lifestyle as long-term solutions, it is opposed to short-term solutions of nationalization and rationing of health care equipment and procedures. There is limited support for short-term solutions of regulation and competition. While there is public support for the Medicaid program, it is linked to state welfare programs and the public does not favor additional spending for welfare. It is concluded that public leaders will have to move away from a search for a single solution and build a cost-containment program that incorporates those elements that have public support.

AHCMS 28539 HC

Block, James A.; Regenstreif, Donna I; and Shute, Leonard J.
  Experimental Payments Program: It's Working for Rochester-Area Hospitals
Hospital Financial Management, 35:9, 1981, pp. 10 ff.

  The authors of this article describe the Rochester-Area Hospitals Experimental Payments (HEP) Program, which encourages hospital cost containment through the introduction of appropriate incentives in the hospital financing system that affect both inpatient and outpatient services. These incentives are the result of the following two features of the HEP system. (1) Payments to each hospital are based, after the first year of the program, on that hospital's preceding year's payments without regard to its incurred costs. Cost savings realized by a hospital accrue to its benefit. (2) Total revenue available to community hospitals is determined in advance of each year of that program. This revenue covers all hospital expenses including incremental operating expenses associated with approved certificate-of-need (CON) projects, increases in volumes of services, and costs associated with unforeseen events. This feature provides incentives for hospitals to work together to avoid unnecessary duplication of services while preserving autonomy. HEP addresses two causes of hospital cost inflation: volume problems caused by incentives in traditional reimbursement schemes to reward high rates of admission, long length of stay, and increasing resource use per admission; and planning problems—planning agencies' approval of projects under CON neither reflects an accurate assessment of financial reasonableness nor links projected expenses with actual experience. The article describes HEP incentive mechanisms that deal with these problems and illustrates how a hospital's allowable cost base is computed. First year results under HEP show an improved financial situation for the participating hospitals and an increase in expenditures almost half that of the national averages for 1980.

AHCMS 25359 FM

Boldt, Ben I., Jr.
  Financial Modeling: A Must for Today's Hospital Management
Hospital Care Management Review, 3:3, 1978, pp. 7–13.

  The article describes and illustrates the use of various types of computerized financial models as tools for the detailed and thorough planning required in hospital management today. Among the various models discussed are structured and unstructured general models that produce income statements, balance sheets, and statements of cash flow or change in working capital. It is concluded that financial modeling is a valuable planning tool that can determine consequences quickly when financial decisions are needed.

AHCMS 21775 FM

Boston University Health Policy Institute
Control of Hospital Costs by Rate Setting
Boston University Health Policy Institute, 53 Bay State Rd., Boston, MA

This report presents an overview of the mandatory rate setting programs under state commissions, describing both operational and philosophical differences. The salient features of prospective reimbursement and the budget review process are described.

AHCMS 20071 HC

Breslow, Lester; Fielding, Jonathan E.; and Lave, Lester B.
Annual Review of Public Health, Vol. 2
Annual Reviews Inc., 4139 El Camino Way, Palo Alto, CA 94306, 1981, 505 pp.

This volume, the second in a series that documents trends and developments in the field of public health, presents selected papers highlighting advances in the knowledge and care for the perinatal period and infancy, as well as control of infectious and certain parasitic diseases. Other topics discussed include: recent trends in cardiovascular disease, especially the significant decline in ischemic heart disease; prevention of dental disease; health effects of air pollution and low level exposure to lead; technological and economic issues in public health; health hazard appraisal; health indicators and information systems for the future; new and continuing problems in ambulatory and other aspects of health care; and behavioral factors in health improvement and health services.

AHCMS 23059 HE

Brown, M.; McMann, K.; and Cadle, L.
Medical Equipment Inventory and Service Scheduling by Computer: Experience with a Working Scheme
Journal of Medical Engineering and Technology, 7:5, 1983, pp. 228–33.

The computerized inventory management system used by Liverpool Health Authority now holds records of 7,500 items of equipment (past and present) and provides information and instructions to 13 separate service sections located in various hospitals in the district. A detailed service history for each item of equipment is retained on the original service and safety-test record card, and the computer inventory forms a summary. Entry is via a single operator console at authority headquarters and consists of 22 items of information. Service units receive up-to-date lists of equipment under their care and a weekly service demand showing items due or overdue for service. Workload, average costs of servicing, future capital costs to replace equipment, and trends in equipment use can all be estimated from relatively simple search programs, and listed information on equipment can be provided for each hospital, department, service unit, and manufacturer. After four years' experience, it is concluded that the costs of the system are justified by the benefits to the equipment servicing programs and to the management of equipment.

AHCMS 27363 EN

Bruton, Deirdra
Uniform Reporting for Case Mix
Topics in Health Care Financing, 6:2, 1979, pp. 79-96.

A discussion of the emergence of uniform case-mix reporting as a means for regulatory bodies to obtain comparable cost data among hospitals.

AHCMS 22339 HC

Buchanan, Robert J.
  Health-Care Finance: An Analysis of Cost and Utilization Issues
Lexington Books, 1981, 174 pp.

  This study is concerned with Medicaid and nursing homes for old people in the United States at a time when over half the funds for nursing home care come from public expenditure. The author compares proprietary and nonprofit nursing homes and concludes that the rates charged by the former are generally no higher than those of the latter. The various methods of reimbursement under Medicaid are described and analyzed in three categories: (1) the reasonable-cost-related method; (2) the fixed-rate method; and (3) the negotiated-rate method. The merits of prospective versus retrospective reimbursement are also debated. The author next uses cost and utilization indexes to investigate whether differences in reimbursement methods affect costs and access to health care under Medicaid. A section of the book is devoted to the legislative history and effects of a law enacted in 1972, PL 92–603 (Section 249), which requires state Medicaid programs to reimburse long-term care facilities on a reasonable-cost-related basis as of July 1976. The author concludes by recommending prospective reimbursement and proposing a system of payment by this method. Numerous statistical tables and a list of references are included.

                                                                        AHCMS 25501 HC

Buchanan, Robert J.
  Medicaid Cost Containment: Prospective Reimbursement for Long-Term Care
Inquiry, 20:4, 1983, pp. 334–42.

  This study analyzes the impact of prospective rate setting by state programs on Medicaid payment and utilization rates for long-term care. For each year between 1975 and 1982, the use of prospective reimbursement was always associated with lower Medicaid payments for long-term care without adversely affecting recipient access to care.

                                                                        AHCMS 27162 HC

Burcke, James M.
  Employers Cut Healthcare Spending, But Few Use Most Successful Methods
Modern Healthcare, 14:6, 1984, p. 56.

  A survey of 602 industrial and financial service firms, utilities and retailers, government entities, universities, and hospitals on how they contain health care costs shows that employers all reported taking measures to cut their health spending per employee. However, the survey shows that administrative actions like hospital utilization reviews or claims processing controls, which could result in significant savings, were used by few employers.

                                                                        AHCMS 27666 HC

Campbell, James G. and Serway, Gay D.
  Cost Benefit Analysis User's Manual
Pacific Health Resources, 1982
Available from Center for Hospital Management Engineering, American Hospital
  Association, Chicago, IL
  This manual provides a step-by-step process for cost-benefit analysis.
                                                                        AHCMS 27118 HC

Cannedy, Lloyd L.
An Inquiry into the Utilization of Money-Market Investments by Non-Federal General Hospitals in the United States Exceeding 500 Beds
University of Alabama, Birmingham, AL, 1968, 114 pp.
Available from University Microfilms
    An inquiry of utilization for investments by hospitals of nine representative types of short-term securities over three time periods.

                                        AHCMS AC0022

Caper, Phillip and Zubkoff, Michael
Managing Medical Costs Through Small Area Analysis
Business and Health, 1:9, 1984, pp. 20–25.
    Small area analysis measures the use of medical resources by comparable populations residing in different hospital markets and documents the variation among hospitals in performance rates for many common medical and surgical procedures. It can be used in managing medical costs. Small area analysis shows sizable differences in the per capita rates of hospital admission for surgical and medical care among hospital service areas. These variations exist because physicians tend to compare their own practice with treatment choice. When provided information about how their own practices compare with those of their colleagues in other geographic locations, physicians would modify their practice styles which would result in the reduction of performance rates for many procedures. The population-based analysis of medical practice patterns also provides a powerful tool for understanding the elasticity of demand and the role of physician-induced demand for hospital and other medical services. These techniques can be used to promote selective reduction in the utilization rate of hospitals and of medical services that are of uncertain value.

                                        AHCMS 28500 HC

Catholic Hospital Association
Guides to Hospital Administrative Planning and Control Through Accounting
The Association, Saint Louis, MO, 62 pp.
Available from University Microfilms
    A manual for administrators which presents the uses of accounting and statistical data in specific but nontechnical terms. Reports recommended by administrator, how they should be interpreted by him, and what uses he can make of them are discussed in considerable detail.

                                        AHCMS 1

Chawla, Marshall and Steinhardt, Bruce J.
Episode of Care Accounting Methodology For a Cost-Effectiveness Approach to Quality Assurance in a Health Maintenance Organization
Group Health Association of America, Inc., Washington, DC, 1975, 323 pp.
    A methodology is described for evaluating and promoting cost-effectiveness in health maintenance organizations (HMOs), using an episode of care accounting framework. Methods for reallocating constrained resources, based on an analysis of cost-effectiveness, are detailed. A technical description of a standard accounting and statistical information system, required for analyzing the quality of care provided by HMOs and their cost-effectiveness, is presented. Costs of constituent elements of an episode of care, particularly professional medical services, are identified. The results of time studies of two ambulatory health care settings are

presented. It is concluded that a significant amount of variations in professional resources consumed by patients can be attributed to their different diagnoses or medical problems and may be predictable. The methodology is considered useful for internal HMO management, cross-HMO comparisons, and the implementation of uniform cost-reporting requirements. Appendixes contain narrative information and tabular data on HMO cost-effectiveness.

AHCMS 18867 IN

Clark, Bliss B. and Lamont, Gwynn X.
Accurate Census Forecasting Leads to Cost Containment
Hospitals, 50:11, 1976, pp. 43–48.

The article presents a model that helped achieve accurate hospital census forecasts for eight medical-surgical units. Seven steps used in developing the model included obtaining and evaluating a historical data base, classifying discrete events affecting the census, and projecting the potential impact of future discrete events on the census. The forecast was used in planning personnel and bed utilization, with resulting savings. Accuracy of the forecast is illustrated.

AHCMS 16786 HE

Cleverley, William O.
Capital Management: Accounting Return on Equity in the Nonprofit Hospital
Hospital Financial Management, 35:7, 1981, pp. 26–38.

In this article, the author describes a number of financial ratios that influence accounting return on equity (ROE) values in the hospital industry, compares ROE of the tax-exempt sector with the Hospital Corporation of America between 1977 and 1979, and suggests ways in which accounting ROE might be improved.

AHCMS 24172 FM

Cleverley, William O.
Evaluation of Alternative Payment Strategies for Hospitals: A Conceptual Approach
Inquiry, 16:2, 1979, pp. 108–18.

The article evaluates alternative payment systems for health care institution providers according to their perceived attainment of defined criteria.

AHCMS 21451 HC

Cleverley, William O.
An Input-Output Model for Hospital Costing
Bulletin of the Operations Research Society of America, 22:1, 1974.

The basic objective of this paper is to apply input-output methodology as a cost-finding system in a hospital. Simple regression analysis is used to develop estimates of the technological coefficients.

AHCMS 13221 AC

Cleverley, William O.
Minimizing Price Exposure Risk Through the Commodities Markets
Hospital and Health Services Administration, 27:4, 1982, pp. 55–66.

In this article, the author describes the technique of hedging in the futures commodities market as a means of reducing a hospital's exposure risk to unanticipated increases in prices of needed resources. The mechanics of trading in the futures market are illustrated through an example of purchasing six-month contracts for silver in the commodities market (hospitals are fairly large indirect purchasers of silver because of its substantial content in X ray film). Important considerations in the technique of hedging include the timing of the purchase date with hospital rate establishment, the quantity to be hedged, and the historical price relationship between the price of the commodity (for example, silver) and prices of purchased items that are made of the commodity (for example, X ray film). The author also discusses alternative hedging strategies, such as buying long or selling short, reimbursement and financial reporting treatment of hedging, and application of the hedging technique to other commodities, such as foodstuffs of importance to dietary departments.

AHCMS 26945 FM

Cleverley, William O.
One Step Further: The Multi-Variable Flexible Budget System
Hospital Financial Management, 30:4, 1976, pp. 33–44.

Describes a method for developing a multivariable, flexible budget system using existing data of a nursing cost center for budgeting RN, ancillary, and total hours to illustrate how a system can be developed and what level of improved accuracy might be expected.

AHCMS 19039 AC

Cleverley, William O.
Return on Equity in the Hospital Industry: Requirement or Windfall?
Inquiry, 19:2, 1982, pp. 150–59.

Discusses the need for a return on equity in the nonprofit health care industry and defines the amount needed. The author addresses return on equity from a financial requirements or "components" perspective (that is, return on equity capital is a function of present and prospective financial needs). This approach is in contrast to the "owner's equity" approach which argues that a return is essential not for present and future needs, but as payment for the cost of equity capital used at the present time. The owner's equity approach is retrospective and based on market factors.

AHCMS 25543 FM

Cleverley, William O.
Valuation: Its Impact on Accounting Measures of Income and Return on Capital
Health Care Management Review, 8:2, 1983, pp. 51–63.

This article examines the potential impact that a change in the basis of accounting for income would have on the determination of required returns on and returns on capital. The author recommends that hospitals begin to experiment with preparation of supplementary reports based on principles defined in FASB Statement 33, because it will give governing boards a more realistic perception of the true capital position of hospitals and may create some movement in third party payment policy.

AHCMS 26948 FM

Cleverley, William O. and Felkner, Joseph G.
FAS Subscribers Surveyed: Hospitals Increase Use of Capital Budgeting Process
Healthcare Financial Management, 38:6, 1982, pp. 70 ff.

Reports the results of a survey on capital budgeting practices used in the hospital industry over a five-year period. Some of the major conclusions follow. (1) Sample hospitals are rapidly improving almost every facet of the capital budgeting process; respondents showed a trend toward application of capital methods to a larger percentage of capital expenditures. The use of discounted cash flow methods, however, is still below industry standards, but great progress is being made. (2) Respondents believed project definition and estimation of cash flows to be the most critical phase in the capital budgeting process. (3) A greater number of hospitals appear to be developing long-range plans in a strategic planning process. In 1980, 79% of the respondents prepared long-range plans. (4) Eighty-seven percent of the respondents said that alternatives to major investment proposals were searched and considered.

AHCMS 25377 FM

Cleverley, William O. and Nutt, Paul C.
The Decision Process Used for Hospital Bond Rating—And Its Implications
Health Services Research, 19:5, 1984, pp. 615–37.

Investigation of the process of hospital bond rating related the ratings assigned by Moody's and Standard and Poors to indicators of hospital financial condition (such as debt per bed and peak debt coverage), institutional factors (including size, occupancy, and local market competition), indenture provisions (such as reserves), and contextual factors. The criteria used by Moody's and Standard and Poors to rate hospital bonds were revealed to be similar but not identical. Criteria used in the bond rating process have several important implications (for example, the rating approach provides strong financial incentives for increases in hospital size and complexity), and hospitals that rely on extensive amounts of public financing appear to be penalized in the rating process.

AHCMS 28357 FM

Cohen, David I.; Jones, Paul; Littenberg, Benjamin; and Neuhauser, Duncan
Does Cost Information Availability Reduce Physician Test Usage? A Randomized Clinical Trial with Unexpected Findings
Medical Care, 20:3, 1982, pp. 286–92

Four similar teams of physicians associated with similar inpatient units and randomly assigned patients were used to study the effect of providing physicians with cost information about their use of laboratory tests and X rays. Two teams received information about test costs, and two teams received X ray cost information. Test and X ray usage fell during the experimental conditions and continued to fall after the experimental period ended in teams in which there was an interested leader.

AHCMS 25738 HC

Conrad, Douglas A.
Returns on Equity to Not-for-Profit Hospitals: Theory and Implementation
Health Services Research, 19:1, 1984, pp. 41–63.

It is argued that not-for-profit hospitals can be assumed to generate a return on equity capital due, in principle, to competition in the final product market for hospital services and in the capital market. Practical difficulties in identifying claimants to the net income of the firm, as well as the incentive problems of cost-based reimbursement, suggest that a competitive pricing approach is likely to be the appropriate means to provide a reasonable return on equity for the not-for-profit and for-profit hospital. Implications of the analysis for the correct discount rate in investment decisions are outlined.

AHCMS 27572 FM

Conyard, Shirley J.
  An Exploratory Study of Professional Standards Review Organization (PSRO)
  Effectiveness on Economic Costs and Social Costs
Adelphi University, Garden City, NY, 1980
Available from University Microfilms

This study explored the effect of PSROs on economic costs and on social costs (diminished quality of care) of Medicaid and Medicare patients in ten short-term voluntary hospitals in New York City. The study used two types of controls: a control group, non–Medicare-Medicaid, and time (before and after PSRO). Economic costs were measured by the length of stay (LOS), and social costs were measured by changes in admission rates (AR) and opinions of hospital administrators. The study findings were as follows. (1) The LOS declined post-PSRO for Medicare and Medicaid (experimental groups) but not for non–Medicare-Medicaid patients (control group). However, by the second year, PSRO effectiveness in reducing LOS had begun to decline. (2) The AR for the three groups increased post-PSRO; however only Medicare's AR increased significantly. (3) There was a significant correlation between decreased LOS and increased AR for Medicare and non–Medicare-Medicaid, but not for Medicaid patients. (4) The experimental group continued to have availability to beds and access to inpatient services post-PSRO. It was the opinion of some administrators (40%) that premature discharges had increased post-PSRO. The study findings suggest that PSRO has a significant effect on reducing LOS without diminishing the quality of care.

AHCMS 24325 HC

Cooper, Barbara S.; Worthington, Nancy L.; and Piro, Paula A.
  National Health Expenditures: Calendar Years 1929–1972
Research and Statistics Note, No. 3, February 1974, 14 pp.

Report presents data on health spending in the United States for 1972. Tables include data on national health expenditures by source and percentage of gross national product for selected years 1929–72; national health expenditures by type of expenditure and source of funds 1970–72; expenditures for health services and supplies under public programs 1970–72; distribution of personal health care expenditures for selected years 1950–72; aggregate and per capita national health expenditures for selected years 1929–72; and the amount and percent of personal health care expenditures met by third parties 1972.

AHCMS 12136 HE

Copeland, Ronald and Jacobs, Philip
  Cost of Capital, Target Rate of Return, and Investment Decision Making
Health Services Research, 16:3, 1981, pp. 335–41.

Recent attempts to develop an investment decision criterion for nonprofit hospitals that follows the for-profit criteria have resulted in little agreement. Terminology is much to blame for the lack of consensus. Attempts have been made to identify a "cost of capital" for nonprofit institutions, and to employ this concept in a manner similar to the way it is employed in a for-profit setting. In fact, the application of this concept to nonprofit institutions has resulted in confusion. The use of "target rate of return" in its place would orient the debate more properly toward institutional ends and the means required to achieve them.

AHCMS 25013 FM

Council of State Governments
Health Cost Containment: The Connecticut, Maryland, and New Jersey Responses
The Council, Lexington, KY, 1976, 74 pp.

Report describes health care cost containment programs in Connecticut, Maryland, and New Jersey, three states that have chosen to intervene directly by regulating hospital rates. Their experiences suggest they are making some progress in limiting the rise in medical care costs. Report also outlines important considerations in creating a health cost regulatory commission.

AHCMS 17720 HE

Cranshaw, Jane F.
The Computer-Assisted Budget
Topics in Health Care Financing, 10:1, 1983, pp. 9–26.

Computer modeling in the hospital budgetary process helps to develop three separate yet integrated plans for the overall budget: capital budget, operating budget, and cash flow budget. It is pointed out that the integrated storage features, accuracy, and processing speed of computerized budgeting systems are of great assistance during each of the steps in budgeting. Capital budget development involves definitions of the project, cash flow projections, and financial analysis of alternative proposals. The operations budget is the most tedious and time-consuming of the three budgets and requires projecting year-end activity; projecting utilization statistics; distributing budget worksheets; budgeting staff hours, salary expense, nonsalary expense, and revenue; and fine-tuning. The cash flow budget converts the accrual-based revenue and expense information contained in the operating budget to a cash basis. It is concluded that using a computer system for these activities will provide the user with accurate and organized information as well as increased time and flexibility to analyze and evaluate alternative financial plans.

AHCMS 27473 FM

Cromwell, J. and Burstein, P.
Impact of State Hospital Prospective Reimbursement Programs on Hospital Capital Formation, Competition and Industrial Structure: An Evaluation
Abt Associates, Inc., Cambridge, MA, 1984
Available from National Technical Information Service (PB84–181445)

Discusses the effects of prospective payment programs on hospital investment and competition during the 1970s. Capital formation incentives of nine major state programs are reviewed, models of investment under regulation are developed, and extensive descriptive and econometric analysis is presented on each program.

AHCMS 27820 FM

Cromwell, J. and Hewes, H.
Impact of State Hospital Prospective Reimbursement Programs on Medicare Hospital and Non-Hospital Costs
Abt Associates, Inc., Cambridge, MA, 1984
Available from National Technical Information Service (PB84–181544)

Using the Health Care Financing Administration Medicare 5% Medical History Sample File, hospital and nonhospital utilization and expenditures were analyzed on a county-year basis. The sample included 1,300 counties in 15 PR and all non-PR states for the 1974–78 period. Extensive descriptive and econometric analysis is performed using a quasi-experimental design. A literature review of hospital-nonhospital substitution is included, along with general modeling of Medicare reimbursement and cross-subsidization effects. Among the seven states with statistically significant results, six (including Connecticut and New York) showed reductions in total Medicare spending; only New Jersey was positive. No evidence was found of "cost-shifting" to Medicare where it does not participate.

AHCMS 27843 HC

Cummings, K. Michael; Frisof, Kenneth B.; Long, Michael J.; and Hrynkiewich, George
The Effects of Price Information on Physicians' Test-Ordering Behavior: Ordering of Diagnostic Tests
Medical Care, 20:3, 1982, pp. 293–301.

This research evaluated the effects of providing physicians with information about the prices of diagnostic tests on their subsequent test-ordering behavior. The study population consisted of 36 second- and third-year residents and 23 clinical faculty in three family practice centers affliated with the Department of Family Medicine at Wayne State University School of Medicine, Detroit, Michigan. Study participants were asked to review four case studies, each describing a patient with ambiguous symptoms, and to indicate on an attached test order form the tests they would order for each patient. Subjects were randomly assigned either to a group that received test order forms on which the prices of diagnostic tests were printed (price-information group) or to a group that received test order forms with no prices indicated (control group). The study results show that for each of four cases, the average number of diagnostic tests ordered was significantly lower in the price-information group than in the control group. Findings also show an average reduction in the cumulative cost of tests ordered per patient of 31.1% related to the provision of price information. The feasibility of regularly providing physicians with price information is discussed and reviewed in light of other approaches that have been developed to modify physician behavior in ordering diagnostic tests.

AHCMS 25737 HC

Davidson, Stephen M. and Wacker, Ronald C.
Community Hospitals and Medicaid
Medical Care, 12:2, 1974, pp. 115–30.

The study examines Medicaid utilization patterns, determining the extent to which Medicaid recipients in a Chicago community use hospitals in their own community. Data from the February 1970 Hospital Discharge Study show that substantial numbers of Medicaid patients bypass nearby community hospitals and receive care instead in more distant teaching hospitals. In addition to possible harmful medical consequences, this pattern turns out to be much more expensive to the state's Medicaid program than care in closer community hospitals would be. Possible reasons for these patterns are suggested, implications for planning are discussed, and questions for further research are identified.

AHCMS 11937 IN

Davis, Karen
Medicaid Payments and Utilization of Medical Services by the Poor
Inquiry, 13:2, 1976, pp. 122–35.

Summarizes the major benefits provided and persons served by Medicaid and assesses the impact of medical services and financial hardship inflicted on the poor by high medical bills. Analysis indicated that the rural, black, and nonwelfare poor have not received a proportionate share of medical benefits and that the Medicaid program overall has not reduced the percentage of their income the poor must spend on medical care.

AHCMS 19125 IN

Davis, Karen
National Health Insurance: Benefits, Costs and Consequences
The Brookings Institution, Washington, DC, 1975, 194 pp.

Seven major national health insurance proposals introduced in Congress are analyzed. The approaches taken by the proposals to financing health care vary from tax subsidies for the purchase of private insurance, through a combination of private and public insurance, to coverage that is predominantly publicly financed. Each proposal is examined against a set of questions derived from three basic goals: (1) to ensure that all Americans have access to adequate medical care; (2) to eliminate the financial hardship of large medical bills; and (3) to limit the rise in health care costs.

AHCMS 17407 IN

Davis, Karen
Relationship of Hospital Prices to Costs
Applied Economics, 4, 1971, pp. 115–25.

The ratio of hospital prices to average costs of providing hospital care is studied. Empirical evidence presented here contradicts the prevailing view that hospitals merely attempt to recover costs in their pricing policy. In addition, the view that the excess of price over average cost is merely an attempt on the part of the hospital to accumulate sufficient revenue to make needed investment is not substantiated. Instead, price-average cost ratios are found to be sensitive to certain demand and supply conditions.

AHCMS 09128 HE

Deason, James M. (ed.)
Flexible Budgeting
Topics in Health Care Financing, 5:4, 1979.

This article describes the implementation and evaluation of the flexible budgeting system (FBS). An overview of the steps in the budget preparation process is presented, and the development of performance standards which give meaning to this process is also described. Applications of the FBS for both day-to-day management and for long-term decision making are presented.

AHCMS 21450 FM

Deets, M. King and Krentz, Susanna E.
Hospital Debt Capacity in a Competitive Environment
Healthcare Financial Management, 36:7, 1982, pp. 26 ff.

In this article, the authors discuss the impact of increased competition in the hospital sector in terms of business risk (threats that can negatively affect cash flow and are a function of the industry as a whole), enterprise risk (threats that affect only an individual hospital or multihospital group), and financial risk (exclusive risk associated with borrowing money).

AHCMS 25372 FM

Detsky, Allan S.; Strider, Steven C.; Mully, Albert G.; and Thibault, George E.
Prognosis, Survival, and the Expenditure of Hospital Resources for Patients in an Intensive-Care Unit
New England Journal of Medicine, 305:12, 1981, pp. 667–72.

To define more precisely the factors determining the allocation of resources to critically ill patients, the authors asked physicians to estimate at the time of admission the short-term prognosis of patients who accounted for 1,831 admissions to a medical intensive-care and coronary-care unit. The relations between this prognosis, the actual outcome, and the resource expenditure during a single hospitalization were then examined, revealing that the care of nonsurvivors involved a significantly higher mean expenditure than did the care of survivors. Among nonsurvivors, expenditure positively correlated with the probability of survival estimated at the time of admission. Among survivors, expenditure negatively correlated with the probability of survival. Among both nonsurvivors and survivors, total expenditure per day was greatest for patients whose outcomes were most unexpected. The authors conclude that prognostic uncertainty is important in determining resource expenditures for the critically ill.

AHCMS 25121 HC

Dittman, David A. and Ofer, Aharon R.
  The Effect of Cost Reimbursement on Capital Budgeting Decision Models
Topics in Health Care Financing, 3:1, 1976, pp. 35–50.

Article illustrates the effect cost-based reimbursement has on four basic capital budgeting models: accounting rate of return; payback; internal rate of return; and net present value. The usefulness of the various models is discussed.

AHCMS 17069 AC

Dittman, David A. and Ofer, Aharon R.
  The Impact of Reimbursement on Hospital Cash Flow
Topics in Health Care Financing, 3:1, 1976, pp. 27–31.

Article illustrates the effect third party reimbursement has on the investment decision process of health care institutions. Two examples are outlined: the hospital makes a cost saving investment in labor-saving equipment; and the hospital purchases revenue-generating equipment. In both instances it is shown that cost-based reimbursement affects the net cash flow realized.

AHCMS 17070 AC

Donabedian, Avedis
  A Review of Some Experiences with Prepaid Group Practice
School of Public Health, The University of Michigan, Ann Arbor, MI, 1965, 80 pp.

Analyzes available published information on expenditures, utilization, and quality of prepaid plans, together with surveys of subscriber attitudes. Two tables describe member physician attitudes. The author notes that "only those studies which permit fairly valid comparison" are included. References are described in an annotated bibliography and data are presented in detailed appendix tables.

AHCMS HE0123

Donabedian, Avedis and Thorby, Jean A.
  The Systematic Impact of Medicare
Medical Care Review, 26:6, 1969, pp. 567–85.

Bibliography of 67 items and review article discussing the impact of Medicare on use, prices, voluntary health insurance and provider agencies, and individuals. There is brief reference to the degree of protection, quality of care, the impact on public welfare, and civil rights aspects. Public health departments are among the provider agencies discussed.

AHCMS IN4084

Dowling, William L. (ed.)
  Prospective Rate Setting
Topics in Health Care Financing, 3:2, 1976, 167 pp.

This issue of *Topics in Health Care Financing* is concerned exclusively with prospective rate setting (PR), presenting seven papers that explore how to provide administrators and financial managers with up-to-date information about the nature of PR and how it might affect their institutions.

AHCMS 18086 AC

Dowling, William L.
  Prospective Reimbursement of Hospitals
Inquiry, 11:3, 1974, pp. 163–80.

Develops a framework for examining different approaches to prospective reimbursement, identifies areas of hospital performance that might be affected by prospective reimbursement, suggests changes in hospital performance that might occur under different approaches to prospective reimbursement, and discusses alternative methods that can be used to set budgets or rates prospectively. The acceptability to hospitals of any rate setting method, assuming participation is not mandated, probably depends more on expected payment level than on method used to determine rates.

AHCMS 13263 IN

Dowling, William L.; House, Peter J.; Lehman, Jeffrey M.; Mead, Gary L.; Teague, Nancy; Trivedi, Vandan; and Watts, Carolyn A.
  Prospective Reimbursement in Downstate New York and Its impact on Hospitals: A Summary
Center for Health Services Research, University of Washington, Seattle, WA, 1976, 93 pp.

Study evaluates the impact of New York Blue Cross and Medicaid prospective reimbursement systems begun in 1970 on hospital costs and operations in downstate New York.

AHCMS 17525 IN

Drucker, William R. et al.
  Towards Strategies for Cost Containment in Surgical Patients
Annals of Surgery, 198:3, 1983, pp. 284–300.

A study of high-cost surgical patients as a possible source of hospital cost containment is described. In 1980, at Strong Memorial Hospital, Rochester, New York, 261 surgical patients from a total of 3,935 had total charges of over $20,000 each. They made up 32% of total surgical charges and patient days. Eighty-five high-cost patients from a subset of 2,021 surgical patients were studied in more detail. These patients were responsible for a disproportionate share of surgical charges and hospital days. Average total charges were eight times those of the subset. Nineteen of the 85 patients died in hospital, and 42 were dead within three years. Forty were "complex" patients, usually elderly and with multiple illnesses and admissions. A study of hospital ancillary procedures disclosed a similar pattern of high costs. Means of cost containment can be applied to these high-cost, complex patients. Strategies to help in this should include: (1) a system that gives physicians the incentive to reduce costs, (2) an accurate means of identifying potential high-cost and complex patients, and (3) an awareness of the need to withhold expensive intervention in certain cases.

AHCMS 28065 HC

Dunham, Andrew B. and Morone, James A.
The Politics of Innovation: The Evolution of DRG Rate Regulation in New Jersey
Health Research and Educational Trust of New Jersey, Princeton, NJ, 1983, DRG Evaluation, Vol. IV-A

This volume examines the political evolution of New Jersey's diagnosis-related group (DRG) reimbursement system for reimbursing hospitals equally on a payer per case basis. It presents a detailed "chain-of-events" account of DRG development, an analysis of the roles played by different actors from various institutions, and a discussion of the potential. By 1983, all acute care hospitals in New Jersey were reimbursed by DRGs. The report finds that there are several factors that militate against the diffusion of the DRG concept to other states: (1) huge data requirements; (2) the technical complexity of the system; and (3) some unfavorable publicity about the problems that characterized the early stages of implementation. It is felt, however, that if the Health Care Financing Administration determines the New Jersey experiment is a promising one, some form of diffusion will become more likely. It is concluded that government, health care institutions, and third party payers have become increasingly intertwined in reimbursement systems such as DRG. The likely result of this will be an enhanced government role at the center of the health care system.

AHCMS 26440 HC

Dunkelberg, John S.; Furst, Richard W.; and Roenfeldt, Rodney L.
State Rate Review and the Relationship Between Capital Expenditures and Operating Costs
Inquiry, 20:3, 1983, pp. 240–47.

It is commonly assumed that an increase in capital expenditures leads to increased operating costs and a subsequent increase in rates, and thus that state rate review systems must incorporate certificate-of-need type controls over capital expenditures. The results of this study indicate that in those states with comprehensive rate review systems, increased capital expenditures may not lead to higher operating costs and rates; rather, increased wage rates are reflected in higher operating costs and rates. This pass-through of wages, and not capital costs, may have important policy implications.

AHCMS 26892 HC

Economic Stabilization Program
Acute Care Hospitals: Planning and Executing Capital Projects Under Cost Controls
U.S. Government Printing Office, Washington, DC, 1974, Stock Number 4114-00032, 26 pp.

The purpose of this document is to facilitate the planning and implementation of capital expenditure projects while meeting the cost control objectives of planning agencies, hospitals, and programs, such as Phase IV.

AHCMS 12346 AC

Edwards, Arch B.
Capitation Budgeting: An Idea Whose Time Has Come
Topics in Health Care Financing, 7:3, 1981, pp. 1–8.

This article discusses how the concept of capitation care financing used in health maintenance organizations can be adapted to hospitals as a means of providing incentives for cost containment. The experience of the Military Health Service System (MHSS) in developing and testing a capitation budgeting system is described. Three key steps were followed in developing the capitation budget system: (1) determination of actual costs for the current year; (2) development of a capitation budget target that has two components—one built on costs that will not vary significantly with the size of the hospital's service population and one adjusted for inflation and for changes in the service population size and characteristics; and (3) development of management actions that permit the hospital to operate within the targeted capitation budget (for example, staffing ratios and mix, utilization rates, rates and charges). The MHSS test of capitation budgeting showed that this approach can create incentives for managers to improve efficiency and effectiveness of care.

AHCMS 23683 FM

Eggers, Paul W.
Trends in Medicare Reimbursement for End-Stage Renal Disease: 1974–1979
Health Care Financing Review, 6:1, 1984, pp. 31–38.

This article presents detailed analyses of the trends in Medicare expenditures for persons with end-stage renal disease. Program expenditures increased at an annual rate of 30.5% from 1974 to 1981. Three-fourths of this increase was a result of increases in enrollment. Per capita reimbursements for dialysis patients increased at a 5.2% annual rate and per capita reimbursements for transplant patients increased at a 10.5% annual rate. In 1979, per capita reimbursements for home dialysis patients were $5,000 less than for in-unit dialysis patients. Patient characteristics such as age, sex, race, and cause of renal failure were, for the most part, unrelated to the costs of dialysis and transplantation.

AHCMS 28288 HC

Eilers, Robert D.
Postpayment Medical Expense Coverage: A Proposed Salvation for Insured and Insurer
Blue Cross Association, Chicago, IL, 1969, 15 pp.

The author proposes postpayment medical expense coverage as the most realistic method of overcoming present inadequate insurance payments for a large portion of families' total health care expenditures. Postpayment provides credit for medical care. The carrier pays provider's total bill with provision for periodic repayment by the individual to the carrier of the noninsured portion. The author discusses services to be included, repayment time periods and interest rates. Governmental repayment might be arranged for the indigent. Despite unsettled aspects such as legal difficulties, risk and eligibility, the author believes the plan should be given exhaustive study for its many advantages to society.

AHCMS IN1036

Eisenberg, John M. and Williams, Sankey V.
Cost Containment and Changing Physicians' Practice Behavior: Can the Fox Learn to Guard the Chicken Coop?
Journal of the American Medical Association, 246:19, 1981, pp. 2195–2201.

Six different strategies have been used in an effort to improve physicians' awareness of the costs of health care and to reduce medical expenditures: education; peer review with feedback; administration changes; participation; penalties; and rewards. This paper reviews the literature on experience with these approaches, emphasizing their application to physicians' use of ancillary services such as laboratory tests and diagnostic X ray examinations.

AHCMS 26420 HC

Elnicki, Richard A.
Effect of Phase II Price Controls on Hospital Services
Health Services Research, 7:2, 1972, pp. 106–17.

Nonmaternity cost data from three Connecticut hospitals are analyzed to determine the contribution to total costs per discharge made by increases in cost per unit of service and by increases in units of service per discharge between 1960 and 1969.

AHCMS 09220 HE

Enthoven, Alain C.
Consumer-Choice Health Plan: A Rational Economic Design for National Health Insurance
Center for Health Administration Studies, University of Chicago, Chicago, IL

This lecture addresses the problem of escalating costs in health care economy and the implications of this inflationary trend for designing a national health insurance (NHI) scheme that will result in effective utilization of health resources. The advantages and disadvantages of four alternative NHI plans are described: Health Security Act (Kennedy-Corman); Comprehensive Health Insurance Plan (Nixon Administration) and Publicly Guaranteed Health Plan (HEW); Target Plan (Long-Ribicoff); and Consumer-Choice Health Plan (CCHP), which is patterned after the Federal Employees Health Benefits Program. Rational economic incentives and fair market competition under CCHP are cited as the most viable methods for reducing costs and improving the efficiency of resource allocation; CCHP allows consumers to choose between competing alternatives. CCHP is not proposed as an immediate radical replacement of the present financing system, but as a set of "mid-course corrections" whose cumulative impact would alter the delivery system radically, but gradually and voluntarily.

AHCMS 20481 IN

Ernst & Whinney
Accounting for Medicare Prospective Payments
Ernst & Whinney, Cleveland, OH, 1984

Although Medicare has shifted from a cost-based reimbursement system to a fixed rate per DRG, outpatient costs continue to be reimbursed on a reasonable cost basis as well as certain inpatient costs (for example, capital-related costs, certain kidney acquisition costs, bad debts of Medicare patients, and direct approved medical education costs). This report discusses major issues in accounting for revenue earned from services to Medicare patients that have not been discharged, Medicare in-house accounts, and losses of Medicare in-house accounts at the end of an accounting period. Other issues—can expected profits and losses on Medicare in-house accounts be offset, how should hospitals measure losses on Medicare in-house accounts, should hospitals continue to record contractual adjustments under PPS, how should Medicare timing differences be treated, and how should hospitals account for outliers—are also discussed. The report provides an explanation of accounting for Medicare inpatient revenues under periodic interim payments and claim-submitted methods of payment under PPS.

AHCMS 28021 FM

Ernst & Whinney
Reporting Practices Concerning Hospital-Related Organizations
Ernst & Whinney, Cleveland, OH, 1981

This report analyzes the various sections of the Statement of Position (SOP) 81–2 issued by the American Institute of Certified Public Accountants as a clarification of a section in its *Hospital Audit Guide* entitled "Other Related Organizations." This section was vague about how hospitals should account for such related organizations as auxiliaries, foundations, and guilds in their financial statements. SOP 81–2 is effective for fiscal years beginning on or after July 1, 1981. The SOP gives no new guidance on whether a hospital should consolidate or combine its financial statements with those of a related organization, but does provide new guidance on what disclosures a hospital should make if it is related to another organization and does not issue consolidated or combined statements. A not-for-profit organization is considered related to a not-for-profit hospital if the hospital "controls" it or if the hospital is, for all practical purposes, its sole beneficiary. In such cases, the hospital is required to disclose in a footnote a description of the relationship between the organizations and a summary of the financial information about the separate organizations' assets, liabilities, results of operations, and changes in fund balance. If related organizations do not meet both control and sole beneficiary criteria, but the hospital receives material amounts of funds from the organization or the two have material transactions, the hospital should disclose this in notes to its financial statements.

AHCMS 24534 FM

Ernst & Whinney
The Revised DRGS: Their Importance in Medicare Payments to Hospitals
Ernst & Whinney, Cleveland, OH, 1983

The purpose of this report is to provide health care executives with an understanding of the diagnosis-related group (DRG) classification system which has been revised recently and to identify its new significance to hospital management. The original DRG system was based on the International Classification of Diseases Adopted–8th Revision (ICDA–8). However, because ICD–9–CM replaced ICDA–8 as the primary disease classification system used in the United States, a new set of DRGs had to be developed. Report explains factors that led to revision of the original DRG system, identifies limitations of DRGs, and reviews Medicare's current use of DRGs to adjust for differences in hospital case mix. An outline of reimbursement strategies is included which hospitals can use to improve their operations under cost-per-case payment systems. Appendix lists the 467 DRGs with their descriptions. Passage of the Tax Equity and Fiscal Responsibility Act of 1982 signals some changes in Medicare reimbursement. These changes are based on a case-mix index which was constructed using a slightly modified version of the ICD–9–CM DRGs; thus, it is considered essential that hospital executives understand the DRG system and its use in hospital payment systems.

AHCMS 26585 HC

Esmond, Truman H., Jr.
Budgeting Procedures for Hospitals, 1982 Edition
American Hospital Association, Chicago, IL, 1982

A step-by-step illustration of the procedures a community hospital can follow in developing a sound annual budget. Emphasis is on understanding the interrelationship of the strategic planning cycle and the control cycle of operational planning and budgeting. A timetable for accomplishment of each step in the budgeting process is presented. The book describes how to prepare the various elements of the operating budget, for example, revenue and expense budget, cash budget, capital budget, projected balance sheet and related statements, and supplementary explanations, schedules, and exhibits. It discusses the use of statistics in developing utilization forecasts of patient days and ancillary services, and includes 50 sample schedules or worksheets that can be used in developing a budget. Appendix includes a sample operating budget which can serve as a model for final budget documentation to be presented to a hospital's governing board.

AHCMS 28658 FM

Esposito, Alfonso; Hupfer, Michael; Mason, Cynthia; and Rogler, Diane
Abstracts of State Legislated Hospital Cost-Containment Programs
Health Care Financing Review, 4:2, 1982, pp. 129–59.

This report summarizes state legislated efforts to control rising hospital costs and the status of these efforts in May 1982. The abstract for each of the 17 state programs summarizes key legislative features and operating aspects. The states included in this report are: Arizona, California, Connecticut, Florida, Illinois, Maine, Maryland, Massachusetts, Minnesota, New Jersey, New York, Oregon, Rhode Island, Virginia, Washington, West Virginia, and Wisconsin. The abstracts focus on programs requiring the disclosure, review, or legislation of hospital rates and budgets.

AHCMS 25558 FM

Evans, Robert G.
Efficiency Incentives in Hospital Reimbursements
Harvard University Library, Cambridge, MA, 1970

Thesis analyzed the effect of reimbursement plans on incentives for efficiency in the hospital industry. Study begins with the premise that hospitals produce too much care too expensively and the present means of payment of hospitals encourage waste. Data are presented to show that the rapid increase in resource utilization by hospitals in the last two decades is not related to any equivalent measurable increase in health and that health can be maintained with a much lower level of hospital activity input. An explicit model of hospital management is constructed to explain hospital technical and economic inefficiency.

AHCMS IN0–6252

Evans, Robert G.
Health Care in Canada: Patterns of Funding and Regulation
Journal of Health Politics, Policy and Law, 7:1, 1983, pp. 1–43.

During the 1970s the share of health care expenditures in Canadian GNP remained roughly stable, in the range of 7% to 7.5% of GNP, in marked contrast to its escalation in most other countries (the U.S. in particular) and to previous Canadian experience. The shift to a stable pattern coincided with the completion of the Canadian system of universal comprehensive public hospital and medical care insurance. This paper explores how and why the public insurance system served to contain cost escalation. The author then discusses the inadequacy of expenditure experience per se as a basis for health system evaluation—the same data will support claims of both "underfunding" and "spiralling costs." More serious questions involve the influence of alternative patterns of health care funding and delivery on the effectiveness and efficiency of care provision, and the resulting distributional patterns of care and income. A brief sketch is given of the present situation and future possibilities of Canadian health care under these heads.

AHCMS 26932 HC

Federation of American Hospitals
  Study Indicates Slower Rise in Costs in Non–Rate Setting States
The Review, 14:4, 1981, p. 54.

Findings from a study of hospital costs conducted for the Federation of American Hospitals are reported in this article. The study compared costs in 7 states with mandatory rate-setting programs to those in the other 43 states and the District of Columbia, plus the national average for all 51 jurisdictions. Data reveal that the gap in the annual rate of increase between regulated and nonregulated states is narrowing. Although the states without mandatory rate setting have a higher annual rate of increase, their 1979 performance indicates a slower rise than those with mandatory rate setting. The rate of increase in per capita expenditures rose only 0.3% in unregulated states between 1978 and 1979, compared to 2.1% in the regulated states. There were similar findings in expenditures per case. Regarding community hospital expenditures for 1979, per capita and per case expenditures for community hospital services were higher in states with mandatory rate review or control than the national average.

AHCMS 24194 HC

Feldstein, Martin S.
  The Rising Cost of Hospital Care
Information Resources Press, Arlington, VA, 1971, 88 pp.

The author makes the point that one factor that should be considered as causing the rising costs of hospital care in addition to sharply increased wages and other costs is the change in the product, the hospital care itself. Rising income and more comprehensive insurance coverage have changed the patient's expectation of care; through present methods of financing care the hospital can provide more expensive care than the patient may need or want; and technical change in care may not necessarily be technical progress though costs can be increased per day of hospital care. And, almost as an afterthought: "The current approach to medical research may be biased toward producing information that favors cost-increasing innovations."

AHCMS 09092 HE

Feldstein, Martin and Taylor, Amy
  Rapid Rise in Hospital Costs
Harvard University, Cambridge, MA, 1977, 76 pp.
Available from National Technical Information Service (HRP–0016527/4WW)

An analysis of causes contributing to inflation in hospital costs is presented. It focuses on the cost of a day of inpatient care in short-term general hospitals, and makes use of statistics from the Bureau of Labor Statistics, Department of Labor, and from the American Hospital Association. The major conclusion is that the rapid, continuous increase in hospital costs results from the fundamental and continuously changing character of the service provided by the hospitals and that this change has been induced by a growth of insurance. The effect of prepaying for health care through insurance has been to encourage hospitals to provide a more expensive product than most consumers actually wish to purchase. The explanation of rising hospital costs lies not so much in changing wage rates or other input prices as in a changing product and the increased rate at which that product is consumed.

AHCMS 18741 HE

Feldstein, Paul J.
An Analysis of Reimbursement Plans in *Reimbursements for Medical Care*
Office of Research and Statistics, Social Security Administration, Washington, DC, 1968, pp. 23–54.

A study of reimbursement plans in terms of lower cost incentives, greater efficiency in hospital procedures and accounting methods, and maintaining quality care. Various payment plans are discussed as to their long- and short-term marginal costs, and as to their ability to strike a balance between efficiency, low cost, and quality. Conclusions suggest: relative reimbursement, capitation, group prepayment, incentives aimed at results rather than means, reimbursement based on relative performance, effective use of a variety of health facilities all within a plan that counterchecks for levels of quality, should be elements of a reimbursement plan.

AHCMS IN0012

Feldstein, Paul J.
An Empirical Investigation of the Marginal Cost of Hospital Services
University of Chicago, Chicago, IL, 1961, 77 pp.

Report from a doctoral dissertation of a study at Methodist Hospital of Gary, Indiana, from January 1956 to December 1958 examines short-run marginal costs in separate hospital departments on a monthly basis. Independent variables used to estimate costs were adult patient-days, staff days off with pay, and changes or substitution in techniques or production.

AHCMS ACIO, No. 56

Feldstein, Paul J.
Prepaid Group Practice: An Analysis and Review
The University of Michigan, Ann Arbor, MI, 1971, 147 pp.
Available from University Microfilms

Study presents a framework for analysis of prepaid group practices and a comparison of these with alternative delivery systems.

AHCMS IN2–6952

Feldstein, Paul J.
A Proposal for Capitation Reimbursement to Medical Groups for Total Medical Care in *Reimbursement Incentives for Medical Care*
Office of Research and Statistics, Social Security Administration, Washington, DC, 1968, pp. 87–103.

A proposal to develop a capitation reimbursement system under Medicare that pays organized groups of doctors who share facilities and expenses. Increased efficiency, decreased costs, and methods of implementation are discussed, as well as the maintenance of quality care and freedom of choice for patients.

AHCMS IN0011

Feldstein, Paul J. and Waldman, Saul
Financial Position of Hospitals in the Early Medicare Period
Social Security Bulletin, October 1968.

Data on prices, expenses, and utilization for community short-term hospitals are presented and analyzed for the years from 1960 to 1967. Implementation of Medicare, expansion of Medicare and other government programs, an above-average rise in hospital charges, substantial increases in hospital expenses, and moderate increases in hospital utilization and occupancy rates are among the developments affecting hospitals in the period since June 1966. Authors conclude that in the period following the start of Medicare, the financial situation of most hospitals improved.

AHCMS IN4–6097

Ferguson, Carl; Lee, Maw Lin; and Wallace, Richard
Effects of Medicare on Hospital Use: A Disease Specific Study
University of Missouri, Columbia, MO, c. 1975, 20 pp.

Paper presents an analysis of the impact of Medicare on hospital use for 23 disease categories, using data from Missouri hospitals for the period 1965–71. Comparison of utilization data from the period 1965–66 (pre-Medicare) with data after Medicare was implemented indicated the proportion of patients age 65 and over increased from 20% to 24%, number of total patient days for this group increased from 34% to 40%, and length of stay increased from an average of 12 days to over 13 to 15 days. Analysis of utilization by age group shows impact of Medicare on hospital use was greater for the 75 and over group than for the 65 to 74 age group. Analysis of disease categories shows largest increases in utilization occurred where risk of dying and degree of severity of medical problem were relatively low. Paper points out these findings are consistent with Feldstein's suggestion that greatest impact of Medicare was on use of discretionary types of medical service.

AHCMS 12144 HE

Fetter, Robert B.; Mills, Ronald E.; Riedel, Donald C.; and Thompson, John D.
The Application of Diagnostic Specific Cost Profiles to Cost and Reimbursement Controls in Hospitals
Center for Study of Health Services, Yale University, New Haven, CT, 38 pp.

Describes a cost and reimbursement control system for hospitals that was developed to generate hospital budgets based on type of patient served.

AHCMS 17294 HE

Finkler, Steven A.
The Pyramid Approach: Increasing the Usefulness of Flexible Budgeting
Healthcare Financial Management, 36:2, 1982, pp. 30 ff.

This article presents an approach to facilitate understanding of a flexible budgeting system. Flexible budgets take into account the budgeted amount and the actual amount, focusing on what the budget would have been had the output or workload been forecast perfectly. A three-tiered pyramid approach to the concept of flexible budgeting is described which will help the health manager maximize the information content derived from a flexible budgeting system. The pyramid approach offers a method for determining three key types of variance that cause actual costs to differ from budgeted expenses: price, quantity, and volume. Examples are provided for how to analyze these variances at each of the three pyramid levels for a combination of variable and mixed costs.

AHCMS 26022 FM

Fitz, Thomas E., Jr.
Assessing Financial Capabilities: Debt Capacity Analysis is Critical to Planning
Healthcare Financial Management, 37:1, 1983, pp. 52 ff.

This article discusses the basic components of debt capacity analysis, a technique for assessing the financial capabilities of an institution as part of the long-range planning process. To demonstrate the application of debt capacity analysis, a hypothetical hospital's financial capability to undertake a $6.5 million expansion and renovation program is analyzed and evaluated.

AHCMS 26312 FM

Folsom, M. B.; Weaver, W.; Kernan, F.; Molony, J. P.; Park, R. H.; Straus, J. I.; and Willis, W.
  Governor's Committee on Hospital Costs: Summary of Findings and Recommendations
New York State Journal of Medicine, August 1, 1965, pp. 2030–44.

A committee appointed by Governor Nelson Rockefeller and headed by Marion B. Folsom, former Secretary of Health, Education, and Welfare, was commissioned to study the causes of rising costs of hospital care in New York and make recommendations for action. This article summarizes findings and conclusions. These included: more effective use of hospitals over weekends; pooling of maternity beds in multihospital communities; joint purchasing; and the elimination of duplication of highly specialized facilities. Preadmission testing, self-care, home care, long-term care, and drug formularies were all recommended as means of reducing patients' bills. Medical review procedures and better hospital management were called for to ensure better patient care and more efficient use of facilities. It was also suggested doctors could use the hospital for ambulatory diagnostic services and thus increase the institution's revenues.

AHCMS HE 0107

Foster, Richard W.; Phillip, P. Joseph; Hai, Abdul; and Jeffers, James R.
  The Nature of Hospital Costs: Three Studies
Hospital Research and Educational Trust, Chicago, IL, 1976, 268 pp.

These three papers commissioned by the AHA Board of Trustees concern various aspects of hospital costs: (1) "The Financial Structure of Community Hospitals: Impact of Medicare" by Richard W. Foster presents results from a study of financial statements of a stratified sample of 462 community hospitals certified as Medicare providers for the period 1962 to 1970. (2) "Hospital Costs: An Investigation of Causality" by P. Joseph Phillip and Abdul Hai is a cross-sectional investigation of causal links between hospital cost behavior and external, product, and input factors. A systhesis of factor analysis and regression analysis developed to minimize problems of multicollinearity and interaction effects was used. The sample included all but 581 hospitals of the 5,789 community hospitals registered with the AHA in 1973. (3) "Indexes of Factor Input Price, Service Intensity and Productivity for the Hospital Industry" by P. Joseph Phillip, James R. Jeffers, and Abdul Hai reviews the background, development, and results from a study of the impact of changes in these three factors on changes in the cost of the patient day.

AHCMS 19796 HE

Foyle, William R.
  Evaluation of Methods of Cost Analysis
Unpublished, c. 1964, 18 pp.
Available from University Microfilms

The author evaluates five cost methods available to hospitals for cost determinations.

AHCMS AC1001

Frank, Frederick and George, Michael P.
Capital Management: Funding Strategy Among Multi-Hospital Systems
Hospital Financial Management, 35:9, 1981, pp. 24 ff.

This article outlines strategies that are available to investor-owned and tax-exempt multihospital chains for attracting capital. The authors point out that attracting capital at a reasonable cost will be difficult throughout the 1980s and that chains must reformulate their strategies to treat capital like other scarce resources.

AHCMS 25360 FM

Freeland, Mark S. and Schendler, Carol E.
Health Spending in the 1980s: Integration of Clinical Practice Patterns with Management
Health Care Financing Review, 5:3, 1984, pp. 1–68.

Health care spending in the United States more than tripled between 1972 and 1982, increasing from $94 billion to $322 billion. This growth substantially outpaced overall growth in the economy. National health expenditures are projected to reach approximately $690 billion in 1990, which would be roughly 12% of the gross national product. Government spending for health care is projected to reach $294 billion by 1990, with the federal government paying 72%. The Medicare prospective payment system and increasing competition in the health services sector are providing incentives to integrate clinical practice patterns with improved management practices.

AHCMS 28036 HC

Freeland, Mark S. and Schendler, Carol E.
National Health Expenditures: Short-Term Outlook and Long-Term Projections
Health Care Financing Review, 3:2, 1981, pp. 97–138.

This article presents projections of national health expenditures by type of expenditure and source of funds for 1981, 1985, and 1990. Rapid growth in national health expenditures is projected to continue through 1990.

AHCMS 23909 HC

Freeland, Mark S.; Schendler, Carol E.; and Anderson, Gerard
Regional Hospital Input Price Indexes
Health Care Financing Review, 3:2, 1981, pp. 25–48.

A description of the development of regional hospital input price indexes consistent with the general methodology used for the National Hospital Input Price Index. The regional indexes incorporate variations in cost-share weights (the amount an expense category contributes to total spending) associated with hospital type and location, and variations in the rate of input price increases for various regions. Between 1972 and 1979 none of the regional price indexes increased at average annual rates significantly different from the national rate. For the period 1977 through 1979, however, the increase in one census region was significantly below the national rate. Further analyses indicated that variations in cost-share weights for various types of hospital produced no substantial variations in the regional price indexes relative to the national index. Findings are considered preliminary because current, relevant, and reliable data are limited.

AHCMS 26344 HC

Freeman, Gary and Allcorn, Seth
  Examine the Balance Fraction Method. Improving Receivables Management
Healthcare Financial Management, 38:5, 1984, pp. 76 ff.

   Traditional methods of managing accounts receivable have been shown to have deficiencies that compromise their utility and worth. The 1980s challenge hospitals to use all their resources to their best competitive advantage. With 75% of current hospital assets held in receivables, an improvement in control and monitoring can have a substantial positive fiscal effect for hospitals. The authors in this article demonstrate that the balance fraction method of managing hospital receivables is worth serious consideration. The method, which combines attributes of traditional receivable monitoring methods and effectively controls for the problems and distortions of these methods, has two important benefits. Aside from improving monitoring accuracy, the method is very sensitive to fluctuations that may occur in any period and can promptly detect the changes when payments slow or accelerate in any given month. The second benefit is more aggressive cash management as it is relatively easy to calculate expected payment patterns if receivables balance fractions are known. The authors conclude that these two benefits can provide substantial fiscal rewards that will offset implementation costs when the magnitude of the sums of money and effort involved in accounts receivable are considered.

AHCMS 27588 FM

Friedman, Bernard and Pauly, Mark V.
  A New Approach to Hospital Cost Functions and Some Issues in Revenue Regulation
Health Care Financing Review, 4:3, 1983, pp. 105–14.

   This article reviews the regulatory issues and choices involved in retroactive hospital revenue allowances for changes in volume of service. In an attempt to clarify them, new econometric work is used that explicitly allows for the effects of transitory as well as expected demand changes on hospital expense, and length of stay is treated as an endogenous variable in cost functions. Cost variation was analyzed for a panel of over 800 hospitals that reported monthly to Hospital Administrative Services between 1973 and 1978. Marginal cost of unexpected admissions was revealed to be about half of average cost, while marginal cost of forecasted admissions was about equal to average cost. Relatively low estimates of the cost of an "empty bed" were obtained. The study tends to support proportional volume allowances in revenue regulation programs, with perhaps a residual role for selective case review.

AHCMS 26598 HC

Friedman, Lawrence A. and Neumann, Bruce R.
  Replacement Cost Accounting: An Alternative to Price Level Indexes
Hospital and Health Services Administration, Fall 1979.

   Replacement cost accounting is recommended as a superior accounting technique for health care organizations to use in correcting for the effect of inflation. The article demonstrates how replacement cost data can be used for several important decisions: for reimbursement or rate review hearings, for financial statement disclosure, and for decision making within the hospital.

AHCMS 22368 FM

Fuller, Norman A.; Patera, Margaret W.; and Koziol, Krista
  Medicaid Utilization of Services in a Prepaid Group Practice Health Plan
Medical Care, September 1977.

  To provide medical services at lower costs without diminishing either quality
or coverage, the District of Columbia enrolled approximately 1,000 Medicaid beneficiaries, voluntarily, in a prepaid group practice (PGP). The project was evaluated
over a three-year period (1971–74) with regard to: (1) rates of utilization of medical
care before and after enrollment; (2) costs of care per capita as compared with
those of the 160,000 beneficiaries in the Medicaid fee-for-service universe; and
(3) patient satisfaction with the PGP.

                                                                    AHCMS 19990 IN

Furst, Richard W. and Markland, Robert E.
  How Hospital Capital Investment and Operating Costs Relate
Inquiry, 17:4, 1980, pp. 313–17.

  This article presents preliminary results of a research study designed to explore the relationship between investment and operating costs in the hospital,
using data from *Hospital Statistics* and the *AHA Guide to the Health Care Field*.
Total plant assets, operating costs, and payroll costs data were gathered for all U.S.
short-term general and other special hospitals on a yearly basis from 1955 through
1977. The change in plant assets became a measure of net capital investment in
each period, while changes in total operating costs, payroll costs, and other operating costs became measures of changes in operating costs. Simple and multiple
regression techniques were used to investigate relationships between changes in
plant assets and costs over time, with focus on lead/lag relationships. Overall
results seem to support the demand-pull theory of relationships between plant
assets and operating costs; that is, hospital costs rise in response to increased
demand and when capacity is reached, assets must be expanded. Little support
was found for the popular theory that an increase in supply leads to changes in
operating costs. Implications of findings for cost containment policies and regulatory programs, such as certificate of need, are discussed.

                                                                    AHCMS 23538 FM

Furst, Richard W. and Roenfeldt, Rodney L.
  Capital Management: Estimating the Return on Equity Capital
Hospital Financial Management, 35:6, 1981, pp. 34–35, 38, 40, 42, 44.

  The discussion in this article focuses on three methods of estimating the cost
of equity capital that have been widely used in the for-profit sector in order to
illustrate the application of these methods to proprietary hospitals, and to show
how each of these methods might be adapted to estimate the cost of equity capital
for nonprofit hospitals. The methods are: (1) debt rate plus equity premium model,
(2) capital asset pricing model, and (3) dividend valuation model. Since each method
requires estimates of key variables, the authors suggest that using more than one
approach is useful in developing a range of estimates. It is concluded that although
all three methods require estimation, each approach is substantially superior to
the current method employed by Medicare to determine the cost of equity capital
for proprietary hospitals. Further, if health care institutions are to survive, they
must earn the rate of return required by the providers of equity capital. The authors
cite the deterioration of many hospitals in urban areas as a clear example of the
financial policy that ignores this fact.

                                                                    AHCMS 23426 FM

Gabel, J. R. and Monheit, A. C.
Will Competition Plans Change Insurer-Provider Relationships?
Milbank Memorial Fund Quarterly, 61:4, 1983, pp. 614–40.

It is believed that inefficiency in the health care sector is more than the problem of excess consumer demand or "moral hazard" from overinsurance. This article examines whether competition proposals are likely to provide sufficient stimuli to change existing payment relationships between insurers and providers and thereby effectuate a fundamental change in health care delivery. The authors hypothesize that unless insurers change their reimbursement methods so that providers bear some financial risk for their resource decisions, the health care system is likely to retain much of its inherent inefficiency.

AHCMS 27641 HC

Garret, Sharon D.
Hospital Failure in California: An Investigation
University of California, Los Angeles, CA, 1984
Available from University Microfilms

A study of data from 1976 through 1980 for small California hospitals indicates that hospitals that failed were generally smaller, had lower occupancy rates (under 50%), had smaller numbers of medical staff in relation to available beds, and depended more heavily on Medi-Cal patients than did nonfailed hospitals.

AHCMS 27934 FM

Gartside, Foline E.
Causes of Increase in Medicaid Costs in California
Health Services Reports, 88:3, 1973, pp. 225–35.

This study analyzes the fivefold increase in the costs of California's public welfare medical care program over a six-year period. Price increases, growth in the eligible population, and increased use of services due to expanded benefits and per capita changes in utilization all contributed to the rise in expenditures.

AHCMS 12140 IN

Gartside, Foline E.; Hopkins, Carl E.; and Roemer, Milton I.
Medicaid Services in California Under Different Organizational Modes
School of Public Health, University of California, Los Angeles, CA, 1973, 99 pp.

This is a comparative study to determine if the organizational mode of delivery affects volume, costs, quality, and outcomes of services to Medicaid beneficiaries in California. Six organizational modes were selected for the study: three open market (free choice, fee-for-service) modes; and three organized delivery modes. Each set of three included one prepaid or capitation health plan operating as a demonstration pilot project of the Medi-Cal program and two other modes without Medi-Cal capitation agreements and differing in objectives, controls, and financing. Each mode served at least 3,000 Medi-Cal beneficiaries. Major findings of the study are: organizational differences were found to be associated with measurable differences in nature of services accessible to and received by Medi-Cal beneficiaries, their volume and costs and, to the limited extent observable, in their quality and outcomes.

AHCMS 12141 IN

Gavin, Thomas A.
Financial Accounting and Internal Control Functions Pursued by Hospital Boards
Healthcare Financial Management, 38:9, 1984, pp. 26 ff.

The article presents findings from a survey of 526 hospital chief financial officers regarding the manner and extent to which financial accounting and internal control functions are undertaken by boards of trustees of voluntary short-term general hospitals.

AHCMS 28208 FM

Gibbs, James O.; Newman, John F.; Long, Stephen; and Cooper, David
Study of Health Services Used and Costs Incurred During the Last Six Months of a Terminal Illness
Blue Cross and Blue Shield Association, Chicago, IL, 1982
Available from National Technical Information Service (PB83–170506)

The purpose of this study was: (1) to locate Blue Cross and Blue Shield subscribers who had died of cancer, (2) to backtrack in their claims histories for six months prior to death, and (3) to summarize costs and claims histories for this period. Revealed from 1,054 cases from three Blue Cross and Blue Shield plans was a mean expenditure of $15,836, of which 78% was for hospital inpatient care. Mean number of hospital admissions during the last six months was 2.6, and mean number of inpatient days was 37.7. Disaggregations and distributions are included.

AHCMS 26738 HC

Gibson, Lorrie
Employers Lean on Employees in Fight Against Rising Healthcare Costs
Modern Healthcare, 14:6, 1984, pp. 50 ff.

The article discusses the results of a recent survey of managers' ideas of the most effective measures employers can take to control their health care costs. Employers generally think that the most effective cost-containment measure is the redesigning of benefit plans to make employees share more costs and educating employees to be wise health care consumers. Employers also think that developing a wellness program to help employees keep healthy is essential in curbing unnecessary doctors' visits and medical bills.

AHCMS 27665 HC

Gilbert, R. Neal
Hospital Capital Budgeting System Development
Coopers and Lybrand, Philadelphia, PA, 1975, 28 pp.

Develops a mechanism to help insure that the capital resources of the health care institution are allocated in the most efficient and effective manner possible consistent with the delivery of high quality health care.

AHCMS 13659 AC

Gilbert, R. Neal
The Hospital Capital Financing Crisis
Coopers and Lybrand, Philadelphia, PA, 1974, 26 pp.

Paper examines the capital financing situation in the hospital industry and how cost-based reimbursement figures in the task of obtaining sufficient capital.

AHCMS 13656 AC

Gilbert, R. Neal
Hospital Priorities and Criteria for Selecting a Method of Financing
Blyth, Eastman, Dillon Health Care Funding, Inc., San Francisco, CA
Available from University Microfilms

This paper discusses the factors that have the greatest influence on the method and type of financing used by a hospital. These factors include: timing—how soon the money is available; cost—interest rate, insurance premiums, and financing fees; equity requirements, including reimbursement implications of debt versus equity capital; cost of capital; hospital policy toward government intervention; prepayment provisions; loan terms; loan amortization method; security—first deed mortgage, gross revenues, or negative pledge; ability to issue additional debt in the future; and maintaining flexibility in the selection of financing alternatives because of the time lag between conception of a project and construction and the changing market conditions. It is concluded that selection of the most appropriate and advantageous financing technique necessitates an in-depth understanding by the hospital of all the available methods of financing and the short- and long-range ramifications of utilizing each method. Assistance can be provided by the hospital's financing committee, architect, attorney, fiscal director, and administrator.

AHCMS 19618 FM

Gilbert, R. Neal
The Principles of Capital Budgeting for Hospitals
Coopers and Lybrand, Philadelphia, PA, 1974, 12 pp.

Paper develops principles for efficient and effective allocation of capital resources in hospitals. Essential elements of an ideal hospital capital budgeting system are outlined and discussed: cost containment; planning; coordination; control; assessment of future financial support requirements; communication; and acceptability.

AHCMS 13658 AC

Gilbert, R. Neal
Refinancing, Refunding and Restructuring Long-Term Debt
Saint Mary's Hospital and Medical Center, San Francisco, CA, 1981
Available from University Microfilms

Author examines possible advantages of change in a hospital's long-term debt structure and discusses three methods available to effect such change: restructuring, refinancing, and refunding. This paper also discusses accounting and reimbursement issues related to advance refunding.

AHCMS 13680 FM

Ginsburg, Paul B. and Sloan, Frank A
Hospital Cost Shifting
New England Journal of Medicine, 310:14, 1984, pp. 893–98.

The article analyzes the issue of hospital cost shifting (payment differentials) and sources of payment differentials, and presents estimates of their magnitude. It also discusses whether cost shifting is justified and assesses the effects of payment differentials on hospitals, insurers, and the public at large. Three aspects of policies of insurers that pay on a cost or prospective basis are found to be responsible for most payment differentials: limitations in cost-funding accounting systems that are used to allocate costs among different groups of patients; costs of hospital activities that are not directly attributable to the care of paying patients such as charity care and unfunded research; and prudent purchasing policies of insurers. The analysis indicates that payment differentials have grown over time; nonrecoverable charges as a percentage of billed charges increased from 14% in 1975 to 23% in 1981. A likely explanation for this is that hospitals raised charges faster than costs increased. Some justifications for the payment differentials are the need to cover bad debts and charity care and the need to reimburse for capital costs. The merits of three policy options available to alter payment differentials and their effects are presented: grants to hospitals for bad debts and charity care; use of state-level commissions to set hospital rates; and an antitrust exemption to permit commercial insurers to negotiate as a group with hospitals. It is concluded that the problem of cost shifting is a complex one to analyze and difficult to resolve, and its resolution may not be found in specific changes in reimbursement policy, but in dealing with broad policy issues such as using greater reliance on market forces or increased regulation to constrain the growth of medical care costs and deciding how to finance the care of the indigent.

AHCMS 28676 HC

Ginzberg, Eli and McClure, Walter
The Coming Struggle for the Health Care Dollar. Two Perspectives
Mount Sinai School of Medicine, Department of Health Care Management, One Gustave L. Levy Place, New York, NY 10029, 1983

A report of a two-part seminar held to identify and examine critical issues facing medical care providers and consumers. Ginzberg suggests a struggle is inevitable in view of the growing number of physicians and the nonexpansion of the health care industry (in terms of services). The consequences, as he sees them, will be a lowering of physicians' incomes, state budgetary control, and keen competition. He concludes that in this period of turmoil, the needs of the poor and the near poor will be at greatest risk. To counteract that he suggests that the rest of the population pay more for their health care out of their own pockets. McClure suggests that, to assure adequate medical coverage for everyone at an affordable cost, there is a 75% chance of strong government control. McClure thinks that the way to save money is to improve productivity and thereby put inefficient institutions out of business. He concludes that when the hospital industry shrinks, the survivors will be the very powerful and capable hospitals and medical care organizations.

AHCMS 27008 HC

Glenn, Edward M.
The Effect of Copayment Provisions in Hospitalization Insurance
Available from University Microfilms

This dissertation attempts to ascertain the efficacy of cost-sharing provisions as contractual features designed to control health care costs. The principal finding was that cost-sharing provisions are capable of lowering the demand for medical services, thereby lowering health care utilization and costs. Copayment had a strong statistical relationship to an observed reduction in the overall level of demand for inpatient hospital care, other factors remaining the same. Of three measures of hospital utilization and costs used in this study, two (admission rates and the amount of covered charges on a per capita basis) were found responsive to the cost-sharing device, while a third measure (length of stay) was not affected.

AHCMS 21249 IN

Go, Robert and Fox, John N., Jr.
Capital Formation: An Ongoing Strategic Development Process
Michigan Hospitals, 19:2, 1983, pp. 17–21.

This article reviews factors and trends in the marketplace that provide impetus for the increasing demand for capital by hospitals whose capital or equity sources have decreased with the reduction in contributions from public and government sources.

AHCMS 27038 FM

Gold, Marsha
Hospital-Based versus Free-Standing Primary Care Costs
Journal of Ambulatory Care Management, February 1979, pp. 1–20.

This article discusses the differences in costs between hospital-based versus freestanding primary care.

AHCMS 20853 HC

Gorin, Gloria J.
Internal Controls and Auditing in Hospitals
Xavier University, Cincinnati, OH, 1982
Available from University Microfilms

As the health care industry becomes more complex and difficult to manage, and undergoes closer scrutiny by government and consumers, internal controls increase in importance. Within this concept, the author outlines current issues for hospitals, defines operational terms, and traces the historical development of internal controls, auditing, and the profession of accounting. The author, after surveying 16 hospitals and businesses in the Cincinnati area, compares national and local hospital utilization of internal auditing with that of industry. Finally, audit results of the internal control program at The Christ Hospital, Cincinnati, Ohio, are reported.

AHCMS 25621 FM

Gravelle, H. S. E. and Williams, Alan
Health Service Finance and Resource Management
King's Fund Centre, 126 Albert St., London NW1 7NF, 1980

This book presents five papers prepared in connection with the Royal Commission on the National Health Service (NHS). The first paper discusses alternative models of financing health services. The second describes one of those models as used in Britain's NHS, namely health service charges. A third paper discusses efficient management of resources in the NHS. The last two papers deal with specific resource management issues relevant to hospitals: clinician budgeting and the costs of training doctors and nurses.

AHCMS 23844 FM

Greenberg, Warren and Southby, Richard McK. F. (eds.)
Health Care Institutions in Flux: Changing Reimbursement Patterns in the 1980s
Information Resources Press, 1984

The book presents proceedings of a September 1983 conference sponsored by the Institute of Health Policy Administration. The conference consisted of 18 experts representing government, Blue Cross and commercial insurers, health care institutions, and academia who addressed the issue of how much the nation can afford to pay for health care. Some of the major topics discussed were: current medical cost reimbursement methods, including Medicare and Medicaid; all-payer systems; the new DRG payment mechanism for Medicare; cost-containment reforms; cost shifting; roles of insurers; effects of technological innovations; and competition and regulation in the marketplace. The potential effects of changing reimbursement patterns were examined from five perspectives: federal government; state government; private sector (for example, Blue Cross); supply side (for example, acute care institutions); and academic viewpoint. All participants agreed that profound changes in reimbursement had surfaced in the early 1980s, but it is unclear what the effects will be on health care costs, quality, and access. They also agreed that the DRG reimbursement method is not the only system that will make an impact. Systems in California (selective contracting with hospitals for the provision of Medicaid inpatient services) and Massachusetts (case management system and all-payer prospective reimbursement) are expected to affect strongly the health care institutions. The participants felt that the relationship between health care institutions in flux and changing reimbursement patterns may be a circular one: higher health care costs engender new reimbursement patterns and initiatives by third parties which in turn may cause further turmoil among health care institutions and result in formation of multihospital systems to diversify into nonacute care or reduce the size of the health work force.

AHCMS 28295 HC

Greene, Joshua E.
Tax Subsidies for Medical Care: Current Policies and Possible Alternatives
U.S. Government Printing Office, Washington, DC

A paper analyzing the impact on the medical cost spiral of three federal tax subsidies that cost the federal government about $14.5 billion in lost tax revenues: exclusion from taxable income of employer contributions to employee health insurance plans; deductibility of health insurance premiums and large out-of-pocket medical expenses; and use of tax-exempt bonds to finance capital projects at private hospitals and medical institutions. Alternatives to each of these subsidies are proposed and evaluated.

AHCMS 22337 HC

Greenman, Barbara W.
Altering Incentives in Health Care Delivery
Institute for Health Planning, Madison, WI, 1982

This document presents three strategies for modifying underlying incentives in the health care delivery and financing system to achieve cost containment. The three approaches are prepaid health care, self-insurance, and preferred provider organizations. Prepaid health care forces the health care delivery system to work within a budget fixed by a periodic, prepaid fee. Self-insurance requires employers rather than third party insurers to assume the risk of providing health care benefits. Preferred provider organizations offer discounted health care to groups of beneficiaries. The analysis explores the effect each strategy has on incentive mechanisms and provides case examples of all three approaches.

AHCMS 26289 HC

Greenman, B. W.
Cost Shifting—A Public Policy Debate
Institute for Health Planning, Madison, WI, 1984
Available from National Technical Information Service (HRP–0904785/3)

Cost shifting refers to the hospital practice of charging one group of patients more because another group of patients does not pay an appropriate share of the costs incurred to provide care. It is alleged that payment under Medicare, Medicaid, and even Blue Cross does not cover the full costs of hospital operations. The result is that hospitals must shift unreimbursed costs to other patients, namely the private-paying or commercially insured patients who pay full charges. As a consequence, one class of patients—privately insured or charge-paying—subsidizes the hospital care provided to publicly insured, cost-paying patients. This reviews the issue of cost shifting from a variety of perspectives. Much of the debate has focused on whether or not the practice exists, whether pricing differentials are justified, and how to end payer inequities. This paper touches on these issues and analyzes the sources of the cost-shifting problem, recent reimbursement policy changes and their effects on cost shifting, and possible solutions to cost shifting within the context of cost containment. The paper also addresses two important considerations in the cost-shifting issues: who currently bears the burden of cost shifting through the tax system and what the impact of proposed solutions might be. Special attention is focused on the public policy issue of financing health care services for the elderly and the poor and the relation of this issue to cost shifting.

AHCMS 27779 HC

Griffith, John R.; Hancock, Walton M.; and Munson, Fred C.
Practical Ways to Contain Hospital Costs
Harvard Business Review, 51:6, 1973, pp. 131–39.

The basis of this article stems from four years of close study in different cities of two medium-sized hospitals that have been unequally successful in tightening control over costs. Concentrating on what can be realistically expected, the authors focus on four areas: planning of facilities and services, scheduling of patients and patient services, medical control of facilities utilization and quality of service, and administrative control of manpower and expenditures. An essential ingredient of cost containment is measures by which trustees and administrators can gauge their performance according to norms and standards. Also essential, the authors maintain, is communitywide planning.

AHCMS 12223 HE

Grooms, Ferris L.
An Analysis of the Impact of Medicare on Hospital Financial Reporting Practices
Texas Tech University, Lubbock, TX, 1971
Available from University Microfilms

The author concludes that Medicare has imposed sophisticated accounting and reporting practices upon hospitals, which are generally resolved within the framework of accepted accounting principles.

AHCMS 08776 AC

Grossman, Randolph M.
A Review of Physician Cost-Containment Strategies for Laboratory Testing
Medical Care, 21:8, 1983, pp. 783–802.

This article reviews the role of the physician as a contributor to the health care cost problem and the state of physician cost-control strategies relative to laboratory testing in confronting this national problem.

AHCMS 27255 HC

Gulinson, Sheldon K.
A Study of the Direct Cost to the Hospital of Processing Duplicate Coverage Third Party Claims
Duke University, Durham, NC, 1969, 21 pp.
Available from University Microfilms

A study to determine the problem posed by processing duplicate coverage third party claims at Wilson Memorial Hospital, a 254-bed community general hospital.

AHCMS AC3016

Hadley, Jack; Mullner, Ross; and Feder, Judith
  The Financially Distressed Hospital
New England Journal of Medicine, 307:20, 1982, pp. 1283–87.

The prevalence and sources of short-term and long-term hospital deficits are examined in this paper. The focus was on urban hospitals in the 46 largest U.S. cities.

AHCMS 26954 FM

Hagan, Michael M.
  Medical Equipment and Supplies: Purchases and Rental, Expenditures, and Sources of Payment
U.S. Dept. of Health and Human Services, Washington, DC, 1982

This data preview from the National Health Care Expenditures Study presents population estimates for the component of health services use that involves the purchase or rental of wheelchairs, crutches, corrective shoes, supportive devices, hearing aids, syringes, and similar items. Differences among selected population characteristics in the likelihood and frequency of purchases and rentals of medical equipment and supplies are established. The mean charge per purchase and the average proportion of this charge paid by various sources of payment are shown, as well as the distribution of persons by out-of-pocket expenditures for such items. Also, estimates of annual expenditures per person are presented. All findings are from final household data reported for the period January 1 to December 31, 1977, in the National Medical Care Expenditure Survey.

AHCMS 26253 HC

Hall, Charles P., Jr.; Flueck, John A.; and McKenna, William F.
  Medicaid and Cash Welfare Recipients: An Empirical Study
Inquiry, 14:1, pp. 43–50.

The primary objective of this article is to determine the proportion of Medicaid eligibles receiving health care services and the method of financing, type of service, and place of receipt of care for this population. The paper also attempts to determine utilization effects and, to the extent possible, the perceived health status of the eligibles. Data on Medicaid eligibles were collected in 1973 through household interviews conducted in four geographically distinct metropolitan areas.

AHCMS 20918 IN

Havighurst, Clark C.
  Controlling Health Care Costs: Strengthening the Private Sector's Hand
Journal of Health Politics, Policy and Law, 1:4, pp. 471–98.

This article examines the limitations on private-sector cost-control efforts and suggests actions that would permit and encourage private decision makers to be more effective. In particular, the private health insurer's potential role in cost control is explored.

AHCMS 19142 HC

Havighurst, Clark C.
  Professional Restraints on Innovation in Health Care Financing
Duke Law Journal, 2, 1978.

This article discusses the resistance of the medical profession to economizing innovations in the organization and administration of private plans for financing health care, contending this resistance is an important contributor to the crisis caused by the rapid escalation of health care costs. In addition to examining professional restraints on the growth of recognized innovations such as HMOs, the article seeks to establish the importance of de facto disciplinary power exercised by organized medicine over third party payers, which it contends has slowed the pace of developing private sector cost containment capabilities. The article also discusses the potential utility of antitrust laws to reduce the threat posed by organized medicine to innovations in health care financing.

AHCMS 21860 HC

Health Research and Educational Trust of New Jersey
DRG Evaluation, Vol. II: Economic and Financial Analysis
Health Research and Educational Trust of New Jersey, Princeton, NJ, 1984

The report examines the economic and financial impacts of the diagnosis-related group (DRG) reimbursement system during its first year of operation in New Jersey. Overall, the analysis revealed that more money was injected into the hospital system than would have been the case under SHARE. Each hospital received additional revenue of nearly $2.3 million on average, due partly to the generous allowance for working cash, depreciation of capital facilities, uncompensated care, and costs incurred to meet data and administrative requirements of the new system. Analysis of financial ratios indicates that DRG reimbursement has proven beneficial to hospitals. What is unclear is whether the financial strength of hospitals in the early years of the program was achieved at the expense of cost containment efforts. In 1982 expenses outstripped revenues. Possible reasons for this are discussed. The study also found that teaching status has a significant effect on costs and length of stay in the DRGs studied. The report's analysis of the components of the rate-setting formula indicated the following consequences. (1) When the mode labor market cost was substituted for the mean, all hospitals realized a disincentive. (2) Manipulation of the sharing factor, which was originally used with the degree of confidence in determining the mix between actual cost and standard cost, had only marginal effects on revenue. (3) Changes in the degree of confidence produced directly proportionate changes in the rate of reimbursement. (4) When patient volume is increased, there is an increase in the amount of revenue over expenses. When volume is decreased, the deficit is increased.

AHCMS 27689 FM

Heath, Lloyd C.
Let's Scrap the "Funds" Statement
Journal of Accountancy, October 1978.

This article discusses confusion arising from use of the funds statement, contending that the confusion does not stem from lack of a proper definition of the term "funds," but from what the objectives of the funds statement should be.

AHCMS 09592 FM

Heaton, Harley L.; Johnson, Stephen P.; Fox, Kathryn E.; Koontz, Michael D.; and Rhodes, John H.
Analysis of the New Jersey Hospital Prospective Reimbursement System: 1968 – 1973
Geomet, Inc., Gaithersburg, MD, 1976, 337 pp.
Available from National Technical Information Service (PB 272 058/9WW)

The analysis of the prospective reimbursement system utilized in 89 short-term, general, acute care hospitals in New Jersey from 1968 through 1973 is dis-

cussed. No statistically significant relationships between prospective reimbursement as practiced in New Jersey and hospital cost, productivity, or quality of care
were demonstrated.

AHCMS 18897 IN

Hedinger, Frederic R.
The Social Role of Blue Cross: Progress and Problems
Inquiry, 5:2, 1968, pp. 3–12.

This article traces the historical background and philosophical roots of Blue
Cross and discusses the influence exerted by the entrance of the commercial insurance industry into the field of hospital care financing. Local control, community
rating, and full-service benefits are explored from the philosophical and competitive viewpoint. Author concludes that Blue Cross is closer to the commercial
insurance model than the social insurance model and suggests two points of view:
(1) that Blue Cross has fulfilled its original mission with the acceptance of a new
field of service or (2) that Blue Cross is a failure because many of its social points
of philosophy have been discarded or modified.

AHCMS IN2019

Hellinger, Fred. J.
*Prospective Reimbursement through Budget Review: New Jersey, Rhode Island,
and Western Pennsylvania*
Inquiry, 13:3, 1976, pp. 309–20.

Analyzing prospective reimbursement programs through budget reviews in
three states, the author finds that the programs are ineffective in controlling hospital cost escalation.

AHCMS 19056 AC

Helms, L. J.; Newhouse, J. P.; and Phelps, C. E.
Copayments and Demand for Medical Care: The California Medicaid Experience
Rand Corporation, Santa Monica, CA

This study holds that copayments for ambulatory care among welfare recipients as a method of controlling medical care costs may well be ineffectual or even
self-defeating. Data obtained from the 1972 California Copayment Experiment,
showed that while charging for office visits decreased demand there (by about
8%), it increased the demand for hospital inpatient services by 17%, and there was
an overall program cost increase of 3% to 8%.

AHCMS 19666 IN

Herkimer, Allen G., Jr.
Patient Account Management
Aspen Systems Corporation, Gaithersburg, MD, 1983

This text is written for the patient accounts manager and defines the knowledge, information, and skills required by the professional manager of patient accounts. The various chapters discuss the following topics: (1) organizing patient
business services department—describes manager's role, department missions,
organizational design, delegation of authority, and job functions; (2) use of standard plans—policies, procedures, and methods; (3) hospital accounting process—
outlines basic concepts and principles of hospital accounting and key financial
reports; (4) management accounting and application; (5) developing a productivity
improvement program; (6) budgetary control systems; (7) application of variable

budgeting; (8) cost finding; (9) financial requirements and rate setting; (10) cash forecasting; (11) financial statement analysis including use of financial ratios and types of ratio analysis; (12) payment systems; and (13) internal audit and control of receivables.

AHCMS 26361 FM

Herrera, Olga B.
Information Feedback and Budget-Related Behavior: An Investigation of the Budgeting Process in Non-Profit Hospitals
Claremont Graduate School, Claremont, CA, 1984
Available from University Microfilms

This research aims to investigate the impact of budgeting process characteristics on human behavior in an effort to address the issue of budget effectiveness as a planning and control tool. The focus of this investigation was an analysis of the budget process in terms of its informational content, based on the supposition that information can serve as an instrument of social and intellectual control.

AHCMS 28095 FM

Herzlinger, Regina
Can We Control Health Care Costs?
Harvard Business Reviews, 56:2, 1978.

This article examines the causes of the escalating costs of health care and the growth of government financing of these costs, evaluates various attempts to control the problem, and outlines the most fruitful approaches. Major causes are seen as: increases in quality and quantity of services; maldistribution of health resources; and inefficiencies in the system, i.e., price elasticity and production inefficiency. Analysis of government regulations, such as certificate-of-need laws and reimbursement schemes, and devices such as HMOs indicates that they have curbed some abuses but not helped health organizations control costs; in some instances they have contributed to higher costs. It is suggested that we need to focus our attention on the three elements that can do something about curbing health expenditures: health care administration; physicians; and business organizations (corporations and unions) that provide insurance benefits.

AHCMS 19435 HC

Hill, Frank and Oliver, Christine
Hospice—The Cost of In-Patient Care
Health Trends, 16:1, 1984, pp. 9–11.

This paper reports an in-depth survey of the cost of providing inpatient care in 20 of the major hospices, all of them independent freestanding units. The results show that costs per bed per week are highest in the smaller units and fall to a minimum in the range of 25 to 30 beds, rising again thereafter. On average, medical salaries account for 7.5% of salary costs and nursing salaries for 66.2%. The largest source of income (68.7%) is donations; and National Health Service support averages 23.2% in 18 of the hospices. It is estimated that total expenditure, excluding capital developments, on hospice care in the United Kingdom is now in excess of £25 million a year.

AHCMS 27949 HC

Hoey, John; Eisenberg, John M.; Spitzer, Walter O.; and Thomas, Duncan
Physician Sensitivity to the Price of Diagnostic Tests: A U.S.–Canadian Analysis
Medical Care, 20:3, 1982, pp. 302–7.

A questionnaire containing 11 patient management problems was completed by 495 physicians and medical students at an American and a Canadian medical school. Respondents indicated whether they would order a particular diagnostic test in each case, given five different prices for the test. Approximately 25% of the attending staff and a higher proportion of residents, interns, and clerks responded that they would order the test depending on the price. Approximately 50% of attending staff and smaller proportions of residents, interns, and clerks indicated that they would not order the test even if there were no price. Respondents in Montreal were more likely than those in Philadelphia to select a price-sensitive response, the reverse of the expected tendency. Since some tests may be ordered on the basis of price, education of physicians regarding the price of diagnostic tests may alter their use of these services, but a large proportion of tests are ordered because of clinically absolute reasons, which may be insensitive to price.

AHCMS 25739 HC

Holder, William W.
 Hospital Budgeting: State of the Art
Hospital and Health Services Administration, Spring 1978.

This study examines a sample of general short-term nonfederal institutions to assess the usefulness, accuracy, and completeness of preparing a one-year operating budget and a three-year capital budget as required by PL 92–603.

AHCMS 20695 FM

Holder, William W.
 The Impact of Selected Third Party Reimbursement Policies on Capital Expenditure Decisions for General Hospitals
University of Oklahoma, Norman, OK, 1974, 184 pp.
Available from University Microfilms

This study was concerned with the effects the advent of Medicare and Medicaid had upon the capital expenditure decisions of short-term, general, nonfederal, not-for-profit hospitals in the state of Oklahoma. The study concludes that hospital administrations significantly altered the methods of capital expenditure planning and evaluation in response to Medicare and Medicaid. In general, hospitals now plan for longer periods of time and in much greater detail than in 1966.

AHCMS 13882 AC

Hopkins, David S. P.; Heath, Dan; and Levin, Peter J.
 A Financial Planning Model for Estimating Hospital Debt Capacity
Public Health Reports, 97:4, 1982, pp. 363–72.

This paper describes a model formulated during the early stages of planning for a major renovation and construction program at Stanford (California) University Hospital. It was specifically designed to project cash flow, the buildup of reserves, gift receipts, and debt requirements under a variety of planning assumptions. Operating as an interactive forecasting device, the model specifically incorporates all the major effects of a substantial capital project on the hospital's net cash flow. It was used to examine the net financial impact of specified facility plans, and to test whether and under what circumstances the institution could afford the amount of debt that would be required for such a project. Use of the model showed that the proposed modernization plan was financially feasible under a reasonable (that is, not unduly optimistic) set of assumptions and facilitated the examination of the major sources of risk.

AHCMS 26571 FM

Horn, Susan D.
Measuring Severity of Illness: Comparisons across Institutions
Center for Hospital Finance and Management, Johns Hopkins University, Baltimore, MD, 1982

Reviews a new severity of illness index that is generic to most medical and surgical conditions in a hospital, and that has been found to produce subgroups of patients that are more homogeneous with respect to hospital resource use (as assessed by total charges, length of stay, routine charges, and laboratory charges) than diagnostic-related groups, staging, and generalized patient management paths. The severity of illness groups are used to compare total charges and length of stay across hospitals. Results reveal that charges and length of stay in an academic teaching hospital are similar to those in community hospitals with and without teaching programs when severity of illness is controlled for.

AHCMS 26059 HC

Horn, Susan D.
The Role of Severity-Adjusted Case Mix in Hospital Management
Center for Hospital Finance and Management, Johns Hopkins University, Baltimore, MD, 1982

Conventional methods for classifying patients with respect to utilization of health care resources are based almost exclusively on diagnostic criteria. This article reviews hospital case-mix grouping systems in use or under development, and describes advantages and disadvantages of each. It also describes a new method of grouping patients based on a severity of illness index. It is generic to most medical and surgical conditions in a hospital and has been found to produce more homogeneous case-mix groups than other case-mix grouping systems. A demonstration of how this new method may resolve some known problems with current case-mix grouping methods is offered.

AHCMS 26432 HC

Horn, Susan D.; Chan, Cynthia; Chachich, Bette; and Clopton, Cathy
Measuring Severity of Illness: A Reliability Study
Center for Hospital Finance and Management, Johns Hopkins University, Baltimore, MD, 1982

This paper describes a severity of illness index that is generic and applicable to almost all hospital patients. The reliability of the index and the time required for different types of raters to apply it are examined. It is suggested this index be used in conjunction with case-mix groupings to examine hospital output and compare patients reliably across hospitals.

AHCMS 26434 HC

Horn, Susan D.; Schumacher, Dale N.; Bertram, Dennis A.; and Sharkey, Phoebe D.
Measuring Severity of Illness: Homogeneous Case Mix Groups
Center for Hospital Finance and Management, Johns Hopkins University, Baltimore, MD, 1982

This paper evaluates a new severity of illness index for use in defining case-mix groupings of hospitalized patients. The index takes severity of illness into account and produces groups that are more homogeneous than those produced by four other case-mix grouping methods that do not reflect the total burden of a patient's illness. Implications of these results for programs of prospective reimbursement and for cross-hospital comparison studies are presented.

AHCMS 26435 HC

Hosek, James R. and Palmer, Adele R.
Teaching and Hospital Costs: The Case of Radiology
Journal of Health Economics, 2:1, 1983, pp. 29–46.

This article investigates the production and cost effects of teaching in radiology departments. If students are substitutes for physicians, production costs may be less in teaching hospitals than in nonteaching hospitals for a given level of output. Empirical results for Veterans Administration hospitals suggest that teaching reduces cost for most radiology procedures. If teaching can reduce costs of primary products, teaching hospitals may be able to provide a given program of patient care at lower costs than nonteaching hospitals. However, costs might still be higher at teaching hospitals than at nonteaching hospitals because of differences in case mix, medical techniques, or quality of care.

AHCMS 26927 HC

Hospital Survey Committee
Debt Financing Alternatives for Hospital Construction
Hospital Survey Committee, 7 Benjamin Franklin Pkwy., Philadelphia, PA, 19103
1973, 48 pp.

Report is a systematic study of hospital financial planning. Rapid inflation in construction costs has created a financial crisis in many hospitals. Study explains the implications of this crisis and offers several alternative means of debt financing as a means of ameliorating the situation.

AHCMS 12742 AC

ICF, Inc.
Assessment of Recent Estimates of Hospital Capital Requirements
ICF, Inc., Washington, DC, 1983
Available from National Technical Information Service (PB83–244871)

During the last several years, different authors have estimated potential community hospital capital requirements during the 1980s at between $80 billion and $193 billion. This study analyzes 11 of those estimates to determine the causes of the variation and presents new normative estimates of hospital capital requirements that reflect a range of values for the key assumptions underlying the methodologies of previous estimates.

AHCMS 26873 FM

ICF, Inc.
Background Data on Changes in Hospital Expenditures and Revenues 1979–80
Federation of American Hospitals, Washington, DC, 1982

Trends in community hospital expenditures and revenues are presented for the period 1970–80. In addition to examining trends in total expenditures and revenues, the authors examined these trends on a per person and per case basis for each state over the period, as well as the differences between states with mandatory rate controls and other states. The data presented are based upon the results of annual surveys made by the American Hospital Association.

AHCMS 25289 HC

Iglehart, John K.
Cutting Costs of Health Care for the Poor in California: A Two-Year Follow-Up
New England Journal of Medicine, 311:11, 1984, pp. 745–48.

This article discusses the consequences of 1982 legislative changes that California adopted at the height of a state fiscal crisis, over the objections of the hospital and physician lobbies. California was one of only two states to adopt statewide Medicaid reforms. Changes adopted involve selective contracting or payment based on capitation rather than fee-for-service. Legislators, however, are concerned about the quality of the health system for the poor if California moves to a capitation-only Medi-Cal program. The California public hospital system, which provides a large amount of free or subsidized care to the working poor and the unemployed, also fears that the state's steps toward reducing health care spending will only place greater strains on their limited resources.

AHCMS 28645 HC

Inquiry
Cost Containment in the Voluntary Sector
Inquiry, 20:2, 1983, pp. 101–41.

A special section of this issue of the journal is devoted to reports on selected cost-containment experiments in the private sector. Earlier versions of the papers were presented at the 1982 annual meeting of the American Public Health Association. Following an introduction by John E. Craig, Jr., the papers are: (1) "The Decline in the Blue Cross Plan Admission Rate: Four Explanations," by Monroe Lerner, David S. Salkever, and John F. Newman; (2) "The Hospital Capitation Payment Project: New Incentives and Tools for Cost Containment," by William B. Elliott, Helen M. Strand, Fred H. Meyers, Jacob R. Getson, Calvin Paulson, Jane E. Hill, Mary N. Hennings, John F. Newman, and Theodore M. Raichel; (3) "The INSURE Project on Lifecycle Preventive Health Services: Cost Containment Issues," by Donald N. Logsdon, Matthew A. Rosen, and Michele M. Demak; (4) "Community Programs for Affordable Health Care," by Donna L. Gerber; and (5) "The Providence Plan: Prepaid Health Care for a Voluntarily Enrolled Population," by John F. Newman, Mark Schreiber, and James O. Gibbs.

AHCMS 27234 HC

Institute for Health Planning
Business/Health Care Coalitions in Profile
Institute for Health Planning, Madison, WI, 1983

This paper describes factors that have contributed to the development of coalitions, some employer-only, some including representatives, and presents an overview of membership, sponsorship, objectives, staffing, structure, finances, representation, projects, and accomplishments of coalitions in general. Eighteen coalitions formed by 1982 are profiled in the document. An annotated bibliography contains entries on publications by and about coalitions and supplements an earlier Institute for Health Planning bibliography on business and health care coalitions.

AHCMS 27078 HC

Institute for Health Planning
Competition in Health Care: Basic and Supplemental Readings
Institute for Health Planning, Madison, WI, 1981
Available from National Technical Information Service (HRP–0903065/1)

Serious consideration is now being given to restructuring the health care financing system to promote competition in the industry. This bibliography has been prepared to enhance understanding of the issues at stake in such a major policy shift. Both basic and supplemental readings published within the last five years are cited. Abstracts are included for 23 basic works on competition theory and its application, discussions of competition's role vis-à-vis regulation, and information on Congressional advocates and their proposals. An unannotated listing of 145 additional titles covers all aspects of the competition question.

AHCMS 24423 HC

Institute for Health Planning
Federal Tax Policy: Implications for Hospitals
Institute for Health Planning, Madison, WI, 1983

This report examines the likely effects on the hospital sector of two recent pieces of tax legislation: Economic Recovery Tax Act of 1981 and Tax Equity and Fiscal Responsibility Act of 1982. This legislation is used to illustrate how tax policies have a differential effect on nonprofit and for-profit hospitals, in the hope that future tax policy development will take into account the effect of tax policy on hospitals.

AHCMS 27974 FM

Institute for Health Planning
Strategies for Controlling Health Costs
Institute for Health Planning, Madison, WI, 1982

This report identifies and summarizes a wide range of solution strategies to deal with the components of the health care cost problem. It indicates which external control and market improvement strategies have been suggested for the public sector and which for the private sector. These individual strategies represent the building blocks for a coordinated approach to the problem of health care costs.

AHCMS 26346 HC

Joint Commission on Accreditation of Hospitals
Special Issue: Cost Containment
QRB/Quality Review Bulletin, September 1983, pp. 252–74.

Collection of articles related to cost containment and some of its effects. The articles are: (1) "Quality Assessment of Medical Care: An Economist's Perspective," by Uwe E. Reinhardt; (2) "Payment Source as a Variable in Utilization Research: A Selected Literature Review," by James Studnicki and Dorothy Honemann, which presents the study focus and unit analysis, the dependent/independent variables used, and a brief summation of results and conclusions of 55 study report articles published primarily during 1968–83; (3) "A Hospital Association's Efforts to Reduce Costs," by Karen M. Sandrick, which deals with experience in Saint Louis; (4) "Importance of the Medical Record Process in a DRG-Based System," by Richard J. Serluco and Kathleen Johnson, which deals with experience in New Jersey; and (5) "Blue Cross/Blue Shield's PROBE Information Reporting System," by Karen M. Sandrick.

AHCMS 27540 HC

Jones, Craig W.
Sources of Hospital Capital Financing: Shaping Tomorrow's Need by Way of the Past
Available from University Microfilms

The paper discusses the shortage of capital in the health care industry. The author outlines historical sources of capital, the present state of capital financing, and future trends. The data indicate that there is an increasing dependence on hospital operations as the primary source of capital. However, indications are that operating revenue and cost-based depreciation reimbursement will not generate adequate replacement capital.

AHCMS 18923 FM

Jones, Katherine R.
Determination of the Additional Costs Incurred by Patients in a Teaching Hospital due to the Presence of Graduate Medical Education Programs
Stanford University, Palo Alto, CA, 1983
Available from University Microfilms

This study was conducted to determine the incremental charges incurred by patients that are attributable to the graduate medical education programs in teaching hospitals. Hospital charges and hospital stay were compared across three physician groups: private patients with a community attending physician, teaching patients with a community attending physician, and teaching patients with a faculty attending physician. Severity of illness differences were controlled for by selecting patients from surgical diagnostic-related groups, refining these groups by surgical codes and age, identifying prehospital and inhospital severity of illness control variables, and omitting death and transfer cases. The impact of teaching group on hospital charges and hospital stay was analyzed using three regression models: the first included diagnostic control variables, the second included demographic and prehospital control variables, and the third added inhospital control variables. Results indicated that patients on the teaching service with a faculty attending physician incurred significantly higher hospital charges as compared to private, nonteaching patients. The major factors for the higher charges were increased ordering of diagnostic tests, and differential use of supplies and equipment. The patients on the teaching service with a community attending physician did not incur higher hospital charges as compared to the nonteaching patients. The level of resident supervision by attending physicians is significant in determining total charges incurred by teaching patients. Close supervision of the residents resulted in hospital charges for teaching patients that were similar to those for nonteaching patients. Less supervision of residents led to increased use of ancillary services.

AHCMS 27012 HC

Kaitz, Edward M.
Pricing Policy and Cost Behavior in the Hospital Industry
Frederick A. Praeger, Boulder, CO, 1968, 205 pp.

A study to establish and evaluate the relationship between the financial and accounting techniques used by the third party payment system and the price determination, cost control, and capital-budgeting decisions within the individual hospital.

AHCMS AC2012

Kalison, Michael J. and Averill, Richard
The Response to PPS: Inside, Outside, Over Time
Healthcare Financial Management, 38:1, 1984, pp. 78 ff.

This is the first of a five-part series of articles dealing with the prospective payment system (PPS) based on diagnosis-related groups (DRGs) which has been mandated by Congress for Medicare reimbursement. The five-part series provides a framework for responding to the incentives of PPS in terms of product definition, development of a product-oriented approach to management and planning, marketing strategies, control of resource consumption, and strategic planning for the future. This part discusses product definition, describing provisions of the Social Security Act and Tax Equity and Fiscal Responsibility Act which distinguish between physician and nonphysician services (reimbursed under Parts B and A of Medicare, respectively).

AHCMS 27295 FM

Keller, Dina
  Effects of New Jersey's DRG Hospital Reimbursement System on Hospitals' Access to Capital Markets
Health Research and Educational Trust of New Jersey, Princeton, NJ, 1983, Report No. 6
  Author examines and explains the effects that the diagnosis-related group (DRG) hospital reimbursement system has had on New Jersey hospitals' ability to issue bonds for capital investment. It is concluded that the DRG program has tremendous merit in that it encourages cost containment rather than cost shifting, which in turn improves hospitals' financial condition and competitiveness in capital markets.

AHCMS 26943 FM

Kelly, J. V. and O'Brien, J. J.
  Hospital Cost and Utilization Project. Characteristics of Financially Distressed Hospitals
National Center for Health Services Research, Rockville, MD, 1983
Available from National Technical Information Service (PB84–111574)
  This paper identifies and clarifies the roles of hospital case mix, operating characteristics, and other factors that may contribute to financial distress. The effects of chronic deficits on hospital management and operations are discussed. Chronic hospital financial distress is defined and analyzed across hospital locations. Differences in case mix and treatment patterns are examined to test hypotheses regarding causes of chronic deficits. Cost and revenue factors associated with differences in hospital output and operating characteristics are also contrasted. The report concludes with a discussion of policy implications.

AHCMS 27056 HC

Kidder, David; Calore, Kathleen; and Hamilton, Diane
  U.S. Public Health Service Hospital Study
Abt Associates, Inc., Cambridge, MA, 1981
Available from National Technical Information Service (PB82–138553)
  Provides cost comparisons between U.S. Public Health Service (USPHS) hospitals and private sector (nonfederal) community hospitals. The study was undertaken in response to Congressional interest in hospital costs and USPHS interest in reducing direct provision of medical care. The study analyzes the comparative costs of providing patient care in USPHS hospitals and community hospitals, estimates the potential federal reimbursement costs if USPHS primary beneficiaries were treated in community hospitals, and develops estimates for USPHS staff and capital deficiencies. The study showed it would be less costly for the federal government to treat USPHS primary beneficiaries in community hospitals if a cost-based (and cost-shared) reimbursement system like Medicare were used.

The study did not deal with questions concerning ending federal control over the hospitals or termination of the specific entitlement for provision of fully subsidized medical care to primary beneficiaries.

AHCMS 25306 HC

Killian, Michael C.
Patients Are Paying the Bill For Government Regulation
Michigan Hospitals, 14:2, 1978, pp. 2–5.

The study was done to measure hospital costs directly attributable to meeting requirements of government regulations.

AHCMS 19345 HC

Kinkead, Brian M.
Medicare Payment and Hospital Capital: The Evolution of Policy
Health Affairs, 3:3, 1984, pp. 49–74.

The article describes the evolution of hospital capital policy in the 1960s and the federal government's role in shaping it as background for an assessment of hospitals' ability to fund capital investments since the inauguration of the Medicare program in 1966 and the emergence of tax-exempt financing in the early 1970s.

AHCMS 27710 FM

Kinzer, Donna and Warner, Michael
The Effect of Case-Mix Adjustment on Admission-Based Reimbursement
Health Services Research, 18:2, 1983, pp. 209–25.

Addresses two questions: (1) does adjusting for case mix have any effect on prospective admission-based reimbursement? and (2) how does the way in which case type is defined (DRG, ICD–9–CM, age) affect reimbursement systems? Data from 20 Maryland hospitals provide the basis for analysis, and the results illustrate how hospital reimbursement is affected under alternative definitions of case type (including no case type), showing highly significant variation. Implications for cost control and existing and proposed prospective reimbursement systems are discussed.

AHCMS 26685 HC

Klarman, Herbert E.
The Road to Cost-Effectiveness Analysis
Milbank Memorial Fund Quarterly, 60:4, 1982, pp. 585–603.

The empirical literature on cost-benefit analysis in health care concentrates on savings in direct expenditures and averted losses in earnings; valuation of intangible benefits has received little attention. A shift toward cost-effectiveness analysis in health care, although more limited, makes estimates more useful in decision making within the public sector. If well executed, intangibles evaluation can also lay a firm foundation for future cost-benefit analysis.

AHCMS 26619 HC

Kohlman, Herman A.
Determining a Contribution Margin for DRG Profitability
Healthcare Financial Management, 38:4, 1984, pp. 108 ff.

As the health care industry moves toward prospective payment for all inpatient services, hospital financial managers are becoming more interested in profit determination by DRGs. This article demonstrates one of the methods of profit determination by a Medicare step-down process. A ratio of cost-to-charges is developed for each cost center and is obtained from the relationship between revenue and fully allocated (stepped-down) cost for that particular center. The author particularly cautions financial managers to be aware of DRGs that are either unprofitable or are high volume–low profit.

AHCMS 27568 FM

Kominski, Gerald F.; Williams, Sankey V.; Mays, Randall B.; and Pickens, Gary T.
   Unrecognized Redistributions of Revenue in Diagnosis-Related Group–Based Prospective Payment Systems

Health Care Financing Review, 6:1, 1984, pp. 57–69.

   The Medicare prospective payment system, which is based on the diagnosis-related group patient classification system, identified previously unrecognized redistributions of revenue among diagnosis-related groups and hospitals. The redistributions are caused by two artifacts. One artifact results from the use of labor market indexes to adjust costs for the different prices paid by hospitals in different labor markets. The other artifact results from the use of averages that are based on the number of hospitals, not the number of patients, to calculate payment rates from average costs. The effects of these artifacts in a sample data set have been measured, and it was concluded that they lead to discrepancies between costs and payments that may affect hospital incentives—the overall payment for each diagnosis-related group—and Medicare's total payment.

AHCMS 28490 HC

Koretz, Daniel
   Catastrophic Medical Expenses: Patterns in the Non-Elderly, Non-Poor Population
U.S. Congressional Budget Office, Washington, DC, 1982

   High-cost illnesses in the nonelderly, nonpoor population—about 53 million families—are analyzed. Families were designated as high cost if their annual health care expenses exceeded one of four catastrophic thresholds. The report is based on claims data of Blue Cross–Blue Shield Federal Employees Health Benefit Plan for the years 1974–78. Major findings are: (1) In nonelderly, nonpoor population, families exceeding any of the catastrophic thresholds in a single year are relatively rare but account for a sizable proportion of total medical expenses. While the proportion exceeding the thresholds in any one year is small, the proportion exceeding those levels in at least one year during a several-year period is much larger. (2) Families exceeding a threshold in a baseline year have expenses well above average in both previous and subsequent years as well. (3) The proportion of expenditures for high-cost illness to total expenditures has remained relatively stable, but is growing slowly. Policy implications of the findings are discussed. The findings document the need for insurance protection against catastrophic illnesses; however, growth of high-cost illness over time indicates that the cost of such insurance will grow rapidly or the amount of protection provided will fall sharply. Cost-containment efforts aimed at high-cost illnesses will have little impact on overall increase in medical expenditures and will present problems with adverse selection among competing insurance plans.

AHCMS 26376 HC

Kovner, Anthony R. and Lusk, Edward J.
   Effective Hospital Budgeting
Hospital Administration, 18:4, 1973, pp. 44–64.

Article discusses reasons why hospitals have not effectively used capital budgeting, recommends how investment proposals may be more effectively evaluated, and outlines methods for implementing these recommendations.

AHCMS 11795 AC

Langwell, Kathryn M.; Bobula, Joel D.; Moore, Sylvia F.; and Adams, Barbara B.
An Annotated Bibliography of Research on Competition in the Financing and Delivery of Health Services
U.S. Dept. of Health and Human Services, Washington, DC, 1982

This annotated bibliography identifies and summarizes relevant research on competition: its nature, extent, and effects in the market for health services. Literature containing discussions of proposed and/or implemented approaches to improving health services market performance is also included and summarized. A comprehensive bibliography of nearly 1,000 items is presented. More than 200 of the most relevant, useful, and important papers are annotated and cross-classified. Selected data sources that have been, or may be, used to conduct research on competition in the financing and delivery of health services are identified and described.

AHCMS 26242 HC

Langwell, Kathryn M. and Moore, Sylvia F.
A Synthesis of Research and Competition in the Financing and the Delivery of Health Services
U.S. Dept. of Health and Human Services, Washington, DC, 1982

This report provides a comprehensive synthesis of the existing research on the nature and extent of competition in the financing and delivery of health services. The emphasis is on presenting evidence on barriers to competition, price competition, and nonprice competition in the health services market.

AHCMS 26254 HC

Lash, Myles P.
The Development of an Expense Budgeting Procedure
The University of Michigan, Ann Arbor, MI, 1970, 68 pp.
Available from University Microfilms

Report describes procedures undertaken at Annapolis Hospital to develop an expense budgeting program to project the volume and cost of services to be rendered during a future operating period. Regression analysis calculations used for projection of volume of patient days for all nursing units are described in detail.

AHCMS AC1–6955

Lave, Judith R. and Lave, Lester B.
Hospital Cost Functions: Estimating Cost Functions for Multi-Product Firms
School of Industrial Administration, Carnegie-Mellon University, Pittsburgh, PA, 1969, 38 pp.

Describes a method of estimating the cost function of hospitals which takes into account the multiproduct nature of the output (education, research, patient care, and community services). Using data consisting of time series on many firms, two procedures were developed which authors believe can be applied to other multiproduct and multiservice industries as well as to hospitals. Estimation techniques are explained in detail, and the results of testing several hypotheses are discussed.

AHCMS AC1–7051

Lave, Judith R. and Leinhardt, Samuel
  An Evaluation of a Hospital Stay Regulatory Mechanism
  American Journal of Public Health 66:10, 1976, pp. 959–67.
  The results of an evaluation of a predischarge utilization review program (PDUR) for Medicaid patients are presented. A group of hospitals in Allegheny County, Pennsylvania participated in this program on a voluntary basis prior to the program's being mandated statewide. All other hospitals in the county experienced retrospective review of Medicaid cases. The analysis incorporates both types of hospital in a quasi-experimental design. It was found that during the period studied the length of stay of Medicaid patients fell proportionately more than that of the Blue Cross patients in both groups of hospitals; the relative decrease in the length of stay began to occur prior to the introduction of the PDUR program, but no differential effect of the PDUR review process could be demonstrated. The decline in the length of stay was, however, more continuous and smooth in those hospitals participating in the program.

                                                              AHCMS 17745 HE

Leuthauser, Terry A.
  An Analysis of the Extent to which Nonprofit, Voluntary, Acute Care Hospitals Utilize the Bank Term Loan
  University of Iowa, Iowa City, IA, 1973, 168 pp.
  Available from University Microfilms
  Study investigated the extent to which hospitals utilize bank term loans as a means of capital financing. Data were gathered from literature and a questionnaire survey of 497 nonprofit voluntary acute care hospitals in region six of the AHA's list of registered hospitals. Findings indicate 42.1% of large hospitals and 28.5% of smaller hospitals utilized some type of bank term loan.

                                                              AHCMS 14012 AC

Lewin, Lawrence S.; Derson, Robert A.; and Margulies, Rhea
  Investor-Owned and Nonprofits Differ in Economic Performance
  Hospitals, 55:13, 1981, pp. 52–58.
  The authors of this article compare the economic performance of a closely matched sample of 53 hospitals owned by major investor-owned (IO) multihospital systems in California, Florida, and Texas, and 53 not-for-profit (NFP) nonchain community hospitals in the same states, using data drawn from fiscal year 1978 Medicare cost reports. Their purpose was to determine whether there were material differences between IO and NFP hospitals in the sample in cost to purchasers of care and, if so, the extent to which these differences were caused by variations in operating costs of the hospital, the markup of charges over cost, and differences in the use of physicians and human resources. The major findings follow. (1) IO hospitals were more expensive to charge payers. For cost-payers, IO hospitals are slightly more expensive on a per day basis, but essentially comparable on a per admission basis. A substantial portion of this difference for Medicare is the return on equity paid only to IO hospitals. (2) Slightly lower costs per day in NFP hospitals were due to lower costs in ancillary and administrative services and a 5% longer length of stay. IO costs are lower for space-related costs and for routine nursing expense. (3) IO hospitals price their services considerably higher above costs than NFPs—pricing differences are small for routine services, but very large for several ancillary services. (4) IO hospitals use fewer full-time equivalent staff per occupied bed and lower dollar values of fixed assets to produce

comparable volumes of care. Implications of the findings are discussed and areas for further study are outlined.

AHCMS 25067 HC

Lightle, Mary A.
Changes in the Sources of Capital
Hospital Financial Management, 35:2, 1981, pp. 42–47.

This article discusses sources of financing that will be available in the 1980s for private nonprofit hospital construction. Inflation made debt a preferred financing vehicle in the 1970s; today it threatens the very existence of the long-term bond market. Hospital executives must deal with the changing capital financing environment and develop new sources of capital. Two examples of responses to the elusive long-term bond market are the emergence of tax-exempt commercial paper (short-term corporate debts) and experiments with floating interest rates. The increasing leverage of the industry and uncertain prospects for regulation and payment systems suggest the need for new equity to absorb the risks of a changing environment. Aggressive search for private donations and responsible management of scarce resources will be required to meet this need. The article suggests that hospitals which establish pricing policies that recognize future capital needs will have the most capital financing options available to them, since hospitals may be required to make substantial equity contributions to secure financing as uncertain market conditions persist in the 1980s.

AHCMS 23530 FM

Lille, Kenneth and Danco, Walter
Organizing a Cost Containment Committee in the Hospital
American Hospital Association, Chicago, IL, 1976, 47 pp.

A suggested approach for the organization of a hospital cost containment committee is designed to coordinate various methodologies used by hospitals to provide economical and high quality service. The recommendation is made that a cost containment committee must be fully integrated into the total administrative system of a hospital to be effective.

AHCMS 18583 HE

Lindberg, Paul R.
VAV and Heat Recovery in a Medical Center
Heating/Piping/Air Conditioning, 55:8, 1983, pp. 82–88.

The 238-bed Central Maine Medical Center has two patient area air systems. Both are 100% outside air, single duct, multizone systems, with a steam preheater, chilled water coil, steam humidifier, hot water reheat coils, and room terminal induction boxes with hot water coils. A review of the systems was made in search of energy cost saving projects with paybacks of two years or less. This review led to a decision to apply a single variable frequency AC controller to the fans in both systems to reduce the air flows, and to use run-around coil systems for heat recovery. These measures enabled the former annual consumption of 1,200,000 KWH of electricity and 100,000 gallons of fuel oil to be reduced by 300,000 KWH and 60,000 gallons.

AHCMS 27365 EN

Linklater, R. Bruce
Internal Control of Hospital Finances. A Guide for Management
American Hospital Association, Chicago, IL, 1983

The methodology and guidelines presented in this book offer a systematic approach to administering an effective internal control system, monitoring its performance, and identifying and correcting its weaknesses.

AHCMS 28542 FM

Lion, Joanna; Malbon, Alan; Friedman, Robert; and Henderson, Mary G.
Relationship of Physician Medicaid Reimbursement in Private Practice and Hospital Outpatient Departments to Actual Costs of Providing Care
Brandeis University, Waltham, MA, 1983
Available from National Technical Information Service (PB83–212027)

This study compares the mix and cost of patients treated in hospital outpatient departments with those of patients treated in private physicians' offices. Presenting diagnoses do not differ markedly between these settings, but the differences generate costs in one type of setting which differ substantially from those in others.

AHCMS 26613 HC

Long, Hugh W.
Preserving Capital: Asset Choice and Program Selection in a Competitive Environment
Healthcare Financial Management, 36:8, 1982, pp. 34 ff.

This article is the second in a two-part series on preserving capital in both for-profit and tax-exempt institutions. Part I emphasized that the fundamental objective for private organizations should be the preservation of the real value of capital, and that this can be accomplished only if organizations meet the expectations of capital suppliers (expressed as required rates of return on capital). Part I also pointed out that the value of returns received by capital suppliers is not necessarily the same as the cost to the organization of generating those returns; thus, the cost of capital should be distinguished from the required rate of return. The author presents some examples of the cost-of-capital/required-rate-of-return distinction, then considers how implicit and explicit dividends can be viewed within this structure. The second part of the article presents a conceptually sound method of applying these concepts to project evaluation—calculating the net present value of a proposal relative to the organization's weighted average cost of capital (WACC)—and explores some implications of this approach for institutional strategy and national policy. The author suggests that a private sector organization should choose only those assets and participate in only those programs or projects that individually and collectively produce operational cash flows at least of sufficient size to meet the WACC. The article demonstrates that activities meeting the WACC exactly will generate operational cash flows (along with external subsidies through taxation, reimbursement) that allow the organization to meet exactly the expectations of contractual demands of its suppliers of capital, satisfy required rates of return, and insure future access to capital markets.

AHCMS 26226 FM

Long, M. J.; Allen, W. J.; Ament, R. P.; Knop, L. L.; and Kobrinski, E. J.
Profile of the Financial Burden of High Cost Illness
The University of Michigan, Ann Arbor, MI, 1983
Available from National Technical Information Service (PB84–239128)

This report discusses findings of a study of financially catastrophic hospitalization episodes in all 54 Maryland hospitals. Policy implications of findings, including the disproportionate share of catastrophic charges paid by Medicare (for the elderly) and by Medicaid (for the newborn) are discussed.

AHCMS 28304 HC

Loop, Floyd D. et al.
A Strategy for Cost Containment in Coronary Surgery
Journal of the American Medical Association, 250:1, 1983, pp. 63–66.

One of the greatest determinants of total hospital charge is length of stay. A study at the Cleveland (Ohio) Clinic Foundation disclosed that the discharges of coronary bypass patients were rarely postponed unnecessarily, but patients were frequently admitted two days before surgery for routine testing and evaluation or spent several days waiting in the hospital between cardiac catheterization and surgery. In a voluntary cost-containment exercise, patients were examined by outpatient testing and admitted to a staging area on the morning of their operation. Their hospital charges were compared with those of cohorts of coronary surgery patients from 1977 to 1981 who met the same admission criteria. Length of stay was reduced by two days. A 10% saving in hospital charges was realized by the experimental group compared with the 1981 control group. A comparison of total hospital charges, adjusted for inflation, showed that experimental group patients paid 35% less for their hospital room, 45% less for their intensive care period, and 17% less in total charges than the 1977 control group. Interviews indicated that these patients with stable cardiac conditions preferred to stay with their families or friends before surgery.

AHCMS 28000 HC

McCarthy, Carol M.
Cost of Regulation. Report of the Task Force on Regulation
Hospital Association of New York State, West Albany, NY

This report presents findings of a comprehensive study that investigated the costs of regulation in the hospital industry in New York State. It covers the year 1976 and includes data received from 148 acute care facilities.

AHCMS 21131 HC

McCarthy, Carol
Incentive Reimbursement as an Impetus to Cost Containment
Inquiry, 12:4, 1975, pp. 320–29.

This article describes and compares five experimental incentive reimbursement programs that utilize industiral engineering, budgetary, or physician-expander appraoches. It also outlines a number of methods for calculating incentive payments and presents recommendations to stimulate greater success through the incentive reimbursement approach.

AHCMS 19127 IN

MacLeod, Gordon K. and Perlman, Mark (eds.)
Health Care Capital: Competition and Control
Ballinger Publishing Co., Cambridge, MA, 1978

This book is concerned with the capital financing needs of health care institutions and identifies and analyzes available sources of health care capital, particularly in view of the growing impact of new investments on the operating costs for the total industry.

AHCMS 19636 FM

MacLeod, Roderick K.
Program Budgeting Works in Nonprofit Institutions
Harvard Business Review, 49:5, 1971, pp. 46–56.

An exposition of a program budgeting and accounting system for nonprofit institutions, based on the three years' experience of the South Shore Mental Health Center, Quincy, Massachusetts.

AHCMS 08573 AC

Magerlein, David B.; Davis, Rick J.; and Hancock, Walton M.
The Prediction of Departmental Activity and Its Use in the Budgeting Process
Bureau of Hospital Administration, The University of Michigan, Ann Arbor, MI, 1976, 27 pp.

Paper outlines construction of a demand-based flexible operating budget. Emphasis is on describing the methodology used in predicting departmental activity, an essential element in developing such a budget. Predictions of hospital activity measures (admissions, patient days, outpatient visits, budget point) and time-related variables (month, year) are used to predict each departmental activity through application of multiple linear regression. Paper also depicts the use of flexible budgeting to determine cost savings due to hospital resizing and includes an outline of an entire flexible budgeting system.

AHCMS 17888 AC

Magill, Greta
Health Care Vouchers
Institute for Health Planning, Madison, WI, 1982

Procompetitive approaches to cost containment attempt to strengthen market forces through the use of cost sharing; participation in alternative health care delivery systems; the provision of multiple options in health insurance plans; reform in the tax treatment of employee health insurance benefits; and voucher systems for employee groups, the elderly, and/or the poor. Vouchers may provide the poor with the opportunity to participate in the medical care system on equal footing with the more well-to-do and would be likely to encourage the development of a large variety of health care plans and competition among these plans. However, if participation in a Medicare voucher system were voluntary, adverse selections might create problems. High-risk beneficiaries would tend to remain in the traditional Medicare program, thus increasing the costs to Medicare. Private plans may also find it difficult to compete with Medicare because they have to cover departmental, marketing, and administrative costs and higher claims payment rates in their premium prices. Cost shifting by providers may also be reduced under a voucher system, but providers may also be exposed to higher levels of bad debt if a large number of beneficiaries choose plans with cost-sharing arrangements and then find themselves unable to pay their obligations. Because a voucher system would replace open-ended entitlement programs with federally set financial subsidies for purchasing health care benefits, concern has also arisen that vouchers would provide a politically more feasible way to reduce federal commitment to the health care needs of the elderly and poor.

AHCMS 26218 HC

Mankin, Douglas and Glueck, William F.
Strategic Planning
Hospital and Health Services Administration, 22:2, 1977, pp. 6–22.

A study of 15 Missouri hospitals designed to find whether the hospitals used strategic planning, and if those that did were more successful in reaching their objectives. The study found that the hospitals did not formally plan their strategies in detail.

AHCMS 19437 AB

Markel, Gene A.
Pre-Case Reimbursement for Medical Care
Pennsylvania Blue Shield, Camp Hill, PA 17011, 1977, 62 pp.

An experimental program was established to test and evaluate the concept of reimbursing physicians for in-hospital medical care on a case basis, instead of the traditional disaggregated fee-for-service approach. Physician reimbursement amounts were based upon patient's discharge diagnoses, using a schedule of diagnosis categories based upon ICDA classifications. Primary research objectives were to test the effects of per case reimbursement upon inpatient hospital utilization, and to determine any associated changes in medical care costs. Comparisons with cross-sectional and longitudinal control groups indicate some modest favorable changes in average length of stay, with concomitant potential cost savings.

AHCMS 17719 IN

Maryland Health Services
Hospital Rate Setting. Maryland's Experience 1977–1983. Final Report
Maryland Health Services Cost Review Commission, 201 W. Preston St., Baltimore, MD 21201, 1983

The experience of the Maryland Health Services Cost Review Commission's rate-setting system in curbing increases in health care costs is described. The report first discusses events which led to establishment of the commission, its enabling legislation, and its responsibilities. The commission was empowered to set prospective rates using a variety of methods including comparison of one hospital's costs to the costs of similar hospitals, limiting the size of hospital rate increases, and denying high cost hospitals any rate increase. The report explains the reimbursement system and the philosophy and policies behind it. Data indicate that over the past seven years the cost of a day of hospital care in Maryland has been rising at a rate well below the national average and that Maryland has saved an estimated $39.5 million in hospital costs in the fiscal year 1982 and $374 million since regulation started in 1974.

AHCMS 28661 HC

Massell, A. P. and Williams, A. P.
Comparing Costs of Inpatient Care in Teaching and Non-Teaching Hospitals: Methodology and Data
Rand Corporation, Santa Monica, CA, 1977, 71 pp.

This publication identifies and evaluates options for analyzing the costs of inpatient care in teaching and nonteaching hospitals.

AHCMS 19293 AC

May, J. Joel
Diagnosis Related Groups
Topics in Health Care Financing, 8:4, 1982, pp. 1–83.

This special issue is devoted to diagnosis-related groups (DRGs) and the application of this patient classification scheme to hospital planning, utilization review, and hospital reimbursement in New Jersey. The articles are: (1) "Measurement of Case Mix," by James D. Bentley and Peter W. Butler; (2) "Data Systems for Case Mix," by Leo K. Lichtig; (3) "Case Mix and Regulation," by Harold A. Cohen and J. Graham Atkinson; (4) "Diagnosis Related Groups and Management," by John L. Yoder and Robert A. Connor; (5) "Diagnosis Related Groups and Quality Assurance," by John S. Thompson; (6) "One Application of the DRG Planning Model," by John D. Thompson; and (7) "Future Directions for Case-Mix Applications," by John B. Reiss. Appendexes present definitions of case-mix data items, and selected edits used in the New Jersey State Department of Health case-mix data system.

AHCMS 25713 HC

May, J. Joel; Wasserman, Jeffrey
Selected Results from an Evaluation of the New Jersey Diagnosis-Related Group System
Health Services Research, 19:5, 1984, pp. 547–59.

After briefly describing the New Jersey diagnosis-related group (DRG) system and comparing and contrasting it with the Medicare prospective payment plan, selected findings from an evaluation of the New Jersey DRG experience are presented. The discussion highlights the system's effect on ways in which hospitals are organized and managed, and its preliminary economic and financial impact.

AHCMS 28354 HC

Melnick, Glenn A.
The Effects of Certificate of Need and Rate Regulation on Hospital Costs and Utilization, 1975–1979
The University of Michigan, Ann Arbor, MI, 1983
Available from University Microfilms

Evaluates the effects of hospital rate regulation (RR) and certificate of need (CON) on controlling hospital costs. Using a multivariate approach, the independent effects of CON and RR on the annual rate of increase in total hospital expenses, average hospital costs, total admissions, and average length of stay are estimated for the period 1975–79. The results indicate that CON had no effect on any of these measures. Hospital RR programs appear to have been associated with an approximately 2% reduction in the rate of increase in average costs. This reduction did not, however, carry over to total hospital expenses; RR programs appear to have significantly reduced total hospital expenses in only one year (1978) during the five-year study period.

AHCMS 27052 HC

Mennemeyer, S. T.
Evaluation of the Medicare Part B Fixed Price Experiemnts in Maine, Upstate New York, and Illinois
Abt Associates, Inc., Cambridge, MA, 1983
Available from National Technical Information Service (PB84–187657)

This project evaluates the Medicare Part B fixed-price carrier experiments in Maine, Illinois, and upstate New York. The evaluation examines the experiments' effects on program costs and quality of carrier performance. Fixed-price arrangements are compared with the previous systems in the three areas. The performance of each experimental contractor is also compared with the performance of two comparable cost-reimbursed contractors. Findings indicate that the fixed-price contractor experiments resulted in reduced federal costs for carrier services. The decreased costs were achieved by using different processing sites and better processing systems, and through some economies of scale.

AHCMS 27825 HC

MICAH Corporation
The MICAH System for Hospital Cost Analysis
The MICAH Corporation, Ann Arbor, MI, 1968, 30 pp.

Describes a computerized system employing matrix inversion for solving simultaneous equations to compute total departmental costs in a hospital cost finding procedure.

AHCMS AC1032

Michigan Blue Shield
Blue Shield of Michigan Family Health Expenditure Survey 1972–1973
Michigan Blue Shield, Detroit, MI, 1975, 32 pp.

This study investigates how the Blue Cross–Blue Shield population compares with populations having other types of coverage or no insurance at all, and reports on the amount that Blue Cross–Blue Shield subscribers were obliged to spend in utilizing services not covered by their insurance. Data were collected from families living within the city of Detroit first in the year September 1971 through August 1972, then again in the year September 1972 through August 1973. The second sample is compared to the first to observe if any particular trends exist in any of the variables analyzed.

AHCMS 13271 IN

Miller, Irwin
The Health Care Survival Curve: Competition and Cooperation in the Marketplace
Dow Jones–Irwin, Homewood, IL, 1984

The book looks at health care enterpreneurship in a political perspective. The author draws on the experience of HMOs to create a model for affordable, community-based alternative delivery systems—PPOs, IPAs, and primary care networks. The book is organized into three main parts to map out a practical survival plan marked by negotiation, conflict resolution, and compromise. The first part looks at the national health policy framework in terms of turbulence, and offers an approach to managing for survival. The second part addresses the local level of implementing policy—of actual community institution building. The author specifically looks at the prepaid group practice planning process from the perspectives of the three key cooperative role innovators—managers, providers, and consumers. The third part discusses the issue of the industrialization of health, the limits of this process, and the guidance that voluntarism can bring to this transformation.

AHCMS 27500 HC

Morehead, Mildred A.; Zanes, Anne; and Donaldson, Rose
Attitudes, Utilization, and Out-of-Pocket Costs for Health Services
Columbia University, New York, NY, 1967, 170 pp.
Available from University Microfilms

Report of household interviews of selected families participating in the Teamster Comprehensive Care Program (TCP). Study was designed to measure costs, attitudes, and utilization by participating families, and to focus on factors leading families to participate in TCP.

AHCMS IN3019

National Technical Information Service
Control of Health Care Costs. 1980–May 1981 (Citations from the NTIS Data Base)
Available from National Technical Information Service (PB81–806358)

Citations are presented on the studies of various strategies for cost containment in hospitals, long-term care facilities, and ambulatory care. Some topics covered are the effectiveness of shared services and facilities; design and space planning of hospitals; closing of underutilized and substandard facilities; incentives for employee productivity; improvements in personnel staffing; prospective and incentive reimbursement by third party payers; alternative delivery systems, such as health maintenance organizations and ambulatory surgicenters; utilization and rate review; and the roles of state and national government in regulating Medicaid and Medicare expenditures.

AHCMS 26035 HC

National Technical Information Service
Health Care Costs: Health Care Facilities, 1977–May 1981 (Citations from the NTIS Data Base)
Available from National Technical Information Service (PB81–806457)

The selected abstracts of research reports cover construction costs, operation costs, financial management, capital needs, financing, cost effectiveness, incentive reimbursement, health manpower costs, health insurance, and cost-benefit analysis of health care facilities, which include nursing homes, hospitals and mental health facilities.

AHCMS 25186 HC

National Technical Information Service
Health Care Costs: Major Studies. March 1980–June 1982 (Citations from the NTIS Data Base)
Available from National Technical Information Service (PB82–809740)

This volume contains abstracts of research reports covering major studies on health care costs. The bibliography was compiled for professionals interested in the broad range of costs related to health care. Health care facilities, emergency medical services, health manpower, acute care, long-term care, health planning, and health insurance are among the subjects cited.

AHCMS 26313 HC

Nestman, Lawrence J.
Responsibility Accounting: A Tool to Better Planning and Cost Control in the Hospital
Hospital Administration in Canada, 16:2, 1974, pp. 45–48, 50–52.

Article reviews basic concepts of responsibility accounting and discusses advantages and disadvantages of installing and operating a responsibility accounting system in the hospital.

AHCMS 12217 AC

Neuhauser, Duncan
The Large Hospital and the Organization of Medical Care

Presented at the International Conference of Hospital Management in Sao Paulo, Brazil

Available from Duncan Neuhauser, Professor of Epidemiology and Community Health, Case Western Reserve University, Cleveland, OH 44106

Monograph describes the role of the large general hospital in the medical care system. The characteristics of organizational size (volume of demand, economies and diseconomies of scale) are reviewed with a model of hospital organization. This model is based on essential-nonessential and divisible-indivisible services. The role of the tertiary care referral hospital in Sweden, England, and the U.S. Veterans Administration is described, and alternative organizational designs are discussed. Physician education in large hospitals is made difficult by the nonrepresentative nature of referral institutions and the abundance of technological resources. The monograph includes a historical review of the evaluation of medical care in a large hospital and a typology of external forces that regulate hospital performance.

AHCMS 23659 HE

Newhouse, Joseph P.
Income and Medical Care Expenditure across Countries
Rand Corporation, Santa Monica, CA, 1976, 19 pp.

This paper examines the relationship between a country's medical care expenditures and its income. The study covers 13 so-called developed countries. The comparison shows that per capita income can explain much of the cross-national variation in expenditures. The amount of funds spent on medical care is directly proportional to gross domestic product per capita, but the proportion of income spent decreases.

AHCMS 16962 HE

Newhouse, Joseph P. and Taylor, Vincent
Medical Costs, Health Insurance, and Public Policy
Rand Corporation, Santa Monica, CA, c. 1969, 27 pp.

The paper reports on health insurance in relation to excessive medical costs and discusses a number of constructive steps that could be taken to modify the effects of insurance. Variable cost hospital insurance is proposed. By greatly increasing consumer concern with hospital costs, variable cost insurance would slow the rise in these costs. It would also affect inequities in the present insurance system.

AHCMS IN1-5532

O'Donoghue, Patrick
Controlling Hospital Costs: The Revealing Case of Indiana (Summary and Full Report)
Policy Center Inc., Denver, CO

This report analyzes the impact of the prospective rate setting system in Indiana by comparing Indiana hospitals with control hospitals, selected from Michigan, Illinois, Minnesota, and Iowa, which did not have a prospective rate setting program during the main study years, 1968 through 1973.

AHCMS 20787 HC

Ofer, Aharon R.
Third Party Reimbursement and the Evaluation of Leasing Alternatives
Topics in Health Care Financing, 3:1, 1976, pp. 51–67.

Article discusses advantages and disadvantages of leasing hospital equipment and describes the various types of leasing arrangement and how third party payers classify them for reimbursement purposes.

AHCMS 17068 AC

Office of Technology Assessment
The Implications of Cost-Effectiveness Analysis of Medical Technology: Summary
U.S. Government Printing Office, Washington, DC, 1980

This summary presents the findings of an assessment of the use of cost-effectiveness analysis (CEA) and cost-benefit analysis (CBA) in decision making regarding medical technologies. The assessment examines the general role of CEA and CBA in health care decisions, methodological issues, the potential of CEA and CBA for constraining the growth in health care costs, and the past and possible future use of CEA or CBA in six specific health-related programs: Medicare reimbursement, health planning, professional standards review organizations, market approval of drugs and medical devices, research and development, and health maintenance organizations.

AHCMS 24119 HC

Olson, Gary R.
Determining the Debt Capacity of a Voluntary Not-for-Profit Community Hospital
Washington University, St. Louis, MO, 1976, 112 pp.
Available from University Microfilms

This paper describes the method employed for determining the debt capacity of a nonprofit hospital.

AHCMS 18977 FM

Paretta, Robert L. and Lipstein, Robert J.
Internal Control: How Do Hospitals, Industry Compare?
Hospital Financial Management, 33:6, 1979.

The article outlines some of the most commonly recommended methods for exercising internal control over cash, examines current practices of large nonprofit hospitals to alert financial managers to areas of potential weakness, and compares these practices to those of industrial firms.

AHCMS 21358 FM

Paul-Shaheen, Pamela and Carpenter, Eugenia S.
Legislating Hospital Bed Reduction: The Michigan Experience
Journal of Health Politics, Policy and Law, 6:4, 1982, pp. 653–75.

This article presents a case study of one state's effort to deal with health care cost issues, focusing on the formulation and adoption of legislation to reduce the number of hospital beds. The Michigan bed-reduction legislation was the product of a coalition of powerful, organized "professional consumers" of health services who placed hospital cost containment on the political agenda and framed a solution. The provisions of the legislation were reshaped during the legislative process to grant concessions to a variety of interest groups, particularly the Michigan Hospital Association. Cost containment as a goal was, if not subordinated, at least made competitive with other goals—access to care, equity among types of provider, and quality of services. While the initial proposal was attractive as a seemingly simple extension of the certificate-of-need process within the existing regulatory framework, the legislation became increasingly complex in response to new issues raised by political actors who contributed to the shaping of the final version of the legislation.

AHCMS 25106 HC

Pauly, Mark V.
Medical Staff Characteristics and Hospital Costs
Journal of Human Resources 13, Supplement, 1978.

To test the hypothesis that medical staff physicians affect hospital behavior, this paper relates cost data for a sample of nonmajor, teaching, short-term hospitals to information on the characteristics of the medical staffs that treat patients in those hospitals.

AHCMS 21091 HC

Phelps, Charles E. and Newhouse, Joseph P.
Coinsurance and the Demand for Medical Services
Rand Corporation, Santa Monica, CA, 1974, 63 pp.

Paper analyzes consumers' response to changes in the coinsurance rate for various medical services. Using a formal model of utility maximization, a model of demand for medical services is developed for when reimbursement insurance is present and when there are time costs involved in purchasing medical care. A number of data sources are used to estimate elasticities of demand for medical care services, and these results are compared with results of three other studies. Results show services with a relatively high time price exhibit relatively low coinsurance or price elasticities. Services with relatively high money-price to time-price ratio show considerably higher own-price elasticities. Services with coinsurance rates near zero show low-price elasticities. In percentage terms, it is estimated 8% to 17% more services would be demanded at a zero coinsurance rate than at a 25% rate. A pattern of low elasticity for hospital services, greater elasticity for office visits, and greatest elasticity for home visits is developed in the zero to 25% range of coverage. Paper concludes coinsurance is relevant to choice; irrespective of who makes the decision, greater coinsurance implies less use of services and the amount of reduction varies by type of service.

AHCMS 13674 IN

Platou, Carl N. and Rice, James A.
Multihospital Holding Companies
Harvard Business Review, 50:3, 1972.

Article outlines application of the holding company concept to a group of medical care facilities, using information from the Fairview Hospitals, an affiliation of Minnesota hospitals developing a multihospital organization. Major benefits cited of the hospital holding company are: economies of scale resulting from superior management and centralization of certain specialized activities; broader range of services and facilities at the local level; and improved capital resources and operating efficiency that protect the solvency of each local unit.

AHCMS 08756 AC

Plomann, Marilyn P.; Bisbee, Gerald E., Jr.; and Esmond, Truman
Use of Case-Mix Information in Hospital Management: An Overview and Case Study
Healthcare Financial Management, 38:10, 1984, pp. 28 ff.

Based on findings from a three-year project, the article discusses major points hospital management must consider in developing or acquiring a case-mix management system: key characteristics of an effective case-mix system; management responsibilities and strategies to facilitate acceptance and use of data by both administrative and clinical staff; practical considerations regarding the use of case-mix information; and evaluation by hospital managers of the benefits of a case-mix management information system.

AHCMS 28422 FM

President's Private Sector Survey on Cost Control
   President's Private Sector Survey on Cost Control: Report on Federal Hospital Management
President's Private Sector Survey on Cost Control, Washington, DC, 1983
Available from National Technical Information Service (PB84–173228)

The report on federal hospital management contains major recommendations which, when fully implemented, could result in three-year cost savings and revenue generation of $11,912 million. It should be noted, however, that some of the recommendations may require several years for the savings and revenue to be realized. While all facets of federal hospital management could not be surveyed in the time allotted, areas selected for review were considered to offer significant potential for cost control and improved efficiency.

AHCMS 27696 HC

President's Private Sector Survey on Cost Control
   President's Private Sector Survey on Cost Control: Report on Management Office Selected Issues. Vol. 8. The Cost of Congressional Encroachment. Vol. 9. Federal Health Care Costs
President's Private Sector Survey on Cost Control, Washington, DC, 1983
Available from National Technical Information Service (PB84–173426)

Reports on the cost of Congressional encroachment and on federal health care costs. Some of the recommendations in the reports may require several years for the savings to be realized. While all facets of the surveys could not be surveyed in the time allotted, areas selected for review were considered to offer significant potential for cost control and improved efficiency.

AHCMS 27697 HC

Record, Jane Cassels; Vogt, Thomas M.; Penn, Rhesa Lee; and Johnson, Richard E.
   An Episode Approach to Utilization, Costs, and Effectiveness in Health Care
Kaiser Foundation Research Institution, Portland, OR, 1981

Using its exceptional data base for a 5% sample of enrolled members, the Kaiser-Portland Health Services Research Center undertook development of a methodology for identifying, costing, and examining alternative resource bundles used in ambulatory care of defined conditions. Results and detailed analysis are presented for 11 conditions. For 10 of these, distinct treatment bundles (ranging from eight to ten alternatives per condition) emerged which explained between 50% and 70% of the observed cost variation (which for most conditions was quite substantial). Patient and/or provider characteristics explained 29% of cost variations for 5 conditions, between 14% and 19% for others, and less than 10% for the remaining two. There is some indication that laboratory tests and drug orders may substitute for office visits for some conditions. But the authors caution that their results are not yet suitable for use in determining medical policy. They conclude with a description of what further research might be done to strengthen policy applications of their approach, including eight methodological imperatives.

AHCMS 25401 HC

Restuccia, Joseph D. and Chernow, Robert A.
Utilization and Cost of Mental and Health Benefits: A Comparison of Insurance Plans
University of California, Berkeley, CA, 1974, 23 pp.
Available from University Microfilms

This paper provides an insight into the problems surrounding the exclusion of mental illnesses in health insurance and prepayment plans, and describes the emerging public policies that foster benefits for mental illness.

AHCMS 13313 IN

Riedel, Donald C.; Walden, Daniel C.; Singsen, Antone G.; Meyers, Samuel; Krantz, Goldie; and Henderson, Marie
Federal Employees Health Benefits Program Utilization Study
U.S. DHEW Pub. No. (HRA) 75–3125. Public Health Service, Rockville, MD, 1975, 144 pp.

This report is a comparative utilization study of two alternate forms of health maintenance organization. The purpose of the study is to identify the factors that account for the observed lower rate of hospital admissions experienced by beneficiaries of a prepaid group health association in contrast to subscribers of a traditional fee-for-service plan.

AHCMS 14018 IN

Rinaldo, J. A., Jr.; McCubbrey, D. J.; and Shryock, J. R.
The Care-Monitoring, Cost-Forecasting, and Cost-Monitoring System
Journal of Medical Systems, 6:3, 1982, pp. 315–27.

This paper describes the development of and results from an automated system developed by Blue Cross–Blue Shield of Michigan to determine reasons for changes in hospital costs from one year to the next.

AHCMS 26294 HC

Robbins, Jennifer
Uses of Population-Based Data for Rate Setting
Harvard Center for Community Health and Medical Care, Boston, MA, 1976, 35 pp.

The expansion of data bases for rate setting to include information about the population receiving services, the utilization of services, and service outcome is explored.

AHCMS 17774 AC

Rossiter, Louis F. and Wilensky, Gail R.
Out-of-Pocket Expenditures for Personal Health Services
U.S. Dept. of Health and Human Services, Rockville, MD, 1982

This data preview from the National Health Care Expenditures Study (NCHES) presents the financial burden on individuals and families of out-of-pocket expenditures for health care in 1977. While high out-of-pocket expenses were relatively rare, nearly one-tenth of all families in the United States spent 10% or more of their income on personal health care beyond the amounts paid by insurance or other third party payers. In addition, estimates of out-of-pocket expenses for personal health care, exclusive of health insurance premiums, are presented for selected population groups. The distribution of total out-of-pocket expenditures among various types of health service is shown, as is the distribution of persons and families with health expenditures by intervals of annual out-of-pocket expense. Also shown are expenses per person with expense by age, sex, and perceived health status, and by family income according to U.S. census region. All findings are from household data reported for the period January 1 to December 31, 1977.

AHCMS 26244 HC

Ruppel, Ronald W. and Mayo, George E.
   Computerized Financial Modeling: A Way to Improve a Hospital's Economic Position
Hospital Financial Management, 36:2, 1982, pp. 40 ff.

   This article describes the use of computerized modeling in the financial planning process in the hospital. Computer modeling involves definition of the hospital's financial operations in terms of mathematical formulas using revenue, expense, and volume relationships. The authors point out that financial modeling using computer capabilities is particularly applicable to hospitals due to the complex cost reimbursement formulas used by Medicare, Medicaid, and Blue Cross. It is concluded that by using computerized financial modeling, hospitals receive more meaningful and statistical information, have an opportunity to review thoroughly alternative financial plans, have more time for planning, and receive timely information for timely decisions.

AHCMS 26021 FM

Russell, Louise B.
   The Economics of Prevention
Health Policy, 4:2, 1984, pp. 85–100.

   A review of cost-effectiveness studies of prevention supports two conclusions: (1) few prevention programs, if any, reduce medical expenditures; (2) even when prevention costs less per person than acute care, its medical costs per unit of health benefit can be as great or greater. So that future studies will allow comparisons over a wider range of medical choices, the paper proposes some steps toward the greater standardization of cost-effectiveness analyses of medical care.

AHCMS 28395 HC

Sage, Lloyd G.
   Recognition of the Impact of Changing Prices on Conventional Historical Cost Financial Statements of Hospitals
The University of Nebraska, Lincoln, NB, 1984
Available from University Microfilms

   This dissertation investigates the possible application of the FASB's *Statement of Financial Accounting Standards No. 33* (FAS 33) current cost and constant dollar models to the conventional historical cost hospital financial statements, and examine their perceived impact on the financial decisions of selected users of the hospital's financial statements. The study demonstrates that the FAS 33 minimum disclosure requirements and the optional comprehensive financial statement procedures can be feasibly applied to the conventional historical cost financial statements of not-for-profit hospitals.

AHCMS 28556 FM

Sager, Alan
   Learning the Home Care Needs of the Elderly: Patient, Family, and Professional Views of an Alternative to Institutionalization
Levinson Policy Institute, Waltham, MA, 1979
Available from National Technical Information Service (HRP–0902560/2)

This study was designed to improve knowledge of the comparative costs of home and institutional care. It began with a sample of patients about to enter nursing homes, obtained many hypothetical estimates of the cost of an in-home alternative of equal or greater effectiveness, and then compared these costs with those of the institutional care actually provided.

AHCMS 23707 HC

Salkever, David S. and Bice, Thomas W.
Hospital Certificate-of-Need Controls: Impact on Investment, Costs and Use
American Enterprise Institute for Public Policy Research, Washington, DC, c. 1979, 103 pp.

This monograph presents findings from an empirical study of the impact of certificate-of-need (CON) legislation on growth in hospital investment, utilization, and costs over the 1968–72 period.

AHCMS 20933 HC

Sall, L.
NHCES (National Health Care Expenditures Study): Annotated Bibliography of Studies from the National Medical Care Expenditure Survey
National Center for Health Services Research, Rockville, MD, 1983
Available from National Technical Information Service (PB84–145598)

This study examines how Americans use health care services and tries to determine national patterns of health expenditures and insurance coverage.

AHCMS 27504 HC

Sapolsky, Harvey M.; Altman, Drew; Greene, Richard; and Moore, Judith D.
Corporate Attitudes toward Health Care Costs
Milbank Memorial Fund Quarterly (Health and Society), 59, Fall 1981, pp. 561–85.

Most Americans receive their protection against health care costs through benefits provided by employers; the level of corporate concern about the resulting rising costs will inevitably affect national policy. Officials in selected major firms, when interviewed, showed little concern, and even less willingness to risk offending unions, employees, and customers through control of benefit expenditures. It is unlikely that corporations will take a significant role in controlling health care costs.

AHCMS 24940 HC

Sattler, Frederic L.
A Rational Look at the Hospital and Debt Financing
Hospital Topics, 53:1, 1975, pp. 16, 18, 20.

Author discusses debt financing in the nonprofit hospital.

AHCMS 13739 AC

Saward, Ernest W.
The Relevance of Prepaid Group Practice to the Effective Delivery of Health Services
U.S. DHEW, Public Health Service, Health Services and Mental Health Administration, Office of Group Practice Development, Washington, DC, 1969, 24 pp.

The paper discusses five major problems of administering medical services: (1) the rising cost of medical care; (2) absence of quality standards; (3) manpower shortage; (4) technology gap, and (5) expectation gap between patients' expectations and actual treatment. The author proposes the Kaiser Health Plan as an answer to some of these problems and outlines its six basic tenets: (1) prepayment; (2) group practice; (3) medical center facilities; (4) voluntary enrollment; (5) capitation payment; and (6) voluntary coverage. The effectiveness of the Kaiser system is summarized.

AHCMS IN2–6599

Scheffler, Richard M.
The United Mine Workers' Health Plan: An Analysis of the Cost-Sharing Program
Medical Care, 22:3, 1984, pp. 247–54.

This article reports on the introduction of a cost-sharing health care plan to the United Mine Workers. The authors discuss the data base and analyze the impact of the program on the use of health care, the probability of a hospital admission, hospital expenditures and length of stay, the demand for physician services, and the probability of seeing a physician. Hospital admissions and hospital expenditures per stay decreased, as did the probability of seeing a physician. It is suggested that these behavioral adjustments to cost sharing are fairly rapid and long-lasting.

AHCMS 27453 HC

Schneider, Don
A Methodology for the Analysis of Comparability of Services and Financial Impact of Closure of Obstetrics Services
Medical Care, 19:4, 1981, pp. 393–409.

An analysis of seven hospitals in three communities was undertaken to examine the impact on the hospitals and the communities if one hospital in each area closed obstetrics services due to excess capacity in each community.

AHCMS 25145 HC

Schofield, S. and Liebert, S.
Health Cost Management Survey: Fall 1983
Business Coalition on Health, Hartford, CT, 1983
Available from National Technical Information Service (HRP–0904862/0)

The survey was conducted to determine the health care benefit practices and cost-containment techniques being employed in Hartford County, Connecticut. The information from this survey will be used as a baseline to assist local corporations in the development of a model health insurance package.

AHCMS 27800 HC

Senate Subcommittee
Competition in the Health Services Market
Hearings before the Subcommittee on Antitrust and Monopoly of the Committee on the Judiciary, United States Senate, Ninety-third Congress, Second Session, Part I, 1974, 606 pp.
U.S. Government Printing Office, Washington, DC

Report presents the testimony given before the U.S. Senate Subcommittee on Antitrust and Monopoly on May 14 and 15, 1974 regarding the effectiveness of competition in keeping health care costs down and improving the quality of care delivered.

AHCMS 17981 HE

Sheldon, Alan and Windham, Susan
Competitive Strategy for Health Care Organizations
Dow Jones–Irwin, Homewood, IL, 1984

The authors provide a model for comprehensive strategic action and offer information on the techniques for identifying the trends that influence competitive forces, improving competitive positioning, dealing with competitive positioning issues, and preparing and implementing strategy. The book emphasizes strategic action rather than planning.

AHCMS 27693 HC

Shepard, Donald S.
Estimating the Effect of Hospital Closure on Areawide Inpatient Hospital Costs: A Preliminary Model and Application
Health Services Research, 18:4, 1983, pp. 513–49.

A preliminary model is developed for estimating the extent of savings, if any, likely to result from discontinuing a specific inpatient service. By examining the sources of referral to the discontinued service, the model estimates potential demand and how cases will be redistributed among remaining hospitals. This redistribution determines average cost per day in hospitals that receive these cases, relative to average cost per day of the discontinued service. The outflow rate measures the proportion of cases not absorbed in other acute care hospitals, and the marginal cost ratio relates marginal costs of cases absorbed in surrounding hospitals to the average costs in those hospitals. This model was applied to the discontinuation of all inpatient services in the 75-bed Chelsea Memorial Hospital, near Boston, Massachusetts, using 1976 data. As the precise value of key parameters is uncertain, sensitivity analysis was used to explore a range of values. The most likely result is a small increase ($120,000) in the area's annual inpatient hospital costs, because many patients are referred to more costly teaching hospitals. A similar situation may arise with other urban closures. For service discontinuations to generate savings, recipient hospitals must be low in costs, the outflow rate must be large, and the marginal cost ratio must be low.

AHCMS 27311 HC

Shepard, Donald S. and Thompson, Mark S.
Cost-Effectiveness Analysis in Health
Group Practice Journal, 30:2, 1981, pp. 11–13, 23–26, American Group Practice Association, 20 S. Quaker La., Alexandria, VA 22314.

This article discusses application of the principles of cost-effectiveness analysis (CEA) to health care, and to preventive health programs in particular. Strengths and weaknesses of this approach are discussed. CEA requires fewer troublesome steps than does cost-benefit analysis because CEA does not attempt to assign monetary values to health outcomes or benefits. CEA expresses health benefits in more descriptive terms, such as years of life gained. There are five major steps in the formulation of CEA: (1) define the program to be analyzed, its focus, processes, and limits; (2) compute the net monetary cost for prevention and treatment of illness under the proposed program as opposed to the cost of the status quo; (3) compute the health effects or benefits; (4) apply a decision rule based on net costs and net health effects; and (5) perform sensitivity analysis. One hypothetical and two actual applications of CEA are presented.

AHCMS 25537 FM

Shifman, Elliot and Walls, Edward
  Guidelines for Consideration of Capital Financing and Alternative Debt Financing Methods
Metropolitan Health Planning Corporation, 908 Standard Bldg., Cleveland, OH 44113, 1975, 19 pp.

  Guidelines are presented for use by hospitals in determining the most appropriate and effective means for financing necessary capital improvements. The guidelines were developed by the Metropolitan Health Planning Corporation in Cleveland, Ohio.

                                                                    AHCMS 17835 AC

Sigmond, Robert M.
  Capitation as a Method of Reimbursement to Hospitals in a Multihospital Area in *Reimbursement Incentives for Medical Care*
Office of Research and Statistics, Social Security Administration, Washington, DC, 1968

  A plan for reimbursing hospitals on a per capita basis, thus encouraging efficiency and discouraging overextended care. The Yuma County Blue Cross Plan is used as a successful example of the concept. Objections to the idea are also discussed briefly.

                                                                    AHCMS IN0013

Skelli, F. Albert; Mobley, G. Melton; and Coan, Ruth E.
  Cost-Effectiveness of Community-Based Long-Term Care: Current Findings of Georgia's Alternative Health Services Project
American Journal of Public Health, 72:4, 1982, pp. 353–58.

  A study of the cost-effectiveness of community-based, long-term care was conducted with voluntary enrollees eligible for Medicaid reimbursed nursing home care. One year after enrollment, average longevity was greater for the 575 clients in the experimental group, but average Medicaid plus Medicare costs for this group were higher than for the 172 clients in the control group. Among those more at risk of entering a nursing home, costs for persons in the experimental group were somewhat lower than for those in the control group. The results suggest that community-based services targeted to those most at risk of institutionalization may be cost-effective.

                                                                    AHCMS 25141 HC

Sloan, Frank A.
  Studies of Hospital Cost Inflation
Vanderbilt University, Nashville, TN, 1982
Available from National Technical Information Service (PB83–196931)

  This report examines the roles of the physician, the medical staff, employee unionization, and hospital regulation in hospital cost inflation. It presents 13 separate papers on these topics. Some of the findings are that: (1) type of physician compensation is of minor consequence in explaining the increase in hospital costs or the variation of costs among hospitals; (2) no evidence was found that investor-owned hospitals are less expensive than those of other ownership—however, they were similar to comparable nonprofit hospitals with respect to profitability and the proportion of Medicaid patients; (3) the existence of unions raises hospital employee wages by approximately 6% for RNs and 10% for nonprofessionals; (4) mandatory rate-setting programs tend to reduce earnings at the bottom of the wage scale when the occupation is not unionized but have little effect of the top of the scale; (5) mandatory rate-setting programs in effect for more than three years are estimated to reduce hospital costs per adjusted patient day and per admission by about 3% or 4% a year up to about 20% when the program reaches equilibrium; and (6) certificate of need does not appear to affect hospital costs.

AHCMS 26543 HC

Sloan, Frank A. and Becker, Edmund R.
Cross-Subsidies and Payment for Hospital Care
Journal of Health Politics, Policy and Law, 8:4, 1984, pp. 660–85.

This study uses hospital data from the 1979 American Hospital Association Reimbursement Survey in a multivariate framework to assess the impact of discounts and third party reimbursement on hospital costs and profitability. Three central issues are addressed: (1) Is a differential payment justified for Medicare, Medicaid, or Blue Cross on the basis of differential costs? (2) Have the cost-containment efforts of the dominant payers reduced total payments to hospitals? (3) What part of the overall savings in payments to hospitals is in the form of reduced costs rather than reduced profits? The study finds that (1) the differential payment is not justified; (2) the cost-containment efforts of the dominant payers have reduced total payments to hospitals somewhat, but a substantial amount of cost shifting remains; and (3) the savings is in profits, rather than in costs.

AHCMS 27306 HC

Sloan, Frank A.; Feldman, Roger D.; and Steinwald, A. Bruce
Effects of Teaching on Hospital Costs
Journal of Health Economics, 2:1, 1983, pp. 1–28.

This study estimates effects of undergraduate and graduate medical education on hospital costs, using a national sample of 367 U.S. community hospitals observed in 1974 and 1977. Data on other cost determinants, such as case mix, allowed the authors to isolate the influence of teaching with greater precision than most previous studies. Nonphysician expense in major teaching hospitals is, at most, 20% higher than in nonteaching hospitals; the teaching effect is about half this for hospitals with more limited teaching programs. Results for ancillary service departments are consistent with those for the hospital as a whole.

AHCMS 26926 HC

Sloan, Frank A. and Steinwald, Bruce
Insurance, Regulation, and Hospital Costs
Lexington Books, Lexington, MA, 1980

This book examines factors that have influenced hospital costs and employment of inputs during the 1970s. Much of the publication is devoted to empirical analyses of a nationwide sample of 1,228 nonfederal, short-term hospitals; the primary data source was the American Hospital Association's annual surveys of hospitals for the period 1969–75. The more general topics treated are inflation in the hospital industry; policy issues related to health insurance and hospital cost regulation; third party reimbursement for hospital services; and current regulatory trends affecting hospitals.

AHCMS 23776 HC

Sloan, Frank A. and Vraciu, Robert A.
Investor-Owned and Not-for-Profit Hospitals: Addressing Some Issues
Health Affairs, 2:1, 1983, pp. 25–37.

The economic performance of Florida nongovernment, short-term, nonteaching, nonprofit hospitals is compared with that of investor-owned hospitals with fewer than 400 beds in terms of after-tax profit margins, percentage of Medicare and Medicaid patient days, dollar value of charity care, and bad debt adjustments to revenue. Analysis indicated the Florida investor-owned and nonprofit hospitals are virtually identical in terms of the factors studied. There were some differences in services offered by the two groups of hospitals, but no pattern emerged with respect to "profitable" versus "nonprofitable" services. Findings confirm that ownership is a poor predictor of a hospital's willingness to treat low-income patients, cost to the community, and profitability. Findings reinforce those of a national study and are believed to be generalizable.

AHCMS 26477 HC

Smith, Stephen W.
Leasing: An Effective Source of Capital Asset Financing
Hospital Financial Management, 28:9, 1974, pp. 36–41.
   Leasing, as a source of capital asset financing, is discussed.

AHCMS 13531 AC

Social Security Administration
Financing Mental Health Care Under Medicare and Medicaid
Office of Research and Statistics, Social Security Administration, Washington, DC, Research Report No. 37, 1971.
   This report analyzes the use of and expenditures for psychiatric services for the aged under Medicare and Medicaid, especially as these relate to the limitations on mental illness coverage under these programs.

AHCMS 12211 IN

Sorensen, Andrew A.; Saward, Ernest W.; and Stewart, David W.
Hospital Cost Containment in Rochester: From Maxicap to the Hospital Experimental Payments Program
Inquiry, 19:4, 1982, pp. 327–35.
   This article describes the evolution and structure of the prospective reimbursement system underway in Rochester, New York. The Rochester Area Hospital Corporation inaugurated the Hospital Experimental Payments Program (HEPP) on January 1, 1980. Under HEPP, all nine hospitals in Monroe and Livingston counties consented to an individual and regional cap on hospital income derived from contracting payers; Blue Cross, Medicare, and Medicaid agreed to a standard formula based on a ratio of charges to charges applied against costs. Hospital costs are based on 1978 actual costs plus allowances, and trending forward for inflation. There are also provisions for payments based on increases in volume and additional operating costs associated with new equipment or facilities. Under HEPP, hospitals do not lose revenue because of cost reduction efforts. Other attractive features of HEPP are: (1) Control of costs within each hospital was, at the outset of the program, determined locally under voluntary arrangement, giving hospital administrators a direct influence on negotiations of the reimbursement formula in the 1978 base year; (2) HEPP generates a regionwide data base which hospitals and researchers can use to assess utilization and operating efficiency of hospitals; (3) Cash flow has substantially improved because, each week, each hospital receives 1/52 of the annual payment calculations accounting for 90% of each hospital's income from Medicare, Medicaid, and Blue Cross. Although it is too

early to assess the long-term effectiveness of HEPP, substantial progress in reducing hospital expenditures is indicated.

AHCMS 26410 HC

Spiegel, Allen D. (ed.)
The Medicaid Experience
Aspen Systems Corporation, Gaithersburg, MD, 1979, 402 pp.

This book presents a collection of 44 studies and reports that deal with the
entire range of Medicaid problems including funding, administration, and evaluation as well as practical pointers on how to start and manage programs.

AHCMS 21347 IN

Spitz, Bruce
States' Options for Reimbursing Nursing Home Capital
Inquiry, 19:3, 1982, pp. 246–56.

Analyzes the various options states can use in determining capital reimbursement for nursing homes. Under a cost-related system, a state will pay a portion of
a home's property costs (a percentage normally determined by the ratio of Medicaid patient days to total patient days, subject to a minimum occupancy limitation). In determining what those property costs are, four basic approaches can be
used: historic costs, replacement costs, market value, and imputed value.

AHCMS 25442 FM

Sullivan, Sean and Ehrenhaft, Polly M.
Managing Health Care Costs: Private Sector Innovations
American Enterprise Institute for Public Policy Research, Washington, DC, 1984

Case studies of two traditional mid-American manufacturing companies (Deere
and Company and Caterpillar Tractor Company) and two business coalitions, the
Midwest Business Group of Health (MBGH) and the Utah Health Cost Management Foundation, were presented to illustrate the efforts of the private sector in
containing health costs. The two manufacturing companies treated health care as
a managerial function and tried to influence the behavior of employees and providers. Both companies also actively encouraged the development of alternative
health plans and signed contracts with professional standards review organizations
to review the utilization of services by employees who remain in the traditional
insurance plan. The business coalitions focused their efforts on redesigning the
health benefits package and the careful use of comparative data on the cost patterns of health service providers to improve performance of the existing system.
MBGH has developed usable models and standards for its members and local
chapters and user groups to help them deal with providers and insurers. The Utah
foundation has undertaken a major effort to educate consumers by publishing
controversial information on comparative hospital costs, and has played an active
role in championing competition in the health care marketplace.

AHCMS 28588 HC

Taddey, Anthony J. and Gayer, Gordon
Uses and Effects of Hospital Tax-Exempt Financing
Healthcare Financial Management, 36:7, 1982, pp. 10 ff.

This article reports findings from a May 1982 study conducted by Health Care
Financing Study Group to assess the uses and impact of hospital tax-exempt
financing.

AHCMS 25371 FM

Taylor, Humphrey and Paranjpe, Asha
   *The Equitable Healthcare Survey II: Physicians' Attitudes toward Cost
   Containment*
The Equitable Life Assurance Society of the United States, 1285 Ave. of the Amer-
   icas, New York, NY 10019, 1984

   A report of an assessment of physicians' attitudes on the subject of health care
costs and cost-containment policies. It is based on 500 interviews conducted on
a representative cross section of American physicians. Major findings of the survey
include: (1) Less than half of all physicians believe that the American health care
system works well and needs only minor changes. (2) A majority (59%) of physicians think that the cost of hospitalization is unreasonably high. Factors cited as
contributing to the rise in health care costs include the increasing use of expensive
equipment and technology, the aging of the population, the growth of expensive
malpractice suits and malpractice insurance, the ordering of unnecessary laboratory tests, and unnecessary hospitalization. (3) Physicians generally believe that
most policies that would increase cost sharing by patients would be effective and
acceptable; overwhelming majorities endorse changes in the system that would
reduce hospitalization. (4) More than 80% of the physicians find the proposal of
government price control unacceptable, as are HMOs and preferred provider plans.
(5) There is some resistance among physicians to encouraging the use of nurse
practitioners, midwives, and physician's assistants instead of physicians.
                                                              AHCMS 28571 HC

Thompson, C. and LeTouzé, D.
   Hospital Capital Shows Signs of Old Age. Part 2
Dimensions in Health Service, 61:12, 1984, pp. 19–20.

   The authors present estimates on the age of hospital capital assets in Canada
and the cost of replacing those assets by province and type of hospital. It was
determined that the overall replacement value of Canada's hospitals is $20.3 bil-
lion, with the majority of hospital capital in the two most populous provinces,
Ontario and Quebec. The authors find that it will require an investment in the
next ten years of $14.8 billion (in 1984 dollars) to maintain hospital building capital
in its present state. As the average age of major movable equipment is 8.4 years,
which is greater than the recommended 7 years, it will require investment of $9.4
billion to renovate equipment to maximum acceptable age by 1995. The authors
also find there will be a need for more sophisticated hospital capital in the future
because of an aging population and the trend away from the extended family and
its support systems, and yet there are problems just maintaining the present level
of capital investment. These trends support the argument for alternative, less cap-
ital-intensive, systems of care.
                                                              AHCMS 28698 FM

Thompson, C.; Youmans, J.; and LeTouzé, D.
   Hospital Capital Shows Signs of Old Age: Part 1
Dimensions in Health Service, 61:11, 1984, pp. 34–36.

   This first part of a major study of hospital capital and capital funding in
Canada focused on the trends in the age of hospital capital in the country. A ratio
of accumulated depreciation over annual depreciation was applied to financial
information supplied by hospitals to Statistics Canada. This ratio was then adjusted for inflation to arrive at the age of the physical assets of hospitals. The study
found that there is a gradual increase in the age ratio from 1976 to 1980–81 for

the buildings of nonteaching institutions in most provinces; that is, nonteaching hospitals in Canada are wearing out somewhat faster than they are being maintained. Building and building equipment show clear signs of deterioration, and major movable equipment is also aging. The study suggests that the more favorable trend shown for equipment age may be the result of the technological imperative and that hospital decision makers are placing greater emphasis on having up-to-date equipment than on upgrading their physical plant.

AHCMS 28372 FM

Thompson, G. Byron and Pyhrr, Peter A.
ZBB—A New Skill for the Financial Manager
Hospital Financial Management, 33:3, 1979.

This article describes zero base budgeting (ZBB) and its application in the hospital. ZBB views the budget process as part of management—managers must perform ZBB analyses in order to derive a budget.

AHCMS 21291 FM

Thompson, Robert S.; Kirz, Howard L.; and Gold, Robert A.
Changes in Physician Behavior and Cost Savings Associated with Organizational Recommendations on the Use of "Routine" Chest X-Rays and Multichannel Blood Tests
Preventive Medicine, 12:3, 1983, pp. 385–96.

Analyzes the impact of organizational recommendations on the use of routine chest X rays and blood tests by physicians at the Group Health Cooperative of Puget Sound.

AHCMS 27254 HC

Toso, Mark E.; Bergonzi, Albert; and Fisher, Nathaniel S.
Maximization of Net Income Using Procedural Rate Setting
Topics in Health Care Financing, 10:1, 1983, pp. 49–58.

The computer is used in the rate-setting process to maximize third party reimbursement and align charges to costs or to price competition between hospitals.

AHCMS 27476 FM

Towne, David
Case Mix Planning
Topics in Health Care Financing, 10:1, 1983, pp. 1–8.

The author discusses the impetus for case-mix planning in hospitals as a result of the Tax Equity and Fiscal Responsibility Act of 1982 which placed per case limits on the reimbursements hospitals receive for the costs of caring for Medicare patients.

AHCMS 27472 FM

Tripp, Paivi
A Comparative Analysis of Health Care Costs in Three Selected Countries: The United States, The United Kingdom and Australia
Social Science & Medicine, 15C:2, 1981, pp. 19–30, Pergamon Press, Inc., Journals Division, Maxwell House, Fairview Park, Elmsford, NY 10523.

This article compares the health care delivery systems and related costs in the United States, the United Kingdom, and Australia during the period 1950–78. Analysis fails to support the hypothesis that the structure of financing affects in a systematic and predictable way the costs and benefits of health care in a given nation. The evidence, furthermore, does not lend credibility to the argument that the ratio of benefits to costs improves as one moves on a continuum from a decentralized, pluralistic system toward a centralized, monistic system of financing. On the other hand, the opposite statement of no relationship is not entirely accurate. The findings point to differences in several categories in the overall trends of costs and health resources. They also repeatedly rank the selected countries in such a way as to hint at the relative merits a centralized, monistic health care system has over mixed systems of financing.

AHCMS 24948 HC

Tucker, G. Edward, Jr.
Start Small: Computer-Based Financial Modeling Scaled to Size
Healthcare Financial Management, 37:1, 1983, pp. 24 ff.

This article presents, step-by-step, a description of how to use computer-based financial modeling to prepare budgets and analyze costs in a hospital.

AHCMS 26309 FM

U.S. Congressional Budget Office
Containing Medical Care Costs through Market Forces
U.S. Government Printing Office, Washington, DC, 1982

This report analyzes the impact of federal policy alternatives that utilize market forces to control rising medical care costs. The two basic market-oriented strategies involve increasing cost sharing by users of medical care and encouraging enrollment in health maintenance organizations (HMOs) which appear to have lower costs than fee-for-service health plans. Three policy options are evaluated: (1) altering the tax treatment of employment-based health insurance (health benefits would not be excluded from the employee's taxable income or the employer's payroll tax); (2) offering Medicare beneficiaries a voucher to purchase a private health plan which would encourage enrollment in lower-cost plans such as HMOs; and (3) introducing other changes in Medicare's reimbursement and benefit structure, such as applying a tax to premiums of insurance policies that supplement Medicare, altering benefits, or offering a choice of "plan" within Medicare. Analysis of these options indicates that changes in economic incentives can potentially slow the rise in medical costs and reduce federal outlays. The paper finds, however, that use of voluntary Medicare vouchers would not achieve significant savings, because to induce participation, the voucher amount would have to be close to current benefit costs. If low medical care users opted for the vouchers, the costs of the vouchers would exceed what their benefits would cost under Medicare, and federal outlays could even increase. Analysis suggests that the most effective short-term approach would be through cost sharing, but that in the long run, HMOs might play an increasing role. The article also concludes that if the effects of market-oriented options are not large enough in the short run, prospective payment might also be considered as a complement to market-oriented options.

AHCMS 26592 HC

U.S. Congressional Budget Office
Options for Change in Military Medical Care
U.S. Congressional Budget Office, Washington, DC, 1984

The U.S. Department of Defense currently spends over $4 billion a year operating several hundred military hospitals and clinics, and, when necessary, supplements military facilities with civilian medical care under the CHAMPUS program which costs another $1 billion per year. The report discusses options that could save $2 billion in military medical care over the next five years. They are the following: charging outpatients when they visit military physicians; and collecting from private insurers when their military policyholders use military hospitals and clinics; linking CHAMPUS and Medicare to budget within a prospective reimbursement scheme under the DRG system; and "closing" medical enrollments, i.e., restricting sources of medical care so that beneficiaries are assigned to specific facilities for care within a specified geographic area. Implications of these options for reducing waiting lines, the effect on military famililies' out-of-pocket costs, the possible adverse effect on the retention of military personnel and their health status, as well as the impact on private insurance premium rates are discussed.

AHCMS 27702 HC

U.S. General Accounting Office
Need to Eliminate Payments for Unnecessary Hospital Ancillary Services
U.S. General Accounting Office, Washington, DC, 1983
Available from National Technical Information Service (PB84–104991)

Medicare's new prospective reimbursement system will provide an incentive for hospitals to eliminate unnecessary ancillary services. However, the reimbursement rates under the new system are based in part on costs of providing unnecessary care. The General Accounting Office recommends the elimination of the cost of such care from the data base used to establish the rates and notes also that the Medicaid program was vulnerable to payment for unnecessary ancillary services.

AHCMS 27042 HC

U.S. General Accounting Office
Rising Hospital Costs Can Be Restrained by Regulating Payments and Improving Management.
Report to the Congress by the Comptroller General of the United States
The Office of the Comptroller General, Washington, DC, 1980

This is a report of a study to determine whether prospective rate-setting programs have restrained the rise in hospital costs and to evaluate the extent to which prospective rate-setting programs have induced hospital managers to manage with a greater emphasis on operating efficiently by using selected, proven cost-containment management techniques. Information on the success of prospective rate-setting programs was obtained by comparing hospital cost increases in states with programs to cost increases in states without programs, and conducting detailed reviews of prospective rate-setting programs in nine states. Information on the use of management techniques to control costs was obtained primarily from a literature review, an opinion survey of recognized health care authorities, a questionnaire completed by 2,285 hospitals, and site visits to selected hospitals. Findings include the following: (1) States with such programs were more successful in controlling the growth rate in expenditures per case during 1975–77. (2) There appears to be a relationship between the effectiveness of some programs and the elements essential to an effective rate-setting program identified by the Health Care Financing Administration in 1977. (3) Hospital officials in prospective rate-setting states believe they have been able to contain cost increases primarily as a result of improved hospital budgeting practices. (4) Hospitals generally have not yet adopted cost-containing management techniques.

AHCMS 24974 HC

U.S. Office of Technology Assessment
Medical Technology Under Proposals to Increase Competition in Health Care
U.S. Office of Technology Assessment, Washington, DC, 1982
Available from National Technical Information Service (PB83–164046)

This study analyzes the implications for medical technology of two categories of proposals to increase competition: increased cost sharing by patients when they use medical care, and greater competition among plans that provide health insurance and deliver medical care. After describing the provisions of the two strategies, the study examines the likely effects of each approach on the use and innovation of medical technology, the quality of care provided, the needs of consumers for information, and the availability of that information. Policy implications are raised and discussed in each area.

AHCMS 26555 HC

Vaida, Michael L.
The Financial Impact of Prospective Payment on Hospitals
Health Affairs, 3:1, 1984, pp. 112–18.

The study presents estimates of the financial impact of the recently implemented Medicare prospective payment system on hospitals. It is concluded that the analysis casts doubt on the ability of some institutions to adapt to the new reimbursement environment in the relatively short phase-in period, while other hospitals may expect large increases in reimbursement in the next four years.

AHCMS 28111 FM

Valiante, John D.
Forecasting Capital Requirements: Potential Trends in Capital Investment During the 1980s
Healthcare Financial Management, 36:8, 1982, pp. 52 ff.

This article presents estimates of potential hospital capital expenditures by state during the 1980s and the effect these investment patterns will have on occupancy, relative age, and debt capacity of the hospitals. The estimates do not reflect any substantial increase in the use of new technology during the 1980s. They are based upon forecasts of additional bed requirements as well as renovation and replacement requirements, and are reduced by the ability of hospitals to finance these needs. The analysis indicates that capital expenditures will vary considerably by state due to differences in capital requirements and capital availability. Estimates indicate that overall during the 1980s, approximately 150,000 new beds will be added and approximately 600,000 renovated or replaced at a total cost of $130 billion. It is estimated that more than $90 billion of this amount will be financed by long-term debt. The analysis also suggests that capital requirements are rising at a time when capital availability has become an increasing problem. Examination of demographic patterns in the 1980s shows that most states will continue to experience an increase in occupancy rates even with substantial new capital investment.

AHCMS 25513 FM

Van Nostrand, Lyman G.
Capital Financing for Health Facilities
Public Health Reports, November–December 1977.

This article reviews major trends in the supply of hospitals and beds, trends in investments, changing sources of funds for construction, and current federal intervention in capital financing as a framework for considering what our future policy should be with regard to hospital construction and financing.

AHCMS 19405 FM

Vogel, Ronald J.
An Analysis of Structural Incentives in the Arizona Health Care Cost-Containment System
Health Care Financing Review, 5:4, 1984, pp. 13–21.

This article analyzes the financial structures of the prevailing public and private health insurance mechanisms. Based on this analysis, the authors conclude that the financial structures of health insurance mechanisms are deficient in that they generate efficiency in neither the consumption nor the production of health services. On the other hand, closed-ended systems of finance, such as the health maintenance organization or the new Arizona Health Care Cost-Containment System (AHCCCS), give more promise of achieving such efficiencies. The AHCCCS represents an important innovation in the public financing of health care, and, for policy purposes, should be considered a viable national alternative for the reform of Medicare and Medicaid.

AHCMS 28148 HC

Wacht, Richard F.
A Capital Budget Planning Model For Nonprofit Hospitals
Inquiry, 15:3, 1978, pp. 234–45.

Presents a budget model developed to assist nonprofit hospital administrators in achieving financial self-sufficiency for incremental capital investments by coordinating cash flows related to funds acquisition, construction, and operation of long-term health care projects.

AHCMS 20309 FM

Wagner, Judith L.
The Feasibility of Economic Evaluation of Diagnostic Procedures
Social Science & Medicine, 17:3, 1983, pp. 861–69, Pergamon Press, Inc., Journals Division, Maxwell House, Fairview Park, Elmsford, NY 10523.

This paper examines the principles of cost-benefit and cost-effectiveness analysis as applied to diagnostic procedures. Five specific problem areas encountered in the application of economic evaluation to diagnostic procedures are discussed in detail. They are: defining homogeneous patient groups for analysis, specifying the relevant diagnostic alternatives, measuring diagnostic accuracy, measuring diagnostic costs, and specifying the measured outcomes of the diagnostic process. The economic evaluation literature on two diagnostic procedures—the skull X ray and computed tomographic (CT) scanning is also reviewed within the context of a model of economic evaluation. Two studies were found to apply successfully the principles of economic evaluation to CT scanning, but none was found for skull X rays. The most common approaches to evaluating the usefulness of these procedures, and the limitations of these approaches, are summarized.

AHCMS 27232 HC

Wallack, Stanley
Expenditures for Health Care: Federal Programs and Their Effects
U.S. Government Printing Office, Washington, DC, 1977, 67 pp.

This report examines trends in health expenditures and describes the impact of federal programs and policies on rising costs. It evaluates current efforts to contain costs and discusses strategies to curb future growth. Three components of the rise in expenditures are considered: increases in population, prices, and per capita utilization of health services. Federal policies, particularly those of the 1960s, are examined as contributing to growth in expenditures by stimulating demand for health care in their subsidies of private insurance purchases, provision of tax deductions for high medical expenditures, and finance of health care for the aged and poor.

AHCMS 20712 HC

Walls, Edward L.
Estimating Voluntary Hospital Debt Capacity
Harvard University Library, Cambridge, MA, 1970

This thesis proposes a framework for estimating debt capacity of voluntary nonprofit hospitals. More specifically it investigates debt capacity when a major share of revenue is received from cost-based reimbursement not including capital allowances. As a result it analyzes and describes the impact of cost-based reimbursement upon hospital capital financing.

AHCMS AC4-6779

Walters, James E. and Watson, Hugh J.
Building a Budget: Three Generations
Hospital Financial Management, 31:9, 1977, pp. 10–18.

This article illustrates the application of three levels of sophistication in constructing budgets for hospital financial management planning purposes: line item budgeting, deterministic mathematical models, and probabilistic estimates.

AHCMS 19045 AC

Wasserman, Jeffrey
DRG Evaluation: Vol. I. Introduction and Overview
Health Research and Educational Trust of New Jersey, Princeton, NJ, 1982

This is a comprehensive evaluation of the New Jersey diagnosis-related group (DRG) program to provide an understanding of whether the system is properly designed and works as anticipated; whether it makes a difference in terms of hospital performance, effectiveness, and efficiency; what the potential is for regulation, management information, and utilization review; and what advantages and disadvantages there are with DRG reimbursement for hospitals, third party payers, and others. In addition to nine analytical tasks, three hospital surveys were conducted. Survey results indicated that: (1) A larger percentage of the respondents believed that allocating costs to DRGs and using the rate-setting formula was "reasonable" than believed that these factors were "beneficial." (2) There is considerable uncertainty regarding the system's ability to contain costs. (3) The DRG system has led to expansion and automation of data processing systems. (4) Medical staffs were involved in the program's implementation. (5) Administrators are confident that DRG management reports will improve their control over hospital operations.

AHCMS 26341 HC

Watts, Carolyn A. and Klastorin, T. D.
The Impact of Case Mix on Hospital Cost: A Comparative Analysis
Inquiry, 17:4, 1980, pp. 357–67.

This article compares the ability of various measures of case mix to explain the variation in average cost per admission across hospitals. Data are taken from a 1976 sample of 315 short-term, general hospitals in the United States. Regression analysis is used to examine the contribution of ten case-mix variables to the explanatory power of an average cost equation, controlling for other factors that affect average cost. The variables range from a simple univariate proxy (number of beds) to a multidimensional variable based on diagnostic proportions. Results indicate that the detailed variables are able to explain more interhospital cost variation than are the single-valued indexes, and for a given dimension, the direct case-mix variables perform better than do proxy variables. A significant improvement in explanatory power results when a few diagnostic modifiers are added to proxy variables, but they add little to the ability of direct case mix variables to predict average cost. In no case, however, does the proportion of explained variation rise above 70%, which may be inadequate as a basis for reimbursement where reimbursement is required to be reasonably related to cost.

AHCMS 23541 HC

Wennberg, John E.
Should the Cost of Insurance Reflect the Cost of Use in Local Hospital Markets?
New England Journal of Medicine, 307:22, 1982, pp. 1374–81.

Local hospital markets have been shown to vary extensively in per capita expenditures for hospital services and in the reimbursement paid per Medicare enrollee and per Blue Cross subscriber. Insurance premiums do not reflect these differences among local markets, resulting in intermarket subsidies (transfer payments) and distortion of competition between health maintenance organizations and the fee-for-service system. Regulatory strategies to "cap" hospital costs have ignored these market variations and thus perpetuated the established pattern of expenditures and transfer payments. The plans for implementing a voucher system for the Medicare program set the value of the voucher according to average reimbursements at the county or state level. Since several markets can exist within one county's boundaries, the cash value established for the voucher in some low-cost markets will substantially exceed current per capita rates of reimbursements, permitting large profits and an increase in total costs to the Medicare program. If the price of health insurance were adjusted to correspond more closely to local market conditions, transfer payments would be reduced, and more effective regulation, competition, and consumer involvement might result.

AHCMS 26227 HC

Werner, Jack L. and Hu, Teh-Wei
Hospitalization Insurance and the Demand for Inpatient Care
American Medical Association, Chicago, IL, 1977, 18 pp.

The relationship between hospitalization insurance and medical care demand is analyzed. Using multivariate regression analysis, variations in hospital utilization were analyzed with respect to a set of independent variables and the demand for hospital care, economic factors, characteristics of the hospital service area, and characteristics of the hospitals. Hospitalization insurance had a positive impact on the demand for medical care. Insurance had a greater effect on hospital admissions than on patient days. In general, hospital demand patterns did not differ with respect to the composition of insurance receipts.

AHCMS 19956 IN

Western Center for Health Planning
Financial Analysis Workbook
Western Center for Health Planning, San Francisco, CA, 1980
Available from National Technical Information Service (HRP–0902943/0)

The purpose of this workbook is to present techniques of financial analysis that are applicable to the health care industry and that could be used in the context of certificate-of-need and appropriateness review evaluations. Certain techniques of financial analysis that are widely used in the corporate world are not as generally applicable to financial analysis of nonprofit institutions. The emphasis in this workbook is on the techniques most appropriate for financial analysis of hospitals and other health care providers. The examples used in this workbook are primarily nonprofit hospitals; however, the techniques outlined here are equally applicable to skilled nursing facilities, proprietary hospitals, and other providers of health care services.

AHCMS 24739 FM

Wheeler, John R.; Zuckerman, Howard S.; and Aderholdt, John M.
How Management Contracts Can Affect Hospital Finances
Inquiry, 19:2, 1982, pp. 160–66.

Findings from a study conducted to determine how management contracts influence financial viability, organizational stability, and operating performance of hospitals are presented in this paper. The focus is on the financial implications for hospitals managed under contract. Three categories of measures used in the assessment are described: measures of profitability, measures of liquidity, and measures of capital structure. The authors conclude that management contracts can improve the overall financial condition of a hospital in a relatively short time. The study group became financially viable in three years.

AHCMS 25544 FM

Whitted, Gary S.
The Allocation and Management of Direct Health Care Expenses for Employees and Their Dependents: Three Case Studies at Fortune 500 *Corporations*
University of California, Los Angeles, CA, 1983
Available from University Microfilms

This research aims to examine the allocation and management of health care expenses in three large private sector corporations and the principal characteristics and trends in four categories of health expense most important to employers: (1) private health insurance, (2) workers' compensation insurance, (3) non-occupational sickness and disability protection, and (4) governmental health programs. The study focused on the collection of employer health-related expenditure data at both the macro and micro levels of corporate organization during either two or three years. Findings show that the three study firms did not appear to be devoting attention or resources to health care expense management commensurate with its importance. The research also documented that health-related expenditure levels and trends vary markedly. These differences persist over multiple years, and there is a definite pattern for certain organizational subunits, for example, corporate headquarters, to be "high cost" groups, while other groups experience consistently lower health-related expenditures. Evidence from two of the three study sites documented that 1% to 2% of employees or dependents consume one-quarter to one-third of total medical claims.

AHCMS 27979 HC

Wiles, Ann and Horwitz, Ronald M.
PERT Charts Pinpoint Problems in Accounts Receivable Management
Healthcare Financial Management, 38;9, 1984, pp. 38 ff.

The Program Evaluation and Review Technique (PERT) is a charting method useful for pinpointing problems in the timing and sequence of the accounts receivable payment cycle in hospitals. Detailed exhibits are presented with definitions of events in the cycle to illustrate PERT's use, to determine the actions needed to manage accounts receivable efficiently and effectively, to decrease time intervals in the payment cycle, and to facilitate cash flow.

AHCMS 28209 FM

Wirick, Grover
Hospital Use and Characteristics of Michigan Blue Cross Subscribers: An Analytical Interview Survey
Bureau of Hospital Administration, The University of Michigan, Ann Arbor, MI 1972, 208 pp.

A two-stage probability sample of Michigan Blue Cross subscribers was interviewed in depth with the objective of determining whether demographic and social characteristics of subscribers and their families, and knowledge of and attitudes toward hospital insurance and related health subjects influenced the amount of hospital care consumed. Findings failed to support the hypothesis that experience rating (setting insurance rates on the basis of recent experience for particular groups) tends to limit hospital use. A number of variables, including marital status, age, race, occupation, and income, were found to account systematically for a modest amount of hospital use, but numerous complex interactions limit the usefulness of these relationships. Limitations on the model and data gathering instruments were found to confuse the nature of the effect of subscriber opinions about hospitals and doctors on hospital use, and no effect of subscriber opinions about insurance and Blue Cross on hospital use could be found. An interesting finding of the doctor survey was an apparent disinterest on the part of physicians in the problems of rapidly rising hospital costs, especially as these problems affect the hospitals and patients.

AHCMS 09231 IN

Yamilkoski, Lisa A.
Financial Modeling and Payroll Budgeting
Topics in Health Care Financing, 10:1, 1983, pp. 27–36.

The article describes the use of a computerized financial modeling system for payroll budgeting in the hospital. Payroll budgeting systems deal exclusively with staffing (salary dollars and labor hours), focusing on labor areas to improve efficiency, cut costs, and maximize profitability. The system aims to provide a timely and accurate tool to develop a staffing budget, provide an adequate and flexible reporting system to focus on salary and hourly variances, and assist financial managers in assessing the impact of personnel policy changes during the year. The article then describes how to develop a staffing budget using information on numbers and type of personnel required, salary levels, amount of paid unproductive time, and paid benefits contained on the data base. The system is used for monitoring and controlling costs by generating reports that pinpoint specific departments where salary deviations are above specific thresholds. It can also be used to simulate alternative staffing and salary levels to determine budgetary consequences and needs.

AHCMS 27474 FM

Yoder, Arlan R.
Is Being Tax-Exempt Really Better?
Hospital Financial Management, 32:8, 1978.

The advantages and disadvantages of the tax-exempt status of nonprofit hospitals are examined in this article. An analysis of studies comparing proprietary and nonprofit hospitals showed nonfinancial differences between the two becoming less pronounced, and a change of status from nonprofit to proprietary without a change in administration does not create a significant change in the operation of the hospital. Of the utmost importance in evaluating the effects of proprietary versus nonprofit status are the reimbursement formulae.

AHCMS 20482 FM

Young, David W.
Financial Control in Health Care
Dow Jones–Irwin, Homewood, IL, 1984

The book addresses managerial concerns in the areas of accounting, finance, and management control in health and human service organizations. The first chapters of the book are on the concepts and techniques of accounting and financial management. Later chapters address the topic of management control systems, stressing the importance of their relationship to an organization's strategy and structure, and the topic of management information systems and their role in health and human service institutions. The concluding chapter relates the various activities discussed in the preceding chapters not only to each other but to a framework of the organization's strategy and structure.

AHCMS 28503 FM

Young, David W.
"Nonprofits" Need Surplus Too
Harvard Business Review, 60:1, 1982, pp. 124–31.

Traditionally, nonprofit organizations are not allowed a surplus, making it difficult to grow in a climate of scarce long-term financing for asset development and growth. In this article, the author asserts the increasing need to allow nonprofits to keep a surplus, argues for a surplus, and discusses how managers and regulators can determine how much a nonprofit organization should be allowed. A combination of a modified version of the return-on-asset pricing model used in for-profit organizations and a model for assessing working capital needs associated with growth is presented for managers of nonprofit organizations to use to analyze their own surplus needs.

AHCMS 26428 FM

Young, Larry H.
An Analysis of the Utilization of Resources by Various Patient Groups to Establish a Set of Variable Inclusive Rates
Duke University, Durham, NC, 1971, 72 pp.
Available from University Microfilms

Discusses a proposed rate structure for hospitals which uses weighted statistics to reflect differences in the complexity of various patient groups. Ten categories of patients who use hospital resources are defined, and methods for measuring the service or activity of departments are described. The feasibility of a variable-inclusive rate determination is analyzed. Some obstacles to implementation of such a rate structure are discussed, including the problem of physician remuneration.

AHCMS AC2–7715

Young, Mary E.
Control of Health Care Costs (A Bibliography with Abstracts)
Available from National Technical Information Service (PS–79/0358/6WW)

Citations are presented on studies of various strategies for cost containment in hospitals, long-term care facilities, and ambulatory care.

AHCMS 21417 HC

Zaretsky, Henry W.
The Effects of Patient Mix and Service Mix on Hospital Costs and Productivity
Topics in Health Care Financing, 4:2, 1977, pp. 63–82.

The article describes a study that compared costs and productivity among 176 acute care California hospitals, using a cost function that takes into account differences in case mix and service mix.

AHCMS 19339 HC

Zelman, William N.; Neuman, Bruce P.; and Suver, James D.
Managing Rate Adjustments by Health Care Providers
Health Services Research, 18:2, 1983, pp. 165–79.

Explores the implications of adjusting rates for volume and cost changes after the initial budget cycle. A model is developed to aid administrators in adjusting rates to compensate for volume and cost changes.

AHCMS 26683 FM

Zimmerman, Harvey; Buechner, Jay; and Thornberry, Helen
Prospective Reimbursement in Rhode Island: Additional Perspectives
Inquiry, 14:1, pp. 3–16.

Paper describes initiation of prospective reimbursement in Rhode Island during 1971–72 and attempts to evaluate cost control aspects of the program.

AHCMS 20915 HC

Zuckerman, Alan
Cash Flow Modeling
Topics in Health Care Financing, 10:1, 1983, pp. 59–74.

The use of cash fow modeling in health care organizations can forecast cash flows and bank account balances, and allows for manipulations that aid in deciding how best to manage cash resources in future periods. Some of the more widely used statistical techniques used in cash modeling and considerations in selecting the ideal system for a particular institution are described. Statistical techniques used include: educated guessing and controlled cash outflows, linear regression analysis, exponential smoothing, and decay curve analysis. Guidelines for choosing a forecasting model are outlined. Essential functions of a useful cash management system should include data collection and storage, data manipulation, report production, and screen-user orientation. The author concludes that it is preferable to supply the system with a few well-chosen statistical techniques, a clear presentation, and the capability of producing tables and reports that are useful to a wide array of personnel.

AHCMS 27477 FM

List of Publishers and Sources

Abstracts of Health Care Management Studies
1021 East Huron
Ann Arbor, MI 48104

The Accounting Review
5717 Bessie Dr.
Sarasota, FL 33583

The University of Alabama
Graduate Program in Hospital and
Health Administration
Birmingham, AL 35294

American Association of Medical
Clinics
20 South Quaker La.
Alexandria, VA 22314

American College of Healthcare
Executives
840 North Lake Shore Dr.
Chicago, IL 60611

American Enterprise Institute for
Public Policy Research
1150 17th St., N.W.
Washington, DC 20036

American Health Planning Association
1110 Vermont St., N.W., Suite 950
Washington, DC 20005

American Hospital Association
840 North Lake Shore Dr.
Chicago, IL 60611

American Institute of Industrial
Engineering
345 East 47th St.
New York, NY 10017

American Journal of Public Health
1015 15th St., N.W.
Washington, DC 20005

American Management Association
135 West 50th St.
New York, NY 10020

American Medical Association
535 North Dearborn
Chicago, IL 60010

*Annals of the American Academy of
Political and Social Sciences*
Sage Publications, Inc.
275 South Beverly Dr.
Beverly Hills, CA 90212

Annals of Surgery
East Washington Square
Philadelphia, PA 19105

Applied Economics
Chapman & Hall Limited
11 New Fetter La.
London EC4P 4EE, England

Aspen Systems Corporation
1600 Research Blvd.
Rockville, MD 20850

Association of American Medical
Colleges
  One Dupont Circle, N.W.
  Washington, DC 20036

Ballinger Publishing Co.
  54 Church St.
  Harvard Square
  Cambridge, MA 02138

Baylor University–Army
  U.S. Army Medical Field Service
    School
  Brooke Army Medical Center
  Fort Sam Houston, TX 78234

Blue Cross and Blue Shield
Association
  676 North St. Clair St.
  Chicago, IL 60611

Blue Cross Reports
  676 North St. Clair St.
  Chicago, IL 60611

Blue Cross of Western Pennsylvania
  One Smithfield St.
  Pittsburgh, PA 15222

Blyth Eastman Paine Webber, Inc.
  1221 Ave. of the Americas
  New York, NY 10020

The Brookings Institution
  1775 Massachusetts Ave., N.W.
  Washington, DC 20036

*Bulletin of the New York Academy
of Medicine*
  2 East 103rd St.
  New York, NY 10029

*Bulletin of the Operations Research
Society of America*
  290 Westminster St.
  Providence, RI 02903

Business and Health
  922 Pennsylvania Ave., N.W.
  Washington, DC 20003

University of California–Los Angeles
  Program in Health Services
    Management
  School of Public Health
  Los Angeles, CA 90024

Cases in Health Services, see HBS
Case Services

Catholic Health Association of the
United States
  4455 Woodson Rd.
  Saint Louis, MO 63134

University of Chicago
  Center for Health Administration
    Studies
  Walker Museum, Suite 213
  1101 East 58th St.
  Chicago, IL 60637

The University of Chicago Press
  5801 Ellis Ave.
  Chicago, IL 60637

City University of New York
  Center for Social Research
  33 West 42nd St.
  New York, NY 10036

College and University Press
  263 Chapel St.
  New Haven, CT 06513

Columbia University
  Graduate Program in Health
    Administration
  600 West 168th St., 6th Floor
  New York, NY 10032

The Committee for National Health
Insurance
  1757 N St., N.W.
  Washington, DC 20036

Coopers and Lybrand
  1900 Three Girard Plaza
  Philadelphia, PA 19123

Dell Publishing Company, Inc.
  One Dag Hammarskjold Plaza
  New York, NY 10017

Dimensions in Health Service
  Canadian Hospital Association
  17 York St., Suite 100
  Ottawa, Ontario K1N 9J6, Canada

Doubleday & Co., Inc. (Anchor Books)
  245 Park Ave.
  New York, NY 10167

Dow Jones–Irwin
  1818 Ridge Rd.
  Homewood, IL 60430

Duke Law Journal
  Duke University
  Durham, NC 27710

Duke University
  Graduate Program in Health
    Administration
  Box 3018, Duke University
    Medical Center
  Durham, NC 27710

Ernst & Whinney
  National Office Library
  1300 Union Commerce Bldg.
  Cleveland, OH 40115

Federation of American Hospitals,
now Federation of American
Health Systems
  1111 19th St., N.W., Suite 402
  Washington, DC 20036

Financial Management
  University of South Florida
  College of Business
  Tampa, FL 33620

The George Washington University
  Department of Health Services
    Administration
  600 21st St., N.W.
  Washington, DC 20052

University of Georgia Press
  Waddell Hall
  Athens, GA 30602

Group Health Association of
America, Inc.
  1717 Massachusetts Ave., N.W.,
    Suite 203
  Washington, DC 20036

Group Practice Journal
  American Group Practice
    Association
  515 Madison Ave.
  New York, NY 10022

Halsted Press
  605 Third Ave.
  New York, NY 10158

Harvard Business Review
  Soldiers Field
  Boston, MA 02163

Haworth Press
  28 East 22nd St.
  New York, NY 10010

HBS Case Services
  Harvard Business School
  Boston, MA 02163

Health Administration Press
  1021 East Huron
  Ann Arbor, MI 48104

*Health and Society, see Milbank
Memorial Fund Quarterly*

Health Care
  1450 Don Mills Rd.
  Don Mills, Ontario M3B 2X7,
    Canada

Healthcare Financial Management
  1900 Spring Rd., Suite 500
  Oak Brook, IL 60521

Health Care Financing Review
  Superintendent of Documents
  U.S. Government Printing Office
  Washington, DC 20402

Health Care Management Review
  Aspen Systems Corporation
  1600 Research Blvd.
  Rockville, MD 20850

Health Insurance Association
of America
  1850 K St., N.W.
  Washington, DC 20006

Health Insurance Statistics
  Social Security Administration
  Washington, DC 20009

Health Marketing Quarterly
  Haworth Press
  28 East 22nd St.
  New York, NY 10010

Health Policy
  Elsevier Scientific Publishing Co.
  Box 211
  1000 AE Amsterdam, Netherlands

Health Progress
  4455 Woodson Rd.
  Saint Louis, MO 63134

Health Services Reports
  Superintendent of Documents
  U.S. Government Printing Office
  Washington, DC 20402

Health Services Research
  840 North Lake Shore Dr.
  Chicago, IL 60611

Health Trends
Department of Health and Social
Services
Alexander Fleming House
Elephant and Castle
London SE1 6BY, England

D.C. Heath & Co.
125 Spring St.
Lexington, MA 02173

Heating/Piping/Air Conditioning
Penton-IPC, Reinhold Publishing
Division
600 Summer St., Box 1361
Stamford, CT 06904

Holden-Day, Inc.
4432 Telegraph Ave.
Oakland, CA 94609

Holt, Rinehart and Winston, Inc.
521 Fifth Ave., Sixth Floor
New York, NY 10175

*Hospital Administration, see Hospital
& Health Services Administration*

*Hospital Administration in Canada,
see Health Care*

Hospital Association of New York State
15 Computer Dr., W.
Albany, NY 12205

*Hospital Financial Management, see
Healthcare Financial Management*

Hospital Forum
830 Market St.
San Francisco, CA 94102

*Hospital & Health Services
Administration*
840 North Lake Shore Dr.
Chicago, IL 60611

*Hospital Material Management
Quarterly*
Aspen Systems Corporation
1600 Research Blvd.
Rockville, MD 20850

Hospital Research and Educational
Trust
840 North Lake Shore Dr.
Chicago, IL 60611

Hospital Research and Educational
Trust of New Jersey
746–760 Alexander Road, CN–1
Princeton, NJ 08540

Hospital Topics
Box 5976
Sarasota, FL 34277

Hospitals
211 East Chicago
Chicago, IL 60611

Human Resource Management
Graduate School of Business
Administration
The University of Michigan
Ann Arbor, MI 48109

Information Resources Press
1700 N. Moore St., Suite 700
Arlington, VA 22209

Inquiry
Box 527
Glenview, IL 60025

Institute of Gerontology
300 North Ingalls
The University of Michigan
Ann Arbor, MI 48109

Institute for Health Planning, Inc.
702 North Blackhawk Ave.
Madison, WI 53705

University of Iowa
Graduate Program in Hospital and
Health Administration
2700 Steindler Bldg.
Iowa City, IA 52242

Richard D. Irwin, Inc.
1818 Ridge Rd.
Homewood, IL 60430

Johns Hopkins University
Center for Hospital Finance and
Management
615 North Wolfe
Baltimore, MD 21211

Journal of Accountancy
1211 Ave. of the Americas
New York, NY 10036

*Journal of Ambulatory Care
Management*
Aspen Systems Corporation
1600 Research Blvd.
Rockville, MD 20850

*Journal of American Osteopathic
Association*
212 East Ohio St.
Chicago, IL 60611

Journal of Community Health
  Human Sciences Press
  72 Fifth Ave.
  New York, NY 10011

Journal of Health Economics
  North-Holland Publishing Co.
  Box 211
  1000 AE Amsterdam, Netherlands

*Journal of Health Politics, Policy,
and Law*
  Department of Health
    Administration
  P.O. Box 3018, Duke University
  Durham, NC 27710

Journal of Human Resources
  University of Wisconsin Press
  114 North Murray St.
  Madison, Wisconsin 53715

Journal of Medical Education
  One Dupont Circle, N.W.
  Washington, DC 20036

*Journal of Medical Engineering
& Technology*
  Taylor & Francis Ltd.
  Rankin Rd., Basingstoke
  Hants RG 24OPR, England

Journal of Medical Systems
  Plenum Press
  233 Spring St.
  New York, NY 10013

Henry J. Kaiser Family Foundation
  525 Middlefield Rd., Suite 200
  Menlo Park, CA 94025

Kaiser Foundation Research
Institution, see Kaiser-Permanente
Health Services Research Center

Kaiser-Permanente Health Services
Research Center
  4610 S.E. Belmont St.
  Portland, OR 97215

King's Fund Centre (Publications distributed by Oxford University Press)
  200 Madison Ave.
  New York, NY 10016

Law and Contemporary Problems
  Duke University
  School of Law, Room 006
  Durham, NC 27706

Lexington Books
  125 Spring St.
  Lexington, MA 02173

McGraw-Hill, Inc.
  1221 Ave. of the Americas
  New York, NY 10020

Massachusetts Hospital Association
  5 New England Executive Park
  Burlington, MA 01803

Medical Care
  East Washington Square
  Philadelphia, PA 19105

Medical Care Review
  1021 East Huron
  Ann Arbor, MI 48104

Medical College of Virginia
  Virginia Commonwealth University
  Department of Health
    Administration
  MCV Station Box 203
  Richmond, VA 23298

Medical Group Management
  1355 South Colorado Blvd.
  Denver, CO 80222

Mentor Books
  New American Library, Inc.
  1633 Broadway
  New York, NY 10019

The MICAH Corporation
  1521 Harbrooke
  Ann Arbor, MI 48103

Michigan Blue Shield
  600 East Lafayette
  Detroit, MI 48226

Michigan Hospitals
  Michigan Hospital Association
  6215 West St. Joseph Hwy.
  Lansing, MI 48917

Michigan State Department of
Social Services
  P.O. Box 30037
  300 South Capitol Ave.
  Lansing, MI 48926

The University of Michigan
  Bureau of Health Economics
  The School of Public Health
  109 South Observatory St.
  Ann Arbor, MI 48109

The University of Michigan
  Program and Bureau of Hospital
    Administration
  The School of Public Health II
  1420 Washington Hts., Third Floor
  Ann Arbor, MI 48109

The University of Michigan
  The School of Public Health
  109 South Observatory St.
  Ann Arbor, MI 48109

Milbank Memorial Fund Quarterly
  Cambridge University Press
  32 East 57th St.
  New York, NY 10022

Mimir Publishers, Inc.
  P.O. Box 5011
  Madison, WI 53705

University of Minnesota
  The Program in Hospital and
    Health Care Administration
  Box 97, Mayo Bldg.
  Minneapolis, MN 55455

MIT Press
  28 Carleton St.
  Cambridge, MA 02142

Modern Healthcare
  Crain Communications
  740 North Rush
  Chicago, IL 60611

The Modern Hospital, see *Modern Healthcare*

C.V. Mosby Co.
  11830 Westline Industrial Dr.
  Saint Louis, MO 63146

National Center for Health Services
Research and Health Care Technology
Assessment
  U.S. Department of Health and
    Human Services
  Parklawn Bldg., 5600 Fishers La.
  Rockville, MD 20850

National Cooperative Services Center
for Hospital Management Engineering
  840 North Lake Shore Dr.
  Chicago, IL 60611

National Technical Information
Services
  5285 Port Royal Rd.
  Springfield, VA 22161

New England Journal of Medicine
  1440 Main St.
  Waltham, MA 02254

New York State Journal of Medicine
  Medical Society of the State of
    New York
  420 Lakeville Rd.
  Lake Success, NY 11042

Office of Research and Statistics
Social Security Administration
Baltimore, MD 21235

Physicians' Record Co.
  3000 South Ridgeland Ave.
  Berwyn, IL 60402

University of Pittsburgh
  Health Law Center
  Pittsburgh, PA 15261

Policy Center, Inc.
  789 Sherman, Suite 580
  Denver, CO 80203

Frederick A. Praeger
  Westview Press, Inc.
  5500 Central Ave.
  Boulder, CO 80301

Prentice-Hall, Inc.
  Englewood Cliffs, NJ 07632

Pressler Publications
  Bloomington, IN 47401

Preventive Medicine
  Academic Press, Inc., Journals
    Division
  111 Fifth Ave.
  New York, NY 10003

Price Waterhouse
  1251 Ave. of the Americas
  New York, NY 10020

Public Affairs Press
  419 New Jersey Ave., S.E.
  Washington, DC 20003

Public Health Reports
  Superintendent of Documents
  U.S. Government Printing Office
  Washington, DC 20402

Quarterly Journal of Economics
  John Wiley & Sons, Inc.
  605 Third Ave.
  New York, NY 10158

QRB/Quality Review Bulletin
Joint Commission on Accreditation
of Hospitals
875 North Michigan Ave.
Chicago, IL 60611

Rand Corporation
1700 Main St.
Santa Monica, CA 90406

Random House, Inc.
201 East 50th St.
New York, NY 10022

Reinhold Publishing Corporation
430 Park Ave.
New York, NY 10022

Research and Statistics Notes
Social Security Administration
Baltimore, MD 21235

The Review
Federation of American Health
Systems
1111 19th St., N.W., Suite 402
Washington, DC 20036

Rinehart, Winston, see Holt, Rinehart
and Winston

The Ronald Press Co.
P.O. Box 447
Saint Louis, MO 63166

W.B. Saunders Co.
210 West Washington Sq.
Philadelphia, PA 19105

Sloan Management Review
Alfred P. Sloan School of
Management, MIT
50 Memorial Dr.
Cambridge, MA 02139

Social Science & Medicine
Pergamon Press
Maxwell House, Fairview Park
Elmsford, NY 10523

Social Security Bulletin
Superintendent of Documents
U.S. Government Printing Office
Washington, DC 20402

Spectrum Publications, Inc.
979 Casiano Rd.
Los Angeles, CA 90049

Standard & Poor's Corporation
25 Broadway
New York, NY 10004

Charles C. Thomas Publishing Co.
2600 South First St.
Springfield, IL 62717

Topics in Health Care Financing
Aspen Systems Corporation
1600 Research Blvd.
Rockville, MD 20850

Trinity University Press
715 Stadium Dr.
San Antonio, TX 78284

U.S. Department of Health and
Human Services
330 Independence Ave., S.W.
Washington, DC 20201

U.S. Government Printing Office
Superintendent of Documents
Washington, DC 20402

University Microfilms International
300 North Zeeb Rd.
Ann Arbor, MI 48106

The Urban Institute
2100 M Street, N.W.
Washington, DC 20037

Wadsworth Publishing Co.
10 Davis Dr.
Belmont, CA 94002

John Wiley & Sons, Inc.
605 Third Ave.
New York, NY 10158

Xavier University
Graduate Program in Hospital and
Health Administration
2220 Victory Pkwy.
Cincinnati, OH 45207

Yale University
Center for Study of Health
Services
77 Prospect
New Haven, CT 06510

Yale University
Program in Hospital
Administration
School of Medicine
60 College St.
New Haven, CT 06510

Index

About the Authors

HOWARD J. BERMAN became president of Blue Cross and Blue Shield of Rochester, New York, on July 1, 1985. Before that he was Group Vice President of the American Hospital Association and President of the Hospital Research and Educational Trust. He is on the advisory board of the Cooperative Information Center for Health Care Management Studies at The University of Michigan and is a member of the editorial boards of *Inquiry* and *Topics in Health Care Financing*. He is also executive editor of *Health Services Research*. He is a graduate of the University of Illinois in finance and holds a master's degree in hospital administration from The University of Michigan.

LEWIS E. WEEKS was editor of *Inquiry* from 1976 to 1984 and is now conducting oral history interviews of leaders in the health care field for the Lewis E. Weeks Series of the Hospital Administration Oral History Collection housed in the Library of the American Hospital Association, Asa S. Bacon Memorial, in Chicago. Weeks received his master's degree in history from The University of Michigan and his doctorate in communication arts from Michigan State University.

STEVEN F. KUKLA is the manager of hospital finance for the American Hospital Association. He received his bachelor's degree in finance from the Illinois Institute of Technology and his master's degree in business administration from Governors State University. In addition, he has achieved his certificate in public accounting from the University of Illinois. He has served as a member of the Financial Accounting Standards Board task force on nonbusiness entities. He has also designed a test on financial analysis and cost accounting for the hospital administrator.